Core Curriculum for Nephrology Nursing

Sixth Edition

Editor: Caroline S. Counts, MSN, RN, CNN

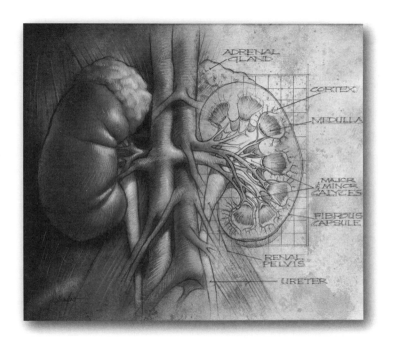

MODULE 2

Physiologic and Psychosocial Basis for Nephrology Nursing Practice

D1289125

ANNA American Nephrology Nurses' Association
www.annanurse.org

Core Curriculum for Nephrology Nursing, 6th Edition

Editor and Project Director
Caroline S. Counts, MSN, RN, CNN

MODULE 2 • Physiologic and Psychosocial Basis for Nephrology Nursing Practice

Publication Management
Anthony J. Jannetti, Inc.
East Holly Avenue/Box 56
Pitman, New Jersey 08071-0056

Managing Editor: Claudia Cuddy
Editorial Coordinator: Joseph Tonzelli
Layout Design and Production: Claudia Cuddy
Layout Assistants: Kaytlyn Mroz, Katerina DeFelice, Casey Shea, Courtney Klauber
Design Consultants: Darin Peters, Jack M. Bryant
Proofreaders: Joseph Tonzelli, Evelyn Haney, Alex Grover, Nicole Ward
Cover Design: Darin Peters
Cover Illustration: Scott M. Holladay © 2006
Photography: Kim Counts and Marty Morganello (*unless otherwise credited*)

ANNA National Office Staff
Executive Director: Michael Cunningham
Director of Membership Services: Lou Ann Leary
Membership/Marketing Services Coordinator: Lauren McKeown
Manager, Chapter Services: Janet Betts
Education Services Coordinator: Kristen Kellenyi
Executive Assistant & Marketing Manager, Advertising: Susan Iannelli
Co-Directors of Education Services: Hazel A. Dennison and Sally Russell
Program Manager, Special Projects: Celess Tyrell
Director, Jannetti Publications, Inc.: Kenneth J. Thomas
Managing Editor, *Nephrology Nursing Journal*: Carol Ford
Editorial Coordinator, *Nephrology Nursing Journal*: Joseph Tonzelli
Subscription Manager, *Nephrology Nursing Journal*: Rob McIlvaine
Managing Editor, *ANNA Update, ANNA E-News*, & Web Editor: Kathleen Thomas
Director of Creative Design & Production: Jack M. Bryant
Layout and Design Specialist: Darin Peters
Creative Designer: Bob Taylor
Director of Public Relations and Association Marketing Services: Janet D'Alesandro
Public Relations Specialist: Rosaria Mineo
Vice President, Fulfillment and Information Services: Rae Ann Cummings
Director, Internet Services: Todd Lockhart
Director of Corporate Marketing: Tom Greene
Exhibit Coordinator: Miriam Martin
Conference Manager: Jeri Hendrie
Comptroller: Patti Fortney

MODULE 2. Physiologic and Psychosocial Basis for Nephrology Nursing Practice
Copyright © 2015 American Nephrology Nurses' Association
ISBN 978-1-940325-07-1

American Nephrology Nurses' Association, East Holly Avenue/Box 56, Pitman, New Jersey 08071-0056
www.annanurse.org ■ Email: anna@annanurse.org ■ Phone: 888-600-2662

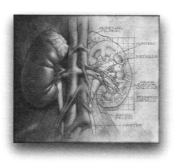

Foreword

The American Nephrology Nurses' Association has had a long-standing commitment to providing the tools and resources needed for individuals to be successful in their professional nephrology roles. With that commitment, we proudly present the sixth edition of the *Core Curriculum for Nephrology Nursing*.

This edition has a new concept and look that we hope you find valuable. Offered in six separate modules, each one will focus on a different component of our specialty and provide essential, updated, high-quality information. Since our last publication of the *Core Curriculum* in 2008, our practice has evolved, and our publication has been transformed to keep pace with those changes.

Under the expert guidance of Editor and Project Director Caroline S. Counts, MSN, RN, CNN (who was also the editor for the 2008 *Core Curriculum*!), this sixth edition continues to build on our fundamental principles and standards of practice. From the basics of each modality to our roles in advocacy, patient engagement, evidence-based practice, and more, you will find crucial information to facilitate the important work you do on a daily basis.

The ANNA Board of Directors and I extend our sincerest gratitude to Caroline and commend her for the stellar work that she and all of the section editors, authors, and reviewers have put forth in developing this new edition of the *Core Curriculum for Nephrology Nursing*. These individuals have spent many hours working to provide you with this important nephrology nursing publication. We hope you enjoy this exemplary professional resource.

Sharon Longton, BSN, RN, CNN, CCTC
ANNA President, 2014-2015

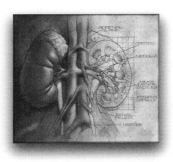

What's new in the sixth edition?

The 2015 edition of the *Core Curriculum for Nephrology Nursing* reflects several changes in format and content. These changes have been made to make life easier for the reader and to improve the scientific value of the *Core*.

1. The *Core Curriculum* is divided into six separate modules that can be purchased as a set or as individual texts. Keep in mind there is likely additional relevant information in more than one module. For example, in Module 2 there is a specific chapter for nutrition, but the topic of nutrition is also addressed in several chapters in other modules.

2. The *Core* is available in both print and electronic formats. The electronic format contains links to other websites with additional helpful information that can be reached with a simple click. With this useful feature comes a potential issue: when an organization changes its website and reroutes its links, the URLs that are provided may not connect. When at the organization's website, use their search feature to easily find your topic. The links in the *Core* were updated as of March 2015.

3. As with the last edition of the *Core*, the pictures on chapter covers depict actual nephrology staff members and patients with kidney disease. Their willingness to participate is greatly appreciated.

4. Self-assessment questions are included at the end of each module for self-testing. Completion of these exercises is not required to obtain CNE. CNE credit can be obtained by accessing the Evaluation Forms on the ANNA website.

5. References are cited in the text and listed at the end of each chapter.

6. We've provided examples of references in APA format at the beginning of each chapter, as well as on the last page of this front matter, to help the readers know how to properly format references if they use citations from the *Core*. The guesswork has been eliminated!

7. The information contained in the *Core* has been expanded, and new topics have been included. For example, there is information on leadership and management, material on caring for Veterans, more emphasis on patient and staff safety, and more.

8. Many individuals assisted in making the *Core* come to fruition; they brought with them their own experience, knowledge, and literature search. As a result, a topic can be addressed from different perspectives, which in turn gives the reader a more global view of nephrology nursing.

9. This edition employs usage of the latest terminology in nephrology patterned after the National Kidney Foundation.

10. The *Core Curriculum for Nephrology Nursing*, 6th edition contains 233 figures, 234 tables, and 29 appendices. These add valuable tools in delivering the contents of the text.

Thanks to B. Braun Medical Inc. for its grant in support of ANNA's *Core Curriculum*.

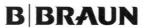

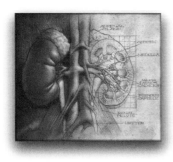

Preface

The sixth edition of the *Core Curriculum for Nephrology Nursing* has been written and published due to the efforts of many individuals. Thank you to the editors, authors, reviewers, and everyone who helped pull the *Core* together to make it the publication it became. A special thank you to Claudia Cuddy and Joe Tonzelli, who were involved from the beginning to the end — I could not have done my job without them!

The overall achievement is the result of the unselfish contributions of each and every individual team member. At times it was a daunting, challenging task, but the work is done, and all members of the "Core-team" should feel proud of the end product.

Now, the work is turned over to you — the reader and learner. I hope you learn at least half as much as I did as pieces of the *Core* were submitted, edited, and refined. Considering the changes that have taken place since the first edition of the *Core* in 1987 (322 pages!), one could say it is a whole new world! Even since the fifth edition in 2008, many changes in nephrology have transpired. This, the 2015 edition, is filled with the latest information regarding kidney disease, its treatment, and the nursing care involved.

But, buyer, beware! Evolution continues, and what is said today can be better said tomorrow. Information continues to change and did so even as the chapters were being written; yet, change reflects progress. Our collective challenge is to learn from the *Core*, be flexible, keep an open mind, and question what could be different or how nephrology nursing practice could be improved.

Nephrology nursing will always be stimulating, learning will never end, and progress will continue! So, the *Core* not only represents what we know now, but also serves as a springboard for what the learner can become and what nephrology nursing can be. A Chinese proverb says this: "Learning is like rowing upstream; not to advance is to drop back."

A final thank-you to the Core-team and a very special note of appreciation to those I love the most. (Those I love the most have also grown since the last edition!) For their love, support, and encouragement, I especially thank my husband, Henry, who thought I had retired; my son and daughter-in law, Chris and Christina, and our two amazing grandchildren, Cate and Olin; and my son-in-law, Marty Morganello, and our daughter, Kim, who provided many of the photographs used in this version of the *Core*. It has been a family project!

Last, but certainly not least, I thank the readers and learners. It is your charge to use the *Core* to grow your minds. Minds can grow as long as we live — don't drop back!

Caroline S. Counts
Editor, Sixth Edition

Module 2

As can be easily seen, Module 2 contains assorted material to assist the nurse in understanding kidney disease, the patient with kidney disease, and interrelated topics. **Chapter 1** begins with an in-depth review of genetics and genomics, since many experienced nurses learned relatively little about the topic when in school. The completion of the Human Genome Project catapulted genetic research that is already transforming health care and has great potential to continue this transformation. It certainly includes nephrology care and requires that nephrology nurses be knowledgeable about the matter. The chapter also covers anatomy, physiology, and pathophysiology. (*Note*: Module 4 deals exclusively with acute kidney injury.) **Chapter 2** focuses specifically on chronic kidney disease and delivers a more detailed approach than the material presented in the previous chapter. **Chapter 3** provides a wide array of material to be considered when caring for an individual patient. One of the new areas includes focus on the veteran. **Chapter 4** concentrates on nutrition, and **Chapter 5** addresses pharmacology. It behooves every nurse to always stay abreast of changes regarding medications, as this is one area that can change rapidly. At all times, be familiar with the package insert and consult with a pharmacist or other reliable source as needed. The foundation of **Chapter 6** is infection control practices and is another area where information can change rapidly. Information from the Centers for Disease Control and Prevention (CDC) was used extensively as a resource.

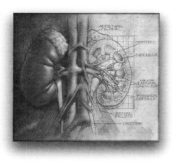

Chapter Editors and Authors

Lisa Ales, MSN, NP-C, FNP-BC, CNN
Clinical Educator, Renal
Baxter Healthcare Corporation
Deerfield, IL
Author: Module 3, Chapter 4

Kim Alleman, MS, APRN, FNP-BC, CNN-NP
Nurse Practitioner
Hartford Hospital Transplant Program
Hartford, CT
Editor: Module 6

Billie Axley, MSN, RN, CNN
Director, Innovations Group
FMS Medical Office
Franklin, TN
Author: Module 4, Chapter 3

Donna Bednarski, MSN, RN, ANP-BC, CNN, CNP
Nurse Practitioner, Dialysis Access Center
Harper University Hospital
Detroit, MI
Editor & Author: Module 1, Chapter 3
Editor & Author: Module 2, Chapter 3
Author: Module 6, Chapter 3

Brandy Begin, BSN, RN, CNN
Pediatric Dialysis Coordinator
Lucile Packard Children's Hospital at Stanford
Palo Alto, CA
Author: Module 5, Chapter 1

Deborah Brommage, MS, RDN, CSR, CDN
Program Director
National Kidney Foundation
New York, NY
Editor & Author: Module 2, Chapter 4
Editor: Module 4, Chapter 3

Deborah H. Brooks, MSN, ANP-BC, CNN, CNN-NP
Nurse Practitioner
Medical University of South Carolina
Charleston, SC
Author: Module 6, Chapter 1

Colleen M. Brown, MSN, APRN, ANP-BC
Transplant Nurse Practitioner
Hartford Hospital
Hartford, CT
Author: Module 6, Chapter 3

Loretta Jackson Brown, PhD, RN, CNN
Health Communication Specialist
Centers for Disease Control and Prevention
Atlanta, GA
Author: Module 2, Chapter 3

Molly Cahill, MSN, RN, APRN, BC, ANP-C, CNN
Nurse Practitioner
KC Kidney Consultants
Kansas City, MO
Author: Module 2, Chapter 3

Sally F. Campoy, DNP, ANP-BC, CNN-NP
Nurse Practitioner, Renal Section
Department of Veterans Affairs
Eastern Colorado Health System
Denver VA Medical Center, Denver, CO
Author: Module 6, Chapter 2

Laurie Carlson, MSN, RN
Transplant Coordinator
University of California –
    San Francisco Medical Center
San Francisco, CA
Author: Module 3, Chapter 1

Deb Castner, MSN, APRN, ACNP, CNN
Nurse Practitioner
Jersey Coast Nephrology & Hypertension
    Associates
Brick, NJ
Author: Module 2, Chapter 3
Author: Module 3, Chapter 2

Louise Clement, MS, RDN, CSR, LD
Renal Dietitian
Fresenius Medical Care
Lubbock, TX
Author: Module 2, Chapter 4

Jean Colaneri, ACNP-BC, CNN
Clinical Nurse Specialist and Nurse
    Practitioner, Dialysis Apheresis
Albany Medical Center Hospital, Albany, NY
Editor & Author: Module 3, Chapter 1

Ann Beemer Cotton, MS, RDN, CNSC
Clinical Dietitian Specialist in Critical Care
IV Health/Methodist Campus
Indianapolis, IN
Author: Module 2, Chapter 4
Author: Module 4, Chapter 2

Caroline S. Counts, MSN, RN, CNN
Research Coordinator, Retired
Division of Nephrology
Medical Unversity of South Carolina
Charleston, SC
Editor: Core Curriculum for Nephrology Nursing
Author: Module 1, Chapter 2
Author: Module 2, Chapter 6
Author: Module 3, Chapter 3

Helen Currier, BSN, RN, CNN, CENP
Director, Renal Services, Dialysis/Pheresis,
    Vascular Access/Wound, Ostomy,
    Continence, & Palliative Care Services
Texas Children's Hospital, Houston, TX
Author: Module 6, Chapter 5

Kim Deaver, MSN, RN, CNN
Program Manager
University of Virginia
Charlottesville, VA
Editor & Author: Module 3, Chapter 3

Anne Diroll, MA, BSN, BS, RN, CNN
Consultant
Volume Management
Rocklin, CA
Author: Module 5, Chapter 1

Daniel Diroll, MA, BSN, BS, RN
Education Coordinator
Fresenius Medical Care North America
Rocklin, CA
Author: Module 2, Chapter 3

Sheila J. Doss-McQuitty, MBA, BSN, RN, CNN, CCRA
Director, Clinical Programs and Research
Satellite Healthcare, Inc., San Jose, CA
Author: Module 2, Chapter 1

Paula Dutka, MSN, RN, CNN
Director, Education and Research
Nephrology Network
Winthrop University Hospital, Mineola, NY
Author: Module 2, Chapter 1

Andrea Easom, MA, MNSc, APRN, FNP-BC, CNN-NP
Instructor, College of Medicine
Nephrology Division
University of Arkansas for Medical Sciences
Little Rock, AR
Author: Module 6, Chapter 2

Rowena W. Elliott, PhD, RN, CNN, CNE, AGNP-C, FAAN
Associate Professor and Chairperson
Department of Advanced Practice
College of Nursing
University of Southern Mississippi
Hattiesburg, MS
Editor & Author: Module 5, Chapter 2

Susan Fallone, MS, RN, CNN
Clinical Nurse Specialist, Retired
Adult and Pediatric Dialysis
Albany Medical Center, Albany, NY
Author: Module 4, Chapter 2

Jessica J. Geer, MSN, C-PNP, CNN-NP
Pediatric Nurse Practitioner
Texas Children's Hospital, Houston, TX
Instructor, Renal Services, Dept. of Pediatrics
Baylor College of Medicine, Houston, TX
Author: Module 6, Chapter 5

Silvia German, RN, CNN
Clinical Writer, CE Coordinator
Manager, DaVita HealthCare Partners Inc.
Denver, CO
Author: Module 2, Chapter 6

Elaine Go, MSN, NP, CNN-NP
Nurse Practitioner
St. Joseph Hospital Renal Center
Orange, CA
Author: Module 6, Chapter 3

Norma Gomez, MSN, MBA, RN, CNN
Nephrology Nurse Consultant
Russellville, TN
Editor & Author: Module 1, Chapter 4

Janelle Gonyea, RDN, LD
Clinical Dietitian
Mayo Clinic
Rochester, MN
Author: Module 2, Chapter 4

Karen Greco, PhD, RN, ANP-BC, FAAN
Nurse Practitioner
Independent Contractor/Consultant
West Linn, OR
Author: Module 2, Chapter 1

Bonnie Bacon Greenspan, MBA, BSN, RN
Consultant, BBG Consulting, LLC
Alexandria, VA
Author: Module 1, Chapter 1

Cheryl L. Groenhoff, MSN, MBA, RN, CNN
Clinical Educator, Baxter Healthcare
Plantation, FL
Author: Module 2, Chapter 3
Author: Module 3, Chapter 4

Debra J. Hain, PhD, ARNP, ANP-BC, GNP-BC, FAANP
Assistant Professor/Lead AGNP Faculty
Florida Atlantic University
Christine E. Lynn College of Nursing
Boca Raton, FL
Nurse Practitioner, Cleveland Clinic Florida
Department of Nephrology, Weston, FL
Editor & Author: Module 2, Chapter 2

Lisa Hall, MSSW, LICSW
Patient Services Director
Northwest Renal Network (ESRD Network 16)
Seattle, WA
Author: Module 2, Chapter 3

Mary S. Haras, PhD, MS, MBA, APN, NP-C, CNN
Assistant Professor and Interim Associate
Dean of Graduate Nursing
Saint Xavier University School of Nursing
Chicago, IL
Author: Module 2, Chapter 2

Carol Motes Headley, DNSc, ACNP-BC, RN, CNN
Nephrology Nurse Practitioner
Veterans Affairs Medical Center
Memphis, TN
Editor & Author: Module 2, Chapter 1

Mary Kay Hensley, MS, RDN, CSR
Chair/Immediate Past Chair
Renal Dietitians Dietetic Practice Group
Renal Dietitian, Retired
DaVita HealthCare Partners Inc.
Gary, IN
Author: Module 2, Chapter 4

Kerri Holloway, RN, CNN
Clinical Quality Manager
Corporate Infection Control Specialist
Fresenius Medical Services, Waltham, MA
Author: Module 2, Chapter 6

Alicia M. Horkan, MSN, RN, CNN
Assistant Director, Dialysis Services
Dialysis Center at Colquitt Regional
Medical Center
Moultrie, GA
Author: Module 1, Chapter 2

Katherine Houle, MSN, APRN, CFNP, CNN-NP
Nephrology Nurse Practitioner
Marquette General Hospital
Marquette, MI
Editor: Module 6
Author: Module 6, Chapter 3

Liz Howard, RN, CNN
Director
DaVita HealthCare Partners Inc.
Oldsmar, FL
Author: Module 2, Chapter 6

Darlene Jalbert, BSN, RN, CNN
HHD Education Manager
DaVita University School of Clinical
Education Wisdom Team
DaVita HealthCare Partners Inc., Denver, CO
Author: Module 3, Chapter 2

Judy Kauffman, MSN, RN, CNN
Manager, Acute Dialysis and Apheresis Unit
University of Virginia Health Systems
Charlottesville, VA
Author: Module 3, Chapter 2

Tamara Kear, PhD, RN, CNS, CNN
Assistant Professor of Nursing
Villanova University, Villanova, PA
Nephrology Nurse, Fresenius Medical Care
Philadelphia, PA
Editor & Author: Module 1, Chapter 2

Lois Kelley, MSW, LSW, ACSW, NSW-C
Master Social Worker
DaVita HealthCare Partners Inc.
Harrisonburg Dialysis
Harrisonburg, VA
Author: Module 2, Chapter 3

Pamela S. Kent, MS, RDN, CSR, LD
Patient Education Coordinator
Centers for Dialysis Care
Cleveland, OH
Author: Module 2, Chapter 4

Carol L. Kinzner, MSN, ARNP, GNP-BC, CNN-NP
Nurse Practitioner
Pacific Nephrology Associates
Tacoma, WA
Author: Module 6, Chapter 3

Kim Lambertson, MSN, RN, CNN
Clinical Educator
Baxter Healthcare
Deerfield, IL
Author: Module 3, Chapter 4

Sharon Longton, BSN, RN, CNN, CCTC
Transplant Coordinator/Educator
Harper University Hospital
Detroit, MI
Author: Module 2, Chapter 3

Maria Luongo, MSN, RN
CAPD Nurse Manager
Massachusetts General Hospital
Boston, MA
Author: Module 3, Chapter 5

Suzanne M. Mahon, DNSc, RN, AOCN, APNG
Professor, Internal Medicine
Division of Hematology/Oncology
Professor, Adult Nursing, School of Nursing
St. Louis University, St. Louis, MO
Author: Module 2, Chapter 1

Nancy McAfee, MN, RN, CNN
CNS – Pediatric Dialysis and Vascular Access
Seattle Children's Hospital
Seattle, WA
Editor & Author: Module 5, Chapter 1

Maureen P. McCarthy, MPH, RDN, CSR, LD
Assistant Professor/Transplant Dietitian
Oregon Health & Science University
Portland, OR
Author: Module 2, Chapter 4

M. Sue McManus, PhD, APRN, FNP-BC, CNN
Nephrology Nurse Practitioner
Kidney Transplant Nurse Practitioner
Richard L. Roudebush VA Medical Center
Indianapolis, IN
Author: Module 1, Chapter 2

Lisa Micklos, BSN, RN
Clinical Educator
NxStage Medical, Inc.
Los Angeles, CA
Author: Module 1, Chapter 2

Michele Mills, MS, RN, CPNP
Pediatric Nurse Practitioner
Pediatric Nephrology
University of Michigan
C.S. Mott Children's Hospital, Ann Arbor, MI
Author: Module 5, Chapter 1

Geraldine F. Morrison, BSHSA, RN
Clinical Director, Home Programs & CKD
Northwest Kidney Center
Seattle, WA
Author: Module 3, Chapter 5

Theresa Mottes, RN, CDN
Pediatric Research Nurse
Cincinnati Children's Hospital & Medical Center
Center for Acute Care Nephrology
Cincinnati, OH
Author: Module 5, Chapter 1

Linda L. Myers, BS, RN, CNN, HP
RN Administrative Coordinator, Retired
Home Dialysis Therapies
University of Virginia Health System
Charlottesville, VA
Author: Module 4, Chapter 5

Clara Neyhart, BSN, RN, CNN
Nephrology Nurse Clinician
UNC Chapel Hill
Chapel Hill, NC
Editor & Author: Module 3, Chapter 1

Mary Alice Norton, BSN, FNP-C
Senior Heart Failure/LVAD/Transplant
   Coordinator
Albany Medical Center Hospital
Albany, NY
Author: Module 4, Chapter 6

Jessie M. Pavlinac, MS, RDN, CSR, LD
Director, Clinical Nutrition
Oregon Health and Science University
Portland, OR
Author: Module 2, Chapter 4

Glenda M. Payne, MS, RN, CNN
Director of Clinical Services
Nephrology Clinical Solutions
Duncanville, TX
Editor & Author: Module 1, Chapter 1
Author: Module 3, Chapter 2
Author: Module 4, Chapter 4

Eileen J. Peacock, MSN, RN, CNN,
   CIC, CPHQ, CLNC
Infection Control and Surveillance
   Management Specialist
DaVita HealthCare Partners Inc.
Maple Glen, PA
Editor & Author: Module 2, Chapter 6

Mary Perrecone, MS, RN, CNN, CCRN
Clinical Manager
Fresenius Medical Care
Charleston, SC
Author: Module 4, Chapter 1

Susan A. Pfettscher, PhD, RN
California State University Bakersfield
   Department of Nursing, Retired
Satellite Health Care, San Jose, CA, Retired
Bakersfield, CA
Author: Module 1, Chapter 1

Nancy B. Pierce, BSN, RN, CNN
Dialysis Director
St. Peter's Hospital
Helena, MT
Author: Module 1, Chapter 1

Leonor P. Ponferrada, BSN, RN, CNN
Education Coordinator
University of Missouri School of Medicine –
   Columbia
Columbia, MO
Author: Module 3, Chapter 4

Lillian A. Pryor, MSN, RN, CNN
Clinical Manager
FMC Loganville, LLC
Loganville, GA
Author: Module 1, Chapter 1

Timothy Ray, DNP, CNP, CNN-NP
Nurse Practitioner
Cleveland Kidney & Hypertension Consultants
Euclid, OH
Author: Module 6, Chapter 4

Cindy Richards, BSN, RN, CNN
Transplant Coordinator
Children's of Alabama
Birmingham, AL
Author: Module 5, Chapter 1

Karen C. Robbins, MS, RN, CNN
Nephrology Nurse Consultant
Associate Editor, *Nephrology Nursing Journal*
Past President, American Nephrology Nurses'
   Association
West Hartford, CT
Editor: Module 3, Chapter 2

Regina Rohe, BS, RN, HP(ASCP)
Regional Vice President, Inpatient Services
Fresenius Medical Care, North America
San Francisco, CA
Author: Module 4, Chapter 8

Francine D. Salinitri, PharmD
Associate (Clinical) Professor of
   Pharmacy Practice
Wayne State University, Applebaum College of
   Pharmacy and Health Sciences, Detroit, MI
Clinical Pharmacy Specialist, Nephrology
Oakwood Hospital and Medical Center
Dearborn, MI
Author: Module 2, Chapter 5

Karen E. Schardin, BSN, RN, CNN
Clinical Director, National Accounts
NxStage Medical, Inc.
Lawrence, MA
Editor & Author: Module 3, Chapter 5

Mary Schira, PhD, RN, ACNP-BC
Associate Professor
Univ. of Texas at Arlington – College of Nursing
Arlington, TX
Author: Module 6, Chapter 1

Deidra Schmidt, PharmD
Clinical Pharmacy Specialist
Pediatric Renal Transplantation
Children's of Alabama
Birmingham, AL
Author: Module 5, Chapter 1

Joan E. Speranza-Reid, BSHM, RN, CNN
Clinic Manager
ARA/Miami Regional Dialysis Center
North Miami Beach, FL
Author: Module 3, Chapter 2

Jean Stover, RDN, CSR, LDN
Renal Dietitian
DaVita HealthCare Partners Inc.
Philadelphia, PA
Author: Module 2, Chapter 4

Charlotte Szromba, MSN, APRN, CNNe
Nurse Consultant, Retired
Department Editor, Nephrology Nursing
   Journal
Naperville, IL
Author: Module 2, Chapter 1

Kirsten L. Thompson, MPH, RDN, CSR
Clinical Dietitian
Seattle Children's Hospital, Seattle, WA
Author: Module 5, Chapter 1

Lucy B. Todd, MSN, ACNP-BC, CNN
Medical Science Liaison
Baxter Healthcare
Asheville, NC
Editor & Author: Module 3, Chapter 4

Susan C. Vogel, MHA, RN, CNN
Clinical Manager, National Accounts
NxStage Medical, Inc.
Los Angeles, CA
Author: Module 3, Chapter 5

Joni Walton, PhD, RN, ACNS-BC, NPc
Family Nurse Practitioner
Marias HealthCare
Shelby, MT
Author: Module 2, Chapter 1

Gail S. Wick, MHSA, BSN, RN, CNNe
Consultant
Atlanta, GA
Author: Module 1, Chapter 2

Helen F. Williams, MSN, BSN, RN, CNN
Special Projects – Acute Dialysis Team
Fresenius Medical Care
Denver, CO
Editor: Module 4
Editor & Author: Module 4, Chapter 7

Elizabeth Wilpula, PharmD, BCPS
Clinical Pharmacy Specialist
Nephrology/Transplant
Harper University Hospital, Detroit, MI
Editor & Author: Module 2, Chapter 5

Karen Wiseman, MSN, RN, CNN
Manager, Regulatory Affairs
Fresenius Medical Services
Waltham, MA
Author: Module 2, Chapter 6

Linda S. Wright, DrNP, RN, CNN, CCTC
Lead Kidney and Pancreas Transplant
  Coordinator
Thomas Jefferson University Hospital
Philadelphia, PA
Author: Module 1, Chapter 2

Mary M. Zorzanello, MSN, APRN
Nurse Practitioner, Section of Nephrology
Yale University School of Medicine
New Haven, CT
Author: Module 6, Chapter 3

STATEMENTS OF DISCLOSURE

Editors

Carol Motes Headley DNSc, ACNP-BC, RN, CNN, is a consultant and/or member of the Corporate Speakers Bureau for Sanofi Renal, and a member of the Advisory Board for Amgen.

Karen E. Schardin, BSN, RN, CNN, is an employee of NxStage Medical, Inc.

Lucy B. Todd, MSN, ACNP-BC, CNN, is an employee of Baxter Healthcare Corporation.

Authors

Lisa Ales, MSN, NP-C, FNP-BC, CNN, is an employee of Baxter Healthcare Corporation.

Billie Axley, MSN, RN, CNN, is an employee of Fresenius Medical Care.

Brandy Begin, BSN, RN, CNN, is a consultant for CHA-SCOPE Collaborative Faculty and has prior received financial support as an injection-training nurse for nutropin from Genentech.

Molly Cahill, MSN, RN, APRN, BC, ANP-C, CNN, is a member of the advisory board for the National Kidney Foundation and Otsuka America Pharmaceutical, Inc., and has received financial support from DaVita HealthCare Partners Inc. [Author states none of this pertains to the material present in her chapter.]

Ann Diroll, MA, BSN, BS, RN, CNN, is a previous employee of Hema Metrics LLC/Fresenius Medical Care (through March 2013).

Sheila J. Doss-McQuitty, MBA, BSN, RN, CNN, CCRA, is a member of the consultant presenter bureau and the advisory board for Takeda Pharmaceuticals U.S.A., Inc., and Affymax, Inc.

Paula Dutka, MSN, RN, CNN, is a coordinator of Clinical Trials for the following sponsors: Amgen, Rockwell Medical Technologies, Inc.; Keryx Biopharmaceuticals, Inc.; Akebia Therapeutics; and Dynavax Technologies.

Elaine Go, MSN, NP, CNN-NP, is on the Speakers Bureau for Sanofi Renal.

Bonnie B. Greenspan, MSN, MBA, RN, has a spouse who works as a medical director of a DaVita HealthCare Partners Inc. dialysis facility.

Mary Kay Hensley, MS, RDN, CSR, is a member of the Academy of Nutrition & Dietitians Renal Practitioners advisory board.

Tamara M. Kear, PhD, RN, CNS, CNN, is a Fresenius Medical Care employee and freelance editor for Lippincott Williams & Wilkins and Elsevier publishing companies.

Kim Lambertson, MSN, RN, CNN, is an employee of Baxter Healthcare Corporation.

Regina Rhoe, BS, RN, HP(ASCP), is an employee of Fresenius Medical Care.

Francine D. Salinitri, Pharm D, received financial support from Otsuka America Pharmaceutical, Inc., through August 2013.

Susan Vogel, MHA, RN, CNN, is an employee of NxStage Medical, Inc.

Reviewers

Jacke L. Corbett, DNP, FNP-BC, CCTC, was on the Novartis Speakers Bureau in 2013.

Deborah Glidden, MSN, ARNP, BC, CNN, is a consultant or member of Corporate Speakers Bureau for Amgen, Pentec Health, and Sanofi-Aventis, and she has received financial support from Amgen.

David Grubbs, RN, CDN, Paramedic, ACLS, PALS, BCLS, TNCC, NIH, has familial relations employed by GlaxoSmithKline (GSK).

Diana Hlebovy, BSN, RN, CHN, CNN, was a clinical support specialist for Fresenius Medical Care RTG in 2013.

Kristin Larson, RN, ANP, GNP, CNN, is an employee of NxStage Medical, Inc.

All other contributors to the *Core Curriculum for Nephrology Nursing* (6th ed.) reported no actual or potential conflict of interest in relation to this continuing nursing education activity.

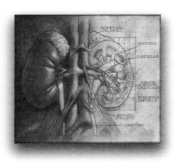

Reviewers

The Blind Review Process

The contents of the *Core Curriculum* underwent a "blind" review process by qualified individuals. One or more chapters were sent to chosen people for critical evaluation. The reviewer did not know the author's identity at the time of the review.

The work could be accepted (1) as originally submitted without revisions, (2) with minor revisons, or (3) with major revisions. The reviewers offered tremendous insight and suggestions; some even submitted additional references they thought might be useful. The results of the review were then sent back to the chapter/module editors to incorporate the suggestions and make revisions.

The reviewers will discover who the authors are now that the *Core* is published. However, while there is this published list of reviewers, no one will know who reviewed which part of the *Core*. That part of the process remains blind.

Because of the efforts of individuals listed below, value was added to the sixth edition. Their hard work is greatly appreciated.

Caroline S. Counts, Editor

Marilyn R. Bartucci, MSN, RN, ACNS-BC, CCTC
Case Manager
Kidney Foundation of Ohio
Cleveland, OH

Christina M. Beale, RN, CNN
Director, Outreach and Education
Lifeline Vascular Access
Vernon Hills, IL

Jenny Bell, BSN, RN, CNN
Clinical Transplant Coordinator
Banner Good Samaritan Transplant Center
Phoenix, AZ

M. Geraldine Biddle, RN, CNN, CPHQ
President, Nephrology Nurse Consultants
Pittsford, NY

Randee Breiterman White, MS, RN
Nurse Case Manager Nephrology
Vanderbilt University Hospital
Nashville, TN

Jerrilynn D. Burrowes, PhD, RDN, CDN
Professor and Chair
Director, Graduate Programs in Nutrition
Department of Nutrition
Long Island University (LIU) Post
Brookville, NY

Sally Burrows-Hudson, MSN, RN, CNN
Deceased 2014
Director, Nephrology Clinical Solutions
Lisle, IL

LaVonne Burrows, APRN, BC, CNN
Advanced Practice Registered Nurse
Springfield Nephrology Associates
Springfield, MO

Karen T. Burwell, BSN, RN, CNN
Acute Dialysis Nurse
DaVita HealthCare Partners Inc.
Phoenix, AZ

Laura D. Byham-Gray, PhD, RDN
Associate Professor and Director
Graduate Programs in Clinical Nutrition
Department of Nutritional Sciences
School of Health Related Professions
Rutgers University
Stratford, NJ

Theresa J. Campbell, DNP, APRN, FNP-BC
Doctor of Nursing Practice
Family Nurse Practitioner
Carolina Kidney Care
Adjunct Professor of Nursing
University of North Caroline at Pembroke
Fayetteville, NC

Monet Carnahan, BSN, RN, CDN
Renal Care Coordinator Program Manager
Fresenius Medical Care
Nashville, TN

Jacke L. Corbett, DNP, FNP-BC, CCTC
Nurse Practitioner
Kidney/Pancreas Transplant Program
University of Utah Health Care
Salt Lake City, UT

Christine Corbett, MSN, APRN, FNP-BC, CNN-NP
Nephrology Nurse Practitioner
Truman Medical Centers
Kansas City, MO

Sandra Corrigan, FNP-BC, CNN
Nurse Practitioner
California Kidney Medical Group
Thousand Oaks, CA

Maureen Craig, MSN, RN, CNN
Clinical Nurse Specialist – Nephrology
University of California Davis Medical Center
Sacramento, CA

Diane M. Derkowski, MA, RN, CNN, CCTC
Kidney Transplant Coordinator
Carolinas Medical Center
Charlotte, NC

Linda Duval, BSN, RN
Executive Director, FMQAI: ESRD Network 13
ESRD Network
Oklahoma City, OK

Damian Eker, DNP, GNP-C
ARNP, Geriatrics & Adult Health
Adult & Geriatric Health Center
Ft. Lauderdale, FL

Elizabeth Evans, DNP
Nephrology Nurse Practitioner
Renal Medicine Associates
Albuquerque, NM

Susan Fallone, MS, RN, CNN
Clinical Nurse Specialist, Retired
Adult and Pediatric Dialysis
Albany Medical Center
Albany, NY

Karen Joann Gaietto, MSN, BSN, RN, CNN
Acute Clinical Service Specialist
DaVita HealthCare Partners Inc.
Tiffin, OH

Deborah Glidden, MSN, ARNP, BC, CNN
Nurse Practitioner
Nephrology Associates of Central Florida
Orlando, FL

David Jeremiah Grubbs, RN, CDN, Paramedic, ACLS, PALS, BCLS, TNCC, NIH
Clinical Nurse Manager
Crestwood, KY

Debra J. Hain, PhD, ARNP, ANP-BC, GNP-BC, FAANP
Associate Professor/Lead Faculty AGNP Track
Florida Atlantic University
Christine E. Lynn College of Nursing
Boca Raton, FL
Nurse Practitioner, Cleveland Clinic Florida
Department of Nephrology
Weston, FL

Brenda C. Halstead, MSN, RN, AcNP, CNN
Nurse Practitioner
Mid-Atlantic Kidney Center
Richmond and Petersburg, VA

Emel Hamilton, RN, CNN
Director of Clinical Technology
Fresenius Medical Care
Waltham, MA

Mary S. Haras, PhD, MBA, APN, NP-C, CNN
Associate Dean, Graduate Nursing Programs
Saint Xavier University School of Nursing
Chicago, IL

Malinda C. Harrington, MSN, RN, FNP-BC, ANCC
Pediatric Nephrology Nurse Practitioner
Vidant Medical Center
Greenville, NC

Diana Hlebovy, BSN, RN, CHN, CNN
Nephrology Nurse Consultant
Elyria, OH

Sara K. Kennedy, BSN, RN, CNN
UAB Medicine, Kirklin Clinic
Diabetes Care Coordinator
Birmingham, AL

Nadine "Niki" Kobes, BSN, RN
Manager Staff Education/Quality
Fresenius Medical Care – Alaska JV Clinics
Anchorage, AK

Deuzimar Kulawik, MSN, RN
Director of Clinical Quality
DaVita HealthCare Partners Inc.
Westlake Village, CA

Kristin Larson, RN, ANP, GNP, CNN
Clinical Instructor
College of Nursing
Family Nurse Practitioner Program
University of North Dakota
Grand Forks, ND

Deborah Leggett, BSN, RN, CNN
Director, Acute Dialysis
Jackson Madison County General Hospital
Jackson, TN

Charla Litton, MSN, APRN, FNP-BC, CNN
Nurse Practitioner
UHG/Optum
East Texas, TX

Greg Lopez, BSN, RN, CNN
IMPAQ Business Process Manager
Fresenius Medical Care
New Orleans, LA

Terri (Theresa) Luckino, BSN, RN, CCRN
President, Acute Services
RPNT Acute Services, Inc.
Irving, TX

Alice Luehr, BA, RN, CNN
Home Therapy RN
St. Peter's Hospital
Helena, MT

Maryam W. Lyon, MSN, RN, CNN
Education Coordinator
Fresenius Medical Care
Dayton, OH

Christine Mudge, MS, RN, PNP/CNS, CNN, FAAN
Mill Valley, CA

Mary Lee Neuberger, MSN, APRN, RN, CNN
Pediatric Nephrology
University of Iowa Children's Hospital
Iowa City, IA

Jennifer Payton, MHCA, BSN, RN, CNN
Clinical Support Specialist
HealthStar CES
Goose Creek, SC

April Peters, MSN, RN, CNN
Clinical Informatics Specialist
Brookhaven Memorial Hospital Medical Center
Patchogue, NY

David J. Quan, PharmD, BCPS
Health Sciences Clinical Professor of Pharmacy
Clinical Pharmacist, Liver Transplant Services
UCSF Medical Center
San Francisco, CA

Kristi Robertson, CFNP
Nephrology Nurse Practitioner
Nephrology Associates
Columbus, MS

E. James Ryan, BSN, RN, CDN
Hemodialysis Clinical Services Coordinator
Lakeland Regional Medical Center
Lakeland, FL

June Shi, BSN, RN
Vascular Access Coordinator
Transplant Surgery
Medical University of South Carolina
Charleston, SC

Elizabeth St. John, MSN, RN, CNN
Education Coordinator, UMW Region
Fresenius Medical Care
Milwaukee, WI

Sharon Swofford, MA, RN, CNN, CCTC
Transplant Case Manager
OptumHealth
The Villages, FL

Beth Ulrich, EdD, RN, FACHE, FAAN
Senior Partner, Innovative Health Resources
Editor, *Nephrology Nursing Journal*
Pearland, TX

David F. Walz, MBA, BSN, RN, CNN
Program Director
CentraCare Kidney Program
St. Cloud, MN

Gail S. Wick, MHSA, BSN, RN, CNNe
Consultant
Atlanta, GA

Phyllis D. Wille, MS, RN, FNP-C, CNN, CNE
Nursing Faculty
Danville Area Community College
Danville, Il

Donna L. Willingham, RN, CPNP
Pediatric Nephrology Nurse Practitioner
Washington University St. Louis
St. Louis, MO

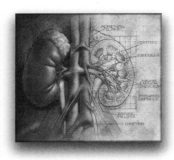

Contents at a Glance

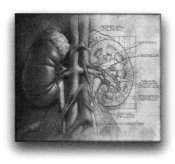

Expanded Contents

The table of contents contains chapters and sections with editors and authors for all six modules. The contents section of this specific module is highlighted in a blue background.

Module 1 Foundations for Practice in Nephrology Nursing

Module 2   Physiologic and Psychosocial Basis for Nephrology Nursing Practice

Module 3   Treatment Options for Patients with Chronic Kidney Failure

Module 4   Acute Kidney Injury

Module Editor: Helen F. Williams

Module 5   Kidney Disease in Patient Populations Across the Life Span

Module 6   The APRN's Approaches to Care in Nephrology

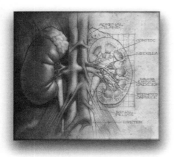

Examples of APA-formatted references

A guide for citing material from Module 2 of the *Core Curriculum for Nephrology Nursing, 6th edition.*

Module 2, Chapter 1

Use authors of the section being cited. This example is based on Section A – Genetics and Genomics.

Greco, K., & Mahon, S.M. (2015). The kidney in health and disease: Genetics and genomics. In C.S. Counts (Ed.), *Core curriculum for nephrology nursing: Module 2. Physiologic and psychosocial basis for nephrology nursing practice* (6th ed., pp. 1-152). Pitman, NJ: American Nephrology Nurses' Association.

Interpreted: Section author(s). (Date). Title of chapter: Title of section. In ...

For citation in text: (Greco & Mahon, 2015) (Use the author of the section you are citing.)

Module 2, Chapter 2

Two authors for entire chapter.

Hain, D.J., & Haras, M.S. (2015). Chronic kidney disease. In C.S. Counts (Ed.), *Core curriculum for nephrology nursing: Module 2. Physiologic and psychosocial basis for nephrology nursing practice* (6th ed., pp. 153-188). Pitman, NJ: American Nephrology Nurses' Association.

Interpreted: Chapter authors. (Date). Title of chapter. In ...

For citation in text: (Hain & Haras, 2015)

Module 2, Chapter 3

Use author of the section being cited. This example is based on Section E – Caring for Veterans.

Brown, L.J. (2015). Individualizing the care for those with kidney disease: Caring for veterans. In C.S. Counts (Ed.), *Core curriculum for nephrology nursing: Module 2. Physiologic and psychosocial basis for nephrology nursing practice* (6th ed., pp. 189-254). Pitman, NJ: American Nephrology Nurses' Association.

Interpreted: Section author(s). (Date). Title of chapter: Title of section. In …

For citation in text: (Brown, 2015) (Use the author(s) of the section you are citing.)

Module 2, Chapter 4

Use authors of the section being cited. This example is based on Section C – Special Considerations in Kidney Disease.

Brommage, D., Cotton, A.B., Gonyea, J., Kent, P.S., & Stover, J. (2015). Foundations in nutrition and clinical applications in nephrology nursing: Special considerations in kidney disease. In C.S. Counts (Ed.), *Core curriculum for nephrology nursing: Module 2. Physiologic and psychosocial basis for nephrology nursing practice* (6th ed., pp. 255-290). Pitman, NJ: American Nephrology Nurses' Association.

Interpreted: Section authors. (Date). Title of chapter: Title of section. In …

For citation in text: (Brommage, Cotton, Gonyea & Kent, & Stover, 2015) (Use the author(s) of the section you are citing.)

Module 2, Chapter 5

Two authors for entire chapter.

Wilpula, E., & Salinitri, F.D. (2015). Foundations in pharmacology and clinical applications in nephrology nursing. In C.S. Counts (Ed.), *Core curriculum for nephrology nursing: Module 2. Physiologic and psychosocial basis for nephrology nursing practice* (6th ed., pp. 291-330). Pitman, NJ: American Nephrology Nurses' Association.

Interpreted: Chapter authors. (Date). Title of chapter. In ...

For citation in text: (Wilpula & Salinitri, 2015)

Module 2, Chapter 6

Six authors for entire chapter.

Peacock, E.J., Counts, C.S., German, S., Holloway, K., Howard, L., & Wiseman, K. (2015). Foundations in infection prevention, control, and clinical applications in nephrology nursing. In C.S. Counts (Ed.), *Core curriculum for nephrology nursing: Module 2. Physiologic and psychosocial basis for nephrology nursing practice* (6th ed., pp. 331-396). Pitman, NJ: American Nephrology Nurses' Association.

Interpreted: Chapter authors. (Date). Title of chapter. In ...

For citation in text: (Peacock, Counts, German, Holloway, Howard, & Wiseman, 2015)

CHAPTER **1**
The Kidney in Health and Disease

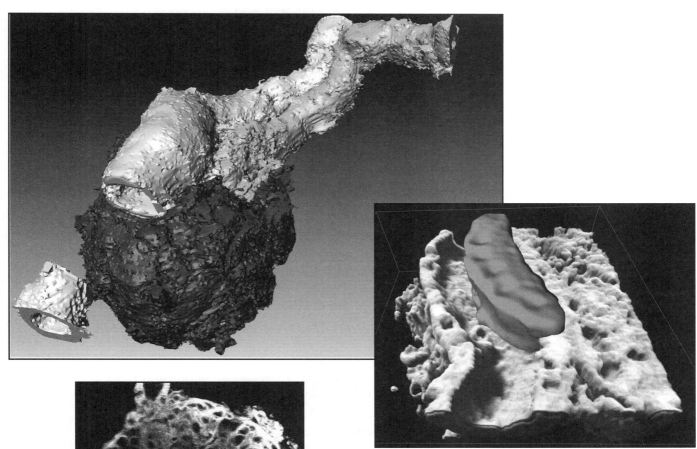

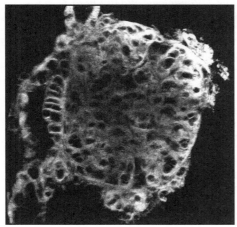

Chapter Editor
Carol Motes Headley, DNSc, ACNP-BC, RN, CNN

Authors
Carol Motes Headley, DNSc, ACNP-BC, RN, CNN
Sheila J. Doss-McQuitty, MBA, BSN, RN, CNN, CCRA
Paula Dutka, MSN, RN, CNN
Karen Greco, PhD, RN, ANP-BC, FAAN
Suzanne M. Mahon, DNSc, RN, AOCN, APNG
Charlotte Szromba, MSN, APRN, CNNe
Joni Walton, PhD, RN, ACNS-BC, NPc

CHAPTER **1**

The Kidney in Health and Disease

This offering for **3.3 contact hours** is provided by the American Nephrology Nurses' Association (ANNA).

American Nephrology Nurses' Association is accredited as a provider of continuing nursing education by the American Nurses Credentialing Center Commission on Accreditation.

ANNA is a provider approved by the California Board of Registered Nursing, provider number CEP 00910.

This CNE offering meets the continuing nursing education requirements for certification and recertification by the Nephrology Nursing Certification Commission (NNCC).

To be awarded contact hours for this activity, read this chapter in its entirety. Then complete the CNE evaluation found at **www.annanurse.org/corecne** and submit it; or print it, complete it, and mail it in. Contact hours are not awarded until the evaluation for the activity is complete.

Example of reference in APA format. Use author of the section being cited. This example is based on Section A – Genetics and Genomics.

Greco, K., & Mahon, S.M. (2015). The kidney in health and disease: Genetics and genomics. In C.S. Counts (Ed.), *Core curriculum for nephrology nursing: Module 2. Physiologic and psychosocial basis for nephrology nursing practice* (6th ed., pp. 1-152). Pitman, NJ: American Nephrology Nurses' Association.

Interpreted: Section author(s). (Date). Title of chapter: Title of section. In ...

Cover photo:

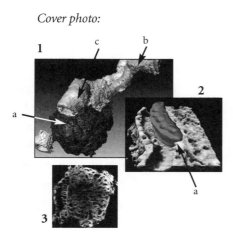

1. Segmented three-dimensional image of the living glomerulus (a). The supplying afferent arteriole (b) and the attached thick ascending limb (c) are also shown.
2. Three-dimensional volume-rendered image of the living juxtaglomerular apparatus with the macula densa (a).
3. Multiphoton confocal micrograph of living glomerulus.

Photos courtesy of P. Darwin Bell, PhD, DCI Professor of Medicine; Director, Renal Biology Research, Division of Nephrology, Medical University of South Carolina, Charleston, SC.

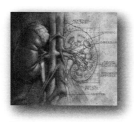

CHAPTER **1**

The Kidney in Health and Disease

Purpose

The standards of nephrology nursing practice first focus on assessment. "The nephrology registered nurse collects comprehensive data pertinent to the healthcare consumer's health and/or the situation." The standard continues by stating that the competent nephrology registered nurse "provides individualized comprehensive assessment of healthcare consumers and their care needs that contribute to the interdisciplinary team assessment" (Gomez, 2011, p. 16). This chapter delivers information on the kidneys in health and disease. It provides material that can assist the RN in understanding the connection between kidney disease and its effects on the individual and in making a thorough assessment.

The fundamental nature of every disease and condition has a genetic and genomic component; kidney disease is no exception. The development and advancement of genomic knowledge and technology has accelerated understanding of the genomic contribution to diseases and clinical capabilities for disease prediction, diagnosis, and treatment. It is also now possible to tailor therapeutics to an individual's genomic profile. It is important to understand that genomic discoveries have led to enhanced clinical capabilities to predict susceptibility to common diseases including hereditary kidney syndromes and diseases with a genetic component that can affect the kidneys such as diabetes, hypertension, and cancer.

This chapter also guides the reader into learning how the unique structure of the kidney facilitates its function. The reader will gain an appreciation for how the kidneys promote homeostasis by excreting waste products within a wide range of urine concentrations. Understanding normal renal physiology leads to understanding the consequences that occur with disease and its pathophysiology whether it is an acute or a chronic issue. This precedes an appreciation of why it is so incredibly difficult to artificially replace the kidneys. The chapter turns to presenting guidance in assessing patients with kidney disease and provides an overview of methods used to evaluate kidney structure and function. Related nursing interventions are summarized.

Objectives

Upon completion of this chapter, the learner will be able to:
1. Describe the importance of genetic/genomic knowledge as it relates to nephrology nursing care.
2. Discuss normal kidney function.
3. Summarize the systemic pathophysiology in acute kidney injury and chronic kidney disease.
4. State typical history and physical assessment findings in patients with kidney disorders.
5. Describe the methods used to assess kidney structure and function.

SECTION A
Genetics and Genomics
Karen Greco, Suzanne M. Mahon

I. The development of genetic/genomic competencies for all nurses.

A. In 2005, a consensus panel of nurse leaders established the *Essential Nursing Competencies and Curricula Guidelines for Genetics and Genomics.*
   1. While these competencies are not meant to replace or re-create existing standards of practice, they are intended to assimilate the genetic and genomic perspective into all nursing education and practice.
   2. Regardless of academic preparation, role, or practice setting, the clinical application of genetic and genomic knowledge has major implications for the entire nursing profession (Consensus Panel on Genetic/Genomic Nursing Competencies, 2009).
   3. In 2006, ANNA endorsed this document and agreed to incorporate this central science into nephrology nursing education and practice.

B. In the spring of 2009, a steering committee was convened to provide leadership in developing the *Essential Genetic and Genomic Competencies for Nurses with Graduate Degrees* (Greco et al., 2012).
   1. An advisory board of nursing leaders and genetics experts was created to review and revise the draft document.
   2. Representatives from a diverse number of nursing and advanced practice nursing organizations were later added to create a consensus panel to refine and validate these 38 competencies, which have subsequently been endorsed by 20 nursing and professional organizations.
   3. These graduate-level genetic/genomic nursing competencies are complementary to existing nursing competencies and standards of practice and are intended to provide structure as graduate-level nurses incorporate genetics and genomics into clinical and nonclinical roles.
   4. The primary purpose of this document is to identify essential genetic and genomic competencies for individuals prepared at the graduate level in nursing.
   5. These competencies apply to anyone functioning at the nursing graduate level, including but not limited to APRNs, nurse educators, nurse administrators, and nurse scientists.

C. Specialty genetics nursing practice.
   1. Nurses have been involved in genetics since the 1960s, when nurses provided services to children with genetic disorders and their families.
   2. The International Society of Nurses in Genetics (ISONG) was incorporated in 1988.
   3. ISONG has been instrumental in the development of genetics nursing as a specialty practice.

D. Largely through ISONG's efforts, in 1997 the American Nurses Association (ANA) established genetics nursing as an official specialty of nursing practice.
   1. In 2001, the Genetic Nursing Credentialing Commission was established.
   2. In 2001, the first Genetics Advanced Practice Nurses were credentialed followed by credentialing of the first Genetics Clinical Nurses in 2002 (Greco & Mahon, 2003).
   3. Nurses specializing in genetics/genomics have an expanded scope and practice which includes genetic counseling and testing for genetics nurses in advanced practice (ANA/ISONG, 2007).
   4. ISONG continues to foster the professional growth of nurses in genetics/genomics worldwide.

E. Although establishing genetics nursing practice as a clinical specialty is an important milestone, the real issue for nursing in the 21st century is genetics and genomics as it relates to the fundamental practice of every nurse (Greco, 2003).

II. Historical milestones in genetics and genomics nursing.

A. Background information.
   1. There is reason to believe that the concept of genetics was contemplated by the first human beings.
      a. As specific traits were noted to be shared by parent and child, questions were raised about inheritance.
      b. The sharing of specific traits was then applied to other areas such as plant cultivation and animal husbandry.
   2. And thus, the foundation was laid for the modern genetics that is practiced today.

B. 1865 – Austrian monk, Gregor Mendel, first traced inheritance patterns in pea plants and is considered the founding father of modern genetics.

C. 1953 – DNA structure was determined to be a double helix by James Watson and Francis Crick, using data from Rosalind Franklin. Their discovery heralded a new age of discovery in genetics and laid the foundation for the sequencing of the human genome.

D. 1956 – Jo Hin Tjio and Albert Levan established the number of chromosomes in humans to be 46.

E. 1958 – Crick proposed what was to become the central dogma of molecular biology: DNA is transcribed into RNA, which is translated into protein.

F. 1977 – Fred Sanger, Walter Gilbert, and Allan Maxam, working independently, developed techniques to determine the nucleic acid sequences for long sections of DNA.

G. 1984 – Genetics Nursing Network was formed, which later became the International Society of Nurses in Genetics (ISONG).

H. 1986 – The term *genomics* was coined by Thomas Roderick.

I. 1988 – ISONG was incorporated as a global nursing specialty organization dedicated to fostering the profession of nurses in human genetics and genomics worldwide.

J. 1989 – Francis Collins and Lap-Chee Tsui sequenced the first human gene. It encodes the CFTR protein; defects in this gene cause cystic fibrosis.

K. 1990 – The Human Genome Project was initiated. It is an international effort with scientists from 20 research centers in six countries: China, France, Germany, Japan, the United Kingdom, and the United States.

L. 1996 – The National Human Genome Research Institute, the American Nurses Association, and the American Medical Association form the National Coalition for Health Professional Education in Genetics (NCHPEG). The mission of NCHPEG is to promote health professional education and access to information about advances in human genetics to improve the health care of the nation.

M. 1997 – Genetic Nursing designated an official nursing specialty by the American Nurses Association.

N. 1998 – *Statement on the Scope and Standards of Genetics Clinical Nursing Practice* published by ISONG and ANA.

O. 2001 – The first draft sequences of the human genome are released simultaneously by the Human Genome Project and Celera Genomics.

P. 2002 – Genetic Nursing Credentialing Commission officially incorporated and established credentialing for genetic clinical nurses (GCN) and advanced practice nurses in genetics (APNG).

Q. 2003 – Successful completion of the Human Genome Project with 99% of the genome sequenced to a 99.9% accuracy.

R. 2006 – *Essential Nursing Competencies and Curricula Guidelines for Genetics and Genomics*, created in 2005 by an independent panel of nurse leaders from clinical, research, and academic settings, was published to establish genetic and genomic competencies for all nurses.

S. 2012 – *Essential Genetic and Genomic Competencies for Nurses with Graduate Degrees*, established by an independent panel of nurse leaders from clinical, research, and academic settings, was published to establish genetic and genomic competencies for all nurses with graduate degrees.

T. 2014 – Credentialing for genetic nurses is transferred to the American Nurses Credentialing Center (ANCC).

III. Theoretical background.

A. Genetics is the study of biologically inherited traits determined by genes that are passed from parent to offspring (Gunder & Martin, 2011).

B. Human genomics is the systematic study of all genes in the human genome, which includes genetic analysis and expression (Gunder & Martin, 2011).

C. DNA, or deoxyribonucleic acid, is the hereditary material. It is a macromolecule composed of polynucleotide chains in a double helix that contains all of the genetic material in a cell. Most DNA is located in the cell nucleus, but a small amount may be found in the mitochondria.
   1. The order, or sequence, of the information in DNA is stored as a code made up of four nitrogenous bases: adenine (A), guanine (G), cytosine (C), and thymine (T) (see Figure 1.1).
   2. The billions of nucleotides are organized in a linear fashion along the double helix in functional units known as genes.
   3. The DNA contains a specific set of instructions for making the proteins needed by the body's cells for their proper functioning.
   4. DNA bases pair up with each other to form units called base pairs. Each base is also attached to a sugar molecule and a phosphate molecule.
   5. A nucleotide is the combination of this base, the sugar, and the phosphate. Nucleotides are arranged in two long strands that form a spiral called a double helix (see Figure 1.1).
   6. An important property of DNA is its ability to replicate. This is critical when cells divide, as each new cell needs to have an exact copy of the DNA present in the old cell.

D. RNA, or ribonucleic acid, is a chemical similar to a single strand of DNA (Gaff & Bylund, 2011).
   1. RNA contains ribose rings and uracil, unlike

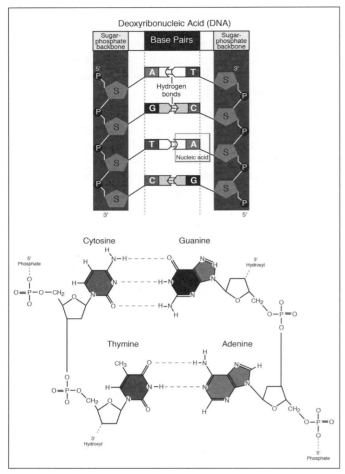

Figure 1.1. Model of deoxyribonucleic acid (DNA). A base pair is two chemical bases bonded to one another forming a "rung of the DNA ladder." The DNA molecule consists of two strands that wind around each other like a twisted ladder. Each strand has a backbone made of alternating sugar (deoxyribose) and phosphate groups. Attached to each sugar is one of four bases – adenine (A), cytosine (C), guanine (G), or thymine (T). The two strands are held together by hydrogen bonds between the bases, with adenine forming a base pair with thymine, and cytosine forming a base pair with guanine.

Public domain image obtained from
http://www.genome.gov/dmd/img.cfm?node=Photos/Graphics&id=85272
Courtesy of National Human Genome Research Institute.

DNA, which contains deoxyribose and thymine. It is composed of four bases: uracil, adenine, guanine, and cytosine (see Figure 1.2).

2. RNA is transcribed from DNA by enzymes called RNA polymerases and is further processed by other enzymes.

3. RNA serves as a template for translation of genes into proteins. It delivers DNA's genetic message to the cytoplasm of a cell where proteins are made.

E. Genes are the basic physical and functional units of heredity. A gene is an ordered sequence of nucleotides located in a particular position on a particular chromosome that encodes for a specific functional product (i.e., a protein or RNA molecule) (see Figure 1.3).

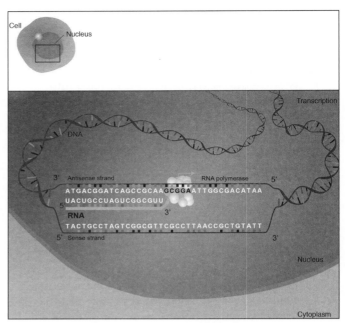

Figure 1.2. Model of ribonucleic acid (RNA). RNA is a molecule similar to DNA. Unlike DNA, RNA is single-stranded. An RNA strand has a backbone made of alternating sugar (ribose) and phosphate groups. Attached to each sugar is one of four bases – adenine (A), uracil (U), cytosine (C), or guanine (G). Different types of RNA exist in the cell: messenger RNA (mRNA), ribosomal RNA (rRNA), and transfer RNA (tRNA). More recently, some small RNAs have been found to be involved in regulating gene expression.

Public domain image obtained from
http://www.genome.gov/dmd/ img.cfm?node=Photos/Graphics&id=85237
Courtesy of National Human Genome Research Institute.

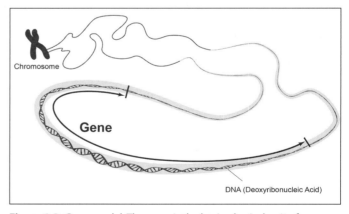

Figure 1.3. Gene model. The gene is the basic physical unit of inheritance. Genes are passed from parents to offspring and contain the information needed to specify traits. Genes are arranged, one after another, on structures called chromosomes. A chromosome contains a single, long DNA molecule, only a portion of which corresponds to a single gene. Humans have approximately 23,000 genes arranged on their chromosomes.

Public domain image obtained from
http://www.genome.gov/ dmd/img.cfm?node=Photos/Graphics&id=85170
Courtesy of National Human Genome Research Institute.

1. Genes are made up of DNA, the code for a specific protein or RNA.
2. It is estimated that humans have between 20,000 and 25,000 genes.
3. Genes vary in size and range from a hundred DNA bases to more than 2 million bases.
4. Most genes are the same in all people. Less than 1% of the total is slightly different and account for each person's unique physical characteristics.
5. Alleles are variants of the same gene with slight differences in their sequence of DNA bases (e.g., at a locus for eye color, the allele might result in blue or brown eyes) (see Figure 1.4).

F. Chromosomes are the microscopic, thread-like structures in the cell nucleus into which the DNA molecule is packaged (see Figure 1.5) (Brown, 2009).
   1. Each chromosome is made up of DNA tightly coiled many times around proteins called histones that support its structure.
   2. Distinct chromosomes are only visible under a microscope when the cell is dividing.
   3. Each chromosome has a constriction point called a centromere that divides the chromosome into two sections or arms.
      a. The shorter arm is called *p*; the longer arm is called *q*.
      b. The centromere gives the chromosome its characteristic shape and can be used to help describe the location of specific genes in a genetic map (see Figure 1.5).
   4. The telomere is a repetitive segment of DNA found on the ends of the chromosomes.

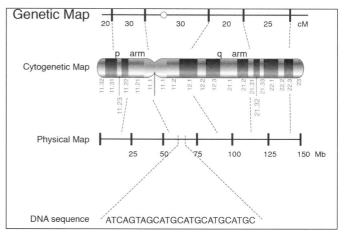

Figure 1.5. Structure of a chromosome. A genetic map is a type of chromosome map that shows the relative locations of genes and other important features. The map is based on the idea of linkage, which means that the closer two genes are to each other on the chromosome, the greater the probability that they will be inherited together. By following inheritance patterns, the relative locations of genes along the chromosome are established.

Public domain image obtained from:
http://www.genome.gov/ dmd/img.cfm?node=Photos/Graphics&id=85174
Courtesy of National Human Genome Research Institute.

      a. With each mitotic division, parts of the telomeres are lost.
      b. A theory of cellular aging proposes that the telomeres act as a biologic clock. When they are depleted, the cell dies or becomes less active (see Figure 1.6).
   5. Each human cell normally contains 23 pairs of chromosomes, for a total of 46.

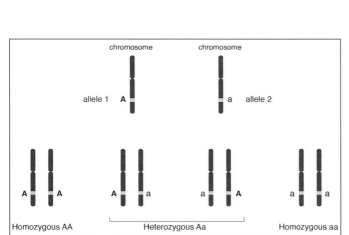

Figure 1.4. Model of allele. An allele is one of two or more versions of a gene. An individual inherits two alleles for each gene, one from each parent. If the two alleles are the same, the individual is homozygous for that gene. If the alleles are different, the individual is heterozygous. Though the term *allele* was originally used to describe variation among genes, it now also refers to variation among noncoding DNA sequences.

Public domain image obtained from http://www.genome.gov/ dmd/img.cfm?node=Photos/Graphics&id=85261
Courtesy of National Human Genome Research Institute.

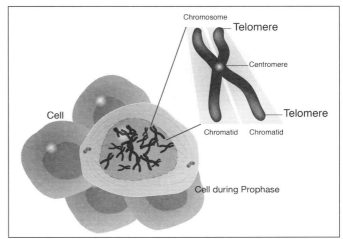

Figure 1.6. Model of telomere. A telomere is the end of a chromosome. Telomeres are made of repetitive sequences of non-coding DNA that protect the chromosome from damage. Each time a cell divides, the telomeres become shorter. Eventually, the telomeres become so short that the cell can no longer divide.

Public domain image obtained from http://www.genome.gov/ dmd/img.cfm?node=Photos/Graphics&id=85248
Courtesy of National Human Genome Research Institute.

a. Twenty-two of these pairs are known as autosomes and are the same in males and females.
b. The 23rd pair differs between males and females and comprises the sex chromosomes.
   (1) Females have two copies of the X chromosome.
   (2) Males have one copy of the X chromosome and one copy of the Y (see Figure 1.7).
6. The 22 autosomes are numbered by size from 1 to 22.

G. Formation of protein.
1. Most genes contain the information to make proteins that are required for the structure, function, and regulation of the body's tissues and organs.
2. Twenty different amino acids can be combined to make a protein. The sequence of amino acids determines each protein's structure and function (See Figure 1.8) (Brown, 2009).

H. A gene mutation is a permanent change in the DNA sequence that makes up a gene. Mutations range in size from a single DNA base to a large segment of a chromosome. Through natural selection, advantageous mutations will be preserved and disadvantageous mutations will be eliminated. This is the process that drives evolutionary change. Most often mutations are thought to be deleterious (see Figure 1.9.) (Gunder & Martin, 2011).

1. Gene mutations can be inherited from a parent or acquired during a person's lifetime.
2. Hereditary (germline) mutations are present throughout a person's life in virtually all cells in the body.
   a. Mutations that occur only in an egg or a sperm or occur just after fertilization are called de novo (new) mutations.
   b. De novo mutations may explain genetic disorders that appear with no family history of the disorder.
3. Somatic mutations are acquired and can be caused by environmental factors such as ultraviolet radiation from the sun.
   a. These changes can also occur if a mistake is made during cell replication.

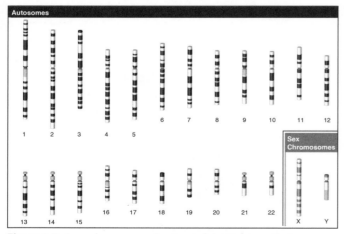

Figure 1.7. A sex chromosome is a type of chromosome that participates in sex determination. Humans and most other mammals have two sex chromosomes, the X and the Y. Females have two X chromosomes in their cells, while males have both X and a Y chromosomes in their cells. Egg cells all contain an X chromosome, while sperm cells contain an X or Y chromosome. This arrangement means that it is the male that determines the sex of the offspring when fertilization occurs.

Public domain image obtained from http://www.genome.gov/ dmd/img.cfm?node=Photos/Graphics&id=85238 Courtesy of National Human Genome Research Institute.

RNA codon table					
1st position	2nd position				3rd position
	U	**C**	**A**	**G**	
U	Phe Phe Leu Leu	Ser Ser Ser Ser	Tyr Tyr stop stop	Cys Cys stop Trp	U C A G
C	Leu Leu Leu Leu	Pro Pro Pro Pro	His His Gln Gln	Arg Arg Arg Arg	U C A G
A	Ile Ile Ile Met	Thr Thr Thr Thr	Asn Asn Lys Lys	Ser Ser Arg Arg	U C A G
G	Val Val Val Val	Ala Ala Ala Ala	Asp Asp Glu Glu	Gly Gly Gly Gly	U C A G
Amino Acids					

Ala: Alanine
Arg: Arginine
Asn: Asparagine
Asp: Aspartic acid
Cys: Cysteine
Gln: Glutamine
Glu: Glutamic acid
Gly: Glycine
His: Histidine
Ile: Isoleucine
Leu: Leucine
Lys: Lysine
Met: Methionine
Phe: Phenylalanine
Pro: Proline
Ser: Serine
Thr: Threonine
Trp: Tryptophane
Tyr: Tyrosisne
Val: Valine

Figure 1.8. Genetic code. The instructions in a gene tell the cell how to make a specific protein. A, C, G, and T are the "letters" of the DNA code; they stand for the chemicals adenine (A), cytosine (C), guanine (G), and thymine (T), respectively, that make up the nucleotide bases of DNA. Each gene's code combines the four chemicals in various ways to spell out three-letter "words" that specify which amino acid is needed at every step in making a protein.

Public domain image obtained from http://www.genome.gov/ dmd/img.cfm?node=Photos/Graphics&id=85173 Courtesy of National Human Genome Research Institute.

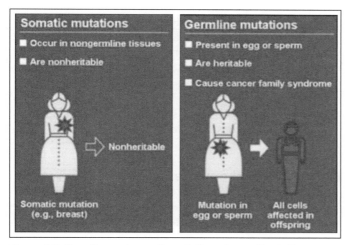

Figure 1.9. Germline and somatic mutations. A germline is the sex cells (eggs and sperm) that are used by sexually reproducing organisms to pass on genes from generation to generation. Egg and sperm cells are called *germ cells*, in contrast to the other cells of the body that are called *somatic cells*.

Most cancers arise from several genetic mutations that accumulate in cells of the body over a person's life span. These are called *somatic mutation*s, and the genes involved are usually located on autosomes (nonsex chromosomes).

Cancer may also have a germline mutation component, meaning that they occur in germ cells, better known as the *ovum* or *sperm*. Germline mutations may occur de novo (for the first time) or be inherited from parents' germ cells. An example of germline mutations linked to cancer are the ones that occur in cancer susceptibility genes, increasing a person's risk for the disease.

Courtesy of National Cancer Institute.

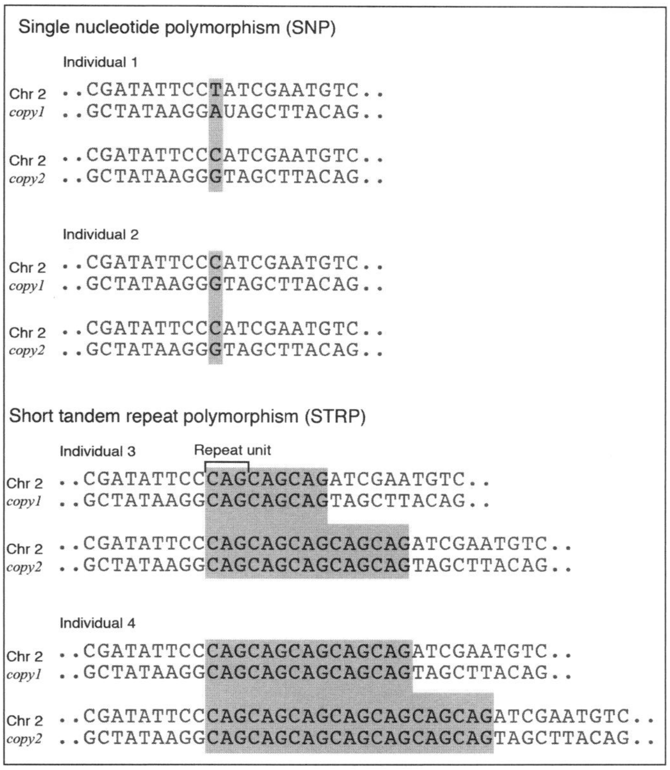

Figure 1.10. A polymorphism involves one of two or more variants of a particular DNA sequence. The most common type of polymorphism involves variation at a single base pair. Polymorphisms can also be much larger in size and involve long stretches of DNA. Called a single nucleotide polymorphism, or SNP (pronounced "snip"), scientists are studying how SNPs in the human genome correlate with disease, drug response, and other phenotypes.

Public domain image obtained from http://www.genome.gov/dmd/img.cfm?node=Photos/Graphics&id=85228
Courtesy of National Human Genome Research Institute.

    b. Somatic mutations cannot be passed on to the next generation.
4. Germline mutations are inherited genetic mutations that are transmitted in the egg or sperm.
5. Polymorphisms are genetic variations that occur in all individuals.
    a. They are responsible for many of the normal differences among people such as eye color, blood type, etc.
    b. Some of the variations may influence the risk of developing certain disorders (see Figure 1.10).
6. Gene mutations can prevent one or more of the thousands of proteins that are responsible for correct cell function from working properly.
    a. A mutation can cause the protein to malfunction or to be missing entirely.
    b. This can disrupt normal development or cause a medical condition – a genetic disorder.
7. Only a small percentage of mutations cause genetic disorders.
    a. Gene mutations are often repaired by certain enzymes before the gene is expressed as a protein.
    b. DNA repair is an important process by which the body protects itself from disease.

8. Gene mutations have varying effects on health depending on where they occur and whether they alter the function of essential proteins (see Figure 1.11). The types of mutation include:
    a. Missense (one amino acid substituted for another).
    b. Nonsense (a premature signal stops the process of building the protein).
    c. Insertion (a piece of DNA is added).
    d. Deletion (a piece of DNA is removed).
    e. Duplication (a piece of DNA is abnormally copied one or more times).
    f. Frameshift (the addition or loss of DNA bases changes a gene's reading frame that codes for one amino acid). Insertions, deletions, and duplications can all result in frameshift mutations.
I. Chromosomal disorders are caused by a change in the number or structure of chromosomes. This can occur during the formation of reproductive cells, in

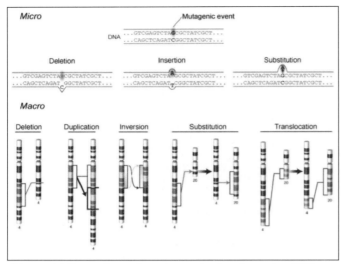

Figure 1.11. Types of mutations. A mutation is a change in a DNA sequence. Mutations can result from DNA copying mistakes during cell division, exposure to ionizing radiation, exposure to chemicals (carcinogens), or infection by viruses.

Public domain image obtained from http://www.genome.gov/dmd/img.cfm?node=Photos/Graphics&id=85206 Courtesy of National Human Genome Research Institute.

early fetal development, or at other times during the life of an individual (Gunder & Martin, 2011).

1. Aneuploidy is the gain or loss of chromosomes from the normal 46.
   a. Trisomy is the most common form of aneuploidy and is the presence of an extra chromosome in each cell. Down syndrome is an example of a condition caused by trisomy.
   b. Monosomy is another form of aneuploidy and is the presence of one copy of a particular chromosome instead of two. Turner syndrome is a condition caused by monosomy.
2. Translocation is the breaking and removal of a large segment of DNA from one chromosome, followed by the segment's attachment to a different chromosome. This can potentially alter gene expression.
3. Loss of heterozygosity is the loss of one parent's contribution to the genome through the loss of a gene copy (or copies) due to chromosomal rearrangement or point mutations.

J. Researchers are discovering that nearly all conditions and diseases have a genetic component. Conditions caused by many contributing factors are called complex or multifactorial disorders.

1. Diabetes, cardiovascular disease, and obesity are examples of complex or multifactorial disorders. They do not have a single genetic cause but are associated with the effects of multiple genes in combination with lifestyle and environmental factors.

2. While complex disorders often cluster in families, they do not have a clear-cut pattern of inheritance.
   a. With complex disorders it becomes difficult to determine the risk of inheriting or passing the disorder on as well as difficult to study and treat the disorders.
   b. This is because the specific factors that cause most of these disorders have not yet been identified.

IV. Mendelian inheritance is defined as the manner in which genes and traits are passed from parents to children. Examples of Mendelian inheritance include autosomal dominant, autosomal recessive, and sex-linked genes.

A. Autosomal dominant is a pattern of inheritance whereby an affected individual possesses one copy of a mutant allele and one normal allele (see Figure 1.12).
1. Individuals with autosomal dominant diseases have a 50–50 chance, with each pregnancy, of passing the mutant allele and hence the disorder onto their children if one parent is heterozygous and the other is homozygous normal.
2. Paternal to male transmission can be observed.
3. Key characteristics include (Gunder & Martin, 2011):
   a. Vertical transmission with multiple affected generations.
   b. Males and females are affected with equal frequency and severity for nonsex conditions.

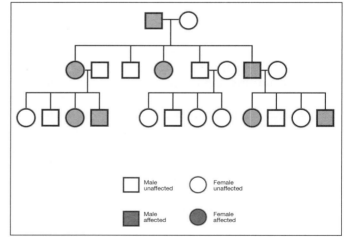

Figure 1.12. Autosomal dominant inheritance. Autosomal dominance is a pattern of inheritance characteristic of some genetic diseases. "Autosomal" means that the gene in question is located on one of the numbered, or non-sex, chromosomes. "Dominant" means that a single copy of the disease-associated mutation is enough to cause the disease. This is in contrast to a recessive disorder, where two copies of the mutation are needed to cause the disease. Huntington's disease is a common example of an autosomal dominant genetic disorder.

Public domain image obtained from http://www.genome.gov/dmd/img.cfm?node=Photos/Graphics&id=85267 Courtesy of National Human Genome Research Institute, Darryl Leja.

c. Only one parent must be affected for an offspring to be affected.
4. An example of such a disease is autosomal polycystic kidney disease (ADPKD).

B. Autosomal recessive inheritance refers to disorders that appear only in persons who have received two copies of a mutant gene, one from each parent (see Figure 1.13).
   1. Autosomal recessive diseases are observed more frequently in consanguineous relationships because the individuals are descendants of the same ancestors and are more likely to carry the same genes.
   2. Typically the parents of an affected individual are gene carriers and are not affected themselves.
   3. With each pregnancy there is a:
      a. 25% chance the offspring will inherit two copies of the disease allele and will have the disease.
      b. 50% chance that one copy of the disease allele will be inherited and the person will become a carrier.
      c. 25% chance the offspring will inherit no copy of the disease allele and will not be at risk for passing the disorder on to the next generation (see Figure 1.13).

4. Key characteristics include (Gunder & Martin, 2011):
   a. A horizontal pattern is noted with a single generation being affected.
   b. Males and females are affected with equal frequency and severity in nonsex disorders.
   c. In matings between individuals each with the same recessive phenotype, all offspring will be affected.
5. Examples of such diseases include sickle cell anemia, cystic fibrosis, and autosomal recessive polycystic kidney disease (ARPKD).

C. Sex-linked inheritance (or X-linked) refers to those genes that reside on the X chromosome. Females have two X chromosomes; males have XY (see Figure 1.14).
   1. If a female has a defective trait on one of the X chromosomes, it will be suppressed by the dominant gene for the same trait on the other X chromosome. However, if she has identical defective genes on both of her X chromosomes, she will exhibit the condition and will have a 50% chance with each pregnancy of passing on the disease allele to her offspring.
   2. Since males possess only one X chromosome, if a defective gene is on the X chromosome it will always be expressed because it is unopposed by a normal gene on the other sex chromosome. For this reason, some inherited diseases are almost exclusively diseases of males and some X-linked disorders are lethal in males.

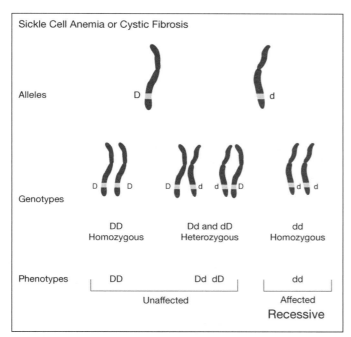

Figure 1.13. Autosomal recessive inheritance. Recessive is a quality found in the relationship between two versions of a gene. Individuals receive one version of the gene, called an allele, from each parent. If the alleles are different, the dominant allele will be expressed, while the effect of the other allele, called recessive, is masked. In the case of an autosomal recessive genetic disorder, an individual must inherit two copies of the mutated allele in order for the disease to be present.

Public domain image obtained from http://www.genome.gov
Courtesy of National Human Genome Research Institute.

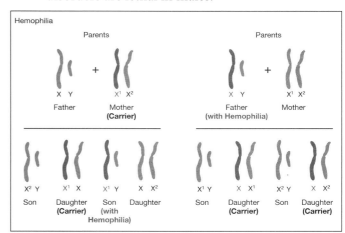

Figure 1.14. Sex-linked inheritance. Sex-linked is a trait in which a gene is located on a sex chromosome. In humans, the term generally refers to traits that are influenced by genes on the X chromosome. This is because the X chromosome is large and contains many more genes than the smaller Y chromosome. In a sex-linked disease, it is usually males who are affected because they have a single copy of X chromosome that carries the mutation. In females, the effect of the mutation may be masked by the second healthy copy of the X chromosome.

Public domain image obtained from
http://www.genome.gov/ dmd/img.cfm?node=Photos/Graphics&id=85239
Courtesy of National Human Genome Research Institute.

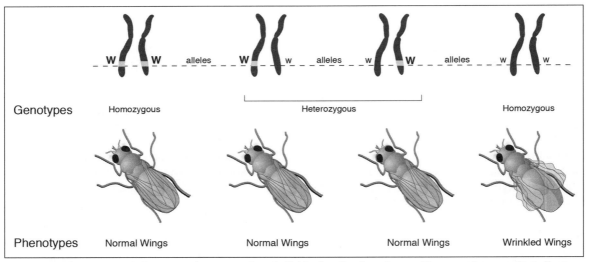

Figure 1.15. Genotype and phenotype. A genotype is an individual's collection of genes. The term also can refer to the two alleles inherited for a particular gene. The genotype is expressed when the information encoded in the genes' DNA is used to make protein and RNA molecules. The expression of the genotype contributes to the individual's observable traits, called the phenotype.

Public domain image obtained from http://www.genome.gov/dmd/img.cfm?node=Photos/Graphics&id=85176
Courtesy of National Human Genome Research Institute.

3. When a male is affected, all of his daughters will gain the diseased allele, but none of his sons.
4. Examples of X-linked diseases or conditions: Anderson-Fabry disease, hemophilia, and color-blindness.

D. Additional terminology.
   1. Genotype – genetic makeup of an individual (i.e., the specific allele makeup of the individual) usually with reference to a specific characteristic under consideration (See Figure 1.15).
   2. Phenotype – the composite of an individual's observable characteristics or traits (See Figure 1.15).
   3. Penetrance – proportion of organisms having a particular genotype that actually express the corresponding phenotype.
      a. If the phenotype is always expressed, penetrance is complete; otherwise, it is incomplete.
      b. Many hereditary cancer syndromes have incomplete penetrance.
   4. Variable expression – many genetic disorders have a wide variety of signs and symptoms, but not all individuals with the disorder will manifest them to the same degree.
      a. Myotonic muscular dystrophy is one such example.
      b. The disease may manifest all of the associated symptoms, while others may have only mild symptoms or symptoms that go unrecognized.
   5. Anticipation – genetic disease that increases in severity or appears at an earlier age with each successive generation. Huntington disease and fragile X disease are examples.
   6. Codominance – a pattern of inheritance in which

neither phenotype is dominant and the person expresses both phenotypes.
      a. For example, the Landsteiner blood types.
      b. The gene for blood types has three alleles: A, B, and i.
      c. The i allele causes O type and is recessive to both A and B.

V. Genetic testing is the analysis of human DNA, RNA, chromosomes, proteins, or certain metabolites to detect alterations related to a heritable disease or condition. Genetic tests have the potential for broad public health impact.

A. Methods. Different genetic test platforms are needed to detect different genetic mutations and abnormalities. An optimal testing strategy for a specific condition may use one or more test methodologies and may include testing various specimens. Some tests are best used for specific patient groups.
   1. Direct testing: directly examining the DNA or RNA that makes up a gene.
      a. Sanger sequencing is original sequencing technology that helped scientists determine the human genetic code.
         (1) Now automated, it is still used to sequence short pieces of DNA.
         (2) It relies on a technique known as capillary electrophoresis, which separates fragments of DNA by size and then sequences them by detecting the final fluorescent base on each fragment.
      b. Polymerase chain reaction (PCR) is a fast and inexpensive technique used to "amplify" – copy

small segments of DNA. Because significant amounts of a sample of DNA are necessary for molecular and genetic analyses, studies of isolated pieces of DNA are nearly impossible without PCR amplification.

    c. Next generation sequencing is sequencing in which many strands of DNA are sequenced at once, generating far more data per instrument run than the Sanger method.

2. Linkage testing: looking at markers co-inherited with a disease-causing gene.

3. Biochemical testing: assaying certain proteins are present or absent. An example is phenylketonuria (PKU) testing, which is routinely done in newborns.

4. Cytogenetic testing: examining the chromosomes using light microscopy.

    a. This technique allows for the identification of chromosomal abnormalities.

    b. A karyotype is an example of cytogenetic testing (see Figure 1.16).

B. Uses for genetic testing.

1. Prenatal testing to determine if a fetus carries a particular trait.

2. Carrier testing to determine if an individual has a specific genotype and the risks of passing to subsequent generations.

3. Predisposition testing to determine if an individual is at risk for developing a particular disease or illness.

4. Genetic testing can also be done on cancer tumor specimens to determine if a specific treatment might be effective.

5. Diagnostic testing to determine if an individual carries a specific trait such as cystic fibrosis, PKU, etc.

VI. Genetic testing process.

A. Collection of family medical history pedigree should include (Riley et al., 2012):

1. At least three generations using standard pedigree nomenclature (National Comprehensive Cancer Network, 2013) (see Figure 1.17). It is best to construct this in a stepwise fashion asking about each relative rather than asking a global question such as "What is the health of your family like?" or "Have any family members been diagnosed with cancer?"

2. Ethnic background. Certain ethnic backgrounds are at increased risk for hereditary syndromes due to the founder effect.

    a. One example is that persons of Ashkenazi Jewish ancestry are at increased risk for three specific mutations associated with hereditary breast and ovarian cancer; this population is also at risk for Tay-Sachs disease and Canavan disease.

    b. The founder effect is the accumulation of random genetic changes in an isolated population as a result of its proliferation from only a few parent colonizers (Gunder & Martin, 2011) (see Figure 1.18).

3. Status of current pregnancies.

4. Current and past health status on all family members.

    a. Age of onset.

    b. Cause of death.

    c. Age at death.

5. This information is confirmed by pathology reports and/or death certificates whenever possible because families often have incomplete or incorrect information about cancer diagnoses.

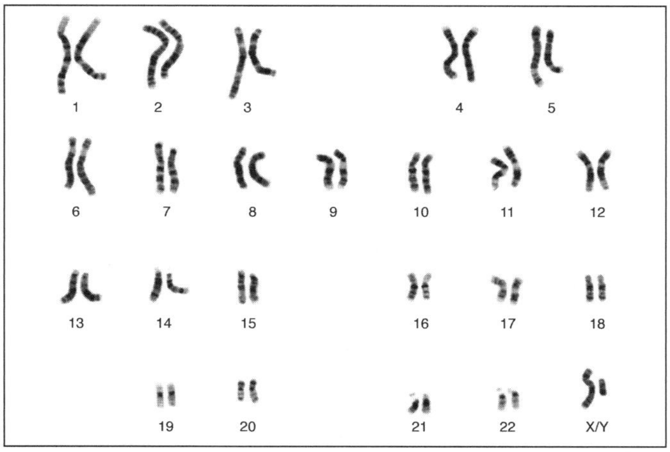

Figure 1.16. A karyotype is an individual's collection of chromosomes. The term also refers to a laboratory technique that produces an image of an individual's chromosomes. The karyotype is used to look for abnormal numbers or structures of chromosomes.

Public domain image obtained from http://www.genome.gov/ dmd/img.cfm?node=Photos/Graphics&id=85192 Courtesy of National Human Genome Research Institute.

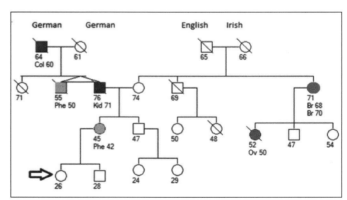

Figure 1.17. Typical pedigree nomenclature. Circles represent females and squares represent males. Vertical lines represent generations. Horizontal lines represent sibship. The arrow points to the proband who is the spokesperson or the person from whom the risks are being calculated. Ancestry is recorded. A slash represents a relative who is deceased. Current age or age at death is recorded. Age at which a cancer was diagnosed is recorded. This pedigree represents four generations.

Figure courtesy of Suzanne M. Mahon.

B. Consideration must be given to consanguinity, or genetic relatedness.
1. First-degree relatives: parents, children, siblings (have approximately half of their genes in common).
2. Second-degree relatives: grandparents, grandchildren, aunts, uncles, nieces, nephews (have about one fourth of their genes in common).
3. Third-degree relatives: a first cousin, great-grandparent or great-grandchild (have about one eighth of their genes in common).

C. The U.S. Surgeon General launched a national public health campaign, called the U.S. Surgeon General's Family History Initiative, to encourage all families to learn more about their family health history (Woodward, 2009).
1. The tool is "My Family Health Portrait" and is available free in English or Spanish from www.hhs.gov/familyhistory
2. The record can be shared with other family members and healthcare providers to help identify common diseases that may run in families.

D. Complete and interpret the risk assessment. Risk of having a mutation or genetic syndrome (Weitzel et al., 2011).
1. For some syndromes, it is possible to calculate a mathematical model estimating the risk of having a mutation.
2. In some syndromes, the decision to offer testing is based on clinical criteria.

VII. Genetic counseling is a communication process that deals with human problems associated with the occurrence or risk of occurrence of a genetic disorder in a family. Due to the complexities involved with genetic testing and the far-reaching effects that the results can have for both the patient and the family, genetic counseling is an integral part of the genetic testing process (Mahon & Crecelius, 2013). Clinical genetic services may be located in a hospital, medical center, or private office. These services may be specialized by age group or by medical condition (Mahon, 2013).

A. Kinds of genetics professionals.
1. Geneticists are physicians with board certification in genetics from the American Board of Medical Genetics.
   a. They complete a fellowship in genetics and pass a board examination.
   b. An active list of board-certified geneticists searchable by name and/or location is available from the American Board of Medical Genetics.

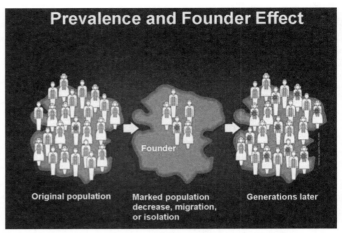

Figure 1.18. Prevalence and founder effect. Some populations have a higher prevalence of specific cancer-associated alleles than others. This may result from a founder effect, which occurs when a population undergoes rapid shrinkage and then expansion in an isolated setting. In a population that is geographically or reproductively isolated, an individual called a founder carries or develops a germline mutation that is rare in the general population. Because of reproductive isolation, later generations of an isolated population will have a higher frequency of a mutation than the original population. For example, Ashkenazi Jews were segregated from the rest of the population and lived in separate communities for hundreds of years. Today, 1% of the Ashkenazi Jewish population – 1 person in 40 – carries a 185delAG mutation in BRCA1, which places them at higher than the average risk for breast and ovarian cancer.

Courtesy of the National Cancer Institute.

2. Licensed genetics counselors are healthcare professionals with specialized graduate degrees in the areas of medical genetics and counseling.
   a. Currently, there are over 30 accredited programs in genetic counseling in the United States.
   b. The American Board of Genetic Counseling certifies genetic counselors.
   c. The National Society of Genetic Counselors maintains an active website in which healthcare professionals and the public can identify credentialed genetics professionals by ZIP code (www.nsgc.org).
3. Credentialed genetic nurses have specialized education and training in genetics credentialed by the ANCC (2014) after evaluation of a portfolio (http://www.nursecredentialing.org/Certification/ExamResources/Eligibility/ECategory/Advanced-Genetics-Eligibilty.html).
   a. Specialty certification in genetics is available for advance practice nurses following submission of an acceptable portfolio (Monsen, 2005).
   b. The portfolio includes:
      (1) Documentation of 1,500 hours of practice hours in genetics.
      (2) At least 30 hours of continuing education in advanced genetics/genomics applicable to nursing in the past 3 years.

(3) Fulfill two additional professional development categories, to be selected from the following list.
  (a) Academic credits.
  (b) Presentations.
  (c) Publication or research.
  (d) Preceptor.
  (e) Professional service.

B. During the first visit with a genetics professional, a patient can expect the following activities to occur (Mahon, 2013; Oncology Nursing Society, 2009; Weitzel et al., 2011):
  1. Make introductions. Discuss purpose of visit and the agenda.
  2. Assess patient concerns, motivations, and expectations regarding genetic testing. Assess psychosocial support including resources from the family, community, and religious affiliation.
  3. Clarify misconceptions about the process or concepts.
  4. Construct pedigree.
  5. Document lifestyle and medical history risk factors.
  6. Perform targeted physical examination for features associated with hereditary syndromes.
  7. Discuss factors that limit interpretation and assessment such as adoption, estrangement from the family, or a small family structure.
  8. Present basic risk information for developing cancer(s) or suspected syndrome. Explain differential diagnosis.
  9. Present risk calculations of having a mutation or discuss clinical criteria that are suggestive of hereditary risk. Discuss expected course of disease.
  10. Discuss principles of genetics such as autosomal transmission, penetrance, founder effect, germline, and somatic mutations.
  11. Identify and discuss the best individual(s) to test in the family. In many cases it is best to begin testing a person who is affected with the disease or cancer because there is a much higher probability of identifying the mutation.
  12. Discuss alternatives to testing, including not testing.
  13. Prioritize order of tests if more than one test or strategy is considered.
  14. Discuss specimen collection. Frequently testing can be done with a buccal (saliva) specimen or a blood specimen.
  15. Discuss potential test outcomes of testing which can include:
    a. True positive – the person carries the mutation.
    b. True negative – the person does not carry a mutation known to be in the family.
    c. Noninformative negative – the person is the first one tested in a family and tested negative

for a particular mutation. This means the person does not carry that particular mutation, but they could have another genetic mutation for which testing has not been completed.
    d. Variant of unknown significance – the person has a change in his/her genetic material, but it is not clear if it is associated with a particular disease or malignancy.
  16. Discuss possible management strategies for each outcome.
  17. Discuss testing costs and insurance issues.
  18. Discuss possible discrimination issues.
  19. Discuss the potential benefits, risks, and limitations of genetic testing.
  20. Discussion of reproductive options, if and when appropriate.
  21. Offer opportunities to ask questions for clarification.

C. Some patients/families will decide not to undergo genetic testing because of psychosocial issues, financial issues, or inability to find an appropriate person to test. These families should anticipate:
  1. Information about strategies to prevent or reduce the risk of developing the disease or malignancy.
  2. Recommendations for screening and surveillance based on the risk assessment.

D. For patients who opt for testing: in posttest counseling sessions the following should be anticipated:
  1. Increased surveillance and screening based on test results.
  2. Prophylactic surgery if indicated in the case of positive test results.
  3. Clinical trials if indicated based on test results.
  4. Chemoprevention and other risk reduction strategies based on test results.
  5. Recommendations for other family members.

E. Points to consider.
  1. Genetic test results in many cases apply not only to the patient, but also to other family members.
  2. Other family members may need to be offered the option of undergoing testing after careful genetic counseling.
  3. Some genetic testing applies only to the individual.
    a. For example, the Oncotype DX test is used to determine the effects of treatment on breast cancer and the chance of its recurrence.
    b. This is quite different from genomic testing that could impact other family members and does not require an informed consent.
  4. Genetic testing should include an informed consent, test interpretation, and appropriate follow-up care, which may require referral to a professional in genetics.

a. The purpose of the informed consent process is to provide individuals with sufficient information so they can make informed choices. It is a dynamic and continuing exchange of information.

b. The informed consent document provides a summary of the information and is often considered the foundation of the process. It does not represent the entirety of the process of informing the patient.

c. Because of the often profound impact of genetic testing, patients should be adequately counseled about the specifics of the test.

d. There is a duty to inform the patient of the test's purpose, medical implications, alternatives, and possible risks and benefits. Patients should also be made aware of their rights to privacy, including if and where their DNA will be stored and who will have access to their personal information.

5. It is important to use a qualified laboratory; however, in the United States, most genetic tests are not currently regulated, which is a good reason to refer to a genetics professional for testing (www.genome.gov/10002335).

6. Interpreting genetic tests can be complex. A good basic resource is *Interpreting the Results of a Genetic or Genomic Test* (NCHPEG, 2014).

F. Ethical considerations of genetic testing.
1. Autonomy is synonymous with the right to choose. The patient must be given enough information to make an informed, reasonable, and independent decision on whether or not to proceed with testing.
   a. Children and adolescents: the issues of consent and confidentiality are of concern.
      (1) Particular attention is given to the implications of predictive testing for onset disorders, carrier testing, and newborn screening.
      (2) Testing of children for adult onset disorders is generally not recommended because management will change until the individual reaches adulthood, and it robs the individual of making the choice of whether or not they want to know if they have genetic predisposition to a disease(s).
   b. Prenatal testing: a diagnosis has the potential of providing early detection of abnormalities, reassuring and reducing anxiety, preparing for optimal management at birth, allowing for prenatal treatment in some cases, or allowing couples to make choices about continuation of pregnancies.
2. Beneficence and nonmaleficence are the principles of "doing good" and "doing no harm." During the

process of obtaining informed consent, the benefits and all possible risks must be disclosed to allow an informed decision by the patient.
3. Justice relates to whether an individual is treated fairly and equitably in the context of society.
   a. Discrimination. There is public concern of potential loss of privacy and resulting insurance or employment discrimination if labeled with a "preexisting condition."
   b. Equitable access to resources. Many people feel as though genetic testing is out of their reach.
4. Confidentiality and privacy imply the assumption of nondisclosure of an individual's genetic information to third parties with the exception of certain situations that require protection of other persons ("duty to warn").
   a. Implications for family members.
      (1) A patient's genetic diagnosis always has to be interpreted in the context of family history.
      (2) A genetic diagnosis never has implications solely for the patient but instead reflects disease probability and risk factors in other blood relatives.
         (a) There may be different reactions among family members.
         (b) Some may not want the information, and healthy relatives who learn they have a predisposition to a disease may have significant changes in quality of life.
      (3) Issues on confidentiality may be raised when a person gives information on an affected family member without that individual's consent.
   b. A key assumption underlying the "duty to warn" is the availability of medical interventions to lessen the risk of developing disease or to lessen harm.
      (1) For some hereditary disorders, effective medical interventions may not be available.
      (2) For other hereditary disorders, there are clear interventions leading to prevention.
5. The reader is referred to Lea, Williams, & Donahue (2005) for an excellent overview of ethical issues in genetic testing.
6. Certain states have enacted statutes that prohibit the release of genetic information without the written consent of the individual.
7. Duty to inform. According to the American Society of Human Genetics (1998), "At a minimum, the healthcare professional should be obliged to inform the patient of the implications of his/her genetic test results and potential risks to family members."
8. Nonpaternity issues.
   a. Detection of misattributed paternity is not a

rare incidence in situations where DNA analysis is carried out.

    b. The situation can become complex (e.g., during testing to become a transplant donor for a sibling).

G. To request or decline genetic testing is ultimately the patient's choice.
1. It is the patient who must consider the risks and benefits of a genetic test while considering his/her own personal and family situation.
2. It is the patient who must make the decision based on his/her own beliefs, values, and priorities.
3. Even though a healthcare provider may see direct benefit to a patient, providing the information regarding genetic testing should be done in a nondirective manner, not with the purpose of encouraging a particular course of action.

VIII. Examples of kidney diseases with known genetic connection.

A. Anderson-Fabry disease (AFD) results from deficient activity of the enzyme alpha-galactosidase (alpha-Gal A) and progressive lysosomal deposition of globotriaosylceramide (GL-3).
1. Alpha-Gal A is an enzyme that normally digests fatty material inside cells throughout the body. In its absence, fatty material is not broken down, and as a consequence, it accumulates, leading to swelling of the cells which then stop working properly.
2. Deposition of glycolipids can be found in the glomerular cells, tubular epithelial cells, and vascular cells. Segmental and ultimately global sclerosis, tubular atrophy, and interstitial scarring lead to kidney dysfunction.
3. The gene is mapped to the X-chromosome and contains 7 exons. Mutations have been described in every exon; 57% are missense mutations, 11% nonsense, 18% partial gene deletions, 6% insertions, and 6% RNA processing defects caused by abnormal processing.
4. It affects more males than females. While 1 in 40,000 males has AFD disease, in the general population the figure is 1 in 117,000.
5. Median survival is 50 years for affected males and 70 years for carrier females. Symptoms generally develop early in childhood and progress with advancing age.
6. AFD disease is inherited in an X-linked recessive manner. In most cases, as de novo mutations are rare, the mother of an affected male is a carrier.
7. A carrier female has a 50% chance of transmitting the mutation in each pregnancy.
8. All daughters of affected males are obligate carriers.
9. Prenatal testing is available.

B. Polycystic kidney disease (PKD) is a genetic disorder characterized by the growth of cysts in the kidneys.
1. The fluid-filled cysts slowly replace much of the mass of the kidneys and compromise kidney function.
    a. The cysts originate in the nephrons but eventually separate and continue to enlarge.
    b. While roughly retaining its shape, the kidney also enlarges and can end up weighing as much as 22 pounds.
2. In the United States, about 500,000 people have PKD.
3. There are two major inherited forms of PKD and a noninherited form.
4. Autosomal dominant PKD (ADPKD) is one of the most common inherited disorders and affects 1 in 400 to 1,000 live births.
    a. If one parent has the disease, there is a 50% chance of passing the mutation to every child conceived.
    b. However, de novo mutations occur in about 10% of affected families.
    c. In some rare cases, the de novo mutation occurs spontaneously soon after conception, and the parents are not the source of the disease.
    d. It is important that parents are adequately screened by imaging methods.
    e. Mutations in the PKD1 gene account for approximately 85% of affected families. Mutations in PKD2 gene account for 15% of affected families.
    f. PKD1 and PKD2 mutations have different prognostic implications, with PKD2 patients developing kidney cysts, hypertension, and CKD stage 5 at a later age than PKD1 patients.
    g. Prenatal testing is possible if the mutation has been identified in an affected family member.
    h. Variability in the disease within families coupled with clustering of the disease's extrarenal manifestations suggests that environmental factors and modifier genes play a role in the clinical severity of ADPKD.
5. Autosomal recessive PKD (ARPKD) affects 1/10,000 to 1/40,000 individuals.
    a. The disease is caused by a particular genetic flaw that both parents must carry and both pass on to their baby.
      (1) There is a 25% chance of this happening.
      (2) If only one parent carries the abnormal gene, the baby cannot get the disease.
      (3) Severity of the disease varies, but in the worst cases the baby can die hours or days after birth.
      (4) Others may have sufficient kidney function for a few years.
    b. If there are other siblings, each child has a:
      (1) 25% chance of inheriting both the disease-

causing alleles (one of two or more versions of a gene) and being affected.
    (2) 50% chance of inheriting the disease causing allele and being a carrier.
    (3) 25% chance of inheriting neither the disease causing allele nor being a carrier.
  c. Mutations are in a single gene on the short arm of chromosome 16.
  d. Prenatal testing for pregnancies at 25% risk is available using molecular genetic testing if both disease-causing alleles have been identified in an affected family member.
6. Acquired cystic kidney disease (ACKD) develops in persons with long-term kidney damage and scarring, especially in those who have been on dialysis for an extended period. About 90% of people on dialysis for 5 years develop ACKD.

C. Medullary cystic kidney disease (MCKD) is a hereditary disorder associated with familial juvenile nephrophthisis (NPH) and with familial juvenile hyperuricemia nephropathy (FJHN). MCKD and FJHN have an autosomal dominant pattern of inheritance. NPH has an autosomal recessive pattern of inheritance.
  1. MCKD is characterized by functionally and morphologically abnormal tubules leading to interstitial inflammation and fibrosis.
    a. MCKD1 was mapped to chromosome 1 and accounts for the minority of cases. MCKD2 was mapped to chromosome 16 and accounts for mutations in most cases.
    b. MCKD occurs in older patients; patients reach CKD stage 5 between 30 and 50 years of age.
    c. When cysts are found, they are located at the corticomedullary junction and in the medulla. The presence of cysts is not universal.
  2. FJHN is an autosomal dominant disorder characterized by elevated serum uric acid concentrations due to low fractional excretion of uric acid, defective urinary concentrating ability, interstitial nephropathy, and progression to CKD stage 5. FJHN has similar features and disease course with MCKD.
    a. The FJHN gene has been identified on chromosome 16 in proximity to the MCKD gene locus, making these two disorders potentially allelic.
    b. Hyperuricemia caused by reduced fractional excretion of uric acid is the hallmark of FJHN and has also been described in some cases of MCKD.
  3. NPH occurs in young children and may have associated extrarenal manifestations. The kidney problems begin at about 4 years of age, leading to CKD stage 5 usually by the second decade of life.
    a. The gene responsible for NPH has been mapped to chromosome 2, making this disease unrelated to MCKD.
    b. MCKD has been traditionally associated with NPH because of similar clinical features and pathologic findings.

D. Alport's syndrome or hereditary nephritis.
  1. The prevalence of the genetic mutation is estimated to be 1 in 5,000 to 1 in 10,000.
  2. In 85% of the cases there is an X-linked inheritance. Carrier mothers may have hematuria due to the random inactivation of one of the X chromosomes.
  3. Of the non-X-linked cases, most are autosomal recessive.
  4. Genetic mutation appears to result in a post-translational defect that prevents the assembly of protomers that are required for the formation of basement membranes.

E. The recent discovery of gene mutations labeled as the apolipoprotein L1 (APOL1) and its link to kidney disease within the African-American population are considered groundbreaking genetic research.
  1. For a long period of time, it was never really clear as to why kidney disease had such a higher prevalence in people of African-American descent.
  2. What was once labeled as hypertensive-associated kidney disease in people of African ancestry now appears to have a genetic link.
  3. From what researchers have found, the APOL1 genetic mutation accounts for what was once called hypertensive-associated kidney disease.
  4. In addition, it also appears to be responsible for idiopathic focal segmental glomerulosclerosis (FSGS) and HIV-associated nephropathy within African-Americans (Pollak et al., 2012; Wasser et al., 2012).

IX. Example of environmental exposure coupled with a genetic component and leading to kidney disease.

A. Primary hypertension (formerly called "essential" hypertension) is by far the most common type of high blood pressure.
  1. Primary hypertension is a multifactorial disease involving interactions among genetic, environmental, demographic, vascular, and neuroendocrine factors.
  2. A number of individual genes and genetic factors have been linked to the development of primary hypertension. However, it is likely that multiple genes contribute to the development of the disease, and it is difficult to accurately determine the relative contributions of each of these genes (Kaplan et al., 2013).
  3. A number of polymorphisms have been associated with differences in blood pressure.

a. Most prominent are the polymorphisms in the angiotensin-renin-aldosterone system.
b. This system evolved millions of years ago to protect early humans during times of drought or stress.
c. Today's high-salt diets and sedentary lifestyles can wreak havoc on this system.
4. Some studies suggest that some people with primary hypertension may inherit abnormalities of the sympathetic nervous system.

B. While researchers are gaining a better understanding by identifying genes that influence the bioaccumulation and susceptibility of a person to an exposure, there are still unanswered questions as to why some people are more susceptible than others to develop the clinical disease.

X. Pharmacogenetics and pharmacogenomics
involve the study of the role of inheritance in individual variation in drug response that can vary from potentially life-threatening adverse drug reactions to equally serious lack of therapeutic efficacy. These new and emerging fields evolved from the convergence of molecular pharmacology and genomics.

A. Pharmacogenetics focuses on specific genes such as drug-metabolizing enzymes. It dates back to the 1950s, when researchers first noted an inherited tendency in the way people react to drugs.

B. Pharmacogenomics deals with the entire human genome, including genes for numerous proteins in the body, such as transporters, receptors, and the entire signaling networks that respond to drugs and move them through the system.
1. The products of this technology would replace the one-formula-fits-all drugs that typically work for only 60% of the population at best.
2. More worrisome and costly are the serious adverse drug reactions that are responsible for 100,000 deaths a year in the United States and cost society approximately $100 billion a year.

C. Significant challenges remain to be overcome if pharmacogenetics and pharmacogenomics are to have a major medical impact.
1. A key task for pharmacogenetics researchers is to pinpoint all of the proteins that medicine will encounter in the body and determine how these proteins vary from person to person.
2. The National Institute of General Medical Sciences (NIGMS) is leading a National Institute of Health (NIH) effort to encourage pharmacogenetics research.
a. They support this research by allocating funds to various research groups and developing a large public database of the results of the studies.
b. The purpose of the database is to match up genetic variations (genotypes) with functional outcomes (phenotypes).
3. The Pharmacogenetics and Pharmacogenomics Knowledge Base (PharmGKB) provides a shared online resource that contains information and analytic tools and is freely available to the scientific community.
a. In addition, it helps researchers identify and fill in knowledge gaps.
b. To protect the privacy of the study participants, names and other identifying information are not stored in the PharmGKB.

D. Application to clinical practice is currently limited, but the technology is steadily moving forward.
1. For example, the Cincinnati Children's Hospital Medical Center launched a genetic pharmacology service that enables MDs and APRNs to test 52 common medications against four well-defined genes.
a. This test, which only has to be done once in a lifetime, will help the clinicians determine how patients will respond to these drugs and thereby improve patient safety.
b. Warfarin.
(1) Researchers have found that differences in a gene influence the dose of warfarin that is the most effective for each person.
(2) The genetic variation in drug metabolizing enzyme gene: CYP2C9, CYP1A2, CYP2C19, CYP3A4.
(3) This information could ultimately help in the quick and precise determination of each patient's dose, without trial and error.
2. Transporter proteins help control responses to antidepressants and other drugs.
a. These proteins not only bring essential material into the cell, but also purge the cell of wastes, drugs, and other chemicals.
b. Researchers have found more than 1,000 genetic differences in 40 of these transporters.
c. The genetic changes may affect the way people respond to a wide variety of drugs.
3. Losartan: an angiotensin II receptor antagonist (ARB).
a. There is a genetic variation in drug metabolizing enzyme gene(s): CYP2C9, CYP3A4, aldosterone synthase.
b. There is also genetic variation in angiotensin II type 1 receptor gene.
4. Within nephrology, there is promise for improvement in the ability to individualize many drugs based on the patient's genetic profile.

For example:
  a. Control of hypertension.
  b. Specific immunosuppressive therapy posttransplant.
  c. Individualized anticoagulation during hemodialysis.

XI. The family health history, if detailed and accurate, provides one of the most powerful "genetic/genomic tools" to identify individuals at risk for inherited disorders when laboratory tests are not available. It can capture the interactions of genetic susceptibility with the environmental, cultural, and behavioral factors shared by family members (refer to Figure 1.15).

A. Alison Whelan and others (2004) developed a mnemonic to help identify indicators that would send up a red flag that may raise a clinician's awareness of possible genetic influences on the patient. It is not 100% sensitive or specific. The mnemonic is Family GENES.
  1. Family history.
    a. Multiple affected siblings or individuals in multiple generations.
    b. It must be remembered, however, that lack of family history does not rule out genetic causes.
  2. G: group of congenital anomalies.
    a. Common anatomic variations are not unusual.
    b. Two or more are more likely to indicate the presence of a syndrome with genetic implications.
  3. E: extreme or exceptional presentation of common conditions. Examples:
    a. Early onset cardiovascular disease.
    b. Cancer.
    c. Kidney failure.
    d Unusually severe reactions to infectious or metabolic stress.
    e. Recurrent miscarriage.
    f. Bilateral primary cancers in paired organs.
    g. Multiple primary cancers of different tissues.
  4. N: neurodevelopmental delay or degeneration. Suspicion should be raised in developmental delay in the pediatric age group, or in developmental regression in children or early onset dementia in adults.
  5. E: extreme or exceptional pathology. Examples include unusual tissue histology, such as:
    a. Pheochromocytoma.
    b. Acoustic neuroma.
    c. Medullary thyroid cancer.
    d. Multiple colon polyps.
    e. Plexiform neurofibromas.
    f. Most pediatric malignancies.
  6. S: surprising laboratory results. Examples include variants of unknown significance or results not consistent with family history.

B. Implications for nursing care.
  1. Recognition and discussion of the emotional responses of family members to the information given. This could include shock, disbelief, relief, fear, guilt, sadness, shame, acceptance, etc.
  2. Review of the normal grief responses and signs that indicate further psychosocial support is needed.
  3. Listening to the whole story and hearing what the situation has meant to the family.
  4. Exploring strategies for communicating information to others, especially family members who might be at risk.
  5. Providing written materials and referrals to support groups, local and national service agencies, etc.

C. Follow-up means maintaining ongoing communication.
  1. Arranging for follow-up diagnostic testing or management appointments, or this information is communicated to the referring healthcare provider.
  2. Documentation of the content of the consultation for the referring healthcare provider and for the patient if appropriate.
  3. Contacting the patient to assess level of understanding and response to decisions made.
  4. Encouraging the family to contact the clinic again when considering pregnancy or for updated information.
  5. Being available for future questions.

Genetics and Genomics
Case Studies

I. **Case study: Von Hippel Lindau syndrome.** Von Hippel Lindau syndrome (VHL) is an inherited disorder characterized by the formation of both benign and malignant tumors and cysts in various parts of the body (Lindor et al., 2008).

A. Case study (see Figure 1.19).

B. Inheritance pattern: Autosomal dominant.

C. Gene and chromosomal location: VHL on chromosome 3p25-p26.

D. Common associated tumors (average age of onset and risk) are shown in the following chart.

Tumor	Average Age of Diagnosis	Average Lifetime Risk
Central nervous system hemangioblastoma	30	79%
Renal (Clear Cell) Cancer	40	75%
Retinal Hemangioblastoma	21	70%
Epididymal cystadenoma	14	27%
Pancreatic islet cell carcinoma	25	25%
Pheochromocytoma	25	17%
Endolymphatic sac tumors	16	16%

Based on information from Lindor et al., 2008; Shehata et al., 2008; Wilding et al., 2012.

E. Clinical indicators of VHL (Coleman, 2008; Frantzen et al., 2012; Lindor et al., 2008; Pilarski & Nagy, 2012). Nephrology nurses who identify these criteria or think a genetic evaluation is indicated should refer the patient to a genetics specialist for risk assessment, evaluation, and coordination of genetic testing.
1. Two or more central nervous system (CNS) or retinal hemangioblastomas. No additional family history is needed.
2. A single CNS or retinal hemangioblastoma with one of the following:
   a. Multiple renal, pancreatic, or hepatic cysts.
   b. Pheochromocytoma.
   c. Clear cell renal cancer.
   d. Endolymphatic sac tumor.
   e. Papillary cystadenoma of the epididymis or broad ligament.
   f. Neuroendocrine tumor (pancreas).
3. Definite family history of a VHL tumor with one of the following in the individual:
   a. CNS or retinal hemangioblastoma.
   b. Multiple renal, pancreatic, or hepatic cysts.
   c. Adrenal or extra-adrenal pheochromocytoma.
   d. Renal cancer prior to age 60.
   e. Epididymal or broad ligament cystadenoma.
4. A known VHL mutation in the family.

F. Recommended management (Frantzen et al., 2012; Inglese, 2007; Teplick et al., 2011). Nephrology nurses should be familiar with these guidelines so they can facilitate appropriate referrals and provide appropriate education.
1. Annual ophthalmologic examination (start at age 5).
2. Annual physical examination, including blood pressure to assess for pheochromocytoma, and neurologic evaluation for signs of cerebellar or spinal cord lesions starting at age 5.
3. Audiologic evaluation for hearing loss associated with endolymphatic sac tumors starting at age 1.
4. Imaging of the central nervous system and the spinal cord by magnetic resonance imaging (MRI) with gadolinium starting at around age 12.

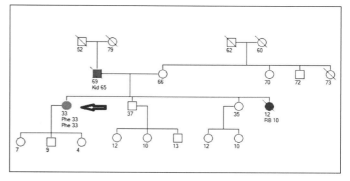

Figure 1.19. Case study.

A 33-year-old female presented to her primary care provider for follow-up of severe, uncontrolled hypertension for the past 3 months. She had also recently begun experiencing palpitations. Urine studies revealed elevated catecholamines. Magnetic resonance imaging showed large bilateral adrenal masses. At surgery, bilateral pheochromocytomas were resected. She was referred to a genetics professional for further evaluation because the presence of bilateral pheochromocytomas is suggestive of a hereditary cancer syndrome.

Her mother was 66 years old with a history of arthritis. Her father died at age 69 from complications of clear cell renal cancer diagnosed at age 65. She has two healthy siblings, three healthy offspring, and a sister who died from complications of a retinoblastoma diagnosed at age 10.

During her visit with the genetics professional, she was questioned about any personal or family history of vision problems. She stated that she had been experiencing some blurry vision in her right eye. She was then referred to an ophthalmologist and was found to have a unilateral retinal angioma. Genetic testing of the VHL gene was performed and a deleterious mutation was detected, confirming the clinical diagnosis of VHL. Imaging was negative for renal cell carcinoma or additional hemangioblastomas.

Her mother and two siblings underwent genetic testing for the same mutation and all were found to be negative. Her two daughters tested positive for the mutation, and her son tested negative for the mutation.

Figure courtesy of Suzanne M. Mahon.

5. Annual complete blood count seeking evidence of polycythemia (caused by erythropoietin secretion from renal cysts and cerebellar hemangioblastoma) starting about age 5.
6. Annual urinalysis to check for microscopic hematuria and abnormalities starting about age 5.
7. Annual urine and/or plasma fractionated metanephrines starting at ages 2 to 5 years when relatives have pheochromocytomas or, otherwise, at age 16.
8. Annual ultrasound imaging of the kidneys and pancreas, beginning no later than age 16. MRI (in children) or computed tomography (in adults) should be performed to evaluate any abnormalities detected by ultrasound.

II. **Case study: Birt-Hogg Dubé syndrome.** Birt-Hogg-Dubé syndrome is a rare disorder that affects the skin with multiple benign lesions and the lungs with spontaneous pneumothorax, and increases the risk of certain types of tumors including renal tumors. Its signs and symptoms vary among affected individuals (Coleman, 2008; Morrison et al., 2010; Toro, 2008).

A. Case study: A 36-year-old female was referred to a genetics professional because of the development of small, skin-colored papules across her forehead, neck, and upper torso. The patient also reports that her brother and father have similar papular lesions, and her father has had two pneumothoraces in the past, necessitating chest tube placement. A paternal uncle has been diagnosed with renal cancer and multiple renal cysts. A skin biopsy obtained confirmed the presence of fibrofolliculomas. Genetic testing demonstrated a mutation in the FLNC gene. Following the identification of the mutation, testing was offered to her siblings and paternal relatives.

B. Inheritance pattern: autosomal dominant.

C. Gene and chromosomal location: FLCN (folliculin) on chromosome 17p11.2.

D. Common associated tumors with average age of onset are shown in the following chart.

Tumor	Average Age of Diagnosis	Average Lifetime Risk
Cutaneous lesions angiofibroma perifollicular fibromas fibrofolliculomas	30 to 40 years	Women tend to have fewer and small lesions
Pulmonary cysts and spontaneous pneumothorax	25 to 40 years	89% cysts (mean = 16 cysts) 38% pneumothorax
Kidney tumors (most common tumors are a hybrid of oncocytoma and chromophobe histologic cell types)	30 to 70 years (median age is 48 years)	29–34%
Based on information from Gupta et al., 2013, & Stamatakis et al., 2013.		

E. Diagnostic criteria. Birt-Hogg-Dubé should be suspected in persons with one major criteria or two minor criteria (Menko et al., 2009). Nephrology nurses who identify these criteria or think a genetic evaluation is indicated should refer the patient to a genetics specialist for risk assessment, evaluation, and coordination of genetic testing.
  1. Major criteria.
     a. At least five fibrofolliculomas or trichodiscomas, at least one histologically confirmed.
     b. Pathogenic FLCN germline mutation.
  2. Minor criteria.
     a. Multiple lung cysts.
     b. Bilateral basally located lung cysts with no other apparent cause, with or without spontaneous primary pneumothorax.
     c. Renal cancer at an early age.
     d. Multifocal or bilateral renal cancer, or renal cancer of mixed chromophobe and oncocytic histology.

F. Management and screening recommendations. Nephrology nurses should be familiar with these guidelines so they can facilitate appropriate referrals and provide appropriate education.
  1. If normal at baseline or clinical diagnosis, abdominal/pelvic CT scan with contrast or MRI (if CT is not possible) every 2 to 3 years are the optimal studies for complete assessment of kidney lesions beginning about age 25 (Garg & Herts, 2012; Stamatakis et al., 2013).
  2. Monitor tumors.
     a. Tumors less than 3 cm in diameter by periodic imaging; they may not require surgical intervention yet.
     b. Tumor reaches 3 cm in maximal diameter, at which point nephron-sparing surgery should be ideally pursued.
     c. Ideally these lesions should be managed by a urologic surgeon with expertise in managing these high risk families.
  3. Rapidly growing lesions and/or symptoms including pain, blood in the urine, or atypical presentations require a more individualized approach.
  4. Periodic pulmonary function testing if profusion of cysts sufficient to impair lung function (Gupta et al., 2013).
  5. Pneumococcal vaccination and annual influenza vaccination.
  6. Action plan for pneumothorax (symptoms to recognize, tunneled pleural catheters [TPC]/pleurodesis after first event).
  7. Dermatologic consultation for disfiguring skin lesions.

G. Prevention measures include avoiding:
  1. Cigarette smoking.
  2. High ambient pressures, which may precipitate spontaneous pneumothorax, including air travel and scuba diving.

III. Case study: Cowden syndrome. Cowden syndrome is a hereditary syndrome associated with an increased risk of developing cancers of the breast, thyroid, and endometrium. Other cancers that have been identified in people with Cowden syndrome include colorectal cancer, kidney cancer, and melanoma. Compared with the general population, people with Cowden syndrome develop these cancers at younger ages, often beginning in their 30s or 40s. Other diseases of the breast, thyroid, and endometrium are also common in Cowden syndrome. Additional signs and symptoms can include an enlarged head and developmental delays, including those on the autism spectrum.

A. Case study (see Figure 1.20 and Figure 1.21).

B. Inheritance pattern – autosomal dominant.

C. Gene and chromosome location – PTEN 10q23.3.

D. Common associated tumors are shown in the following chart.

Tumor	Average Age of Diagnosis	Average Lifetime Risk
Macrocephaly	Usually in late 20s	Frequently present
Trichilemmomas	Usually in late 20s	Frequently present
Papillomatous papules	Usually in late 20s	Frequently present
Benign cancer	Age 38-46	25–50%
Thyroid cancer	Age 37	10%
Endometrial cancer	Late 30s to early 40s	28%
Benign breast disease	Usually early 30s	67%
Benign thyroid disease	Usually early 30s	75%
Gastrointestinal polys – frequently harmatomas	Usually early 40s	90%
Colon cancer	Late 30s	9%
Based on information from Eng, 2012; Lindor et al., 2008.		

E. Diagnostic criteria: 2 or more major criteria; 1 major and 2 minor criteria; or 4 minor criteria (Eng, 2012). Nephrology nurses who identify these criteria or think a genetic evaluation is indicated should refer the patient to a genetics specialist for risk assessment, evaluation, and coordination of genetic testing.
  1. Major criteria.
     a. Breast cancer.
     b. Epithelial thyroid cancer (nonmedullary), especially follicular thyroid cancer.
     c. Macrocephaly (occipital frontal circumference ≥ 97th percentile).
     d. Endometrial carcinoma.
  2. Minor criteria.
     a. Other thyroid lesions (e.g., adenoma, multinodular goiter).
     b. Intellectual disability (IQ ≤ 75).
     c. Hamartomatous intestinal polyps.
     d. Fibrocystic disease of the breast.

  e. Lipomas.
  f. Genitourinary tumors (especially renal cell carcinoma).
  g. Genitourinary malformation.
  h. Uterine fibroids.

F. Management and screening guidelines. Nephrology nurses should be familiar with these guidelines so they can facilitate appropriate referrals and provide appropriate education.
  1. Pediatric (age <18 years) (Eng, 2012).

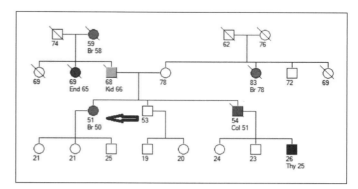

Figure 1.20. Pedigree Cowden (PTEN) mutation. The proband has already undergone testing for BRCA1/2 mutations because she was diagnosed with triple negative breast cancer at age 50. She tested negative for these mutations. Her nephew was recently diagnosed with an aggressive thyroid cancer and she asked her oncologist if there was a connection. She was referred to a genetics professional who reviewed the family history which was significant for several different types of cancer. The proband had a head circumference of 59 cm, a lipoma on her arm, oral papillomas, and a history of a thyroid nodule. She had a colonoscopy that was negative for gastrointestinal polyps. Her 25-year-old son was developmentally disabled with autism.

Figure courtesy of Suzanne M. Mahon.

Based on the information provided, the estimated probability of a PTEN gene mutation for the adult subject is 19%. PTEN gene testing is recommended for patients with an estimated probability of 3% and up.

Due to statistical variation, the precise estimate varies between 10.3% and 32.7%.

This estimate is based on a total risk score of 18.

▨ Head circumference ≥ 59 cm

▨ Breast cancer at age 50

▨ Thyroid goiter or thyroid nodules or thyroid adenomas or Hashimoto's thyroiditis

▨ Oral papillomas

▨ Skin lipomas

Figure 1.21. Risk of having a Cowden syndrome mutation. The genetics professional considered the family history, personal history, and clinical evalutation of the proband and made the calculation above. This family history is suggestive of Cowden syndrome because of the history of breast, uterine, colon, thyroid, and kidney cancers, as well as the history of autism in the proband's son. The proband underwent genetic testing and was found to have a mutation in the PTEN gene.

Table 1.1

Genomics Resources for Nephrology Nurses

International Society of Nurses in Genetics http://www.isong.org/	● Information ISONG educational conferences, webinars, and resources. ● Links to other genetics related websites. ● Online genomics resources for nurses in clinical practice, education and research.
National Institutes of Health: Genetics Home Reference Locating a Genetics Health Professional http://ghr.nlm.nih.gov/handbook/consult/findingprofessional	● Links with searchable databases for finding genetics professionals in your area.
National Coalition of Health Professionals in Genetics http://nchpeg.org/	● Family History Tool: Information on family history collection and a family history collection form. ● Genetic Red Flags: Six genetic red flags that indicate there might be increased genetic risk in an individual or family. ● GeneFacts provides decision support for non-geneticist clinicians at the point-of-care by providing concise, accurate, fact sheets on genetic conditions.
National Institutes of Health: National Human Genome Research Institute http://www.genome.gov	● Health section provides resources for the Public and for Health Professionals. ● Education section provides genetics/genomics educational materials. Some resources are available in Spanish.
National Institutes of Health: Genetics Home Reference http://ghr.nlm.nih.gov/	● A description of genes and how they work. ● An alphabetical listing of genetic conditions and diseases that nurses can look up. ● An overview of the Human Genome Project, genetic testing, and gene therapy.
National Genetics Education and Development Centre http://www.geneticseducation.nhs.uk/	● Genetics education resources for learning genetics, teaching genetics, and genetics in practice.
National Genetics Education and Development Centre: Telling Stories http://www.tellingstories.nhs.uk/index.asp	● Telling stories about an individual with a genetic condition is used as the framework to teach real life genetics to patients, family members, and professionals.
World Health Organization Human Genetics Programme http://www.who.int/genomics/en/	● Online resources and educational tools for health professionals. ● Information on the genetics of common diseases. ● Ask the Expert is a resource that allows an individual to query a group of health professionals in genetics and related disciplines about genetics and related issues.

    a. Yearly thyroid ultrasound examination.
    b. Yearly skin check with physical examination.
  2. Adult – beginning at age 20.
    a. Yearly thyroid ultrasound (Hall et al., 2013).
    b. Yearly dermatologic evaluation (Aslam & Coulson, 2013; Gabree & Seidel, 2012).
  3. Women beginning at age 30 years (NCCN, 2013):
    a. Breast self-examination.
    b. Yearly breast mammogram; MRI may also be incorporated.
    c. Yearly transvaginal ultrasound or endometrial biopsy with pelvic examination (Daniels, 2012).
  4. For men and women:
    a. Colonoscopy beginning at age 35 to 40 years; frequency dependent on degree of polyposis identified (Paparo et al., 2013).

    b. Biennial renal imaging (CT or MRI preferred) beginning at age 40 years (Chan-Smutko, 2012).
  5. For those with a family history of a particular cancer type at an early age, screening may be initiated 5 to 10 years prior to the youngest diagnosis in the family. For example, in a woman whose mother developed breast cancer at age 30, breast surveillance may begin at age 25 to 30 years.

IV. Case study: Type 1 diabetes mellitus. Also called juvenile diabetes or insulin-dependent diabetes and is thought to be an autoimmune disorder. Presents before age 40 and often occurs in children. About 30% of patients with type 1 diabetes mellitus will eventually suffer from kidney failure.

A. Genetics. Most cases of type 1 diabetes are associated with the HLA DR3, DR4, DR7, or DR9 genes (American Diabetes Association [ADA], 2013a). The genetics of diabetes is not well understood, and genetic testing is currently thought to be of limited value in the evaluation and management of patients with type 1 diabetes.

B. Siblings of persons with type 1 diabetes have a significant increased risk of the disease (about 6% risk compared to 0.3% to 0.5% in the general population) (Jorde et al., 2000).

C. Clinical presentation. Signs and symptoms of the disease include albumin in the urine, hypertension, frequent urination, excessive thirst, weight loss, elevated BUN and creatinine, fatigue, and blurred vision.

D. Case study: John is a 19-year-old Caucasian college student who presents to his primary care provider for a checkup.
  1. Medical history. No significant medical history, although his blood pressure was a little high (138/90) when his neighbor checked it on his home blood pressure unit 3 months ago.
  2. He has one sister, age 15, who is healthy. His mother was diagnosed with diabetes and hypertension in her early 30s and has been on insulin since then. John's maternal grandfather may have also had diabetes, but John does not know his age of diagnosis or if he was on insulin. His paternal grandfather was diagnosed with diabetes in his late 60s and was managed with diet, exercise, and medication.
  3. Review of systems. John admits to getting up two to three times a night to go to the bathroom, and he seems to have less energy than he used to. He reports a healthy appetite but has trouble keeping weight on.
  4. Vital signs. BP 148/96, apical pulse 84 regular rate and rhythm, weight 140, height 5 foot 10 inches. The physical exam is unremarkable.
  5. Lab results. Complete blood count (CBC) normal; chemistry panel normal except fasting blood glucose is 160mg/dL; HbA1C is 7%, glomerular filtration rate (GFR) is 88 mL/min/1.73 m^2.
  6. A complete workup is conducted, and John is subsequently diagnosed with type 1 diabetes and stage 2 kidney disease.
  7. John is concerned about his sister's diabetes risk. John's nurse recently attended a genetics conference. Because of John's young age and family history, he is referred to a genetics specialist for genetic risk assessment and to determine if genetic testing would be beneficial.
  8. The genetics specialist takes a complete family history and constructs a three-generation pedigree. John is informed that the genetics of diabetes is not well understood and that genetic testing would not be informative. His sister does have an increased risk for diabetes and close follow-up is recommended.

V. **Additional genomics resources for the nephrology nurse can be found in Table 1.1.**

SECTION B
Anatomy and Physiology
Carol Motes Headley

I. **Anatomy of the renal system.**

A. Overview (see Figure 1.22).
  1. The kidneys function as the primary excretory organ.
    a. The bowel, skin, and lungs also function as excretory organs, but the renal system is the major system responsible for getting rid of waste through the formation and excretion of urine.
    b. Excretion of metabolic wastes includes getting rid of urea (generated from protein), creatinine (generated from muscle), uric acid (byproduct of purines), bilirubin (from hemoglobin), metabolites (from hormones), and drugs.
    c. In one day, the kidneys will filter almost 200 liters of fluid from the blood.

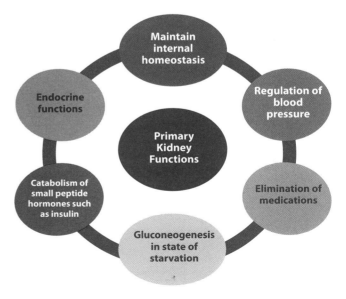

Figure 1.22. Primary functions of the kidney.

d. Metabolic waste products, toxins, and excess ions are excreted through the urine.

2. As this large amount of filtrate makes its way through the system, the kidneys will selectively conserve what is needed and return it back to the blood.

3. Each kidney is made up of a large mass of nephrons that are the functioning units and do the work.
   a. That work involves so much more than elimination of waste products.
   b. Nephrons function as the principal regulators of the body's internal environment.
      (1) They help to maintain extracellular and intercellular fluid volumes.
      (2) The nephrons also help maintain electrolyte concentrations within a remarkably narrow range.

4. Other kidney functions include regulation of acid/base balance, hormone synthesis, and in certain circumstances, generation of glucose, termed *gluconeogenesis* (Schrier et al., 2012).

B. The gross anatomy of the renal system (see Figure 1.23).
   1. Location.
      a. The kidneys can be found in the posterior abdominal wall in the retroperitoneal space.
      b. They are in front of and on both sides of the vertebral column between twelfth thoracic and third lumbar vertebrae.
   2. The right kidney is slightly lower than the left because the liver is above the right kidney.
   3. The kidneys have several protective facets that provide protection from blunt force trauma as well as preventing the spread of any infection that might occur from traveling outside the kidney.
      a. The renal fascia is the outer layer of connective tissue that holds the kidney in place. This tissue

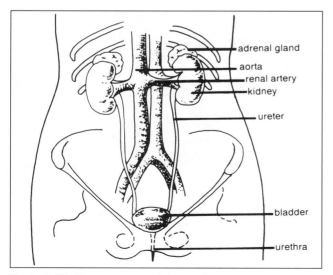

Figure 1.23. Gross anatomy of the renal system.

serves to anchor the kidney to surrounding structures.
   b. The perirenal fat capsule encases the kidney to provide a cushion of support.
      (1) If there is a reduction in body fat, such as in the case of severe malnutrition, then this can result in the kidneys becoming displaced and actually dropping.
      (2) This is called renal ptosis. Renal ptosis can result in a ureter becoming kinked.
   c. Another capsule, a transparent fibrous capsule, acts to prevent the spread of any infection.

4. Gross structure of the kidneys.
   a. Weight of adult kidney: 120 to 160 grams (about 5 ounces).
   b. Size of adult kidney: 5 to 7 cm wide, 11 to 13 cm long, and approximately 2.5 cm thick, about the size of an adult fist.
   c. Kidney size is not influenced by body mass.

5. Renal blood vessels, lymphatics, nerves, and ureter enter or exit through an area called the hilum of each kidney (Taal et al., 2012).

C. The adrenal gland is located on top of each kidney but functions independently. Even blood flow and nerve innervation is separate (Taal et al., 2012).

II. Internal structure of the kidney (see Figure 1.24).

A. The cortex is the outer rim of the kidney.
   1. It receives a tremendous amount of blood; approximately 90% of the renal blood flow goes to the cortex.
   2. It is the most highly perfused tissue per gram of any organ in the body.

B. The medulla is the inner portion of the kidney and extends to the renal pelvis. It receives 10% of the renal blood flow (about average tissue perfusion).
   1. The medulla contains pyramids and renal columns (Bertin's columns), loops of Henle, vasa recta, and medullary collecting ducts.
   2. Pyramids are triangular-shaped structures composed of nephrons and their blood vessels. Renal columns are cortical tissue between the pyramids.
   3. The calyces are branches enclosing the papilla or points of the pyramids.
   4. The calyces collect urine. The tip (apex) of each pyramid, called the papilla, opens into a minor calyx. Several minor calyces form a major calyx. The major calyces join to form the common ureter, which exits the renal pelvis and transports urine to the ureters, then bladder, and finally the urethra.

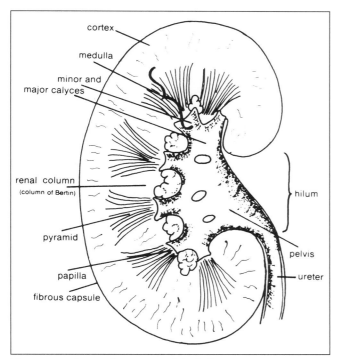

Figure 1.24. Internal structure of the kidney.

C. Nephrons are the workhorses of the kidney (see Figure 1.25).
   1. There are generally two major categories of nephrons.
      a. The cortical nephrons make up 85% of total nephron mass and the juxtamedullary nephrons make up the remaining portion.
      b. Cortical nephrons are shorter and do not extend into the inner portion of the kidney, called the medulla.
   2. The juxtamedullary nephrons are longer.
      a. Their loops of Henle travel deep into the medulla.
      b. This is important because their structure with the longer tubules allows the kidney to produce concentrated urine.

D. Collecting system.
   1. The collection system of the nephron is composed of structures that collect and transport urine but do not alter its composition or volume.
   2. Once urine flows through the papilla at the tip of the pyramid, the urine composition is unchanged (Schrier et al., 2012).

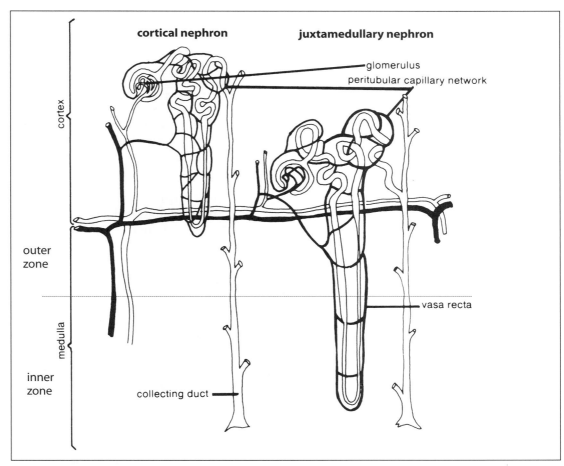

Figure 1.25. Arrangement of a cortical and juxtamedullary nephron. Note the relationship between vascular and tubular components.

<table>
<tr><td>

Mini Exercise of Understanding

1. Jim is a triathlete and has developed a large muscle mass. Would you expect him to have a larger nephron mass than someone else his same age? If so, why? If not, then why not? *Nephron endowment is fixed after birth. Nephron mass is not independently impacted by body mass.*

2. Bill plays college basketball and was hit in his upper back during a game. What supports and protects his kidneys from injury? *The position of the kidneys in the retroperitoneal space, the renal fascia and a perirenal fat capsule protect and support the kidneys from injury.*

3. The fibrous connective tissue that surrounds each kidney is called the:
   a.   Cortex.
   b.   Hilum.
   c.   *Renal capsule.*
   d.   Renal medulla.

</td></tr>
</table>

III. Kidney blood supply, lymphatic drainage, and innervation.

A. Overview.
  1. Normal kidney function is highly dependent upon receiving adequate blood supply. The blood provides oxygen and glucose for energy.
  2. Each nephron is composed of highly metabolic cells (e.g., basal cells full of mitochondria that line the loop of Henle).
     a. These cells are responsible for creating pumps that require energy.
     b. As a consequence, the kidneys do not tolerate a low blood flow or low oxygen state.
  3. Preservation of blood flow is maintained and highly well-orchestrated by neurohormonal reflexes that react to even the slightest reduction in blood flow.
  4. Disease-states develop when circumstances prevent the kidneys from maintaining adequate blood flow and alter the pressure/volume status (Cupples, 2007; Eaton, & Pooler, 2013).

B. The renal blood supply.
  1. The kidneys receive approximately 20–25% (about 1200 mL/min) of the cardiac output under normal physiologic conditions.
  2. The body's total blood supply circulates through the kidneys approximately 12 times per hour.
  3. Approximately 90% of the renal blood supply circulates through the cortex at a rate of about 4.5 mL/min, and 10% circulates through the medulla at about 1 mL/min.
  4. Each kidney has one renal artery that branches from the abdominal aorta and enters the kidney at the hilum (see Figure 1.26).
  5. The renal hilum is a cleft where the ureters, renal blood vessels, lymphatics, and nerves enter the kidneys.

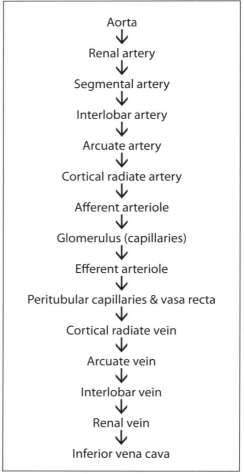

Figure 1.26. Renal blood flow tracked from origination off the abdominal aorta to its venous return, emptying into the inferior vena cava (Kestenbaum & Drueke, 2012).

  6. The renal artery divides into segmental arteries that further divide into interlobar arteries that travel alongside the pyramids into the cortex.
  7. At the junction of the cortex and medulla, the interlobar arteries bend at right angles.
  8. The arcuate arteries begin at this point. The arcuate arteries branch into interlobular arteries, which travel further into the cortex.
  9. In the cortex, the interlobular arteries divide into afferent arterioles.
  10. Each afferent arteriole divides into tufts of capillaries called the glomerulus.
  11. The glomerular capillaries rejoin to form the efferent arteriole, which then becomes the peritubular capillary network (and vasa recta for the juxtamedullary nephrons).
  12. The vasa recta ascend off the efferent arteriole.
     a. It is a capillary bed that wraps around the tubular network of the juxtamedullary nephron.
     b. Usually a capillary network has a venous

portion (venule) leading away from the capillary system, but not in the glomerulus.
  c. The efferent arteriole is still oxygenated or has arterial blood.
  d. When the blood reaches the interlobular veins, it becomes a venous system (Schrier et al., 2012).
  13. The interlobular veins join the segmental veins, which empty into the renal vein.
  14. The renal vein exits through the hilum and joins inferior vena cava, which returns blood to the right atrium.

C. Lymphatic drainage from the kidneys and upper ureters flows into the aortic and paraaortic lymph nodes and then into the thoracic lymph duct.

D. The kidneys are innervated by sympathetic branches from the celiac plexus, upper lumbar splanchnic and thoracic nerves, and intermesenteric and superior hypogastric plexus. These join to form a surrounding renal nerve plexus (Eaton & Pooler, 2013).

IV. Microscopic anatomy of the nephron.

A. Overview.
  1. An individual's nephron endowment refers to the number of functioning nephrons that a person has at birth. Nephrons are not generated after birth.
  2. People that are born with a single kidney (renal agenesis) in all likelihood will be able to maintain adequate kidney function through their lifespan.
  3. Nephron endowment can range anywhere from 300,000 to 2 million per kidney, but average is around 1 million (Luyckx & Brenner, 2010).
  4. Each nephron has an afferent arteriole that is made up of smooth muscle cells that allow it to dilate and contract.
  5. The efferent arteriole has valves.
  6. The glomerulus sits between these two arterioles.
  7. Filtration through the glomerulus is dependent upon the amount of pressure that is physiologically generated by these two arterioles.
  8. Glomerular filtration is also dependent upon the glomerular capillary membrane.
    a. This highly specialized membrane is selective in its filtration capacity.

  b. From the electrical charge generated by the proteins to the junctions between the podocytes, all work together to create a filtrate that is relatively free of protein and cells (Taal et al., 2012).

B. The function of the nephron is to make a filtrate that will eventually become urine. Each nephron consists of two components (see Figure 1.27).
  1. The vascular component includes the afferent arteriole, glomerulus, efferent arteriole, peritubular capillary network, and vasa recta (for juxtamedullary nephrons only).

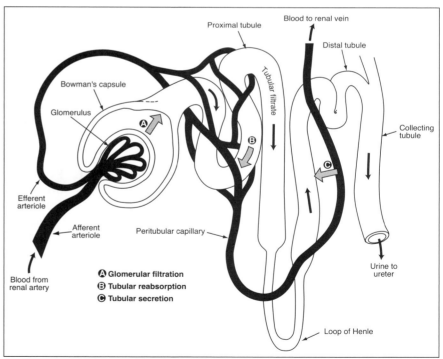

Figure 1.27. Summary of nephron structure and function. The plasma portion of blood flowing into the glomerular capillaries is filtered into Bowman's capsule (A). As the filtrate flows through the lumen of the tubule, some substances are reabsorbed from the filtrate into the peritubular capillaries (B), and other substances are secreted from the peritubular capillaries into the lumen of the tubule (C).

2. The tubular component includes Bowman's capsule, proximal tubule (PT), descending and ascending limbs of the loop of Henle, distal tubule (DT), cortical collecting tubule, and medullary collecting duct.
3. The nephron produces concentrated or dilute urine through several processes including filtration, reabsorption, secretion, and excretion. These processes also help to maintain homeostasis of the body's internal environment (see Figure 1.28).

C. Each nephron consists of a glomerulus surrounded by a series of tubules lined by a layer of epithelial cells.
   1. The glomerulus is a tuft of capillaries set between the afferent and efferent arterioles (note: oxygenated blood is in both afferent and efferent arterioles).
   2. Vascular component (see Figure 1.29).
   3. Each afferent arteriole divides into a tuft of capillaries called the glomerulus, which is surrounded by Bowman's capsule.
   4. Blood in the glomerulus is separated from fluid in Bowman's capsule only by its capillary membranes. Bowman's capsule fits like a glove around the glomerular capillary bed.
   5. The space between both layers of Bowman's capsule is the urinary space.

D. Permeability of the glomerular capillaries is about 100 to 500 times greater than capillaries in other parts of the body. The glomerular capillaries are highly selective for the types of molecules that can pass through.

Recognize and Remember

The glomerular capillary allows for a much larger amount of filtration than other capillaries because there is higher hydrostatic pressure.

This high hydrostatic pressure within the glomerulus changes very little over the entire capillary bed.

The lower hydrostatic pressure and lower oncotic pressure (protein-free) within Bowman's capsule contribute further to filtration.

Last, there is the higher permeability factor associated with the fenestrated membrane of the glomerulus.

E. Glomerular capillary membrane permeability and selectivity are related to the size, structure, and charge of molecules. The membrane has three major layers (see Figure 1.29).
   1. The endothelial layer of the glomerular capillaries is perforated by thousands of holes called fenestrae.

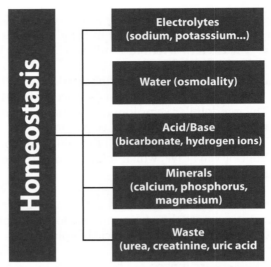

Figure 1.28. Kidneys' role in maintaining homeostasis. The kidneys are able to maintain homeostasis of body fluids despite extremes in dietary intake or changes in metabolism. This diagram includes examples of several homeostatic mechanisms, but it is not meant to be totally inclusive.

---

   a. Thus, glomerular capillaries are often called fenestrated capillaries.
   b. The large fenestrae allow filtration of water and small solutes with diameters up to about 100 nanometers.
   2. The basement membrane layer is composed of collagen and proteoglycans that have large spaces through which water and some solutes can pass.
   3. A layer of epithelial cells (called podocytes) line the outer surface of the glomerulus and also serves as the inner layer of Bowman's capsule.
   a. These cells have structures called foot processes that are not continuous but have slit pores about 25 to 60 nanometers wide.
   b. The pores allow water and some solutes to pass.

F. Reasons for selectivity of molecules that can filter through glomerular capillaries.
   1. The glomerulus will freely filter uncharged molecules with a radius diameter up to 1.8 nanometers. As molecule size progresses, their filtration capacity becomes more and more restricted as indicated by their fractional clearances.
   2. All three layers of the glomerular membrane have negative charges. Plasma proteins and other solutes with negative charges are therefore repelled by the negative charges and are not filtered by the membrane.
   a. For example, albumin has a molecular diameter of about 6 nanometers. Therefore, based on size, it should filter through the glomerular membranes.

b. Yet, almost no albumin is present in the glomerular filtrate because albumin has a strong negative electrical charge.

c. The pores in the glomerular membrane have a strong negative electrical charge.

d. Thus, electrostatic forces from both will repel each other to keep almost all the albumin from filtering across the glomerular membrane.

3. Glomerular capillaries are separated by mesangial cells, which provide support for the capillaries.

4. Glomerular capillaries reunite to form the efferent arteriole, which has two branches.

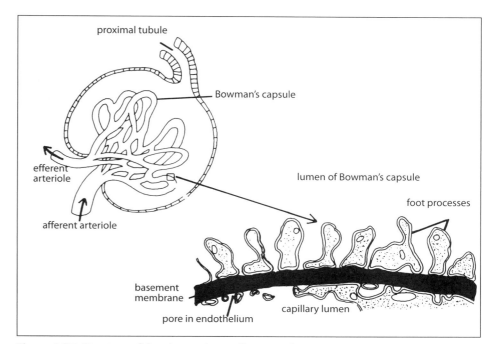

Figure 1.29. Structure of the glomerular capillary membrane.

G. Peritubular capillaries.
1. The peritubular capillaries surround the proximal tubule (PT) and distal tubule (DT), loops of Henle, and collecting tubules of cortical nephrons.
2. These capillaries drain into venules.
3. Vasa recta capillaries are branches of peritubular capillaries, which wrap around and run parallel to the long thin loops of Henle of the juxtamedullary nephrons.

H. Tubular component.
1. Composed of Bowman's capsule, PT, loop of Henle, DT, cortical collecting tubule, and medullary collecting duct.
2. Bowman's capsule is a concave sac that surrounds the glomerular capillaries, creating Bowman's space.
   a. One side of Bowman's capsule shares cells with the glomerulus.
   b. The other side of Bowman's capsule opens into the PT.
3. The PT is composed of columnar epithelial cells with many mitochondria, which provide energy (adenosine triphosphate [ATP]) for active transport of solutes. Hundreds of microvilli (called brush borders) increase the surface area of the PT lumen about 20 times.
4. The PT straightens and narrows to become the descending limb of the loop of Henle.
   a. It is composed of squamous epithelial cells with few organelles (e.g., mitochondria) and few microvilli.

b. Because the walls of the descending segment are very thin, it is called the thin segment or concentrating segment of the loop of Henle.
5. The loop of Henle makes a sharp U-turn and ascends through the cortex parallel with the descending limb.
   a. The early segment of the ascending limb is thin and is called the passive diluting segment.
   b. About halfway up the ascending limb, the diameter of the limb increases and the cells change to cuboidal epithelial, with more mitochondria and microvilli. This is called the thick ascending segment or active diluting segment of the loop of Henle.
6. The loop of Henle empties into the DT.
   a. Several DTs join to form the cortical collecting tubule, which descends downward through the cortex into the medulla where it is then called first the outer and then the inner medullary collecting duct.
   b. The cortical collecting tubule and medullary collecting duct run parallel to the descending and ascending limbs of the loops of Henle.
   c. The early part of the DT functions in concert with the thick ascending limb of the loop of Henle, and the late part of the DT functions in conjunction with the cortical collecting tubule.

I. Several collecting ducts join and open into the papilla of the pyramid (duct of Bellini) and then into a minor calyx of the ureter.

V. Interstitium.

A. Nephrons are separated by interstitial cells.
1. More are located in the medulla than in the cortex.
2. The function of these interstitial cells is not well delineated.
3. They are probably phagocytic and secrete hormones or hormone precursors.

B. Juxtaglomerular complex or apparatus (JGA).
1. Each nephron has a region of cells called the juxtaglomerular apparatus.
   a. This area of the nephron contains two specialized groups of cells (granular and extraglomerular mesangial cells).
   b. The cells help to regulate the rate of filtrate formation and blood pressure.
2. The juxtaglomerular apparatus is located at the distal portion of the thick ascending limb of the loop of Henle adjacent to the afferent arteriole and sometimes the efferent arteriole.
   a. These specialized cells are granular cells that act as mechanoreceptors.
   b. The cells sense changes in the blood pressure (like a vessel sphygmomanometer).
3. The macula densa, meaning "dense spot," is a group of tightly packed cells that are contained within the wall of the ascending limb of the loop of Henle.
   a. These cells are chemoreceptors (similar to a test strip) and are in close proximity to the granular cells.
   b. These chemoreceptor cells detect changes in the salt content of the filtrate (Eaton & Pooler, 2013; Hall, 2011).

Mini Exercise of Understanding

1. The glomerulus is normally a high-pressure capillary bed compared to other capillaries in the body. This high pressure contributes to large volumes of filtrate. What prevents blood cells and large proteins from being filtered? *Molecule size, molecular charge, Starling forces, membrane characteristics.*

2. Some molecules are relatively small, but are still not filtered. Why? *Molecular charge; the negative charge of proteins will repel like-charged molecules, other negatively charged molecules.*

3. Based upon what you have learned thus far, the loss of glomerular basement membrane integrity, and thus functionality, would be one of the first or last signs of abnormal kidney function? *A first sign of kidney dysfunction is often proteinuria (glomerular membrane dysfunction), with a normal glomerular filtration rate.*

VI. The ureters.

A. The ureters are a pair of retroperitoneal, mucosa-lined, fibromuscular tubes that transport urine from the renal pelvis to the urinary bladder.
1. The ureters are 30 to 33 cm long.
2. Their diameter is 2 to 8 mm, with narrowest diameter at the ureteropelvic junction and ureterovesical junction (bladder).

B. The walls of the calyces, pelvis, and ureter contain smooth muscle cells that contract to move urine along its course to the bladder.

C. Their oblique entrance into the bladder creates a mucosal fold. Pressure in the bladder creates a sphincter-like effect that prevents backflow of urine from the bladder into the ureters and renal pelvis.

VII. The urinary bladder.

A. The bladder is a pouch composed of thick, smooth muscle that is lined with epithelial cells.

B. The bladder is located in the pelvis anterior and inferior to the peritoneal cavity and posterior to the pubic bones.

C. Bladder capacity.
1. The adult's bladder capacity is about 300 to 500 mL.
2. A child's bladder capacity can be calculated by adding the child's age + 2 = bladder capacity in ounces.
   a. Remember that an ounce has 30 mL.
   b. Thus, a 5-year-old child's bladder capacity would be 5+2 = 7 and 7 x 30 mL = 210 mL (Kaefer et al., 1997).

D. The ureteral orifices join the urethra that connects to the bladder to form an exit route for urine. These three orifices form a triangular area called the *trigone.*

VIII. The urethra.

A. The urethra is a tube that carries urine from the bladder to the urinary meatus for excretion.
1. An internal urinary sphincter, formed by bladder smooth muscle, is located at the junction of the urethra with the bladder.
2. An external urinary sphincter is formed by skeletal muscle surrounding the urethra as the urethra passes through the pelvic floor.
3. Sphincters control movement of urine through the urethra.

B. Length of the urethra.
   1. The male urethra is about 20 cm long.
      a. Much of it is external to the body.
      b. The meatus opens at the end of the penis.
   2. The female urethra is about 3 to 5 cm long.
      a. It lies within the body.
      b. The female meatus opens superior to the vaginal orifice (VanPutte et al., 2013).

IX. Embryonic and fetal development.

A. Overview.
   1. Three successive types of kidneys develop in the embryo: pronephros, mesonephros, and metanephros.
   2. The urinary system develops in a three-stage process.
      a. Formation and evolution of the pronephros, mesonephros, and the ureteric bud during normal embryologic development occur sequentially.
      b. The adrenal glands and gonads develop from mesodermal tissue.

B. Conception to 8 weeks.
   1. Pronephros develop during the 4th week after conception and are transient, nonfunctioning structures. The pronephros are replaced by the mesonephros at 5 weeks, developing from the paravertebral mesoderm of the upper thoracic or lumbar region.
   2. The mesonephros are also nonfunctional. They evolve from the urogenital ridge, then degenerate.
   3. The mesonephros develop at the end of the 4th week and give rise to the ureteral bud, then degenerate. The mesonephros function through 8th week of development.
   4. The ureteral bud gives rise to metanephros and metanephric blastema from which the kidney develops during the 5th week.
      a. Metanephros becomes a functional structure (definitive kidney) at the end of the 8th week (beginning of fetal period).
      b. The paired metanephros form urine during fetal development; the urine is expelled through the urinary system into amniotic fluid.
   5. Bladder development is separate from kidney development. The bladder develops from a structure called the urogenital sinus.

C. The 5th to 14th or 15th weeks.
   1. The metanephros gives rise to the permanent kidney; it contains glomeruli and a tubular system.
   2. A fully functioning kidney that produces urine is established by approximately the 11th week of gestation.
   3. After development, kidneys migrate from the caudal position to their permanent position near the lumbar spine.
   4. Kidneys can be visualized in-utero using transvaginal ultrasound at the 10th to 12th week of gestation.
   5. Risk factors for renal agenesis include a body mass index over 30 prior to pregnancy, smoking during the preconception period, and binge drinking during the second month of gestation (Slickers et al., 2008).

D. The 14th or 15th to 20th or 22nd weeks.
   1. The collecting system matures.
   2. New nephrons develop.

E. 20th or 22nd to 32nd or 36th weeks.
   1. Collecting ducts grow toward renal capsules and gather nephrons.
   2. Cortical nephrons originate.

F. 32nd or 36th week, kidneys are fully developed.
   1. Nephrons lengthen and become tortuous.
   2. Glomeruli enlarge.
   3. Kidney surface becomes smooth during neonatal period.
   4. The kidneys reach maturity by second year of life.

G. The kidneys are fully developed by the 36th week of gestation.
   1. People are born with a variable number of nephrons; nephrons do not develop after birth. The kidneys continue to mature after birth and obtain adult function by the age of 2 years.
   2. The ureter begins to form from a portion of ureteral bud.
   3. Anterior bud dilates and gives rise to the renal pelvis, which grows and differentiates into calyces and collecting ducts.
   4. Metanephric blastema differentiate into nephrons.
   5. DT joins the end of the collecting ducts. Subsequently the loop of Henle, PT, Bowman's capsule, and glomerular capillaries form.
   6. Kidneys originate in lower pelvic region. During first growth period, they rotate 90° medially and start ascent for adult position (Little et al., 2010; Reidy & Rosenblum, 2009; Schrier et al., 2012).

X. Physiology of the kidney (see Figure 1.30).

A. Urine formation involves an intricate process of filtration, reabsorption, secretion, and excretion that occur within the nephron. Each nephron functions independently from other nephrons because each nephron has its own blood supply.

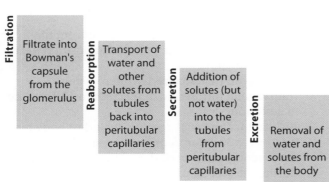

Figure 1.30. Renal physiology essential concepts (Brenner & Rector, 2012).

Recognize and Remember

The primary function of the glomerulus is formation of a filtrate from plasma.

The proximal tubule reabsorbs over 50% of the filtered sodium chloride and 90% of the filtered bicarbonate.

The loop of Henle functions as a countercurrent multiplier and reabsorbs sodium chloride in excess of water.

The distal tubule reabsorbs about 5% of filtered sodium chloride and is the major site for calcium excretion.

B. Primary purposes of the kidney.
1. Regulate body fluid volume and osmolality.
2. Regulate electrolyte balance of body fluids.
3. Regulate acid-base balance of body fluids, in conjunction with body buffer systems and the respiratory system.
4. Remove metabolic wastes from the body fluids, such as urea, creatinine, uric acid, beta-2 microglobulin, and many others.
5. Regulate blood pressure.
6. Regulate bone marrow production of red blood cells.
7. Synthesize vitamin D to its physiologic active form.
8. Perform gluconeogenesis (in a fasting state).
9. Synthesize hormones, such as prostaglandins, endothelin, and nitric oxide.
10. Excrete drugs and toxins from the body fluids.

C. Basic concepts (see Tables 1.2 and 1.3 for summaries).
1. Nephron regulation of blood and body fluid composition.
2. The plasma portion of blood is filtered as it flows through the glomerulus. The process of forming urine:

a. Begins with the passive process of filtration of water and other small molecules from the plasma into Bowman's capsule.
b. The filtrate enters Bowman's space and the lumen of the tubule.
 (1) The filtration process, although passive, occurs under pressure, which is generated by blood pressure.
 (2) The process is similar to fluid being forced through a fine sieve.
 (3) Fluid within Bowman's capsule is termed *filtrate* and ultimately becomes urine, although urine is markedly different from the initial filtrate.
c. Typically, about 180 liters of filtrate is made in one day (i.e., the glomerular filtration rate).
 (1) Only 1 to 2 liters are excreted as urine.
 (2) This means that 99% of the filtrate is reabsorbed.
3. As the filtrate moves along and through the tubule:
a. Some substances, such as amino acids and glucose, are completely reabsorbed.
b. Other substances, such as urea, creatinine, and excess water and electrolytes, are either not reabsorbed or only partially reabsorbed depending on the body's need for the substance.
4. Other substances may be secreted into the tubule as the filtrate moves through the tubule.

XI. Glomerular filtration rate (GFR) and its regulation.

A. Glomerular filtration begins as blood enters the glomerulus from the afferent arteriole under high pressure.
1. This pressure is known as the glomerular hydrostatic pressure and is estimated to be 60 mmHg.
2. Note: These pressures have never been measured in the human kidney. They have been measured in dogs and have been extrapolated to estimate human kidney pressures.
3. Ultimately, it is the balance between Starling forces, glomerular permeability, capillary surface area, and plasma flow rate that determines GFR. Starling forces include the resistance of the afferent and efferent arteriole, arterial blood pressure, venous pressure, and osmotic pressure.
4. Hydrostatic pressure within the glomerular capillary is opposed by glomerular capillary colloid osmotic pressure, also called oncotic pressure.
a. It is caused by plasma proteins (especially albumin) that do not filter from the capillary into the tubule.

<table>
<tr><td>

Recognize and Remember

Urine output is **not** autoregulated.

Increases in perfusion pressures result in an increase in urinary flow termed *pressure natriuresis.*

Thus, isolated urinary output is not a good overall index of kidney function.

The best index of kidney function is glomerular filtration rate.

</td></tr>
</table>

b. This pressure is estimated as 30 mmHg.

5. Hydrostatic pressure in the glomerular capillary is also opposed by Bowman's capsule hydrostatic pressure, estimated to be 20 mmHg.

6. The colloid osmotic pressure in Bowman's capsule is normally 0 mmHg because plasma proteins do not filter from the glomerular blood into Bowman's capsule.
   a. If plasma protein (e.g., albumin) does filter into Bowman's capsule, it creates a colloid osmotic pressure.

Table 1.2

Summary of Physiologic Concepts Related to Renal Regulation of Water and Electrolyte Balance

GLOMERULAR FILTRATION RATE (GFR): volume of plasma filtered from the glomerular capillaries into Bowman's capsule each minute, expressed in mL/min. Average GFR for a young adult in 100–125 mL/min.

DIFFUSION: passive (does not require ATP) movement of particles from an area of higher to an area of lesser concentration of particles; diffusion ceases when equilibrium is reached.

ACTIVE TRANSPORT: movement of substances against an electrochemical or pressure gradient; requires energy from ATP.

OSMOSIS: movement of water across a semipermeable membrane from an area of lower concentration of solutes to an area of higher concentration of solutes. Osmosis ceases when concentration (osmolality) on the two sides of the semipermeable membrane equilibrates.

COLLOIDAL OSMOTIC (ONCOTIC) PRESSURE: the osmotic pressure related to proteins, especially albumin.

HYDROSTATIC PRESSURE: the pressure exerted by a fluid in a closed system.

OSMOLE (Osm): unit of osmotic pressure created by one mole of atoms or molecules in solution. Milliosmole (mOsm): one-thousandth of an osmole.

OSMOLALITY: concentration of a solution in terms of osmoles or milliosmoles per kilogram of water (osm/kg H_2O or mOsm/kg H_2O). In a solution, the fewer the number of particles in proportion to the volume of water, the less concentrated, or the lower the osmolality, of the solution.

OSMOLARITY: the concentration of solution in terms of osmoles or milliosmoles per liter of water (osm/L H_2O or mOsm/L H_2O).

HYPOSMOTIC: decreased osmolarity or osmolality of a solution.

HYPEROSMOTIC: increased osmolarity or osmolality of a solution.

ISO-OSMOTIC: solution with an osmolarity or osmolality equal to that with which it is compared.

TUBULAR REABSORPTION: process by which substances move from the tubular filtrate into the plasma of peritubular capillaries.

TUBULAR SECRETION: process by which substances move from the plasma of peritubular capillaries into the tubular filtrate.

TRANSPORT MAXIMUM (Tm): the point at which the tubular membrane transport proteins for a specific substance become saturated and cannot accept more. Reabsorption of a substance that has a Tm (e.g., glucose and amino acids) ceases when its Tm is exceeded, and the excess substance is excreted in the urine.

CLEARANCE (Cl): volume of plasma that is cleared of a specific solute by the kidneys per unit of time, expressed in mL/min. Renal clearance of a specific substance depends on several factors, including:

• if a substance is filtered at the glomerulus and is not reabsorbed or secreted in the tubule, then clearance of that substance equals the amount filtered.

• if a substance is filtered at the glomerulus and partially or completely reabsorbed from the tubule, then clearance of that substance equals the amount filtered minus the total amount reabsorbed.

• if a substance is filtered at the glomerulus and secreted into the tubule, then clearance of that substance equals the amount filtered plus the total amount secreted.

• if a substance is filtered at the glomerulus and both reabsorbed and secreted in the tubule, then clearance of that substance equals the amount filtered minus the total amount reabsorbed plus the total amount secreted. The amount cleared may be less than, equal to, or greater than the amount filtered, depending on the rates of filtration, reabsorption, and secretion.

Table 1.3

Summary of Major Functions of Nephron Components in Water and Electrolyte Regulation

GLOMERULUS
- filtration of plasma-like substance (filtrate) into Bowman's capsule.
- RBCs, WBCs, and plasma proteins normally not filtered.

PROXIMAL TUBULE (PT)
- 65% of sodium actively reabsorbed.
- obligatory passive reabsorption of water with sodium.
- 65% of potassium reabsorbed by cotransport with sodium.
- 25% magnesium actively reabsorbed.
- 65% calcium passively reabsorbed. Increases or decreases as water and sodium reabsorption change.
- most phosphate reabsorbed.
- acid-base balance begins: hydrogen ions secreted; bicarbonate reabsorbed; ammonia synthesized; hydrogen ions buffered with phosphates in filtrate.
- chloride ions reabsorbed along with cations.
- 100% amino acids reabsorbed by cotransport with sodium.
- 100% glucose reabsorbed by cotransport with sodium if Tm not exceeded.
- proteins reabsorbed by pinocytosis.
- some urea reabsorbed.
- exogenous substances (e.g., drugs) secreted.
- volume of filtrate decreased by 65% when it leaves PT, but it is iso-osmotic because equal amounts of water and solutes are reabsorbed.

LOOP OF HENLE
- countercurrent multiplying and exchange mechanism established in long, thin loops of Henle and vasa recta of juxtamedullary nephrons.
- about 25% of sodium, 65% of magnesium, 25% of calcium, and 27% of potassium are reabsorbed; chloride reabsorbed along with cations.

descending limb
- permeable to water; somewhat permeable to sodium, chloride, and urea.
- water moves by osmosis from tubular lumen into hyperosmotic interstitium.
- sodium, chloride, and urea move into tubular lumen from interstitium.
- because water leaves and solutes enter, the osmolality of the filtrate progressively increases.

thick ascending limb
- impermeable to water and urea.
- Na^+-K^+-$2Cl^-$ actively transported into interstitium, which makes the interstitium progressively hyperosmotic from cortex to deep inner medulla.
- because solutes are transported out and water is not, the osmolality of the filtrate progressively decreases and a hyposmotic filtrate leaves the ascending limb.
- the vasa recta act as countercurrent exchangers to maintain the hyperosmotic interstitium.

DISTAL TUBULE (DT)
- early DT functions same as thick ascending limb of loop of Henle; late DT functions same as cortical collecting tubule.

LATE DT, CORTICAL COLLECTING TUBULE, AND MEDULLARY COLLECTING DUCT
- hyposmotic filtrate empties from ascending limb of loop of Henle into collecting tubule.
- sodium is reabsorbed and potassium secreted in presence of aldosterone or vice versa if aldosterone is not present.
- calcium is reabsorbed if parathyroid hormone (PTH) or 1,25-DHCC is present; calcium is not reabsorbed and is lost in urine if PTH or 1,25-DHCC is not present. Calcitonin also decreases calcium reabsorption.
- varying amounts of magnesium reabsorbed or secreted.
- acid-base regulation continues by hydrogen ion secretion, bicarbonate reabsorption, ammonia synthesis, and hydrogen buffering with phosphates in the filtrate.
- ADH determines final urine osmolality.
- if ADH is not present, collecting tubule and medullary collecting duct are impermeable to water and a dilute urine (low osmolality) is excreted.
- if ADH is present, collecting tubule and medullary collecting duct are permeable to water; water is reabsorbed into the hyperosmotic interstitium and a concentrated urine (high osmolality) is excreted.
- when filtrate leaves medullary collecting duct, it is in final form of urine excreted from the body.

(1) When this occurs, glomerular filtration is enhanced.

(2) The plasma protein pulls water from the glomerular capillaries into Bowman's capsule.

   b. This occurs in disease states such as nephrotic syndrome.

B. Normal or effective filtration pressure is around 10 mmHg (see Figure 1.31). The following calculation illustrates the filtration pressure variables:

1. Glomerular capillary hydrostatic pressure +60 mmHg.
2. Pressures opposing glomerular hydrostatic pressure include the glomerular capillary colloid osmotic pressure (-30 mmHg) (it is a pulling back in type of pressure) and the hydrostatic pressure within Bowman's capsule (-20 mmHg). It is a pushing in towards the glomeruli capillary from Bowman's capsule type of pressure.
3. Total opposing pressures = –50 mmHg.
4. Net or effective filtration pressure = +10 mmHg.

C. Effective glomerular filtration pressure forces fluid and some solutes of small molecular size through pores in the glomerular capillaries into Bowman's capsule.
  1. With normal kidney function, filtrate fluid that enters Bowman's capsule has the same ionic composition as blood, but is almost protein free. No cells are filtered.
  2. Filtration is dependent upon pressure and molecular size as well as molecular charges.
  3. Glomerular filtrate (also called tubular filtrate or simply filtrate) is similar to plasma except it lacks proteins (or only in minute quantities) and blood cells.
     a. Proteins have a strong negative electrical charge that is repelled by the negative charge on the pores of the glomerular membranes.
     b. Red and white blood cells are too large to pass through the glomerular capillary pores.

D. Glomerular filtration rate is normally about 125 mL/min in young, healthy adults.
  1. An important concept of GFR is to understand the relationship between renal plasma flow and the filtration fraction. Increases in renal plasma flow (RPF) and/or filtration fraction (FF) ultimately results in an increase in GFR.
  2. GFR = RPF x FF.
  3. Blood is approximately 50% plasma.
  4. Cardiac output (CO) = 5,000 mL/min.
  5. Kidneys receive 20% of the CO.
     a. 20% of 5,000 mL = 1,000 mL/minute of blood travels to kidneys.
     b. 50% of blood is plasma and 50% is cells, mostly red blood cells. In the 1,000 mL of blood traveling to the kidneys, 500 mL is plasma, which is also called the renal plasma flow (RPF).
     c. The filtration fraction (FF) is usually about 25% of plasma.
        (1) The filtration fraction is equal to the amount of plasma that is filtered by the kidney each minute.
        (2) FF = GFR/RPF.

E. Factors that result in an increase in the GFR.
  1. Increased cardiac output.
     a. An increase of CO results in an increase in plasma flow; this results in an increase in glomerular filtration.
     b. An increase can occur in cases such as thyrotoxicosis and pregnancy.
  2. Increases in hydrostatic pressure from dilatation of afferent arteriole or reduction in colloid oncotic pressure (e.g., hypoalbuminemia).
  3. Hypoalbuminemia results in a reduction in colloid osmotic pressure (the "pulling" back into the capillary force).

Recognize and Remember

Starling forces promote filtration from the glomerulus. The hydrostatic pressure is generated by the cardiac output (CO).

Cardiac output is determined by the heart's stroke volume x heart rate = CO.

Oncotic pressure occurs within the interstitium of the glomerulus.

The net flow of filtrate out of the glomerulus is dependent upon the net sum of the hydrostatic and oncotic pressure gradients that occur between the glomerular capillary and Bowman's space.

F. Clearance. The definition of *clearance* is the volume of plasma cleared of a specific solute by the kidneys per unit of time.
  1. Creatinine is not a perfect estimate of glomerular filtration because it is both filtered and secreted; thus, it tends to overestimate calculated GFR.
  2. Renal clearance depends on filtration of the substance by the glomerulus, reabsorption from the tubule, and secretion into the tubule (Cupples, 2007; Taal et al., 2012).

Mini Exercise of Understanding

1. The glomerular filtration pressure is influenced by the hydrostatic pressure within the glomerulus that is generated by _____? *Cardiac output or renal blood flow*

2. How can the GFR be so tightly regulated despite normal blood pressure fluctuations and diurnal changes throughout the day? *Process of autoregulation*

XII. **Tubular reabsorption.** The process of reabsorption is just as incrementally important to nephron function as glomerular filtration. If it were not for tubular reabsorption, volume depletion would rapidly develop. Drinking enough to maintain hydration would be impossible. Water is filtered but almost completely reabsorbed in the tubules. Moreover, most other substances freely (passively) filtered at the glomerulus are subsequently reabsorbed from the tubular system back into the interstitial fluid, then into the blood. Most of what is considered essential to normal body function, such as water, glucose, amino acids, and electrolytes, are ultimately reabsorbed. Reabsorption occurs through passive and active processes. Substances that are not reabsorbed into the blood and those that are secreted into the tubule are then excreted in the urine. Thus, substances in the glomerular filtrate needed by the body are returned to the blood, whereas substances not

...d are not returned and are lost in the urine (Figure 1.31).

A. Water and solutes move from tubular lumen into the plasma of peritubular capillaries.

B. 98–99% of glomerular filtrate is normally reabsorbed from the tubule.

C. Tubular reabsorption involves both passive and active transport mechanisms.

> ### Recognize and Remember
>
> It is important to realize that the amount of daily glomerular filtration for a normal-sized adult is about 150 liters. This is, of course, more than the total body fluid volume. Thus, reabsorption is very important since almost all the original filtrate from the glomerulus is reabsorbed.

1. Passive transport requires no energy as it is based on concentration gradients. Urea, water, chloride, some bicarbonate and phosphates are passively reabsorbed.
2. Active transport (ATP) requires energy to move substances against an electrochemical gradient. Sodium, potassium, glucose, calcium, phosphate, and amino acids are actively reabsorbed.
3. Most reabsorption (about 65%) occurs in the proximal tubule.
4. Variable amounts of the remaining filtrate are

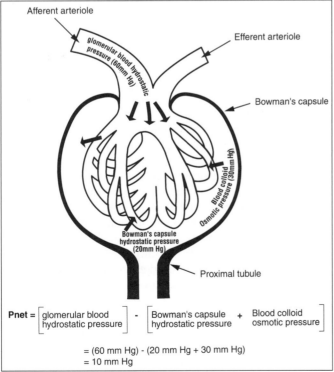

$$Pnet = \left[\begin{array}{c} \text{glomerular blood} \\ \text{hydrostatic pressure} \end{array}\right] - \left[\begin{array}{c} \text{Bowman's capsule} \\ \text{hydrostatic pressure} \end{array} + \begin{array}{c} \text{Blood colloid} \\ \text{osmotic pressure} \end{array}\right]$$

= (60 mm Hg) - (20 mm Hg + 30 mm Hg)
= 10 mm Hg

Figure 1.31. Pressures involved in determining net filtration pressure.

reabsorbed in Henle's loop, DT, cortical collecting tubule, and medullary collecting duct, depending on the body's need to excrete or retain specific substances.

XIII. Tubular secretion.

A. Tubular secretion means that substances move from the peritubular capillary plasma (blood) into the tubular lumen (filtrate). Tubular secretion is essentially reabsorption in reverse.
1. Substances secreted into the tubule include potassium, hydrogen ions, ammonia, uric acid, exogenous substances (e.g., drugs), and other wastes.
2. Tubular secretion helps with the elimination of certain drugs and metabolites that are protein bound. Proteins are not filtered so drugs that are bound to proteins must be actively secreted.
3. Tubular secretion gets rid of extra potassium. Aldosterone drives this process within the collecting ducts and DCT.
4. Tubular secretion is also important in controlling blood pH. If blood pH drops to less than its desired homeostatic threshold, then the renal tubular cells actively secrete more hydrogen ions (H+) into the filtrate and retain as well as generate more bicarbonate ions (HCO_3).

B. Factors that favor reabsorption:
1. Proximal tubule (PT): The bulk of reabsorption occurs in the PT. The distal segments of the tubule do the majority of the fine-tuning of the urine prior to delivery for excretion. Large amounts of the filtrate are reabsorbed through active and passive processes. About 65% of the glomerular filtrate is reabsorbed from the PT.
2. The cells of the PT are large cuboidal epithelial cells with numerous mitochondria, which produce ATP to be used as the energy source for active transport.
3. The luminal border (the cell membrane that faces the tubular lumen) consists of a very extensive brush border that increases the surface area of the luminal membrane about 20 times. The brush border membrane contains numerous protein transport molecules that enhance transport of solutes across the membrane.
4. The basal border (the cell membrane facing the interstitium between the tubule and peritubular capillary) has an active sodium-potassium ATPase pump. This keeps the intracellular sodium concentration low and maintains a negative intracellular charge.
   a. For every three sodium ions that the sodium-potassium pump transports from the interior of the cell, two potassium ions are pumped into the interior of the cell. More sodium ions are

pumped out of the cell than potassium ions are pumped into the cell. This creates an electrochemical gradient between the interior of the cell and the filtrate in the lumen of the tubule.
  b. The pressure in the peritubular capillaries throughout the course of the nephron is less than the pressure inside the tubular lumen, which favors reabsorption of substances back into the capillaries.

C. Sodium regulation in PT.
  1. Because of the active sodium-potassium pump on the basal membrane of the tubular cells, the concentration of sodium inside the cells becomes less than the concentration of sodium in the tubular lumen. The sodium transport proteins on the luminal membrane of PT cells bind with sodium ions and then release them inside the cell, which provides for rapid reabsorption of sodium.
  2. After sodium moves to the interior of the cell, it is pumped across the basal membrane into the interstitium and then reabsorbed into the peritubular capillaries.
  3. 65% of the filtered sodium is reabsorbed from the PT.

D. Amino acid reabsorption in PT.
  1. Amino acids are reabsorbed by cotransport with sodium ions.
  2. On the luminal membrane, both a sodium ion and an amino acid bind with a transport protein that is specific for transporting this combination simultaneously.
  3. The transport protein then releases both the sodium ion and the amino acid to the interior of the cell.
  4. The amino acid is then transported by facilitated diffusion across the basal membrane into the interstitium and absorbed into the peritubular capillaries.
  5. 100% of filtered amino acids are normally reabsorbed.

E. Glucose reabsorption in PT.
  1. Glucose is reabsorbed by cotransport with sodium ions (tags along).
  2. On the luminal membrane, both a glucose molecule and a sodium ion bind with transport proteins that are specific for transporting this combination simultaneously.
  3. The transport proteins release the sodium ion and glucose molecule to the interior of the cell.
  4. The glucose is then transported by facilitated diffusion across the basal membrane into the interstitium and absorbed into peritubular capillaries.

5. 100% of filtered glucose is normally reabsorbed (Hall, 2011; Triplitt, 2012).

F. Substances that are reabsorbed by facilitated diffusion require a specific transport protein. When a transport protein becomes saturated with its specific substance, the remainder of that substance is excreted in the urine instead of being reabsorbed. The maximum rate at which a specific substance can be reabsorbed is called its transport maximum (Tm).

G. Substances that have a Tm include glucose, amino acids, proteins, and phosphate. Sodium does not have a Tm. Its reabsorption depends on its high concentration gradient between the filtrate and the interior of tubular cells.
  1. Tm for a substance depends on the tubular load of that substance. Tubular load is the total amount of a substance that filters through the glomerulus into the tubular lumen each minute.
  2. Proteins are reabsorbed from the PT by pinocytosis. Once the proteins are inside the tubular cell, they are broken down into their constituent amino acids, which are then reabsorbed into the interstitium and peritubular capillaries along with other amino acids. If the tubular load of proteins exceed the Tm, the excess amino acids are excreted.

H. Potassium regulation in PT: About 65% of potassium is reabsorbed from the PT by cotransport with sodium.

I. Magnesium regulation in PT: About 25% of magnesium is actively reabsorbed from the PT.

J. Calcium regulation in the PT: About 65% of calcium is passively reabsorbed from the PT.

K. Calcium reabsorption increases or decreases as water and sodium reabsorption increases or decreases.

L. Phosphate regulation in PT.
  1. Most phosphate is reabsorbed from the PT.
  2. When the tubular load of phosphate exceeds its Tm, the excess phosphate is excreted.
  3. Increased dietary intake of phosphate, parathyroid hormone, and fibroblast growth factor 23 (FGF23) decrease phosphate reabsorption and vice versa.

M. Chloride ions (anions) are passively reabsorbed from the PT along with cations.

N. Metabolic end products.
  1. Most of urea is reabsorbed from the PT.
  2. Filtered creatinine is secreted (about 10%) into the PT.

O. Because of the osmotic gradient created by the reabsorption of solutes from the PT, about 65% of water is passively reabsorbed from the PT. This is called obligatory reabsorption of water. Because solutes and water are reabsorbed at the same rate from the PT, the osmolality of the filtrate does not change, and the filtrate that leaves the PT is iso-osmotic (isotonic). The volume of the filtrate, however, decreases by 65%.

P. The loop of Henle is primarily responsible for producing a concentrated urine. What is interesting is that by the end of the loop of Henle, the osmolality of the filtrate is remarkably low (dilute), ~200 milliosmoles (mOsm)/kg. However, it is this low osmolality within the thick ascending limb of the loop of Henle that essentially sets the stage for the

collecting tubules to produce a concentrated urine. The loop of Henle creates a significant osmotic gradient within the interstitial space that increases from the renal cortex (~290 mOsm/kg) to the tip of the medulla (~1200 mOxm/kg).

Q. The countercurrent multiplying and exchange mechanism is established between the long, thin loops of Henle and vasa recta (peritubular capillaries) of the juxtamedullary nephrons. This mechanism is part of the process involved in regulating body water (see Figure 1.32).
1. About 25% of sodium, 65% of magnesium, 25% of calcium, and 27% of potassium are reabsorbed from the loop of Henle.
2. Chloride is reabsorbed along with the cations.

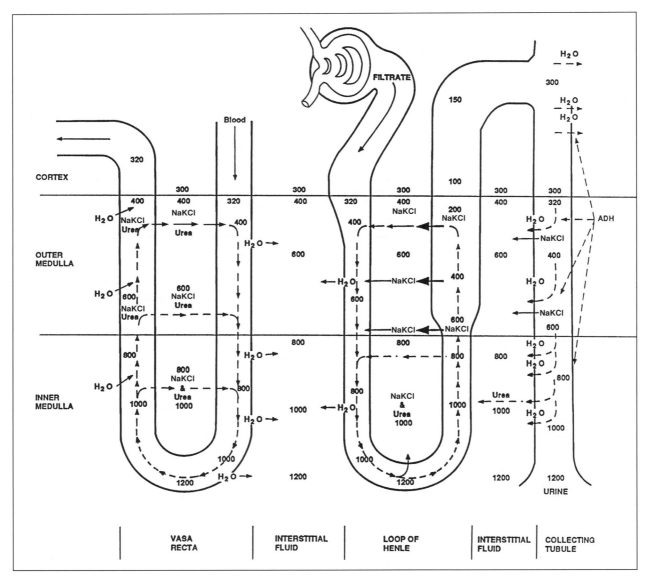

Figure 1.32. Diagram of the countercurrent multiplying and exchange mechanism of juxtamedullary nephrons.

R. Descending limb of the loop of Henle.
1. The epithelial cells of the descending limb of the loop of Henle are very thin and have few mitochondria and rudimentary brush borders.
2. The descending limb is very permeable to water and somewhat permeable to urea, sodium, and other ions. This limb is called the concentrating segment of the loop because water moves out and some solutes move in.

S. Ascending limb of the loop of Henle.
1. The early, thin segment of the ascending limb is much less permeable to water than the thin descending limb. This segment is called the passive diluting segment of the loop.
2. The thick segment begins approximately halfway up the ascending limb. The epithelial cells become thick and have many mitochondria with a rudimentary brush border.
3. The thick ascending limb is called the active diluting segment and is impermeable to water, but the cells are adapted for active transport of sodium, chloride, and potassium ions from the tubular filtrate into the interstitium. Solutes are reabsorbed in excess of water so hypo-osmotic filtrate leaves the ascending limb and empties into the DT. At this point the filtrate has a high concentration of urea.

T. The distal convoluted tubule is where 5–8% of sodium chloride is reabsorbed. The tubule remains impermeable to water and urea, but it is a major site for calcium reabsorption (stimulated by parathyroid hormone, PTH). The DCT is the site for maximal creation of a dilute urine (water excretion).
1. The early part of the DCT functions almost the same as the thick ascending segment of the loop of Henle.
2. Sodium is reabsorbed and potassium is secreted into the tubular lumen (or vice versa) depending on the level of potassium in the presence of aldosterone.
3. When plasma potassium is greater than about 4.0 mEq/L, potassium diffuses from the interstitium into the tubular cell and increases the intracellular potassium. This creates a concentration gradient between the cell and the filtrate in the tubular lumen. As a result, potassium diffuses from the cell into the tubular lumen and is excreted in the urine.
4. Aldosterone is secreted by the zona glomerulosa cells (outer layer) of the adrenal cortex. Angiotensin II is the stimulus for aldosterone secretion.
5. Calcium is reabsorbed in the late distal tubule if parathyroid hormone or 1,25 dihydroxychole-calciferol (1,25-DHCC) is present. Calcitonin decreases calcium reabsorption.

6. The late DCT and the cortical collecting duct are permeable to water if antidiuretic hormone (ADH) is present. Regulation of acid-base balance continues in the late DCT and cortical collecting duct.

U. Medullary collecting duct.
1. The medullary collecting duct is permeable to water and urea if ADH is present.
2. The medullary collecting duct can secrete hydrogen ions into the tubular lumen, an important part of the kidney's regulation of acid-base balance (Eton & Pooler, 2013; Hall, 2011).

Mini Exercise of Understanding

1. The bulk of sodium reabsorption occurs within what portion of the renal tubule? *Proximal tubule*

2. The interstitial space plays a vital role in determining the movement of solutes. Osmolality in the interstitium can reach 4 times that within the renal tubule. Explain the changes in concentration gradients from the cortex to the medulla.

    Sodium without water is actively reabsorbed in the ascending limb of the loop of Henle that result in an interstitial osmolar gradient increase from 285 mosmol/Kg in the cortex of the kidney to 1200 mosmol/Kg in the medulla at the tip of the renal papilla.

3. What portion of the nephron is the primary site for calcium reabsorption? *Distal convoluted tubule*

XIV. Urine concentration.

A. Antidiuretic hormone (ADH).
1. Overview.
    a. ADH is also known as arginine vasopressin.
    b. It is synthesized by the specialized neurons within the supraoptic and paraventricular nuclei contained in the hypothalamus.
    c. Release of ADH is triggered by high osmolality or a reduction in blood pressure.
        (1) However, the primary mechanism that results in release of ADH is an increase in plasma osmolality.
        (2) Osmoreceptors are specialized neurons that are located in the hypothalamus that sense a change in extracellular tonicity rather than osmolarity.
            (a) While sodium ions are the main contributors to fluid tonicity and osmolarity, in certain circumstances tonicity can change independent of sodium (e.g., mannitol infusion).
            (b) The osmoreceptors are very efficient in recognizing and responding to miniscule increases in tonicity (1% to 2%) to trigger the release of ADH.

2. ADH inhibits diuresis or urine output, conserving total body water.
3. ADH assists the kidney in producing more concentrated urine.
    a. This is accomplished by directing a second-messenger system, cyclic adenosine monophosphate (cAMP), to cause insertion of aquaporin channels into the luminal membrane of the principal cells of the collecting ducts, enhancing water reabsorption.
    b. The number of aquaporin channels inserted is directly proportional to the amount of ADH released.
    c. Urine concentration is increased with more water reabsorption.
4. Primary excessive secretion of ADH results in increased water reabsorption in the collecting tubules.
    a. This is called the syndrome of inappropriate ADH secretion, characterized by serum hypo-osmolality and hyponatremia.
    b. Volume expansion does not occur because initial fluid retention leads to spontaneous natriuresis due to an increase in renal perfusion and possibly release of atrial natriuretic peptide.

B. High levels of ADH production result in up to 99% of water reabsorption from the filtrate. The kidneys' ability to produce such a concentrated urine allows people to survive without water for an average of 3 days and in some cases even longer.

C. In contrast, low levels of ADH allows production of a very dilute urine. When aquaporin channels are not introduced into the collecting ducts, urine remains dilute.
    1. When urine filtrate reaches the ascending limb of the loop of Henle, it is dilute.
    2. In order for the kidneys to produce a dilute (hypo-osmotic) urine, it must merely be allowed to continue along the pathway to the renal pelvis for excretion.

D. With little or no ADH production, urine osmolality can drop to as low as 50 mOsm. This is about one-sixth of the concentration of the original glomerular filtrate.

E. Tubular transport maximum (Tm).
    1. Definition: the point at which the tubular membrane transports protein for a specific substance, becomes saturated, and cannot accept more of the substance.
    2. Renal tubules have a different Tm for different substances.
    3. Once the Tm is reached, a substance normally reabsorbed by a particular membrane transport protein is excreted in the urine, and a substance normally secreted by a particular membrane transport protein remains in the plasma.
    4. The most common example of a membrane transport protein that can become saturated and exceed its Tm is the one specific for glucose reabsorption.

F. Clearance is defined as the volume of plasma cleared of a specific solute by the kidneys per unit of time.

Recognize and Remember

The clearance ratio is equal to the clearance of a substance divided by the glomerular filtration rate.

A clearance ratio of 1 means that the solute is fully filtered by the kidney and not excreted or reabsorbed (e.g., insulin).

A clearance ratio of less than 1 means that the solute is freely filtered but also reabsorbed (e.g., sodium).

A clearance ratio of greater than 1 means that the solute is freely filtered but also actively secreted from the peritubular capillaries back into the tubular fluid (e.g., potassium).

A clearance ratio of 0 means that the solute is too large to be filtered (e.g., protein) or it is filtered and fully reabsorbed (e.g., glucose and amino acids).

---

1. Renal clearance depends on filtration of the substance by the glomerulus, reabsorption from the tubule, and its secretion into the tubule.
2. Autoregulation of renal blood flow, glomerular blood flow, and glomerular filtration rate.
    a. Routinely it is thought that vessels will vasoconstrict when the blood pressure is low in order to raise blood pressure, but this is not always the case.
    b. Autoregulation of glomerular filtration rate involves several mechanisms.
    c. In certain systems, a vessel will dilate if the blood pressure is low.
    d. This is done to maintain adequate perfusion, especially of vital organs such as the kidneys.
    e. Myogenic control is what accounts for dilatation of the afferent arteriole when blood pressure is low (hydrostatic pressure is reduced).
    f. Myogenic control is directed by the local chemical conditions of the blood, such as the amount of oxygen, carbon dioxide, or metabolites present (Schrier et al., 2012; Taal et al., 2012).

XV. GFR normally remains constant despite wide variations in mean arterial blood pressure (MAP). For example, a change in MAP from about 70 mmHg to 160 mmHg has little effect on the GFR. This ability of the kidneys to maintain a constant GFR is called autoregulation.

A. Mechanisms responsible for autoregulation.
   1. The process for autoregulation of glomerular filtration is related to myogenic reflex of afferent arterioles and tubuloglomerular feedback.
   2. The myogenic reflex of afferent arterioles relates to the response of the baroreceptors in the walls of the arterioles.
      a. When the MAP increases, the baroreceptors sense the increased vessel stretch and cause afferent arteriole constriction.
      b. This constriction prevents major changes in the glomerular capillary hydrostatic pressure.
      c. The opposite occurs when the MAP decreases; the afferent arteriole dilates and glomerular blood flow increases to preserve glomerular capillary hydrostatic pressure.
   3. A rise in blood pressure will increase capillary hydrostatic pressure within the glomerulus and result in an increase in the GFR.
      a. The built-in tubuloglomerular feedback system causes the afferent arteriole to constrict, thus causing a reduction in hydrostatic pressure within the glomerulus and therefore a reduction in the GFR.
      b. The GFR needs to remain constant in order to maintain delivery of the filtrate at the same constant rate so that reabsorption and secretion are not jeopardized.
      c. If the filtrate moves too quickly through the tubular system, the result is reduced reabsorption; and, if the filtrate moves too slowly, excessive reabsorption may occur (Cupples, 2007; Hall, 2011).

B. Two other areas within the nephron help to maintain the GFR.
   1. The two mechanisms involved in tubulo-glomerular feedback mechanism are the afferent arteriole vasodilator feedback and efferent arteriole vasoconstrictor feedback.
      a. The juxtaglomerular apparatus (JGA) controls most of these feedback mechanisms.
      b. The JGA consists of specialized cells located where the DT of each nephron loops back and comes into contact with the angle of the afferent and efferent arterioles of that nephron.
   2. The cells of the DT located at this junction are called the macula densa, which respond to changes in sodium and chloride concentration (salt).

a. The cells of the afferent arterioles at this point are called juxtaglomerular cells and secrete renin.
b. A decrease in glomerular filtrate decreases sodium and chloride concentration (salt) in the area of the macula densa.
   (1) The macula densa, in turn, sends a message by an unknown mechanism that causes afferent arteriole dilatation.
   (2) As the afferent arteriole dilates, glomerular blood flow and capillary hydrostatic pressure increase, thus maintaining the glomerular capillary pressure and GFR.
c. The opposite occurs if the GFR increases and there is an increased concentration of sodium and chloride at the macula densa. The macula densa stops sending a message to dilate the afferent arteriole, resulting in a relative vasoconstriction.

Recognize and Remember

Autoregulation of filtration is essential to mainlining an acceptable physiologic volume status and blood pressure. When cardiac output is reduced, there is a reduction in plasma flow, but the filtration fraction will increase in order to maintain a constant glomerular filtration rate.

This is accomplished by vasodilatation of the afferent arteriole and vasoconstriction of the efferent arteriole.

The efferent arteriole will have a subsequent lower hydrostatic pressure and a higher oncotic pressure.

This culmination of events results in an increase in the reabsorption of solute and water in the peritubular capillaries, thus helping to preserve an adequate volume status.

C. The macula densa cells sense the "saltiness" of the filtrate. A decrease in sodium and chloride transport at the macula densa also causes renin release from the juxtaglomerular cells.
   1. Renin secretion by these cells also occurs in response to decreased blood flow and pressure in the afferent arteriole and in response to the sympathetic nervous system (SNS) stimulation.
   2. Through a series of several physiologic processes, renin is converted to angiotensin II, which causes efferent arteriole constriction (among other things).
   3. Efferent arteriole constriction impedes the flow of blood from the glomerular capillaries and helps maintain glomerular hydrostatic pressure and a normal GFR.
   4. If the level of circulating angiotensin II is extremely high (as in hemodynamic instability), it also causes afferent arteriole constriction.

a. The arteriole constriction would then decrease glomerular blood flow, hydrostatic pressure, and GFR.
b. This is detrimental to kidney function and can cause serious damage.
c. Regulation of renal blood flow is secondary to the regulation of glomerular blood flow.
d. As blood flow to the glomerular capillaries increases or decreases, blood flow through the arteries and arterioles leading up to the glomerulus increases or decreases accordingly.

D. Other factors.
1. Eicosanoid synthesis. Eicosanoids are vasoactive substances and include prostaglandins, thromboxanes, and leukotrienes.
   a. Produced in almost every body cell by the action of the enzyme phospholipase A2 on fatty acids from the phospholipid cell membrane.
      (1) Arachidonic acid, which is synthesized from the fatty acids in the cell membrane, is acted on by one of two enzymes: cyclooxygenase or lipoxygenase.
      (2) Prostaglandins and thromboxanes are synthesized in the cyclooxygenase pathway.
      (3) Leukotrienes are synthesized in the lipoxygenase pathway.
   b. In the kidney, eicosanoids are produced by the glomerular endothelium, nephrons, and interstitium.
2. Thromboxane and leukotrienes are vaso-constrictors. Their role in the kidney is unclear.
3. Other neurohormonal influences contribute to maintaining appropriate renal blood flow (GFR).
   a. Some prostaglandins, such as PGE1, PGE2, and PGI2 (prostacyclin), are vasodilators.
   b. These substances are released in response to and counteract the effects of vasoconstrictors, such as norepinephrine, epinephrine, and angiotensin II.
   c. Prostaglandins are important in maintaining renal blood flow but have minimal systemic effect.
4. Vasoactive peptides: endothelin, nitric oxide, and atrial natriuretic peptide (ANP).
   a. Endothelin is synthesized in the endothelial cells of kidneys, lungs, cerebellum, and some arteries in response to increased stretch of vessel walls, and is a potent vasoconstrictor. In the kidney, endothelin probably constricts both the afferent and efferent arterioles.
   b. Nitric oxide is released from vascular smooth muscle in response to vasodilators, and is probably the mediator of the vasodilatation caused by these substances. In addition, nitric oxide may inhibit renin secretion.
   c. ANP is secreted by cardiocytes in the atria and large veins in response to atrial distention and elevated atrial pressure, which occurs with increased volume states.
      (1) ANP causes dilatation of the afferent arteriole and constriction of the efferent arteriole, thus maintaining glomerular pressure.
      (2) ANP inhibits the effects of ADH, angiotensin II, and aldosterone.
      (3) The overall effects are diuresis (increased sodium and water excretion), natriuresis (decreases sodium reabsorption by the collecting ducts), decreased extracellular volume, vasorelaxation, and decreased blood pressure.

E. In summary.
1. Through the process of autoregulation, renal blood flow, glomerular blood flow, and the GFR are maintained within a narrow range despite wide fluctuations in mean arterial pressure (MAP).
2. Once the MAP falls and is sustained below 70 to 80 mmHg, the renal autoregulatory processes are no longer able to maintain adequate renal blood flow and the GFR.
3. As a result, in states of prolonged hypotension and renal hypoperfusion, kidney injury often occurs.
4. Kidney injury is in some cases irreversible. However, if recognized and treated early, kidney injury may possibly be reversed (Cupples, 2007; Schrier et al., 2012; VanPutte et al., 2013).

XVI. Regulation of body water with formation of a dilute or a concentrated urine.

A. Recall that blood pressure is equal to cardiac output x peripheral vascular resistance.
1. And, cardiac output is determined by heart rate and stroke volume. Stroke volume is largely determined by the extracellular fluid volume, which is regulated by the kidneys through excretion of sodium and water.
2. Of the 125 mL/min (180 L in 24 hours) filtered from the glomeruli into the tubules, approximately 98–99% of the filtrate is reabsorbed from the tubular lumen of the nephrons into the plasma of the peritubular capillaries and returned to the systemic circulation.
3. Thus, of the 180 L of glomerular filtrate each 24 hours, only about 1.5 to 2 L is excreted as urine.
   a. A smaller amount of concentrated urine is excreted in states of water deficit (increased extracellular osmolality).
   b. A larger amount of dilute urine is excreted in states of water excess (decreased extracellular osmolality).

B. Excretion of a dilute or concentrated urine facilitates return of the body's water volume and extracellular osmolality to normal.
   1. Total body water (TBW) is estimated to be 0.6 L/kg of body weight.
   2. The majority (two thirds) of TBW is contained in the cell (intracellular).
   3. The remaining one third is contained in the extracellular fluid space (plasma and interstitial compartments).

Recognize and Remember

Excretion of water is highly regulated by the excretion of solute.

Solute excretion obligates water excretion.

Natriuretic diuretics increase solute excretion by inhibiting reabsorption of salt.

Osmotic diuretics enhance water filtration by creating an oncotic pressure gradient (e.g., hyperglycemia and mannitol).

---

   4. Osmolality = total body solute ÷ TBW.
   5. Normal plasma osmolality (POSM) = 275 to 290 mOsm/kg.
      a. Urea and blood glucose are considered ineffective solutes (osmoles) under normal conditions.
      b. Ultimately, serum sodium concentration is the primary determinate of osmolality.
   6. Two x (2x) the plasma sodium concentration ≈ its plasma osmolality.
   7. The kidneys are able to produce either a highly dilute urine with an osmolality as low as 50 mOsm/kg to a very concentrated urine with an osmolality of 1200 mOsm/kg.
   8. In situations where sodium intake is markedly reduced, blood flow and tissue perfusion is preserved by sodium retention in the kidneys.
      a. The kidneys have a set point at which sodium excretion is virtually halted.
      b. The body tends to hang onto salt, although not forever.
      c. In situations where the diet is rich in salt, urinary sodium excretion will transiently increase but does not equal dietary intake until positive sodium balance is achieved and ECF volume is increased.

C. Osmoregulatory pathways involve the brain (hypothalamic osmoreceptors) that senses a change in plasma osmolality. Relatively minor changes in osmolality result in stimulation of a response. A change of approximately 2 mOsm/L change is all that is needed to invoke a response. Several barometers (regulators) exist throughout the body.
   1. The macula densa in the kidney detects saltiness (chemoreceptor).
   2. The afferent arteriole detects changes in pressure (mechanoreceptor).
   3. The atria in the heart detect increase or decrease in stretch (mechanoreceptors).
   4. The carotid sinuses detect pressure changes (mechanoreceptor).
   5. The body responds by releasing effectors (hormones).
      a. Arginine vasopressin (AVP).
      b. Renin-angiotensin-aldosterone (RAA).
      c. Atrial natriuretic peptide.

D. The body also responds by causing or eliminating the sensation of thirst.
   1. The thirst center is located in the anteroventral wall of the third ventricle (organum vasculosum of the lamina terminalis, third ventricle) and the preoptic nucleus in the brain.
   2. The thirst center is stimulated by an increase in the ECF osmolality (cellular dehydration), volume depletion, or if there is an increase in release of angiotensin II (Taal et al., 2012).

E. The syndrome of inappropriate ADH secretion.
   1. Other stimuli, besides volume depletion or an increase in ECF osmolality, cause the release of AVP.
   2. Many times these triggers are pathologic and result from abnormal responses or pathologies (termed syndrome of inappropriate ADH).
      a. Pain.
      b. Diseases (e.g., cancer, brain tumor, or other pathologies).
      c. Nausea and vomiting.
      d. Medications (e.g., antipsychotics, inhaled nicotine, and others).
   3. A state of hyponatremia (low serum sodium, less than 135 meq/L) means that there is excess TBW relative to total body sodium.
      a. There is too much water relative to salt content in the body.
      b. But, it says nothing about the total body sodium (sodium does not move freely between compartments as does water) (Schrier et al., 2012).

F. The kidneys' processes for regulating body water and extracellular osmolality primarily involve the descending and ascending limbs of the loop of Henle, DT, cortical collecting tubule, medullary collecting duct, and vasa recta of juxtamedullary nephrons.

Recognize and Remember

Total body water is equivalent to 0.5 liters/kilogram of body weight.

Osmolality is a reflection of the amount of extracellular water (total solute divided by total body water).

Too much water is reflected by hyponatremia (low serum sodium concentration).

Too little water is reflected by hypernatremia (high plasma sodium concentration).

G. Osmoreceptors in the hypothalamus and ~~antidiuretic hormone (ADH)~~, which is released from the ~~posterior pituitary gland~~, operate along with the nephrons to regulate body water.

H. Changes in osmolality. The glomerular filtrate has very similar osmolality to plasma (290 to 300 mOsm/L) as it enters Bowman's capsule.

I. In the PT, about 65% of the glomerular filtrate is reabsorbed into peritubular capillaries (described earlier).

J. Due to reabsorption of proportional amounts of solutes and water in the PT, the filtrate leaving the PT and entering the descending limb of the loop of Henle remains at an osmolality of 290 to 300 mOsm/L.

1. In conditions of water deficit, the tubular filtrate can be maximally concentrated to about 1200 mOsm/L before the filtrate leaves the collecting duct as urine. Conversely, in states of water excess, the concentration of the tubular filtrate can be diluted to as low as 50 mOsm/L before it leaves the collecting duct as urine.
2. Regardless of whether a concentrated or a dilute urine is finally excreted, a hyperosmotic medullary interstitium is created by a complex process involving the countercurrent multiplying and exchange mechanism of the juxtamedullary nephrons and vasa recta.

K. Countercurrent multiplying and exchange mechanism.
1. The slow flow of blood in the vasa recta, slow flow of filtrate in the lumen of the juxtamedullary nephrons, and the parallel arrangement of the vasa recta, loops of Henle, cortical collecting tubule, and medullary collecting duct are essential for the formation of both concentrated and dilute urine.
2. This arrangement allows for exchange of solutes and water between the lumen of the tubule, the renal interstitial fluid, and plasma of the vasa recta.

3. As Figure 1.32 shows, the osmolality of the renal interstitial fluid progressively increases from approximately 300 mOsm/L in the cortical-medullary junction, to about 1200 mOsm/L in the deep inner medulla.
4. Creation of this hyperosmotic interstitium is a prerequisite to the nephron's forming either dilute or concentrated urine.

L. Principal mechanisms responsible for creating the hyperosmolality of the medullary interstitium: the countercurrent multiplier.
1. The descending limb (concentrating segment) of the loop of Henle is permeable to water and somewhat permeable to solutes.
   a. Thus, as the filtrate flows down the descending limb, water moves from the lumen into the interstitium; some sodium, chloride, and urea moves from the interstitium into the lumen of the tubule.
   b. The water is removed from the interstitium by the capillary network so it does not dilute the interstitium.
   c. The result is a progressively concentrated (increase in osmolality) tubular filtrate as it moves down the descending limb into the medullary interstitium.
2. The thin ascending segment (passive diluting segment) of the loop of Henle is impermeable to water but is permeable to solutes.
   a. Sodium and chloride move into the interstitium, and urea moves into the lumen of the tubule.
   b. The net movement of sodium and chloride out of the lumen exceeds the net movement of urea into the tubular lumen.
   c. As a result, the filtrate becomes progressively dilute (decreased osmolality) as it moves up the ascending limb.
   d. Because only passive transport is involved, the osmolality of the tubular fluid can decrease only to the osmolality of the surrounding interstitium.
3. The thick ascending segment (active diluting segment) of the loop of Henle is impermeable to water, but actively transports sodium, potassium, and chloride ions from the lumen of the tubule into the interstitium.
   a. As a result, sodium, potassium, and chloride become concentrated in the interstitium, and the osmolality of the interstitium increases.
   b. Because solutes are actively pumped from the thick segment and because it is impermeable to water, the osmolality of the tubular filtrate progressively decreases (is more dilute) and is less than 100 mOsm/L by the time it reaches the late DT.

4. Small amounts of sodium ions are also actively transported from the collecting duct into the interstitium. This further increases the osmolality of the interstitium.
5. In the presence of high concentrations of ADH, urea diffuses from the medullary collecting duct into the interstitium. This also increases the osmolality of the interstitium.
6. The constant transport of sodium, potassium, and chloride from the thick ascending limb and continuous inflow of new sodium and chloride from the proximal tubule constitute the countercurrent multiplier mechanism.

M. The above mechanisms create an osmolality of about 1200 mOsm/L both at the sharp U-turn of the loop of Henle and in the deep medullary interstitium.
   1. Recta processes: the countercurrent exchanger.
      a. The arrangement of the vasa recta and the slow blood flow through the vasa recta limit the removal of the solutes from the interstitium and maintain the interstitial hyperosmolality.
      b. As Figure 1.32 shows, the descending and ascending limbs of the vasa recta are arranged parallel to each other.
      c. Thus, as blood flows down the descending limb, it is concurrently flowing up the ascending limb.
      d. This arrangement allows the vasa recta to operate as countercurrent exchangers.
   2. As blood flows down the descending limb of the vasa recta, sodium, potassium, and chloride ions and urea diffuse from the interstitium into the blood.
      a. At the same time, water diffuses from the blood into the hyperosmotic interstitium.
      b. Because of influx of solutes and outflux of water, the osmolality of the blood in the vasa recta progressively increases from approximately 320 mOsm/L as it enters the vasa recta to about 1200 mOsm/L at the tip of the vasa recta, which is about the same as the osmolality of the interstitium at each point.
   3. As blood flows up the ascending limb of the vasa recta, sodium, potassium, and chloride ions and urea diffuse out of the blood into the interstitium, and water diffuses back into the blood. As the blood in the ascending vasa recta leaves the renal medulla, its osmolality is almost the same as that of the blood that flowed into the descending limb of the vasa recta (i.e., ~320 mOsm/L).
   4. As a result, the osmolality of the medullary interstitium has been maintained because only a small amount of solutes was removed from the interstitium by the blood flow in the vasa recta.

N. Role of the osmoreceptor–antidiuretic hormone system.
   1. Antidiuretic hormone (also called vasopressin) controls the formation and excretion of either a dilute or a concentrated urine through its effect on the cortical collecting tubule and medullary collecting duct.
      a. ADH is formed in neurons of the hypothalamus (specifically the supraoptic and paraventricular nuclei).
      b. After synthesis, ADH is packaged into vesicles, which are transported into synaptic bulbs at the tips of the neurons. The bulbs terminate in the posterior pituitary gland.
      c. Release of the contents of the vesicles in the synaptic bulbs results in release of ADH into the interstitium surrounding the posterior pituitary gland.
      d. The hormone then diffuses into the surrounding capillaries and is transported in the systemic circulation.
   2. Other neurons, called osmoreceptors, are located in the hypothalamus near the supraoptic and paraventricular nuclei.
      a. These are extremely responsive to slight changes in extracellular osmolality.
      b. The osmoreceptors are stimulated by an increase in serum sodium (increased osmolality) and inhibited by a decrease in serum sodium (decreased osmolality).
      c. Serum sodium concentration can increase as either the result of increased sodium or decreased water.
      d. Conversely, serum sodium concentration can decrease as either the result of decreased sodium or increased water.
   3. The osmoreceptors signal the supraoptic and paraventricular nuclei to increase or decrease the secretion of ADH, depending on extracellular osmolality.
   4. Osmoreceptor–ADH–renal system integration.
      a. An increase in serum sodium (or a decrease in water) specifically, and other ions to some extent, increase the extracellular fluid osmolality.
      b. The increased extracellular fluid osmolality stimulates the osmoreceptors.
      c. The stimulated osmoreceptors, in turn, stimulate the supraoptic and paraventricular nuclei.
      d. The supraoptic and paraventricular nuclei then cause release of ADH from the posterior pituitary gland.
      e. ADH causes increased permeability of the cortical collecting tubule and medullary collecting duct to water.

f. ADH binds with receptors on the basal membrane (interstitial side) of the collecting tubule and duct cells.

g. ADH's binding with its receptors causes activation of the enzyme adenyl cyclase, which, in turn, causes the formation of cyclic adenosine monophosphate (cAMP) in the cell cytoplasm; cAMP acts as the second messenger to activate the enzyme protein kinase A.

h. Protein kinase A regulates the insertion of preformed water channels (called aquaporins) from the luminal membrane (the side of the tubular cell that faces the tubular lumen) to the basal membrane (the side of the membrane facing the interstitium).

i. Water is reabsorbed across the luminal membrane through these channels and exits the basal membrane into the interstitium from where it is reabsorbed into the vasa recta and returned to the systemic circulation. As the tubule becomes more permeable to water, urea is also reabsorbed into the interstitium, which enhances the interstitial hyperosmolality.

j. Although increased permeability of the tubules leads to increased reabsorption of water from the tubular lumen, most solutes are not reabsorbed and are excreted in the urine.

k. With reabsorption of water, the extracellular osmolality is returned to normal. Hypothalamic osmoreceptors sense the decrease toward normal in extracellular osmolality and decrease release of ADH.

5. In conditions of decreased serum sodium (or excess water), the osmoreceptors sense the low extracellular osmolality and decrease ADH release. With decreased circulating ADH, less water is reabsorbed from the renal tubules until the extracellular osmolality returns to normal (Eaton & Pooler, 2013; Hall, 2011; Triplitt, 2012).

XVII. Kidney regulation of acid-base balance.

A. Overview.
   1. The kidney's mechanisms for regulating acid-base balance are HCO3- reabsorption and H+ secretion, excretion of H+ with urinary phosphates, and excretion of H+ by synthesis of ammonia and excretion of ammonium chloride.
   2. The processes primarily occur in the PT, DT, and collecting duct.
   3. Formulas:
      a. Bicarbonate buffer system:
         $H_2O + CO_2 \leftrightarrow H_2CO_3 \leftrightarrow H^+ + HCO_3^-$.
      b. Phosphate buffer system:
         $HPO_4^- + H^+ \leftrightarrow H_2PO_4$.
      c. Ammonia buffer system: $NH_3 + H^+ \leftrightarrow NH_4^+$.

B. The kidneys regulate the HCO_3^- portion of the Henderson-Hasselbalch equation. This equation allows you to estimate the pH of a buffer solution, like blood plasma.

C. Acid urine is formed if the pH of body fluids is in the acid range. Then the kidneys excrete more H^+ than HCO_3^-.

D Alkaline urine is formed if the pH of body fluids is in the alkaline range. Then the kidneys excrete more HCO_3^- than H^+.

E. The kidneys can excrete urine with a pH between 4.5 and 8.

F. Reabsorption of filtered bicarbonate.
   1. Basic rule. For every H^+ secreted into the tubular lumen, a HCO_3^- and a Na^+ ion are reabsorbed into the plasma of peritubular capillaries.
   2. HCO_3^- cannot be reabsorbed from the renal tubules directly because it is a large ion and has a negative electrical charge. Therefore, HCO_3^- must be broken down and then regenerated and reabsorbed.

G. Na^+ and HCO_3^- are filtered from the glomerulus into the filtrate of the tubular lumen.

H. In the PT and DT, Na^+ is reabsorbed and H^+ is secreted into tubular filtrate.

I. H^+ ions react with HCO_3^- (carbonic acid) to form H_2CO_3 (bicarbonate ion).

Recognize and Remember

The body senses osmolality in order to correct serum sodium.

The serum osmolality is regulated by water balance and not the concentration of sodium.

Therefore, the serum sodium is a surrogate marker for serum osmolality.

When there is an increase in sodium intake (e.g., salt), then there is a reduction in sodium reabsorption by the kidney; the result is a higher urinary sodium excretion.

However, sodium intake does not immediately equal sodium output (there is a certain amount of lag time) by the kidney.

A positive sodium balance is allowed to occur, and along with it, an increase in extracellular fluid volume.

J. Under influences of carbonic anhydrase (CA) that is present in the PT and DT cell membrane, H_2CO_3 breaks down into H_2O and CO_2.

K. H_2O and CO_2 enter the cell at the PT.

L. In cell cytoplasm, CO_2 and H_2O in the presence of carbonic anhydrase form H_2CO_3.
1. H_2CO_3 dissociates into H^+ and HCO_3^-.
2. HCO_3^- is also reabsorbed into the plasma of peritubular capillaries.
3. H^+ ions are secreted into tubular lumen and Na^+ is reabsorbed from the tubular lumen.

M. Although not the original HCO_3^- that was filtered into the tubular lumen, an equivalent amount is regenerated and reabsorbed by the above process.

N. The basic rule holds true: when a H^+ ion is secreted, a sodium ion and bicarbonate ion are then reabsorbed.

O. In the late DT and collecting tubule, specialized cells (intercalated cells) actively secrete hydrogen ions into the tubular lumen against a high concentration gradient.
1. These cannot be transported as free H^+ ions.
2. They first combine with buffers in the tubular filtrate and are excreted in the urine in this form.

3. The two important buffers of the tubular filtrate are the phosphate buffer system and the ammonia buffer system. Both these processes allow for synthesis of new bicarbonate.

P. Transport of H^+ by phosphate buffers.
1. The phosphate buffer system is composed of HPO_4^{-2} (base phosphate) and $H_2PO_4^-$ (acid phosphate). HPO_4^{-2} can accept H^+ and $H_2PO_4^-$ can donate H^+.
2. Na_2PO_4 is filtered from the glomerulus into the tubular filtrate (see Figure 1.33).
3. One of the Na^+ ions is reabsorbed and a H^+ ion is secreted by countertransport.
4. H^+ ions bind with HPO_4^{-2} to form $H_2PO_4^-$.
5. The other Na^+ ions bind with the $H_2PO_4^-$ to form NaH_2PO_4, which is excreted in the urine. (Note that this involves excretion of H^+.)

Q. In the renal cell, CO_2 binds with H_2O to form H_2CO_3, which dissociates to H^+ and $H_2CO_3^-$.
1. The HCO_3^- is reabsorbed and H^+ is secreted into the tubular lumen.
2. As an outcome, for each H^+ that binds with HPO_4^{-2}, a new HCO_3^- is formed and transported into the blood along with Na^+. The secretion and excretion of H^+ and the reabsorption of HCO_3^- contribute to acid-base regulation.

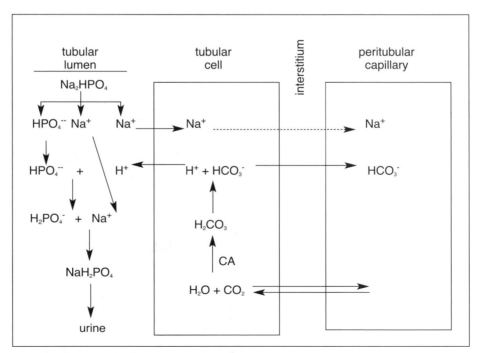

Figure 1.33. Diagram of excretion of hydrogen ions with phosphate buffers. Note that a hydrogen ion is secreted and excreted and a new bicarbonate ion is reabsorbed.

R. Transport of H^+ by the ammonia buffer system.
1. Ammonia (NH_3) is synthesized in the epithelial cells of the proximal tubule.
    a. The NH_3 is synthesized primarily from the amino acid glutamine in the presence of the enzyme glutaminase, which is present in the proximal tubular cell.
    b. The NH_3 is secreted into the tubular lumen.
2. In the filtrate of the tubular lumen, NH_3 binds with H^+ to form ammonium (NH_4^+), a cation.
3. The NH_4^+ combines with Cl^- to form NH_4Cl, which is excreted in the urine. (Note this involves excretion of H^+.)
4. At the same time H^+ ion is secreted, Na+ and a new HCO_3^- are reabsorbed.
5. As an outcome, H^+ ion is secreted and excreted and a new HCO_3^- is reabsorbed, which contributes to acid-base regulation.

S. The synthesis of NH_3 increases in acidosis and decreases in alkalosis.

T. The kidney's response to acidosis.
1. HCO_3^- reabsorption increases.
2. H^+ ion secretion increases, so H^+ excretion increases.
3. NaH_2PO_4 production increases.
4. NH_3 synthesis and NH_4Cl excretion increase.
5. Active secretion of H^+ by DT and collecting tubule increases.
6. The pH of urine decreases to as low as 4.5 as acid urine is produced as excess H^+ is excreted and HCO_3^- is reabsorbed into body fluids.

U. Summary of the kidney's response to alkalosis.
1. HCO_3^- reabsorption decreases, so HCO_3^- excretion increases.
2. NH_3 synthesis decreases.
3. Active secretion of H^+ by DT and collecting tubule decreases.
4. The pH of urine increases to as high as 8.0 as alkaline urine is produced as excess HCO_3^- is excreted and H^+ is retained in the body fluids.

XVIII. Ureter and bladder function and micturition, otherwise known as the act of urination.

A. Overview.
1. Tubular filtrate becomes urine when it reaches the renal pelvis.
2. It is not subject to further alteration.
3. It must travel to the urinary bladder for excretion.

B. Hydrostatic pressure in the renal pelvis averages 0 mmHg. There is no pressure gradient to force urine to flow to the urinary bladder through the ureters.

C. Ureters are made of primarily smooth muscle.
1. Peristaltic contractions of the smooth muscle, which occur about every 2 to 3 minutes, progress from the renal pelvis to the urinary bladder.
2. This forces urine to flow through the ureters at a velocity of about 3 cm/sec.
3. Parasympathetic stimulation increases, and sympathetic stimulation decreases the frequency of these contractions.

D. Micturition.
1. When urine is not in the urinary bladder, the internal pressure is about 0 mmHg. As urine collects in the bladder, there is a slow pressure increase until the volume reaches about 400 to 500 mL. Above this volume the pressure rises rapidly.
2. As the bladder fills, stretch receptors in the bladder wall are stimulated.
3. Afferent nerve signals are sent from the bladder to sacral segments of spinal cord through the pelvic nerves.
4. Reflex integration takes place in the spinal cord. Efferent nerve impulses are conducted from the spinal cord to the urinary bladder through the parasympathetic portion of pelvic nerves.
5. A conscious desire to urinate occurs when the ascending tracts in the spinal cord conduct nerve impulses to the brain.
6. Bladder muscles contract while the internal and external urinary sphincters relax as a result of efferent nerve impulses.

E. In normal adults and children over age 2 or 3, the reflex can be voluntarily inhibited or stimulated by higher brain centers.

F. During voluntary urination, the higher brain centers send impulses to the spinal cord to enhance the micturition reflex and inhibit contraction of external urinary sphincter (Schrier et al., 2012; Tall et al., 2012; VanPutte et al., 2013).

*some drugs (trimethoprim + cimetidine) inhibit creatinine secretion by kidney tubules → ↑ creatinine

24° urine collection is best done to determine a Cl in cachectic/pt BMI < 18.5, pt c cirrhosis + ascites, pt c amputations (MDRD + Cockcroft v Gault over estimate also very obese pts c BMI > 30.

Putting It All Together

1. Alex joined a fraternity in the 1970s. He recalls one night of hazing where he was forced to consume 1 gallon of water over 2 hours. Other than being easily manipulated, Alex was and is otherwise healthy.

a. Besides the need for frequent urination, what do you think might have happened?
1. Total body water increased, serum osmolality increased.
2. Total body water increased, serum osmolality did not change.
3. Total body water did not change, serum osmolality did not change.
4. Total body water did not change, serum osmolality decreased.

Answer: 3. Total body water did not change, serum osmolality did not change.

b. Was ADH increased or decreased?

Answer: Normally, it is difficult for someone to develop water intoxication because the kidneys are highly adept at creating dilute urine even when people consume several liters of water a day. However, if large volumes of water are consumed without food, then it becomes dangerous. If someone is fasting, then water intoxication becomes a potential risk. In the above scenario, ADH will be appropriately suppressed (decreased) in an otherwise healthy person due to their excess water intake that results in an expansion of total body water. In someone with the syndrome of inappropriate secretion of ADH (SIADH), they will develop a picture similar to water intoxication due to the increased release of ADH from the pituitary gland. When ADH is high, more water is reabsorbed in the urine (creating a more concentrated urine). ADH stimulates the insertion of aquaporin channels into the epithelial lining of the collection duct, thereby making them more permeable to water.

c. Was the urine osmolality closer to 800 mOsm/L or 100 mOsm/L?

Answer: The urine osmolality would be low because of a higher amount of water excretion in the urine. Urine osmolality would be closer to 100 mOsm/L.

d. Did serum sodium change significantly?

Answer: The serum sodium would not be significantly impacted due to Alex having normal kidney function and the ability to excrete dilute urine. It would take a significantly larger amount of water over a short period of time to induce water intoxication. An example would be a marathon runner that consumes 5 to 6 liters of pure water without salt replacement over a short period of time (4 to 5 hours). Women are at higher risk for water intoxication due to smaller body mass distribution.

2. A 76-year-old female had an acute myocardial infarction and as a consequence developed congestive heart failure. Her cardiac filling pressures are increased and cardiac myocytes are stretched, but her cardiac output is reduced.

a. What do you think will happen to sodium handling in this patient?
1. The kidneys will excrete more sodium than ingested.
2. The kidneys will retain more sodium leading to an increase in volume.
3. The kidneys will excrete more sodium and water.
4. The kidneys will not be impacted by this change in hemodynamics.

Answer: 2. The kidneys will retain more sodium leading to an increase in volume.

b. What happens to GFR with reduction in cardiac output?

Answer: Reduction in blood pressure leads to a reduction in renal blood flow and a lower hydrostatic pressure within the glomerulus. Adaptations will occur in order to maintain GFR. The body will compensate by reducing sodium loss to almost nothing with activation of the renin-angiotensin-aldosterone response system.

c. What will happen to the renal arteriole in response to a reduction in blood pressure? Over time, what happens in congestive heart failure?

Answer: Renal resistance changes in accordance with blood pressure (e.g., blood flow). If blood pressure is reduced by a small amount, then renal blood flow and filtration are not significantly affected. This is due to autoregulatory mechanisms. Small changes in blood pressure (up or down) over a short period of time do not disrupt renal blood flow (protective).

The vasa recta are a specialized peritubular capillary network for the juxtamedullary nephrons of the kidneys. When the kidneys are in a state of desired anti-diuresis (e.g., sustained lower blood pressure), the counter-current arrangement of the vasa recta result in a minimal amount of solute loss in the filtrate. Solute that is filtered from the concentrated ascending limb of the vasa recta is then reabsorbed by the descending limb (counter-current mechanism).

Over time, compensatory mechanisms will ultimately become detrimental. Reduced renal perfusion and activation of neurohormonal pathways like what occurs with congestive heart failure results in an increase in total blood volume.

These mechanisms initially assist with maintaining cardiac output, but over time the increase in venous pressures result in pulmonary and systemic edema. The heart works harder due to the increase in blood volume and neurohormonal stimulation creating a cycle of maladaptation.

Section C
Pathophysiology
Paula Dutka, Charlotte Szromba

I. Acute kidney injury.

A. Background information. The term *acute kidney injury* (AKI) rather than *acute renal failure* (ARF) is now used to refer to the clinical syndrome of acute loss of kidney function.
   1. The syndrome of AKI encompasses both direct injury to the kidney structure and impairment of function (KDIGO, 2012a).
   2. The term implies that the injury to the kidney does not result in "failure" and has significant clinical implications (Okusa & Rosner, 2013).
   3. Clinicians, and even the lay public, recognize the gravity of an acute myocardial infarction, but few associate such risk with AKI.
   4. In spite of this, recent data confirms that AKI is a major contributor to adverse clinical outcomes.
   5. When considering mortality risks, it might be surprising to know that a diagnosis of AKI has a higher death rate than breast cancer, prostate cancer, heart failure, and diabetes combined (Lewington et al., 2013).

B. The clinical definition of AKI includes any of the following:
   1. Increase in serum creatinine (SCr) by $\geq$ 0.3 mg/dL ($\geq$ 26.5 μmol/ L) within 48 hours *or*
   2. Increase in SCr to $\geq$ 1.5 times baseline, which is known or presumed to have occurred within the prior 7 days *or*
   3. Urine volume < 0.5 mL/kg/hr for more than 6 consecutive hours (KDIGO, 2012a).
   4. AKI is preventable, treatable, and potentially reversible.

C. AKI is not associated with specific symptoms. The diagnosis is made based upon changes in laboratory parameters or urine output. Once AKI is identified, it may then be staged for severity using the following KDIGO recommended staging criteria:
   1. Stage 1:
      a. SCr 1.5 to 1.9 times baseline *or*
      b. $\geq$ 0.3 mg/dL ($\geq$26.5 μmol/L) increase and urine output < 0.5 mL/kg/hr for 6 to 12 hours.
   2. Stage 2: SCr 2.0 to 2.9 times baseline AND urine output < 0.5 mL/kg/hr for $\geq$ 12 hours.
   3. Stage 3:
      a. SCr 3.0 times baseline *or*
      b. An increase in SCr to > 4.0 mg/dL (> 353.6 μmol/L) *or*

   c. Initiation of kidney replacement therapy *or*
   d. In patients < 18 years, a decrease in estimated glomerular filtration (eGFR) to < 35 mL/min per 1.73 m^2 and urine output for Stage 3 criteria: < 0.3 mL/kg/hr for $\geq$ 24 hours *or*
   e. Anuria (urine output of less than 100 mL/24 hours) for $\geq$ 12 hours (KDIGO, 2012a).
   4. A rise in SCr is a late finding in AKI.
      a. Alternative biomarkers are gaining credibility for enhancing the capacity to obtain a quicker diagnosis or act as a screening tool.
      b. Some of these investigational biomarkers include neutrophil gelatinase-associated lipocalin (NGAL), Kidney Injury Molecule-1 (KIM-1), interleukin-18 (IL-18), and cystatin C (Lewington et al., 2013).

D. Incidence and outcomes.
   1. Frequently, AKI is a complication of another potentially life-threatening illness or injury.
   2. A recent study from the University of Pittsburgh, which looked at a database of 20,000 patients, suggests that nearly one third of AKI cases are community-acquired (c-AKI), meaning that the process began prior to their hospitalization.
   3. The worldwide incidence of AKI indicates that the majority of AKI cases in developing countries are likely to be community-acquired, but this definitive data is difficult to gather (Prakash et al., 2013).
   4. A meta-analysis of 312 studies was performed to try to determine the global burden of AKI.
      a. Using the KDIGO definition of AKI, 1 in 5 adults and 1 in 3 children worldwide experience AKI during a hospital episode.
      b. In the United States, between 7% and 18% of hospitalized patients develop AKI (h-AKI).
      c. The incidence of AKI is much higher in the critically ill. Between 30% and 70% of patients admitted to an intensive care unit develop AKI (Lewington et al., 2013).
      d. The recognition of the high prevalence of AKI could create a platform to raise public, governmental, and healthcare providers' awareness of the high burden of AKI (Susantitaphong et al., 2013).
      e. In 2005, Chertow and associates reported that an increase of serum creatinine of 0.3 mg/dL was independently associated with mortality (Chertow et al., 2005).

E. Classification systems of AKI (See Figure 1.34).
   1. Classification systems such as RIFLE (Risk, Injury, Failure, Loss, and End-stage kidney failure) and AKIN (Acute Kidney Injury Network) are widely used to assess AKI.
   2. Even small changes in SCr and GFR are associated with increased mortality.

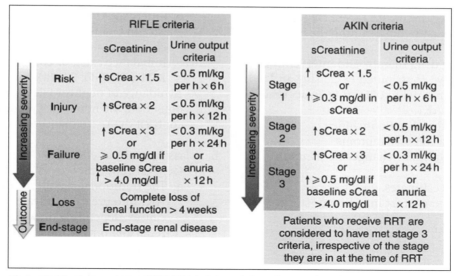

Figure 1.34. Comparison of RIFLE (risk, injury, failure, loss, and end-stage) and Acute Kidney Injury Network (AKIN) Criteria for the diagnosis of AKI.

Open source paper. Used with permission from Seller-Pérez, G., Herrera-Gutiérrez, M.E., Maynar-Moliner, J., Sánchez-Izquierdo-Riera, J.A., Marinho, A., & Luis do Pico, J. (2013). Estimating kidney function in the critically ill patients. *Critical Care Research and Practice*. doi:10.1155/2013/721810

3. AKI contributes to other organ system failures, such as the heart and lungs.
4. Prevention and early diagnosis of AKI is central to clinical management (Macedo, 2010).
5. Mortality for AKI reaches as high as 50% to 60% for patients who require kidney replacement therapy (KRT) (KDIGO, 2012a).
6. Mortality is generally due to the primary illness and/or multiorgan failure rather than kidney failure (Schira, 2008).
7. Although there is no direct relationship between AKI and development of CKD, there is increasing evidence to support a strong association. This finding supports the need to arrange clinical follow-up.

F. General concepts.
1. AKI may be oliguric (< 500 mL/day) or nonoliguric (> 800 mL/day).
2. Azotemia is the retention of nitrogenous waste products (e.g., urea and creatinine) in the blood.
3. Patients affected by AKI usually have diabetes and are older and obese (Lines & Lewington, 2009).
4. The most frequent causes of AKI are renal hypoperfusion, nephrotoxins, or sepsis (Okusa & Rosner, 2013).
5. Signs and symptoms vary and can range from mild azotemia to uremia to failure requiring dialysis to correct fluid and electrolyte imbalances.
6. Failure to recognize AKI results in a delay in treatment, which is associated with higher

morbidity and mortality. Reversible causes include hypotension, volume depletion (seen many times in the elderly), and volume overload.
7. AKI has gone unrecognized in up to 23.5% of patients. It is important to distinguish between AKI and chronic kidney disease because AKI is potentially reversible (Aitken et al., 2013; Yang & Bonventre, 2010).
8. The initial evaluation of the patient with AKI is focused on determining the cause and identifying the most urgent complications (Okusa & Rosner, 2013).
9. Major complications of AKI include volume overload, hyperkalemia, metabolic acidosis (severe pH < 7.1), and hyperphosphatemia.
10. In severe cases, changes in mental status, hyperuricemia, and hypermagnesemia may also be present (Okusa & Rosner, 2013).

G. Patient assessment.
1. The initial assessment should include the careful evaluation of volume status and measurement of serum electrolytes, particularly potassium, bicarbonate, serum phosphate, calcium, and albumin. In addition, serum uric acid, magnesium, and CBC should be assessed.
2. It is important to correlate the findings from the laboratory tests as above with a comprehensive history and physical examination (Yang & Bonventre, 2010).
   a. Obtaining a careful historical account of events

and correlating these with recent trends in SCr levels often assist in determining the etiology for AKI.

b. Incorporating drug therapy and interventions that might have contributed to causing an insult is incremental to obtaining an accurate causation for AKI.

3. Investigative history should include:
a. Type and duration of symptoms.
b. Urinary difficulties or changes in urinary pattern.
c. Urine volume estimates.
d. History of urinary tract infection or stone disease.
e. Recent surgery.
f. Medications.
g. Review of interdisciplinary documentation (Yang & Bonventre, 2010).
h. Prior surgery.
i. Persistent upper and lower G.I. losses (vomiting or diarrhea).
j. Fever.
k. Preparations for multiple diagnostic tests requiring NPO status and/or bowel preps.
l. Acute myocardial infarction.
m. Anaphylactic drug or transfusion reaction.
n. Cardiac resuscitation.
o. Low-sodium diets with fluid restriction.
p. Diuretics and antihypertensives (Schira, 2008).

4. Careful monitoring of daily weights, fluid intake, and urine output are essential to assess daily fluid balance and management goals (Okusa & Rosner, 2013).

5. Differential diagnosis must be considered in a systematic manner to avoid missing multiple factors that may be contributing to the disease process (Jefferson et al., 2010).

H. Major treatment goals.
1. Use of supportive therapy to maintain homeostasis until the kidney injury heals.
2. Prevention of life-threatening complications such as infection, fluid/electrolyte imbalance, acid-base imbalance, and gastrointestinal bleeding.
3. Individualized patient management based on the etiology and degree of kidney injury.
4. Removal of the cause (kidney insult) and contributing factors.
5. Provision of conservative interventions such as rest, volume management, and mild dietary restrictions; these interventions are adequate for many patients.
6. Provision of aggressive interventions such as dialytic therapy and prolonged hospitalization, as necessary.
a. These aggressive interventions are associated with higher mortality.

b. Emergent kidney replacement therapy (KRT) should be initiated when life-threatening changes in fluid, electrolyte, and acid-base imbalance exist, or conditions that necessitate KRT (KDIGO, 2012a).

7. Avoidance of nephrotoxic agents that could potentiate the injury (e.g., iodinated radiographic contrast dye).

I. Classifications of etiology.
1. General concepts.
a. The traditional classification paradigm divides AKI into prerenal, intrarenal, and postrenal causes, depending on which portion of the renal anatomy is most affected by the disorder.
(1) Prerenal AKI may be due to hypovolemia or poor systemic perfusion.
(2) Postrenal obstructive kidney injury is usually diagnosed by urinary tract dilation found by renal ultrasound or computed tomography scanning.
(3) Intrinsic renal etiologies of AKI are categorized by the anatomic components of the kidney (vascular supply, glomerular, tubular, and interstitial disease).
b. In the hospitalized patient, prerenal uremia and acute tubular necrosis (ATN) are the most common causes of AKI (Jefferson et al., 2010).
c. KDIGO recommendations clearly indicate that once AKI is identified, the cause (see Table 1.4) should be determined whenever possible (KDIGO, 2012a).

2. Prerenal AKI.
a. Potential etiologies of prerenal AKI.
(1) Decreased blood flow to the kidneys due to poor systemic perfusion is the most common cause.
(2) Hypovolemia may be related to hemorrhage, burns, shock, renal artery emboli, thrombi or stenosis, aneurysm, trauma, excessive diaphoresis, gastrointestinal losses, peritonitis, or malignancy.
(3) Diminished cardiac output related to congestive heart failure, myocardial infarction, cardiac tamponade, or cardiac dysrhythmias may be present (Schira, 2008).
(4) Prerenal azotemia is the most common cause of AKI in patients with HIV infection (Jefferson et al., 2010).
(5) Altered peripheral vascular resistance may be present from sepsis, antihypertensives, anaphylactic reaction, neurogenic shock, or drug overdose. Hepatorenal syndrome (HRS) is another etiology in which acute or chronic liver disease plays an etiologic role

Table 1.4	
Causes of Acute Kidney Injury	

Prerenal Factors	**Intrarenal Factors**

Hypovolemia
    Hemorrhage, burns, shock, excessive sweating, peritonitis, nephrotic syndrome, gastrointestinal losses, renal losses (e.g., diuretics, diabetes insipidus, malignancies)
 	
Altered peripheral vascular resistance
    Sepsis, antihypertensive medications, drug overdose, anaphylactic reactions, neurogenic shock, nonsteroidal antiinflammatory drugs
 	
Cardiac disorders
    Congestive heart failure, myocardial infarction, cardiac tamponade, cardiac arrhythmias
 	
Renal artery disorders
    Emboli, thrombi, stenosis, aneurysm, occlusion, trauma
 	
Hepatorenal syndrome
	Nephrotoxic agents
	
	Inflammatory processes
	    Bacterial, viral, toxemia of pregnancy
	
	Immune processes
	    Autoimmunity, hypersensitivity, rejection
	
	Trauma
	    Penetrating, nonpenetrating
	
	Radiation nephritis
	
	Obstruction
	    Neoplasm, stones, scar tissue
	
	Intravascular hemolysis
	    Transfusion reaction, disseminated intravascular hemolysis
	
	Systemic and vascular disorders
	    Renal vein thrombosis, malaria, nephrotic syndrome, Wilson disease, multiple myeloma, sickle-cell disease, malignant hypertension, diabetes mellitus, systemic lupus erythematosus
	
	Pregnancy-related disorders

Nephrotoxins	**Postrenal Factors**

Drugs
    Anesthetics, antimicrobials, antiinflammatories, chemotherapeutic agents
 	
Contrast media
 	
Biologic substances
    Toxins: tumor products
    Heme pigments: hemoglobin, myoglobin
 	
Environmental agents
    Pesticides, fungicides
    Organic solvents: carbon tetrachloride, diesel fuel, phenol
 	
Heavy metals
    Lead, mercury, gold, arsenic, bismuth, uranium, cadmium
 	
Plant and animal substances
    Mushrooms, snake venom
	Ureteral, bladder neck, or urethral obstruction
	    Calculi, neoplasms, sloughed papillary tissue, strictures, trauma, blood clots, congenital/developmental abnormalities, foreign object, surgical ligation
	
	Prostatic hypertrophy
	
	Retroperitoneal fibrosis
	
	Abdominal and pelvic neoplasms
	
	Pregnancy
	
	Neurogenic bladder
	
	Bladder rupture
	
	Drugs
	    Antihistamines, ganglionic blocking agents, methysergide

in the renal injury through marked abnormalities in the arterial circulation leading to pronounced renal vasoconstriction.

b. The pathophysiology of prerenal AKI.

(1) The kidneys attempt to adapt to hypoperfusion through autoregulation, including activation of the renin/angiotensin/aldosterone system (see Figure 1.35).

(2) In autoregulation, the afferent arteriole dilates and efferent arteriole constricts to maintain the GFR and creatinine clearance.

(3) The release of renin activates the angiotensin-aldosterone system. This results in peripheral vasoconstriction and

increased sodium reabsorption, reducing urinary sodium.

(4) Increased plasma sodium causes the release of antidiuretic hormone, enhancing vasoconstriction and water reabsorption, resulting in decreased urinary output and increased blood volume.

(5) Prerenal disease due to true volume depletion is most commonly associated with an acute time course.

(6) Prerenal disease due to chronic heart failure or cirrhosis is associated with a persistent reduction in kidney function.

(7) Among patients with chronic kidney disease, the addition of a prerenal process

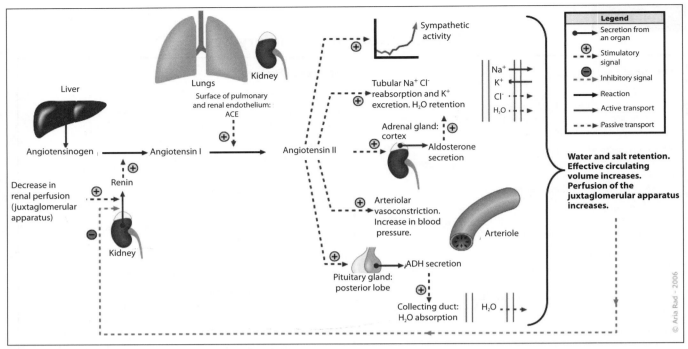

Figure 1.35. Renin-angiotensin-aldosterone system.

Source: "Renin-angiotensin-aldosterone system" by A. Rad (2006). Licensed under Creative Commons Attribution–Share Alike 3.0 via Wikimedia Commons. http://commons.wikimedia.org/wiki/File:Renin-angiotensin-aldosterone_system.png

can further impair kidney function. This is sometimes referred to as *acute-on-chronic disease* (Post & Burton, 2013).

  c. Findings from the physical assessment of a patient with prerenal AKI may include:

    (1) Dry mucous membranes, poor skin turgor, reduced jugular venous pressure, hypotension, weight loss, and oliguria.

    (2) Assessment must be correlated with laboratory findings.

      (a) These are likely to include an increased blood urea nitrogen (BUN), SCr, and SCr to BUN ratio; increased urine osmolality and specific gravity; decreased fractional excretion of sodium (less than 1%); unremarkable urine sediment.

      (b) Diuretics can elevate urine sodium.

    (3) A low fractional excretion of sodium can also be seen with contrast-induced ATN, obstruction, acute glomerulonephritis, and significant proteinuria.

    (4) Laboratory values do not differentiate between acute and chronic kidney disease without knowledge of baseline values.

    (5) Presence of oliguria supports a diagnosis of AKI.

  d. Treatment goals for prerenal AKI.

    (1) The major treatment goal is to improve renal perfusion.

    (2) To accomplish this, fluids will be administered to increase circulatory blood volume. This is generally done with a fluid bolus challenge (e.g., 500 mL over 30 min) which may be repeated if no increase in urine output.

    (3) Monitoring of cardiovascular response must occur simultaneously.

    (4) Cardiac function may need to be increased or supported with medications to improve blood flow to the kidneys.

3. Intrarenal AKI.

  a. Potential etiologies of intrarenal AKI.

    (1) Injury to the renal parenchyma; usually associated with intrarenal ischemia or toxins or both.

    (2) Uncorrected prerenal etiologies will lead to intrarenal injury.

    (3) A transplanted kidney is also susceptible to damage from prolonged low blood flow states or ischemic injury.

    (4) Acute tubular necrosis (ATN) is the most common intrarenal injury.

    (5) Nephrotoxic agents may also be responsible for intrarenal injury. Medications such as chemotherapeutics, amphotericin, NSAIDs and acetaminophen, illicit drug use, and radiographic contrast media (especially iodine-based dyes administered to

someone with preexisting kidney disease), must be considered.

(6) Environmental and occupational agents (e.g., pesticides and organic solvents), as well as heavy metals, some herbal agents, and poison exposure, should be investigated if there is suspicion of exposure.

(7) Older adults are prone to increased nephrotoxicity, both as a consequence of their decline in kidney function and because of their exposure to a higher number of medications.

(a) Clinicians should not assume that a relatively normal serum creatinine indicates normal kidney function in the elderly, as serum creatinine is a less reliable indicator of kidney function in the aging population (Pichler et al., 2010).

(b) Drug dosing needs to be carefully considered in the case of an aging patient (Pichler et al., 2010).

(c) Some inflammatory processes related to bacteria, virus, and pregnancy toxemia may also cause intrarenal injury.

(d) Blood transfusion reactions causing intravascular hemolysis and many vascular disorders result in intrarenal AKI.

(8) Systemic and vascular disorders causing renal injury.

(a) Major disease processes such as diabetes, systemic lupus erythematosus, Wilson disease, malaria, nephrotic syndrome, multiple myeloma, sickle cell disease, and renal vein thrombosis can cause renal injury.

(b) The most common acute renal vascular disease is vasculitis (e.g., Wegener's granulomatosis).

(c) Less common etiologies include thromboembolic purpura (TTP), hemolyticuremic syndrome (HUS), malignant hypertension, and scleroderma (Post & Burton, 2013).

(d) Tumor lysis syndrome or necrosis of large numbers of tumor cells typically occurs after chemotherapy for lymphomas or leukemias (Jefferson et al., 2010).

(e) Pregnancy-related disorders such as septic abortion, preeclampsia, and placenta abruptio may also cause intrarenal AKI.

b. Intrarenal pathophysiology.

(1) Ischemic ATN is caused by an ischemic event resulting from hypoperfusion of the kidneys and is generally the result of a sustained mean arterial pressure (MAP) below 75 mmHg (e.g., vasodilatation from sepsis causing a low flow state).

(2) Prerenal insults (reduced renal perfusion), if severe is a common cause of ATN.

(3) In addition to ischemia, there is a variety of endogenous and exogenous toxins that can lead to acute tubular necrosis (refer to Figure 1.36).

(a) Drugs can cause nephrotoxic ATN (e.g., gentamicin, amikacin, vancomycin).

(b) Chemical agents can cause nephrotoxic ATN (e.g., radiopaque dye administered in radiologic exams).

(c) Sepsis can also result in ATN. This type of ATN is usually associated with decreased renal perfusion and systemic hypotension (e.g., shock). The release of inflammatory cytokines and activation of neutrophils that frequently occurs with sepsis also contribute to development of ATN.

(4) ATN is the most common cause for AKI.

(5) Both ischemic ATN and nephrotoxic ATN result in damage to the kidney tubular epithelium. The pathophysiologies associated with development of ischemic and nephrotoxic ATN are very similar.

(a) With ischemic ATN, renal auto-regulation fails to reestablish adequate blood flow to the kidneys. Prolonged afferent arteriole constriction leads to decreased glomerular blood flow, glomerular hydrostatic pressure, and a reduction in GFR.

i. The amount and degree of cellular damage depends on the length of the ischemic episode and the patient's individual response to the insult.

ii. Patient sensitivity to renal ischemia is highly variable. Some will develop ATN within just a few minutes while others are able to tolerate several hours without developing structural damage. However, eventual injury will occur if sustained.

iii. A prolonged ischemic event can require up to several weeks for recovery of function. Recovery of function is highly variable and sometimes difficult to predict.

iv. Cellular damage continues even

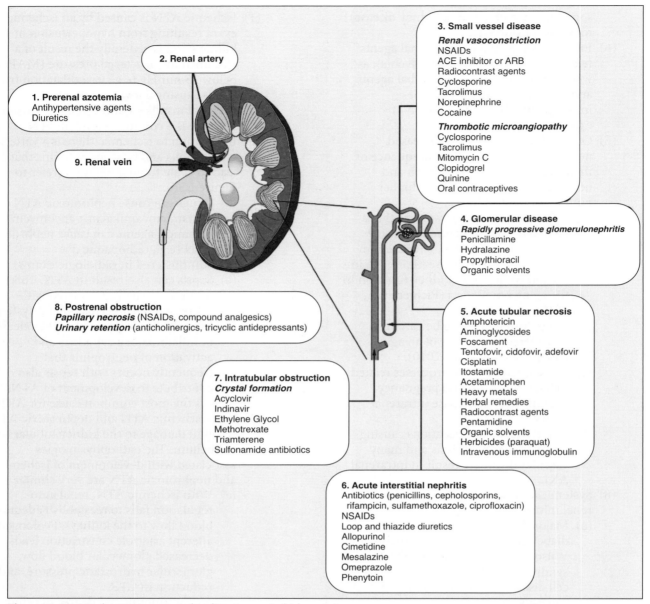

Figure 1.36. Nephrotoxic agents leading to acute kidney injury.

Reprinted from *Comprehensive Clinical Nephrology*, Jefferson, Thurman, and Schrier, Pathophysiology and Etiology of Acute Kidney Injury, p. 804, copyright 2010, with permission from Elsevier.

after reperfusion. Reperfusion results in postischemic vascular congestion that worsens the relative hypoxia leading to cellular injury and death in the predisposed tubular segments.

v. With prolonged ischemia, the kidneys may be unable to produce vasodilating prostaglandins, which tend to exacerbate the injury.

vi. The sympathetic nervous system stimulation redistributes blood flow from the renal cortex to the medulla, thus worsening glomerular capillary flow and tubular ischemia (tubules are located in cortex). This ischemia limits nutrients and oxygen for basic cellular metabolism.

vii. Without adequate oxygen and decreased ATP supply, metabolism changes from aerobic to anaerobic (Schira, 2008).

viii. Prolonged tubular ischemia results in swelling and necrosis of tubular cells, altering the function of the basement membrane. Cell death occurs by both necrosis and apoptosis (programed cell death).

   ix. The reduction in GFR is as much a consequence of cell death as it is from obstruction of the tubular lumen caused by necrotic debris.

   x. Necrotic tubule cells slough causing tubular obstruction and cast formation.

   xi. This increases tubular and Bowman's capsule hydrostatic pressure, thus opposing the glomerular hydrostatic pressure and decreases GFR (Schira, 2008).

(b) Toxic ATN does not frequently result in an oliguric state as occurs with ischemic ATN.

   i. The kidneys are responsible for the concentration and excretion of toxic substances and are therefore exposed to high concentrations of these.

   ii. Blood circulates through the kidneys approximately 1.2 L/min, leading to repeated exposure to the toxins.

   iii. It has been estimated that nephrotoxic drugs account for 20% to 30% of AKI.

   iv. Whenever nephrotoxic agents such as aminoglycosides, amphotericin, and radiopaque contrast dye are given, consider that a patient's risk for development of AKI is increased with dual exposures (KDIGO, 2012a).

   v. Patients with liver disease, causing decreased detoxification of substances in the liver, can potentiate even more renal overload.

c. Differentiation of prerenal AKI from ATN associated AKI.

(1) Evaluation includes first ruling out other causes.

(a) Aminoglycoside exposure resulting in glomerulonephritis; typically has hematuria and dysmorphic red cells (possibly red cell casts).

(b) Acute interstitial nephritis typically associated with pyuria with or without white cell casts or hematuria, but no red cell casts. Or, urinary tract obstruction diagnosed by ultrasound.

(2) Urinalysis is normal or near normal with prerenal etiology of AKI. Classic urinalysis in ATN reveals muddy granular and epithelial cell casts (recall cell death and shedding); might see free renal tubular epithelial cells in the urine.

(3) ATN generally manifests with oliguria (anuria, less than 50 mL/day is rare). However, the decrease in the GFR that occurs with ATN is not always associated with a reduction in urine output. Urine output is highly variable.

(4) Abnormal renal handling of sodium occurs in AKI, and the fractional excretion of sodium test (FENa) helps distinguish prerenal disease from ATN.

(a) A value below 1% suggests prerenal disease, while a value above 2% is usually indicative of ATN.

(b) The FENa is helpful only when there is a marked reduction in GFR. In addition, the FENa will be higher in patients receiving diuretic therapy even with prerenal AKI if someone is receiving diuretics or has any other reason for salt wasting (Post & Burton, 2013).

(5) Another distinguishing factor between prerenal and ATN injury is the response to therapy.

(a) During the correction of a prerenal cause when no actual nephron damage has occurred, there will be a fairly rapid recovery of kidney function. Urine output and blood chemistries will return to normal.

(b) In ATN, which implies nephron damage, the response to treatment is delayed.

(6) ATN requires additional therapy focused on correcting abnormalities stemming from the kidney's inability to maintain regulatory functions.

(7) Another clinical indication of ATN is an inability to concentrate urine, with urine osmolality approximating serum osmolality around 300 to 320 mOsm/L.

(8) The rate of rise of SCr is also helpful in distinguishing between prerenal and ATN.

(a) With ATN, SCr will rise almost daily by 0.3 to 0.5 mg/dL.

(b) A prerenal state has more variability in SCr (characteristic fluctuations are due to the periodic changes in renal perfusion).

d. Treatment goals with intrarenal etiologies.

(1) Prevention of AKI is a primary goal of therapy. This is best done by identifying those at risk for AKI and considering less toxic agents.

(a) To prevent contrast-induced nephropathy (CIN), patients at risk should be maintained at an adequate hydration status prior to procedure (e.g., discontinue diuretics when possible).

(b) Similar precautions should be taken with certain nephrotoxic chemotherapeutic agents.

(2) Assessment of volume status is one of the first steps in management of AKI since amelioration of volume depletion with a fluid bolus has the potential to reverse AKI due to prerenal hypovolemia.

(3) The main treatment goal is maintenance of renal perfusion and avoidance of further kidney injury.

(a) Interventions to preserve kidney function and treat the complications associated with the kidney injury need to occur simultaneously.

(b) Any potentially nephrotoxic agents should be avoided (Macedo, 2010).

(c) Volume status is one of the most difficult parameters to assess, and fluid administration should target a predefined preload, stroke volume, or cardiac output rather than a set mean arterial pressure (Macedo, 2010).

4. Postrenal AKI.

a. The general etiology of this classification of AKI results from the interference with the flow of urine from the kidneys out of the body and is associated with obstruction or disruption of the urinary tract (Schira, 2008).

(1) Possible causes include ureteral, bladder neck, or urethral obstruction from calculi, neoplasms, strictures, trauma, blood clots, foreign objects, or congenital and developmental abnormalities.

(2) Other causes include prostatic hypertrophy, retroperitoneal fibrosis, abdominal or retroperitoneal neoplasms, pregnancy, neurogenic bladder, or bladder rupture.

b. Postrenal pathophysiology.

(1) Unilateral obstruction does not always result in a rise in SCr.

(a) Nevertheless, if not relieved can result in permanent injury and loss of kidney function and eventually result in AKI.

(b) Bilateral obstruction results in anuria as urine flow is unable to pass the obstruction (typically this type of obstruction is located at the level of the bladder or downstream from the bladder).

(c) This type of obstruction is primarily caused by prostate enlargement or tumors in men and urologic or gynecologic tumors in women.

(2) Impedance of urine flow causes backward, retrograde pressure through the collecting system and slows the tubular fluid flow and the GFR.

(a) This results in increased reabsorption of sodium, water, and urea.

(b) As a consequence, there is a decrease in urinary sodium excretion and an increase in urine osmolality.

(c) The BUN will also be increased in the blood.

(3) If the postrenal obstruction is temporary or able to be resolved, there is minimal dilation of the collecting system or loss of renal tissue.

(4) If the postrenal obstruction is prolonged, the collecting system dilates and there is renal tissue loss (damage).

(5) After release of the obstruction, polyuria results as the confined urine flows out.

c. Assessment of postrenal AKI.

(1) Obstructive uropathy is common in elderly men, usually due to benign prostatic hypertrophy, stones, urethral stricture, or prostate cancer.

(2) The incidence in women is at least one third less than in men and is primarily due to malignant neoplasms of the genitourinary tract.

(3) Lower urinary tract obstruction should be excluded by measuring postvoid residual bladder volume by ultrasound or placement of temporary catheter.

(4) Ultrasound is appropriate for diagnosis of upper urinary tract obstruction (Pichler et al., 2010). However, ultrasound is not indicated in all cases of AKI.

(5) A detailed history and physical assessment are essential.

(6) Physical findings vary with etiology and must be correlated with laboratory findings and history.

(7) Nephralgia may be associated with the movement of urinary tract stones or developing hydronephrosis.

(8) Bladder distention may be associated with prostate, bladder neck, or urethral disorders.

(9) Inquiry about changes in urinary patterns is very important in the identification of urinary tract obstructions.

(10) Urine volume may be variable ranging from oliguria, polyuria, or anuria.

(11) Unilateral flank pain is most consistent with obstruction, renal thrombus, or infection (Post & Burton, 2013).

(12) Laboratory findings with postrenal etiology

may reveal variable urine osmolality, specific gravity, and urine sodium.
  (a) Urine osmolality and sodium may be similar to plasma levels.
  (b) Urine urea decreases, while urine sediment may be normal, except if urinary tract infection is present. The BUN and SCr increase with the ratio being normal to slightly increased.
d. Diagnostic considerations in postrenal AKI.
  (1) Renal ultrasound is useful in demonstrating obstruction and/or dilatation of collecting structures, but not necessary in all cases of AKI.
  (2) A CT scan is useful in locating an obstruction such as stones.
  (3) Urinalysis, which involves both the use of a urine dipstick and microscopic examination of the urine sediment, is an essential component of the diagnostic evaluation of AKI in general.
    (a) The dipstick can test for protein, pH, glucose, hematuria, pyuria, and specific gravity.
    (b) Microscopic examination of the urine sediment may reveal characteristic findings suggestive of certain diagnoses.
      i. Muddy brown granular casts and epithelial cell casts in a patient with AKI is highly suggestive of acute tubular necrosis (ATN), but not a definitive diagnosis.
      ii. Red cell cast is suggestive of glomerular hematuria (glomerulonephritis or vasculitis).
    (c) Urinalysis can help subclassify patients with glomerular disease into those with glomerulonephritis and those with a nephritic pattern in which proteinuria is characteristic (Post & Burton, 2013).
e. Treatment goal of postrenal AKI.
  (1) The obstruction or the cause of disruption of urine flow must be relieved and urine flow reestablished.
  (2) Avoidance of nephrotoxic agents in AKI from any etiology is essential to the management because the goal is to remove any offending agent or condition (Jefferson et al., 2010).
5. Vascular causes of AKI.
  a. Atheroembolic kidney disease.
    (1) Seen primarily in older patients with atherosclerotic vascular disease.
    (2) May occur spontaneously or after arteriography, vascular surgery,

thrombolysis (tPA or streptokinase), and anticoagulation.
  b. Destabilization of atherosclerotic plaques results in showers of cholesterol that lodge in small arteries in the kidneys.
    (1) Emboli produce a progressive inflammatory reaction.
    (2) Results in occlusion of the involved vasculature.
  c. Other vascular causes of AKI can also occur from noncholesterol emboli and are more common in older adults.
    (1) Atrial fibrillation is an important risk factor for intrarenal emboli.
    (2) Renal vein thrombosis may occur in the setting of nephrotic syndrome.
6. Scleroderma can lead to severe AKI.
  a. Background information.
    (1) The word scleroderma is derived from the Greek word scleros to describe thickened, hardened skin (Varga, 2013).
    (2) The term scleroderma refers to conditions that affect the skin and connective tissues that support the body's organs.
  b. Pathophysiology.
    (1) Uncontrolled accumulations of collagen and the development of widespread vascular lesions are known to be the hallmarks of the pathophysiologic process.
    (2) "When the characteristic skin disorder is associated with internal organ involvement, the disease is termed systemic sclerosis (SSc)" (Varga, 2013).
    (3) Kidney involvement is common in systemic SSc with most having only mild chronic renal dysfunction.
    (4) In contrast, an acute form of scleroderma called scleroderma renal crisis (SRC) occurs in about 10% to 20% of patients that have the diffuse SSc.
    (5) Morbidity and mortality are high with this form of scleroderma (Guillevin et al., 2012).
  c. Incidence.
    (1) The prevalence rates of systemic scleroderma vary widely from 0.6 to 122 per million persons per year due to geographic variations in occurrence.
    (2) Regional differences are seen, with higher rates in the United States and Australia.
    (3) It appears to be more prevalent in blacks.
  d. Symptoms.
    (1) General symptoms that may be exhibited are fatigue, joint stiffness, loss of strength, sleep difficulties, and skin discoloration (Varga, 2013).
    (2) Scleroderma can have a mild presentation to the extreme of causing debilitating

disease processes resulting in multiorgan failure.

(a) The associated vascular narrowing often results in development of secondary Raynaud phenomenon. Raynaud phenomenon occurs when the blood vessels in the fingers and toes develop an exaggerated vasoconstrictive response to cold temperatures or emotional stress, called vasospastic attacks (Pope, 2007).

(b) Visceral involvement in the systemic form causes interstitial pulmonary fibrosis, diminished esophageal and gastrointestinal motility, restrictive cardiomyopathy, and renal disease (Glassock, 2010).

(c) Renal involvement occurs in approximately 60% of affected patients and can vary from low-grade proteinuria and minimal impairment of GFR to marked reduction in renal blood flow leading to severe AKI.

e. Scleroderma renal crisis (SRC).

(1) Associated with severe hypertension, encephalopathy, diastolic congestive heart failure and oliguric kidney failure.

(2) 20% to 50% of cases progress to kidney failure (Varga & Fenves, 2013).

f. Treatment goals.

(1) Adequate hypertension control is essential to the prevention of renal crisis.

(a) Studies have shown that the optimal class of antihypertensives are ACE inhibitors and are associated with greater efficacy and preservation of kidney function.

(b) The use of medium to high dose of glucocorticosteroids has been associated with a marked increase in the development of renal crisis and doses > 15 mg per day should be avoided (Trang et al., 2012).

(c) Patient education should emphasize the need to maintain physical mobility and optimal nutrition to deter disease progression and potentially alleviate secondary Raynaud manifestations (Varga, 2013).

(d) Plasma exchanges in addition to use of ACE inhibitors are the mainstays of treatment.

i. Plasma exchange has been reserved for patients that develop micro-angiopathy.

ii. Therapeutic plasma exchange uses an automated centrifuge. The filtered plasma is removed; the red blood cells, along with a new replacement colloid (from a donor or albumin), are returned to the patient. Even with plasma exchange, the long-term prognosis remains disappointingly poor (Cozzi et al., 2012).

iii. Extracorporeal photochemotherapy (ECP, photopheresis).

7. Gout as the etiology of AKI.

a. Gout is a metabolic disorder that results in hyperuricemia and urate crystal deposition, causing inflammation.

b. Clinical manifestations may include recurrent attacks of acute inflammatory arthritis, chronic arthropathy, accumulation of urate crystals, uric acid neprolithiasis, and/or a chronic nephropathy most often due to comorbid states (Becker, 2013a).

c. The prevalence of gout in the United States is estimated at between 3 and 8 million individuals and is increasing here and abroad.

d. Predisposing factors.

(1) Numerous circumstances promote acute attacks of gouty arthritis such as trauma, surgery, starvation, fatty foods, dietary overindulgence (i.e., meat and seafood), low-dose aspirin, and increased alcohol consumption (beer and spirits, not wine) (Becker, 2013a).

(2) Hyperuricemia is also relatively common in patients treated with a loop or thiazide diuretic, as they reduce urate excretion and may lead to gouty arthritis (Becker, 2013b).

e. Outcomes and goals.

(1) The typical attack of acute gouty arthritis results in severe pain, redness, swelling, and disability, and resolves within days to several weeks.

(2) Approximately 80% of these attacks involve a single joint, most often the great toe, and is more common in males.

f. Two major complications of chronic hyperuricemia: nephrolithiasis and chronic urate nephropathy.

(1) Uric acid stones are a component of the morbidity seen with gout.

(2) Precipitation of uric acid crystals within the renal nephrons may lead to tubular obstruction and altered renal function.

g. Patient education, in regard to dietary compliance and stone prevention, is very important.

h. The goal of treatment is to reduce hyperuricemia and prevent uric acid crystallization.

(1) This may include a high fluid intake.

(2) Alkalinization of urine.

(3) Administration of urate lowering therapeutic agents such as allopurinol (Schira, 2008).

8. HIV-associated AKI.

  a. Background information.

    (1) The incidence of AKI is higher in HIV-infected patients than in the general population.

    (2) Patients are living longer with HIV due to the evolution and utilization of highly active antiviral therapy (HAART), but this therapy also has a downside.

      (a) Some of the medications are nephrotoxic and, as such, have been associated with development of AKI.

      (b) These HAART therapies have dramatically improved survival and slowed HIV progression.

        i. This has opened the door for other complications such as kidney, liver, and cardiac disease.

        ii. These complications will likely replace opportunistic infections as the leading cause of mortality in HIV infection.

  b. Patients with HIV are at risk for AKI and CKD secondary to three main reasons.

    (1) Medication nephrotoxicity.

    (2) HIV-associated nephrotoxicity.

    (3) Comorbid conditions accompanying aging.

  c. Pathophysiology.

    (1) The two most common etiologies of AKI in HIV-infected patients are prerenal conditions and acute tubular necrosis.

    (2) Underlying causes include volume depletion, heart failure, cirrhosis, ischemia, nephrotoxicity, and obstructive conditions.

    (3) Nephrotoxicity can result from the HAART drugs as well as protease inhibitors and antiviral agents.

      (a) Protease inhibitors such as indinavir and atazanavir can cause crystalluria.

      (b) Tenofovir disoproxil fumarate (TDF), a nucleoside reverse transcriptase inhibitor, can cause AKI.

  d. All HIV-infected patients should be screened for proteinuria and reduced kidney function (Wyatt & Klotman, 2013).

  e. The actual mechanisms behind kidney injury include the following:

    (1) HIV genome present in kidney tissue.

    (2) Leukocyte infiltration of tubular interstitium.

    (3) Viral replication within mesangial cells.

  f. Diagnosis.

    (1) Symptomatology may include proteinuria, edema, and hypoalbuminemia.

    (2) Without HIV treatment, the loss of kidney function may progress rapidly.

    (3) Characteristic large, echogenic kidneys are seen on ultrasound.

  g. Risk factors for progressive kidney injury with HIV infection include:

    (1) Co-infection with hepatitis C virus.

    (2) Low CD4 T cell count and high HIV viral load.

    (3) Presence of other comorbidities, including diabetes and hypertension (Wyatt & Klotman, 2013).

  h. Treatment.

    (1) May include ACE inhibitors to reduce proteinuria and edema, and initiation of antiretroviral agents, if not currently on this therapy, to control viral replication, which may preserve kidney function.

    (2) Standard therapy for kidney disease should also be employed such as blood pressure control with an ACE inhibitor or an angiotensin receptor blocker (ARB) (Kopp et al., 2010).

9. Hepatorenal syndrome refers to acute kidney injury in patients with either acute or chronic liver disease. The onset of kidney failure is generally insidious but can be brought on by an acute insult such as G.I. bleeding or a systemic infection (Runyon, 2013).

  a. Usually seen in patients with portal hypertension due to cirrhosis, severe alcoholic hepatitis, metastatic tumors, or hepatic failure from any cause.

  b. This syndrome is a consequence of reductions in renal perfusion brought about by the progression of severe hepatic dysfunction.

  c. Renal vasoconstriction and systemic vasodilation resulting in renal hypoperfusion are characteristically seen.

  d. The diagnosis of hepatorenal syndrome is associated with a poor prognosis due to combined liver and kidney failure (Schira, 2008).

  e. Clinical presentation. The patient with hepatorenal syndrome may exhibit the following signs and symptoms.

    (1) Progressive rise in SCr.

    (2) Urinalysis is generally unremarkable except possibly having minimal proteinuria or low sodium excretion.

    (3) Oliguria.

    (4) Jaundice, ascites, and portal hypertension.

    (5) Splenomegaly.

    (6) Hypoalbuminemia.

  f. Diagnosis and treatment.

    (1) The diagnosis of hepatorenal syndrome is a clinical diagnosis, and one of exclusion, as

there is no one specific test that can establish a definitive diagnosis.

(2) Other potential etiologies of AKI in patients with liver disease should be ruled out first. Renal biopsy is not routinely performed in patients with cirrhosis and AKI due to the potential for harm.

(3) The treatment goal for hepatorenal syndrome is recovery of liver function.

  (a) The liver is able to improve with abstinence from alcohol in the case of alcoholic hepatitis or with antiviral therapy for treatment of hepatitis.

  (b) In cases where improvement of liver function is not possible in the short term, medical therapy is recommended to reverse the kidney injury.

  (c) It is important to maintain fluid balance, avoid nephrotoxic drugs, and prepare the patient for liver transplant if appropriate (Runyon, 2013).

10. Primary hyperparathyroidism resulting in AKI.
  a. Etiology.
    (1) Hyperplasia and neoplasms of the parathyroid glands, a history of neck irradiation, or parathyroid hormone secreting tumors can all lead to primary hyperparathyroidism.
    (2) Primary hyperparathyroidism is the second most common cause of hypercalcemia.
    (3) Primary hyperparathyroidism can also be inherited either as hyperplasia of the parathyroid glands or as a component in hereditary endocrine glandular disorders (Kestenbaum & Drueke, 2010).
  b. The incidence of primary hyperparathyroidism may be greater in females over 40.
  c. Pathophysiology.
    (1) Normally, hypercalcemia would act as a negative feedback mechanism to control the parathyroid gland to decrease PTH secretion.
    (2) In the presence of primary hyperpara-thyroidism, uncontrolled secretion of parathyroid hormone (PTH) results in elevated serum PTH levels despite hypercalcemia.
  d. The severity of clinical symptoms caused by the resultant hypercalcemia is dependent not only on the degree of calcium elevation, but also on the speed at which the hypercalcemia develops (Kestenbaum & Drueke, 2010).
    (1) The hypercalcemia is responsible for the effects on the kidney.
    (2) Renal related signs include polyuria, urinary tract stones and their

consequences (previously discussed), and occasionally tubulointerstitial disease or nephrocalcinosis (deposits of calcium phosphate in nephrons).

(3) Nephrogenic diabetes insipidus (hypercalcemia interferes with action of ADH on the tubules) may be seen.

(4) Additional potential manifestations of the elevated PTH.

  (a) Hyperphosphaturia and hyper-chloremic metabolic acidosis, due to decreased bicarbonate reabsorption.

  (b) The hydrogen ions are not buffered and chloride is reabsorbed (Schira, 2008).

e. Treatment is aimed at the underlying cause.
  (1) This usually includes partial parathyroid-ectomy and high fluid intake.
  (2) Dietary changes may include calcium restriction and phosphate binders.
  (3) Estrogens may be given, especially in women.
  (4) Calcimetics (Cinacalcet), a new therapeutic class of calcium agonists, can be used to normalize serum calcium along with a reduction of serum PTH (Kestenbaum & Drueke, 2010).

11. The kidney and pregnancy and AKI.
  a. Normal changes in kidney and urinary tract structure and function that occur during pregnancy.
    (1) Kidneys increase 1 to 2 cm in length and up to 70% in volume. This is due to changes in the vascular and interstitial fluid compartments.
    (2) The collecting system (calyces, renal pelvis, and ureters) dilates due to hormonal influences.
      (a) By the third trimester, many women show signs of hydronephrosis termed *physiologic hydronephrosis of pregnancy.*
      (b) A consequence of ureteral dilation is urinary stasis, which increases the risk of an ascending infection (i.e., pyelonephritis).
    (3) The bladder is displaced anteriorly and superiorly, and its capacity is increased.
    (4) Systemic changes of increased cardiac output and peripheral vasodilation leads to increased organ blood flow. Renal blood flow (RBF) increases up to 50% by the second trimester and remains there until just before delivery.
      (a) The increased RBF increases the glomerular filtration rate (GFR).
      (b) The increased GFR (25% increase)

begins at 4 weeks of pregnancy and peaks (up to 50% increase) by midpregnancy (13 weeks), and continues until delivery.

  (c) The increased GFR leads to increased solute clearance.

     i. Plasma solute values are lower in pregnancy than nonpregnant states (e.g., serum creatinine decreases to 0.4 to 0.5 mg/dL in pregnancy, and values of 0.7 to 0.8 mg/dL considered normal in nonpregnancy are concerning in normal pregnancy).

     ii. This increased GFR results in an increased volume of glomerular filtrate, which exceeds tubular reabsorption abilities leading to proteinuria (300 to 500 mg/day) and glycosuria.

     iii. The increased nutrients in the urine can also increase the risk of urinary tract infection.

  (5) In pregnancy, the renal bicarbonate threshold decreases, which results in lower serum bicarbonate level to 10 to 20 mEq/L; thus decreasing the serum pH, causing alkaline urine in the morning.

  (6) Uterine enlargement may cause incomplete bladder emptying, giving yet another factor that increases the risk for pyelonephritis.

    (a) In the third trimester, this enlarged uterus compresses surrounding tissue, and in the supine position there may be partial obstruction of the inferior vena cava and decreased venous return, reducing cardiac output leading to a decrease in blood pressure.

    (b) Attention should be paid to the maternal posture while measuring blood pressure, and keep these postural effects in mind (Baylis & Davison, 2010).

  (7) Total body water increases by 6 to 8 liters, and sodium reabsorption increases, which may lead to dependent edema.

 b. Complications in pregnancy.

  (1) Pyelonephritis is the most common infectious complication in pregnancy, with an incidence of 1 to 2%.

    (a) Asymptomatic bacteriuria that is poorly treated, or not treated, often potentiates its development.

    (b) *E. coli* is the most common pathogen.

    (c) Careful screening of all pregnant women for asymptomatic bacteriuria (> 100,000 colonies/mL) should be done with thorough treatment of all infections.

    (d) Signs and symptoms of pyelonephritis.

     i. Fever (may be high) and chills.

     ii. Nausea and vomiting.

     iii. Flank tenderness/pain and costovertebral angle tenderness.

     iv. Urinalysis is positive for bacteria, red blood cells, white cell casts, leukocyte esterase, and nitrites.

    (e) Blood cultures should be checked.

    (f) Treatment.

     i. Hospitalization may be required for parenteral antibiotics.

     ii. Moderate fluid intake should be maintained.

     iii. Posttreatment urine culture may be warranted with careful monitoring during the remainder of the pregnancy.

    (g) Pyelonephritis is serious and has been associated with preterm labor and fetal death (Schira, 2008).

  (2) Acute kidney failure in pregnancy occurs in 1 out of every 2000 to 5000 cases.

    (a) There are two peak times for occurrence.

     i. The first is in early pregnancy and is associated with septic abortion, shock, or hyperemesis causing electrolyte imbalances.

     ii. The second peak time frame is in the final gestation month and may be associated with one of the following: preeclampsia, hemorrhagic complications or placenta abruption, urinary tract obstruction, or intravascular coagulation.

    (b) Dialysis may need to be initiated early to maintain a normal fetal environment as metabolic waste products cross the placenta (Schira, 2008).

  (3) CKD and pregnancy.

    (a) Pregnancy does not generally affect early CKD if hypertension is not present.

    (b) However, women with early CKD who become pregnant may accelerate kidney dysfunction. Termination of pregnancy may not reverse the situation.

    (c) Women with hypertension and kidney disease are more likely to have complications during pregnancy, such as severe hypertension or a decline in kidney function.

i. These pregnancies are associated with more risk, and fetal surveillance is important.

ii. As kidney function declines, the ability to conceive decreases. Less than 1% of women on dialysis conceive, and 30% of them deliver a live infant, with 20% of infants being born prematurely.

(4) Pregnancy after kidney transplant.

(a) Fertility improves 4 to 6 months after transplant, but it is advisable to wait 1 to 2 years after transplant to conceive to avoid graft rejection.

(b) Kidney function and fetal growth should be monitored throughout pregnancy.

(c) Immunosuppression increases the risk of infection for both mother and fetus. Surveillance for this should be done.

12. Acute and chronic kidney failure with nonkidney organ transplantation.

a. Incidence of acute and/or chronic kidney failure after solid organ transplant or bone marrow transplantation may be as high as 50%.

(1) A major cause of this kidney failure may be the nephrotoxic immunosuppressant agents used after transplant, in particular, cyclosporine and tacrolimus.

(2) Pretransplant factors that contribute to this outcome.

(a) Patients with heart and liver failure.

(b) Patients with hepatorenal syndrome in which accurate determination of kidney function is difficult.

(c) The presence of CKD stages 1 or 2 before transplant is a challenge.

(d) Operative factors may contribute to kidney injury including donor organ from an older person, inherent operative risks, or kidney hypoperfusion intraoperatively.

(e) Posttransplant factors may also come into play, such as prolonged intubation and ventilator support, development of hypertension, development of proteinuria, and hyperlipidemia.

b. Pathophysiology and treatment.

(1) Some antirejection drugs are potentially nephrotoxic. The development of kidney failure is similar, regardless of the transplanted organ. All kidney structures are affected.

(2) The tapering and elimination of the nephrotoxic immunosuppressants may help.

(3) Once CKD stage 5 occurs, any form of

kidney replacement therapy may be initiated, including kidney transplant (Schira, 2008).

13. Acute interstitial nephritis.

a. Etiology.

(1) This acute, often reversible, uncommon cause of AKI is characterized by interstitial inflammatory infiltrates.

(2) Acute interstitial nephritis (AIN) is an immunologically induced reaction to an antigen, usually a drug or an infectious agent.

(3) Prior to antibiotic availability, AIN was most commonly associated with infections, such as scarlet fever and diphtheria.

(4) AIN is now most commonly induced by medications (75% to 90% of all cases), particularly antimicrobial agents, proton pump inhibitors, and nonsteroidal antiinflammatory drugs (NSAIDS).

(5) AIN is identified in only 2% to 3% of all biopsies, but up to 25% of patients undergoing biopsy are doing so for unexplained or drug-induced AKI.

(6) Acute interstitial nephritis can occur at any age, but it is rare in children.

b. Diagnosis.

(1) Most accurately made by renal biopsy.

(2) Testing for eosinophiluria and gallium scanning are both helpful.

(3) If the etiology of AIN is felt to be drug-induced, identification of the causative medication may not be easy if the patient is taking more than one drug capable of inducing AIN. Two biologic tests may help in the identification process.

(a) The lymphocyte stimulation test.

(b) Identification of circulating antidrug antibodies.

c. Treatment begins with removal of the inciting drug.

(1) In addition, a short course of corticosteroids is generally used, but opinions differ on their use.

(2) Improvement in renal function should be seen within 1 week of discontinuing the inciting agent (Rossert & Fischer, 2010).

14. Tumor lysis syndrome.

a. After chemotherapy, when there is necrosis of large numbers of tumor cells, nephrotoxic intracellular contents (uric acid, phosphate, and xanthine) may be released into the circulation (Jefferson et al., 2010).

b. It is more common after the treatment of lymphomas and leukemias.

c. The resulting AKI results in an oliguric – or even anuric – state and should be suspected when high lactate dehydrogenase levels are seen, which is seen with massive cell lysis.

d. Elevated phosphate, urate, and potassium levels may also be found and should be monitored closely.

e. The use of high-dose allopurinol may be started 2 to 3 days before chemotherapy along with either IV or oral fluid loading to ensure a urine output of more than 2.5 L/day (Jefferson et al., 2010).

J. Clinical course of acute kidney injury.
   1. An initiating stage begins when the kidney is injured and may last from hours to days.
      a. Signs and symptoms of kidney function impairment become apparent, such as decreased urine volume.
      b. The etiology of AKI is investigated, and treatment plan for reversal initiated.
      c. The endocrine functions of the kidney are not yet affected.
   2. An oliguric stage follows the initial stage; it usually lasts from 5 to 15 days or may persist for weeks.
      a. Healing may begin with tubular cell regeneration, and the destroyed basement membrane is replaced with scar tissue.
      b. The tubules may be clogged with inflammatory products.
      c. Functional changes at this stage are decreased glomerular filtration, decreased tubular transport, decreased urine production, and decreased renal clearance.
      d. In cases where the acute kidney injury persists for weeks or longer, the kidney's endocrine functions are altered. For example, erythropoietin production is decreased.
      e. Many of these patients are nonoliguric and may have less severe symptoms than oliguric patients.
      f. Hyperkalemia, gastrointestinal bleeding, and infection become morbidity factors at this time.
      g. Daily care is very important to provide supportive and therapeutic interventions to assist in recovery of function (Schira, 2008).
   3. The diuretic stage of recovery usually lasts for 1 to 2 weeks but may persist even longer.
      a. Diuresis is self-limiting as renal tubular patency is restored; retained substances, such as urea and sodium, act as osmotic agents.
      b. Urine concentration has not yet returned, but with continued healing, the kidneys regain most of the lost function.
      c. The patient is at risk for fluid volume deficit during diuresis and must be monitored to prevent reinjury to renal tissue from hypotension and hypoperfusion.
      d. Assessment of fluid balance is achieved through:
         (1) Monitoring of daily weights, vital signs, and intake and output.
         (2) Clinical assessment of edema, skin turgor, and mucous membranes.
         (3) Adjustments to fluid levels can be made as needed.
      e. Fluid needs may increase during the diuresis stage, especially if combined with fever and/or gastrointestinal (GI) losses.
         (1) If there are signs of a fluid volume deficit, the patient must be assessed for hypotension, dizziness, or orthostasis. Safety principles and safety measures to prevent falls must be taught or reiterated.
         (2) Review medications and adjust accordingly per physician, APRN, or PA order.
         (3) Coordinate fluid and nutrition plans with a dietitian and the patient.
      f. Hypokalemia can become a factor at this time related to:
         (1) Increased excretion of potassium.
         (2) Decreased potassium intake.
         (3) Continued administration of diuretics/resin exchanges.
         (4) Intravenous (IV) fluids without potassium.
         (5) Possible GI losses.
      g. Monitor for changes in the plasma potassium and for potential metabolic alkalosis related to hydrogen-potassium cellular exchange.
      h. Many of the physical consequences of the AKI gradually begin to resolve.
         (1) This is the result of the clinical support the patient received that promoted healing.
         (2) The problems related to metabolic acidosis, hyperphosphatemia, and hyperkalemia normalize as kidney function improves.
         (3) The renal regulatory and excretory functions return.
   4. The recovery stage may last for months up to 1 year as the healing process continues.
      a. Contractile scar tissue replaces the basement membrane, nephrons become patent, and tubular cells regenerate.
      b. Scar tissue will remain most times to some degree.
      c. Functional loss is not always clinically significant, and the kidneys usually recover capacity to concentrate the urine.
         (1) Regulatory and excretory functions simultaneously improve.
         (2) This will be seen as urine osmolality increases, urine volume stabilizes, body fluids balance, and uremia resolves.
      d. Patient education should continue regarding

the risk for future episodes of acute kidney injury and preventive measures (Schira, 2008).

K. Daily care considerations with AKI.
1. Infection is always a risk with AKI.
   a. Due to increased susceptibility, especially urinary tract and respiratory infections.
   b. The higher risk has been attributed to hospitalization, an altered immune system, biochemical, and nutritional status.
   c. Preventive steps to avoid infections.
      (1) Avoid urinary catheters.
      (2) Remove catheters when no longer required.
      (3) Ensure that strict aseptic technique is used with all invasive procedures.
      (4) Avoid contact with people with infectious processes.
         (a) Educate the patient and family about increased susceptibility to infection.
         (b) Teach them how to prevent infections as well as the signs and symptoms to report.
      (5) Inspect and assess daily for signs of local or systemic infection, including vital signs, lung sounds, and leukocyte count.
      (6) Maintain skin and mucous membrane integrity.
      (7) Assess changes in wounds, drainage, and body secretions.
         (a) Treat infections promptly to avoid sepsis.
         (b) Use antibiotics and anti-infectives that are specific to the cultured organism, using caution with agents that might be nephrotoxic or excreted by the kidney.
2. Monitor fluid intake and output to minimize fluid volume excess related to decreased excretion and sodium retention.
3. Monitor for ongoing consequences of renal injury (e.g., hyperkalemia and hyperphosphatemia).
   a. These complications are related to impaired renal regulation, diminished excretion, and increased or continued intake of phosphorus and potassium, along with tissue breakdown.
   b. Metabolic acidosis is related to persistent decreased renal excretion of acid and decreased regeneration of bicarbonate, increased tissue catabolism, and endogenous production of acids.
   c. GI bleeding may be potentiated due to physiologic stress, retention of metabolic waste products, platelet dysfunction, and altered capillary permeability.
   d. Nutritional needs must be evaluated, especially protein calories. Consult with a dietitian.
   e. Consider the potential for drug toxicity, adverse reactions, and nephrotoxicity related to the kidneys' inability to excrete drugs and/or drug metabolites, especially with ongoing administration.
4. Cardiovascular complications may ensue.
   a. Anemia occurs due to blood loss, decreased renal production of erythropoietin, and the shortened life span of RBCs in the uremic environment.
   b. Treatment with an erythropoiesis-stimulating agent (ESA) should be considered with decreasing hemoglobin levels.
   c. Cardiac arrhythmias due to electrolyte imbalances and pericardial effusion or tamponade due to uremia are other potential complications.
5. Skin integrity must be monitored and proactively cared for to prevent skin breakdown. Breakdown of the skin can be related to bed rest, inadequate nutrition, fluid/electrolyte imbalances, toxin accumulation, edema, capillary fragility, disrupted hemostasis, and injury from invasive procedures such as repeated venipunctures.
6. Sleep patterns may be disturbed related to biochemical abnormalities, hospitalization, anxiety, and fear regarding disease progression.
7. Self-image and self-concept may be altered due to loss of bodily function, knowledge deficit, fatigue, separation from loved ones, and loss of control.
8. Assess readiness to learn, and provide ongoing patient and family education building on comprehension, using teaching methods suitable for the individual patient needs. Always properly document.

L. Pediatric implications and risk for AKI.
1. The most common causes of AKI in the pediatric population are similar to what occurs in adults. These were previously discussed and include sepsis, nephrotoxic medications, and ischemia (Zappitelli, 2008).
2. The Schwartz formula.
   a. This classification system is specific to the pediatric population.
   b. The RIFLE criteria previously reviewed was modified, applied, and validated in the pediatric population, denoted as the pRIFLE criteria.
      (1) The stratification is still the same with R representing mild AKI and F corresponding to failure.
      (2) Both of these levels of staging are based upon changes in the serum creatinine or estimated creatinine clearance using the Schwartz formula (Schwartz et al., 1987).
   c. This formula takes into account the child's age, height, weight, and serum creatinine.

d. The Schwartz formula:
eGFR = k x (height in cm) ÷ serum Cr
   (1) k = 0.33 in preemie infants.
   (2) k = 0.45 in term infants to 1 year of age.
   (3) k = 0.55 in children to 13 years of age.
   (4) k = 0.70 in adolescent males (females remain at 0.55 after age 13 years).
3. The acronym RIFLE stands for the increasing severity classes: Risk, Injury, and Failure, and the two outcome classes, Loss and ESRD.
   a. The three severity grades are defined by the changes in SCr or urine output, and the two outcome criteria are defined by the duration of loss of kidney function.
   b. This staging and classification system is almost identical to what was previously described for adults, but any pediatric clinician will tell you that children are not just little adults.
   c. Even small changes in a child's volume status can have significant impact in determining their outcome.
   d. The use of this diagnostic tool can assist with achieving an earlier diagnosis of AKI and aid in the development of newer preventive strategies (Yang & Bonventre, 2010).
4. Using the RIFLE criteria or pRIFLE for children to define AKI creates a paradigm for the syndrome that includes a time frame for each classification.
   a. The purpose of setting a time frame for diagnosis of AKI is to clarify the meaning of "acute." Changes in SCr that occur over many weeks is not AKI (KDIGO, 2012a). The RIFLE criteria (GFR criteria on left and urine output criteria on right):
      (1) Three severity grades:
         (a) 1st class – Risk: Increased SCr x 1.5 or GFR decrease > 25% urine output < 5 mL/kg/h times 6 hours.
         (b) 2nd class – Injury: Increased SCr x 2 or GFR decrease > 50% urine output < 5 mL/kg/h times 12 hours.
         (c) 3rd class – Failure: Increased SCr x 3, GFR decrease 75%, or SCr > 4 mg/dL. Urine output < 3 mL/kg/h x 24 hrs or anuria x 12 hrs.
      (2) Two outcome criteria.
         (a) Loss – Persistent ARF: complete loss of kidney function > 4 weeks.
         (b) ESRD – End-stage kidney disease (> 3 months).
5. Refer to Figure 1.34, which depicts the RIFLE criteria and the AKIN criteria.

M. AKIN classification.
   1. The AKIN criteria were devised by the Acute Kidney Injury Network (AKIN), an international network of AKI researchers to modify the RIFLE criteria and capture smaller changes in SCr (> 0.3 mg/dL or 26.5 μmol/L) when they occur within a 48-hour period not captured by RIFLE.
   a. Studies by Joannidis and colleagues (2009) compared the RIFLE criteria with and without the AKIN modification.
   b. The data derived indicate a strong rationale to use both RIFLE and AKIN criteria to identify and define AKI using this stage-based approach (KDIGO, 2012a).
   2. AKIN classification (Joannidis et al., 2009).
      a. Stage 1: ≥ 0.3 mg/ld (26.2 μmol/L) or ≥ 150 to 200% increase from baseline SCr.
      b. Stage 2: ≥ 200% to 299% increase from baseline SCr.
      c. Stage 3: ≥ 300 increase from baseline SCr or absolute SCr ≥ 4.0 mg/dL (354μmol/ L) with an acute rise ≥ 0.5 mg/dL (44 μmol/L) or initiation of KRT.
   3. Future research opportunities.
      a. Genetic research in relation to kidney disease and kidney transplantation is growing rapidly. Preclinical investigations aimed at understanding pathways of kidney disease, disease progression, and biomarkers of risk are underway. This research is leading to a more in-depth understanding of issues in renal transplantation and the pathogenesis of polycystic kidney disease among other etiologies.
      b. The role of biomarkers other than SCr in the diagnosis and prognosis of AKI offers hope for early detection and prevention of AKI (KDIGO, 2012a).
      c. There is a clinical need for earlier intervention and treatment of AKI.
      d. New serum and urine biomarkers have emerged, which will offer improved methods for risk assessment and assist in offering prognostic value.
      e. Two that are being investigated for clinical relevance are urine neutrophil gelatinase-associated lipocalin and serum cystatin.
      f. Other research.
         (1) Focuses on the use of a dipstick to check the pH of saliva that correlates with a person's urea level.
         (2) This novel test strip has the promise of assisting clinicians in detecting AKI in undeveloped countries where there is no access to laboratory facilities (Calice et al., 2013).
      g. Much research remains to be done in this area to validate alternative approaches to the diagnosis of AKI (Coca et al., 2008).

II. Chronic kidney disease.

A. General concepts.
1. The term *chronic kidney disease* (CKD) describes heterogenerous conditions involving the structure and function of the kidneys. There is wide variation in how the disease is described due to differing causes, severities, and rates of progression (Levey & Coresh, 2012).
2. Kidney disease impacts millions of people around the world.
   a. One in every three Americans is at risk for developing kidney disease, and the risk increases with age. It is estimated that one in nine people in the United States have kidney disease, but most do not know it.
   b. Because kidney disease remains asymptomatic until the later stages, many times it is undiagnosed. Diagnosis of CKD sometimes requires a clinician's suspicion of its existence.
   c. Early detection has the potential to slow the progression of kidney disease, so timely diagnosis is important (Grams et al., 2013).
3. CKD is a worldwide public health problem with increasing prevalence and is correlated with increased costs and poor patient outcomes (Fink et al., 2012).
   a. Kidney disease contributes to the death of over 90,000 Americans every year (USRDS, 2014).
   b. In the United States, over 400,000 people require dialysis to sustain their life (USRDS, 2014).
4. CKD is associated with medical diseases such as diabetes, hypertension, and cardiovascular disease (CVD).
5. The aging population and rising obesity and diabetes rates predict a continued increase in prevalence rates in developed as well as undeveloped countries (Levey & Coresh, 2012).

B. Clinical manifestations.
1. CKD, in its early stages, can occur without symptoms and is usually identified while evaluating other comorbid conditions (e.g., diabetes, hypertension, kidney stones).
2. Some etiologies of CKD progress more quickly and result in development of kidney failure within months. The majority of patients diagnosed with CKD progress slowly, over decades. Unfortunately most will die prior to ever reaching CKD stage 5.
3. Symptoms can be attributed to complications of reduced kidney function, and when severe and no longer managed medically, must be treated with kidney replacement therapy (KRT), such as dialysis or transplantation (KDIGO, 2013).
4. Complications of the disease become apparent and more readily identified at the later stages of CKD when GFR is decreased (GFR < 30 mL/min/1.73 m^2).
5. At this later stage, signs of fluid, electrolyte, endocrine, and metabolic derangements can be detected (Fink et al., 2012).
6. Initially, the goal of treatment is to preserve kidney function, control uremic symptoms, prevent complications, and prepare for kidney replacement therapy as the disease progresses (Levey & Coresh, 2012).
7. The major causes of morbidity and mortality in the CKD population are progression to CKD stage 5 and development of cardiovascular disease (CVD). This has resulted in viewing CKD as a global health concern, not just as an end-organ problem that requires KRT (Hallon & Orth, 2010).

C. Background information on clinical practice guidelines regarding CKD. These guidelines are universal declarations that help practitioners and patients make decisions concerning appropriate health care for specific clinical conditions.
1. The guidelines can decrease inconsistency of care, enhance patient outcomes, and improve shortcomings in the delivery of health care (Levey & Coresh, 2012).
2. In 2002, the Kidney Disease Outcomes Quality Initiative (KDOQI) was released by the National Kidney Foundation (NKF). The guidelines examined the evaluation, classification, and stratification of risk factors for CKD.
   a. It offered a conceptual framework for defining and staging CKD, standardized the terminology, and provided treatment guidelines.
   b. The document helped to shift the focus from end-stage renal disease (CKD stage 5) to less advanced stages of CKD with the goal of improving early detection and ultimately outcomes.
   c. The implementation of the 2002 KDOQI guidelines uncovered and brought to light several issues.
      (1) It was found that application of the guidelines to the elderly population resulted in over or misdiagnosis.
      (2) In addition, albuminuria gained a heightened sense of importance because of its correlation with cardiovascular mortality.
      (3) As the 2013 Kidney Disease Improving Global Guidelines (KDIGO) guidelines reflect, albuminuria was added into the categorical classification of CKD in order to denote risk, not only for CKD, but cardiovascular related mortality (KDIGO, 2013).

D. Kidney Disease Improving Global Outcomes (KDIGO).
1. In 2003, KDIGO, an international nonprofit foundation, was formed to improve the care of individuals with kidney disease. Because of international interest and increasing worldwide prevalence of CKD, the need to examine patient outcomes was important.
2. A large amount of data has been created since 2002, and a need was recognized to review, update, and modify the original 2002 KDOQI guidelines (Levey et al., 2010).
3. In 2009, KDIGO conducted a meta-analysis and convened a conference to examine the original definition, assessment, and staging of CKD. The conference studied the association of GFR and albuminuria to patient mortality and outcomes.
4. It was agreed to preserve the current definition for CKD and to alter the classification system by including albuminuria, subdividing stage 3, and stressing clinical diagnosis (Levey et al., 2010).

E. Definition of CKD.
1. "CKD is defined as abnormalities of kidney structure or function, present for > 3 months, with implications for health" (KDIGO, 2013, p19).
2. The definition remains unchanged from KDOQI Clinical Practice Guidelines published in 2002, except for the addition of "with implications for health."
3. The addition indicates that many structural or functional abnormalities may be present and may have consequences for the health of the particular person (KDIGO, 2013).

F. Criteria for the definition of CKD (see Table 1.5).
1. Duration > 3 months on the basis of documentation or inference.
2. Glomerular filtration rate (GFR) < 60 mL/min per 1.73 m².
3. Kidney damage as defined by structural or

Table 1.5

Criteria for Definition of CKD

Criteria	Comment
Duration > 3 months, based on documentation or inference	**Duration is necessary to distinguish chronic from acute kidney diseases.** • Clinical evaluation will often enable documentation or inference of duration. • Documentation of duration is usually not declared in epidemiologic studies.
GFR , 30 mL/min/1.73 m² (GFR categories G3a-G5)	**GFR is the best overall index of kidney function in health and disease.** • The normal GFR in young adults is approximately 125 mL/min/1.73 m². GFR <15 mL/min/ 1.73 m² (GFR category G5) is defined as kidney failure. • Decreased GFR can be detected by current estimating equations for GFR based on SCr or cystatin C but not by SCr or cystatin C alone. • Decreased eGFR can be confirmed by measured GFR, if required.
Kidney damage as defined by structural abnormalities or functional abnormalities other than decreased GFR	**Albuminuria as a marker of kidney damage (increased glomerular permeability), urine AER ≥ 30 mg/24 hours, approximately equivalent to urine ACR ≥ 30 mg/g (≥ 3 mg/mmol).** • The normal urine ACR in young adults is < 10 mg/g (< 1 mg/mmol). • Urine ACR 30–300 mg/g (> 30 mg/mmol; category A3) generally corresponds to "machroalbuminuria," now termed "severely increased." • Urine ACR > 2200 mg/g (220 mg/mmol) may be accompanied by signs and symptoms of nephrotic syndrome (e.g., low serum albumin, edema, and high-serum cholesterol). • Threshold value corresponds approximately to urine reagent strip values of trace or +, depending on urine concentration. • High-urine ACR can be confirmed by urine albumin excretion in a timed urine collection expressed as AER.
(continues)	**Urinary sediment abnormalities as markers of kidney damage.** • Isolated nonvisible (microscopic) hematuria with abnormal RBC morphology (anisocytosis) in GBM disorders. • RBC casts in proliferative glomerulonephritis. • WBC casts in pyelonephritis or international nephritis. • Oval fat bodies or fatty casts in diseases with proteinuria. • Granular casts and renal tubular epithelial cells in many parenchymal diseases (nonspecific).

Table 1.5 continues

Table 1.5 (continued)

Criteria for Definition of CKD

Criteria	Comment
Kidney damage as defined by structural abnormalities or functional abnormalities other than decreased GFR (continued from previous page)	**Renal tubular disorders.** • Renal tubular acidosis. • Nephrogenic diabetes insipidus. • Renal potassium wasting. • Renal magnesium wasting. • Fanconi syndrome. • Nonalbumin proteinuria. • Cystinuria.
	Pathologic abnormalities detected by histology or inferred (examples of causes). • Glomerular diseases (diabetes, autoimmune diseases, systemic infections, drugs, neoplasia). • Vascular diseases (atherosclerosis, hypertension, ischemia, vasculitis, thrombotic microangiopathy). • Tubulointerstitial diseases (urinary tract infections, stones, obstruction, drug toxicity). • Cystic and congenital diseases.
	Structural abnormalities as markers of kidney damage detected by imaging (ultrasound, computed tomography, and magnetic resonance with or without contrast, isotope scans, angiography). • Polycystic kidneys. • Dysplastic kidneys. • Hydronephrosis due to obstruction. • Cortical scarring due to infarcts, pyelonephritis, or associated with vesicoureteral reflux. • Renal masses or enlarged kidneys due to infiltrative diseases. • Renal artery stenosis. • Small and hyperechoic kidneys (common in more severe CKD due to many parenchymal diseases).
	History of kidney transplantation. • Kidney biopsies in most kidney transplant recipients have histopathologic abnormalities even if GFR is > 60 mL/min/1.73 m^2 (GFR categories G1–G2) and ACR is < 30 mg/g (< 3 mg/mmol). • Kidney transplant recipients have increased risk for mortality and kidney failure compared to populations without kidney disease. • Kidney transplant recipients routinely receive subspecialty care.

Abbreviations: ACR – albumin-to-creatinine ratio; AER –albumin excretion rate; CKD –chronic kidney disease; eGFR –estimated glomerular filteration rate; GBM –glomerular basement membrane; GFR –glomerular filtration rate; RBC –red blood cell; SCr –serum creatinine, WBC –white blood cell.

Source: Kidney Disease: Improving Global Outcomes (KDIGO) CKD Work Group. KDIGO 2012 Clinical Practice Guideline for the Evaluation and Management of Chronic Kidney Disease. *Kidney International Supplements 2013*; 3: 1–150 (originally table 3 on page 20). Used with permission.

functional abnormalities other than decreased GFR.

4. Normal GFR in a young adult is about 125 mL/min per 1.73 m^2. GFR < 15 mL/min per 1.73 m^2 is defined as kidney failure (KDIGO, 2013).
5. One common marker of kidney damage is albuminuria, which is also one of the earlier markers of glomerular diseases such as diabetic glomerulosclerosis.
   a. Albuminuria also occurs with hypertensive nephrosclerosis.
   b. Most important, albuminuria needs to be considered as a cardiovascular risk.
6. Other important markers include abnormal

urinary sediment (e.g., microscopic hematuria), red blood and white blood cell casts, granular and renal epithelial cells, and oval fat bodies.
7. Structural abnormalities of the kidney can be detected by imaging such as ultrasound, computed tomography, magnetic resonance, and angiography. This is especially useful in detecting cystic kidneys, renal masses, abnormalities in size, cortical scarring, and renal artery stenosis (KDIGO, 2013).

G. Staging of CKD (see Table 1.6). KDIGO (2013) classified CKD based on cause (C), GFR category (G), and albuminuria category, (A).

Table 1.6

CGA Staging of CKD: Examples of Nomenclature and Comments

Cause	GFR category	Albuminuria category	Criterion for CKD	Comment
Diabetic kidney disease	G5	A3	Decreased GFR, albuminuria	Most common patient in the low clearance clinic.
Idiopathic focal sclerosis	G2	A3	Albuminuria	Common cause of nephrotic syndrome in childhood.
Kidney transplant recipient	G2	A1	History of kidney transplantation	Best outcome after kidney transplantation.
Polycystic kidney disease	G2	A1	Imaging abnormality	Most common disease caused by a mutation in a single gene.
Vesicoureteral reflex	G1	A1	Imaging abnormality	Common condition in children.
Distal renal tubular acidosis	G1	A1	Electrolyte abnormalities	Rare genetic disorder.
Hypertensive kidney disease	G4	A2	Decreased GFR and albuminuria	Usually due to long-standing poorly controlled hypertension, likely to include patients with genetic predisposition – more common in blacks – who should be referred to nephrologist of severely decreased GFR.
CKD presumed due to diabetes and hypertension	G4	A1	Decreased GFR	Should be referred to nephrologist because of severely decreased GFR.
CKD presumed due to diabetes and hypertension	G3	A3	Albuminuria	Should be referred to a nephrologist because of albuminuria.
CKD presumed due to diabetes and hypertension	G3a	A1	Decreased GFR	Very common, may not require referral to nephrologist.
CKD cause unknown	G3a	A1	Decreased GFR	May be the same patient as above.

Abbreviations: CGA – cause, GFR category and albuminuria category; CKD – chronic kidney disease; GFR – glomerular filtration rate.

Note: Patients above the thick horizontal line are likely to be encountered in nephrology practice. Patients below the thick horizontal line are likely to be encountered in primary care practice and in nephrology practice.

Source: Kidney Disease: Improving Global Outcomes (KDIGO) CKD Work Group. KDIGO 2012 Clinical Practice Guideline for the Evaluation and Management of Chronic Kidney Disease. *Kidney International Supplements 2013*; 3: 1–150 (originally table 8 on page 32). Used with permission.

1. Causes of kidney disease were included in the staging because of the importance in predicting outcomes of CKD and to help in selecting cause specific treatments.
2. GFR is considered the best overall index of kidney function and becomes decreased after widespread kidney damage.
3. Albuminuria was included to express risk, severity of kidney injury, and progression. Numerous studies over the years have demonstrated a strong association between albuminuria and cardiovascular related mortality (KDIGO, 2013).

H. Causes of CKD. KDIGO indicated that the cause of CKD is officially designated based on the presence or absence of systemic disease and the location within the kidney of pathologic or anatomical abnormalities (see Table 1.7).

I. GFR categories in CKD (see Table 1.8).
 1. Equations to estimate GFR.
  a. Several factors can affect serum creatinine concentrations, including age, sex, race, diet, body size, and certain medications.
  b. Serum creatinine levels alone are not used to estimate kidney function.

Table 1.7

Systemic Diseases and Primary Diseases Contributing to CKD

	Examples of systemic diseases affecting the kidney	Examples of primary kidney diseases (absence of systemic diseases affecting the kidney)
Glomerular diseases	Diabetes, systemic autoimmune diseases, systemic infections, drugs, neoplasia (including amyloidosis)	Diffuse, focal, or crescentic proliferative GN; focal and segmental glomerulosclerosis, membranous nephropathy, minimal change disease
Tubulointerstitial diseases	Systemic infections, autoimmune, sarcoidosis, drugs, urate, environmental toxins (lead, aristolochic acid), neoplasia (myeloma)	Urinary-tract infections, stones, obstruction
Vascular diseases	Atherosclerosis, hypertension, ischemia, cholesterol, emboli, systemic vasculitis, thrombotic microangiopathy, systemic sclerosis	ANCA-associated renal limited vasculitis, fibromuscular dysplasia
Cystic and congenital diseases	Polycystic kidney disease, Alport syndrome, Fabry disease	Renal dysplasia, medullary cystic disease, podocytopathies

Abbreviations: ANCA – antineutrophil cytoplasmic antibody; CKD – chronic kidney disease, GN – glomerulonephritis. Genetic diseases are not considered separately because some diseases in each category are now recognized as having genetic determinants.

Source: Kidney Disease: Improving Global Outcomes (KDIGO) CKD Work Group. KDIGO 2012 Clinical Practice Guideline for the Evaluation and Management of Chronic Kidney Disease. *Kidney International Supplements 2013*; 3: 1–150 (originally table 4 on page 27, entitled Classification of CKD Based on Presence or Absence of Systemic Disease and Location Within the Kidney of Pathologic-Anatomic Findings). Used with permission.

c. Instead, GFR equations are used that include age, sex, race, and body size along with serum creatinine levels to estimate GFR.
2. The Cockroft–Gault formula is the oldest equation taking into account sex, age, and weight, along with serum creatinine.
   a. Limitations of this formula.
      (1) It is not accurate with GFR ranges above 60 mL/minute.
      (2) Estimates creatinine clearance instead of GFR.
      (3) It tends to overestimate the GFR.
   b. This formula is mainly used to estimate the pharmacokinetic properties of drugs in individuals with decreased kidney function. It remains the standard of drug dosing in this population (Stevens et al., 2010).
3. The Modification of Diet in Renal Disease Study equation (MDRD) is a four-variable equation using serum creatinine, age, sex, and race.
   a. The validity of the equation has been tested in African Americans, individuals with diabetic kidney disease, and recipients of kidney transplants.
   b. In 2004, the National Kidney Disease Education Program of the National Institute of Diabetes and Digestive and Kidney Diseases

Table 1.8

GFR Categories in CKD

GFR category	GFR (mL/min/1.73m^2)	Terms
G1	≥ 90	Normal or high
G2	60–89	Mildly decreased*
G3a	45–59	Mildly to moderately decreased
G3b	30–44	Moderately to severely decreased
G4	15–29	Severely decreased
G5	< 15	Kidney failure

Abbreviations: CKD – chronic kidney disease; GFR – glomerular filtration rate
*Relative to young adult level
In absence of evidence of kidney damage, neither GFR category G1 nor G2 fulfill the criteria for CKD

Source: Kidney Disease: Improving Global Outcomes (KDIGO) CKD Work Group. KDIGO 2012 Clinical Practice Guideline for the Evaluation and Management of Chronic Kidney Disease. *Kidney International Supplements 2013*; 3: 1–150 (originally table 5 on page 27). Used with permission.

(NIDDKD) recommended to clinical laboratories in the United States to report estimates of GFR using this equation (Stevens et al., 2010).

4. One of the newest GFR-estimating equations is the Chronic Kidney Disease Epidemiology Collaboration Equation (CKD-EPI). It has the same four variables as the MDRD equation, but is more accurate across a wider population of individuals.

   a. The terms used to describe the various stages are meant to ensure precision and are descriptors that need to be put into the clinical context of the patient.

   b. For example, stage G2 or mildly decreased function without other markers does not indicate that the patient has CKD.

   c. Data from numerous studies support the division of G3 into a and b categories based on risk profiles and differing outcomes (KDIGO, 2013).

J. Albuminuria in CKD (see Table 1.9).

   1. Definition. Albuminuria refers to an abnormal loss of albumin in the urine.

   a. Recent studies have also indicated that albuminuria is a risk factor not only for CKD but also cardiovascular disease (KDIGO, 2013).

   b. It can be inconvenient to collect urine in a 24-hour sample to calculate the albumin excretion rate (AER).

   2. The recommended method to estimate the level of albuminuria in 24 hours is to obtain an albumin creatinine ratio (ACR) from a random sample of urine.

   3. Albuminuria categories are important because they can help to denote risk, identify pathology, and offer insight into prognosis (see Table 1.10).

   a. The greater quantities are associated with increasing mortality.

   b. Data from worldwide studies suggests the prevalence of CKD to be between 10% and 16%, but there is scarce information about population prevalence by GFR and ACR categories.

K. Risk factors affecting initiation and progression of CKD.

   1. CKD is a process that involves multiple strikes or

Table 1.9

Relationship among Categories for Albuminuria and Proteinuria

Measure	Categories		
	Normal to mildly increased (A1)	**Moderately increased (A2)**	**Severely increased (A3)**
AER (mg/24 hours)	< 30	30–300	> 300
PER (mg/24 hours)	< 150	15–500	> 500
ACR (mg/mmol) (mg/g)	< 3 < 30	3–30 30–300	> 30 > 300
PCR (mg/mmol) (mg/g)	< 15 < 150	15–50 150–500	> 50 > 500
Protein reagent strip	Negative to trace	Trace to +	+ or greater

Abbreviations: ACR – albumin-to-creatinine ratio; AER – albumin excretion rate; PCR – protein-to-creatinine ratio; PER – protein excretion rate.

Albuminuria and proteinuria can be measured using excretion rates in timed urine collections, ratio of concentrations to creatinine concentration in spot urine samples, and reagent strips in spot urine samples. Relationships among measurement methods within a category are not exact. For example, the relationships between AER and ACR and between PER and PCRT are based on the assumption that average creatinine excretion rate is approximately 1.0 g/d or 10 mmol/d. The conversions are rounded for pragmatic reasons. (For an exact conversion from mg/g of creatinine to mg/mmol of creatinine multiply by 0.113.) Creatinine excretion varies with age, sex, race, and diet; therefore the relationship among these categories is approximate only. ACR < 10 mg/g (< 1 mg/mmol) is considered normal; ACR 10-30 mg/g (1–3 mg/mmol) is considered "high normal." ACR > 2200 mg/g (> 220 mg/mmol) is considered "nephrotic range." The relationship between urine reagent strip results and other measures depends on urine concentration.

Source: Kidney Disease: Improving Global Outcomes (KDIGO) CKD Work Group. KDIGO 2012 Clinical Practice Guideline for the Evaluation and Management of Chronic Kidney Disease. *Kidney International Supplements 2013*; 3: 1–150 (originally table 7 on page 31). Used with permission.

Table 1.10		Persistent albuminuria categories Description and range		
Prognosis of CKD by GFR and Albuminuria Categories: KDIGO 2012		A1	A2	A3
		Normal to mildly increased	Moderately increased	Severely increased
		< 30 mg/g < 3 mg/mmol	30–300 mg/g 3–30 mg/mmol	> 300 mg/g > 30 mg/mmol
G1	Normal or high	$\geq$ 90			
G2	Mildly decreased	60–89			
G3a	Mildly to moderately decreased	45–59			
G3b	Moderately to severely decreased	30–44			
G4	Severely decreased	15–29			
G5	Kidney failure	< 15			

GFR categories (mL/min/1.73m²) Description and range

Dark gray, low risk (if no other markers of kidney disease, no CKD); Light blue, moderately increased risk; Light gray, high risk; Dark blue, very high risk.

Abbreviations: CKD – chronic kidney disease; GFR – glomerular filtration rate; KDIGO – Kidney Disease: Improving Global Outcomes.

Source: Kidney Disease: Improving Global Outcomes (KDIGO) CKD Work Group. KDIGO 2012 Clinical Practice Guideline for the Evaluation and Management of Chronic Kidney Disease. *Kidney International Supplements 2013*; 3: 1–150 (originally figure 9 on page 34). Used with permission.

insults to the body and it rarely advances in a straight linear way.

2. Several risk factors for CKD can be in play at the same time.
3. Known susceptibility factors predispose to CKD. Some of the known factors involve genetic and familial aspects such as (Bello et al., 2010):
   a. Race, with a higher incidence in Afro-Caribbeans and Indo-Asians.
   b. Maternal–fetal factors, such as low birth weight.
   c. A higher incidence in the elderly and in males.
4. Other risk factors.
   a. Initiating factors that can directly trigger kidney damage.
   b. Progression factors are connected to deterioration of kidney function.
5. Progression of CKD is variable, and many individuals have stable kidney function over many years or die prematurely of cardiovascular disease before requiring KRT. Disease development is often associated with breakpoints in their progression.
   a. These breakpoints can occur in a spontaneous fashion or can be the result of secondary insults

such as infection, dehydration, exposure to nephrotoxins via drugs or radio contrast medium (RCM), or changes in systemic blood pressure control.
   b. The rate of progression can also be influenced by development of acute kidney injury, sometimes termed *acute-on-chronic kidney disease* (Bello et al., 2010).
6. CKD recognition has improved during the last decade due to identification of risk factors, expanded laboratory testing, application of clinical practice guidelines, and increased awareness of practitioners (Levey & Coresh, 2012).

L. Diseases of the kidney.
1. Developmental/congenital disorders of the kidney.
   a. Congenital anomalies of the kidney and urinary tract appear in approximately 1 in 500 births and are a major cause of morbidity in children. These conditions can occur in the kidneys, collecting system, bladder, or urethra. They account for the majority of pediatric cases of kidney failure (Song & Yosypiv, 2010).

b. Absent kidneys.
   (1) Unilateral renal agenesis is complete absence of one kidney and can be familial, resulting from failure in formation of the ureteral bud. The function of the single kidney should be confirmed by additional testing. This condition occurs in 1 to 500 to 1000 births.
   (2) Bilateral renal agenesis is related to pulmonary hyoplasia and is lethal. The prevalence is approximately 1 in 10,000.
c. Renal malformations include many conditions. Misplaced kidneys include renal ectopia, malrotation, and crossed fused kidneys. *Horseshoe kidney* is a term that describes the joining of both kidneys at the lower pole; they are usually drained by two ureters. This condition is found more commonly in males.
   (1) Renal dysplasia can occur as an isolated anomaly of development.
      (a) Characteristically results in small, irregular kidneys.
      (b) Can also result in cyst formation and development of abnormal structures.
   (2) Renal hypoplasia.
      (a) Defined as significantly reduced renal mass and number of nephrons with no evidence of maldevelopment of the parenchyma.
      (b) Results from arrested development during gestation producing hypertrophy of the glomeruli and tubules of the kidney.
   (3) Renal multicystic dysplasia describes kidneys that are enlarged due to formation of cystic structures; approximately 10% of patients have a family history (Connolly & Neild, 2010).
d. Management of congenital and developmental renal tract abnormalities.
   (1) Educate patient and family regarding clinical condition to promote understanding and encourage adherence. Ensure that the patient, family, and primary care provider are aware that individualized clinical management is required.
   (2) Stress the absolute necessity of long-term follow-up with patients being followed at regular intervals throughout life.
   (3) Obstruction is a common occurrence and must be excluded if there is a change in kidney function. The patient and family members should be taught the symptoms of obstruction and appropriate actions to be taken.
   (4) A urinary tract infection (UTI) is common

with these abnormalities due to urine stagnation, stones, foreign bodies such as stents or catheters, previous infections, and renal scarring. UTIs must be treated in a timely manner after obtaining a urine culture.
   (5) Teach patients and family the signs of infection and emphasize the importance of obtaining early care to prevent progression of CKD.
   (6) Monitor kidney function and check patient for proteinuria and hypertension. Stress the importance of blood pressure measurement to patient and family and encourage home monitoring.
   (7) Observe for signs of progression such as acidosis and bone disease (Connolly & Neild, 2010).
2. Cystic diseases of the kidney.
   a. These disorders are numerous and can be inherited or acquired. They share the common feature of renal cyst formation in the kidney and systemically as well.
   b. The kidneys can develop to the size of a football (possibly up to 30 pounds) because the cysts ultimately destroy the intervening parenchyma of the kidney.
   c. The cysts are filled with fluid that may be clear, turbid, or hemorrhagic. They occur in a broad range of ages and may be single or multiple in nature (Guay-Woodford, 2010).
   d. Autosomal dominant polycystic kidney disease (ADPKD) is a hereditary disease associated with renal cyst formation in the kidneys and other organs such as the liver and pancreas (see Figure 1.37).
      (1) ADPKD is the most commonly inherited type of renal cystic disease. It occurs worldwide and in all races with a prevalence range of 1:400 to 1:1000.
      (2) Kidneys affected by this disease have diffuse cysts and enlargement with sizes varying from normal to weights greater than 4 kilograms (Torres & Harris, 2010).
      (3) Renal ultrasound is safe and relatively low in cost so it can be used for presymptomatic testing. If the results of imaging tests are not conclusive or a precise diagnosis is required, the patient may be referred for genetic testing.
      (4) Structural abnormalities account for some of the clinical manifestations that occur with ADPKD. These may include pain from cyst hemorrhage, kidney stones, or infections.
      (5) Visible hematuria occurs in approximately 40% of patients with ADPKD. Hypertension is a frequent finding in these

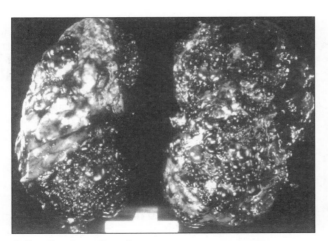

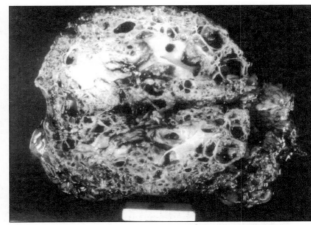

A. Exterior view of two large
cadaveric polycystic kidneys. The
bubble-like structures are cysts.
The ruler is 6 inches in length.

Figure 1.37. Polycystic kidneys.

B. Interior view of a bisected large
cadaveric kidney. Many cysts
are present. The ruler is 6 inches
in length.

patients and contributes to the progression
of kidney disease (Torres & Harris, 2010).
(6) There is a high variability in phenotypes in
ADPKD, and two types have been identified.
 (a) PKD 1 associated disease is severe due
 to the development of more cysts at an
 early age, not to quicker growth of
 cysts, with development of CKD stage
 5 around age 54.
 (b) PKD 2 is less severe, and the average
 age for developing CKD stage 5 is 74
 years old (Torres & Harris, 2010).
(7) Treatment of ADPKD is aimed at the renal
and extrarenal complications of the
disease. Advances have been made in the
understanding of the genetics and system
of cyst development and enlargement.
Current studies are examining the potential
for possible eradication of the disease with
various interventions (Torres & Harris,
2010).
e. Autosomal dominant medullary cystic kidney
disease (ADMCKD) is rarer, with some patients
having parents that are unaffected, but the disease
is noted in a second- or third-degree relative.
(1) The disease is associated with
hyperurecemia and gout.
(2) The diagnosis can be made based on family
history (Guay-Woodford, 2010).
f. Tuberous sclerosis complex (TSC) is an
autosomal dominant syndrome that involves
the formation of tumor-like malformations
called hamartomas, which form in multiple
organ systems incorporating the brain, heart,
lungs, skin, and kidneys.

(1) Neurologic symptoms are usually the
presenting symptoms, and seizures occur in
approximately 90% of affected individuals.
(2) Kidney manifestations are the second most
common finding, with angiomyolipomatas
occurring in up to 80% of affected patients,
and present a risk due to hemorrhage of
these lesions and invasion of normal renal
parenchyma. Renal cystic disease is usually
benign and tends to occur in about 25% of
patients (Dixon et al., 2010).
(3) Diagnosis of this syndrome depends on the
size, location, and number of lesions.
(4) Clinical features of TSC may include
seizures, learning disabilities or autism,
developmental delays, skin lesions, and
interstitial lung disease. Additionally, tumors
may be found in the brain, retina, kidney,
and heart. Annual renal imaging tests are
recommended for patients with TSC.
(5) Treatment of TSC is geared to evaluation
and possible surgical removal of
problematic angiomyolipomas (Guay-
Woodford, 2010).
g. Autosomal recessive polycystic kidney disease
(ARPKD) is an inherited malformation
complex affecting various areas in the kidney. It
begins in utero with the cystic lesion
superimposed on normal renal development.
(1) ARPKD is usually bilateral; cysts can occur
in the liver also.
(2) The estimated perinatal mortality is
approximately 30% (Guay-Woodford, 2010).
h. Juvenile nephronophthisis (NPHP) and
medullary cystic disease complex share many

features including cyst formation, basement membrane thickening, and diffuse interstitial sclerosis.

(1) NPHP is an autosomal recessive disease that occurs in childhood accounting for 5% to 15% of kidney failure in children and adolescents.

(2) The kidneys become contracted with atrophy of tubules and parenchyma.

(3) This condition is associated with retinal atrophy as well (Guay-Woodford, 2010).

i. Medullary sponge kidney gives the kidney a "spongy" appearance due to dilated medullary and papillary collecting ducts.

(1) The disease is relatively asymptomatic unless nephrolithiasis, infection, or hematuria occurs. Symptoms occur at ages 40 to 50 years and include hematuria, stones and granular debris, and hypercalcemia.

(2) The diagnosis is confirmed by imaging testing (Guay-Woodford, 2010).

j. Simple cysts occur more frequently in men, and they originate from the distal convoluted tubules or collecting ducts.

(1) Some risk factors have been identified: smoking, kidney dysfunction, and hypertension.

(2) These cysts are usually asymptomatic and they may be solitary or multiple. Most are found as incidental findings occurring during abdominal imaging studies.

(3) Treatment includes draining under ultrasound guidance or, in larger lesions, laparoscopic surgery (Guay-Woodford, 2010).

k. Acquired cystic kidney disease (ACKD) occurs in patients with kidney failure. Risk increases with time on dialysis. After 10 years of hemodialysis or peritoneal dialysis, prevalence rates reach 80% to 100%.

(1) Patients are usually asymptomatic, and most cysts are discovered during imaging testing. In 25% of kidneys with ACKD, tumors are seen; one third of these undergo a malignant transformation to renal cell carcinoma. Because of the slow growth of the tumors, observation with repeated imaging studies is recommended.

(2) Treatment can range from conservative measures for complications as they occur to nephrectomy depending on patient status (Eitner, 2010).

3. Tubulointerstitial diseases of the kidney.

a. Proximal renal tubular acidosis (Type 2) occurs when the proximal tubule has a decreased ability to reabsorb filtered bicarbonate. There is increased bicarbonate delivery to the loop of Henle and distal nephron that exceeds their capacity.

(1) This results in bicarbonate being lost in the urine, with a resulting decrease in serum bicarbonate levels. Hypokalemia is present due to associated hyperaldosteronism and increased distal nephron sodium reabsorption, resulting in potassium wasting.

(2) This type of renal tubular acidosis (RTA) is associated with Fanconi syndrome (Palmer & Alpern, 2010).

b. Hypokalemic distal renal tubular acidosis (Type 1) results in the patient's inability to acidify the urine in response to metabolic acidosis. There is a decrease in hydrogen secretion in the distal nephron, which results in loss of bicarbonate in the urine and prevents acidification of the urine and urinary ammonia excretion.

(1) Urinary calcium excretion is increased, so nephrolithiasis and nephrocalcinosis are seen with this type of renal tubular acidosis.

(2) Primary distal RTA can be familial or idiopathic in nature. Secondary causes are due to autoimmune disorders, genetic diseases, and drugs such as amphotericin B and toluene, which is inhaled during glue sniffing.

(3) Long-term treatment of this condition involves the administration of sodium and potassium alkali substances (Palmer & Alpern, 2010).

c. Fanconi syndrome is a dysfunction of the proximal tubule resulting in extreme urinary excretion of amino acids, glucose, phosphate, and bicarbonate.

(1) These urinary losses result in metabolic abnormalities such as electrolyte disorders, acidosis, dehydration, and bone problems such as rickets and osteomalacia.

(2) There are numerous inherited disorders associated with Fanconi syndrome, such as cystinosis, Wilson's disease, and galactosemia mitochondrial cytopathies.

(3) Some acquired causes of Fanconi syndrome are related to drugs such as cancer chemotherapy agents and heavy metal intoxication with lead and cadmium.

(4) Treatment is geared to underlying causes and treatment of the secondary biochemical problems. Bone disease should be treated with appropriate therapies (Foreman, 2010).

4. Renal masses.

a. The incidence of renal cancer has increased steadily over the past few decades due to enhanced methods of detection, including cross-sectional imaging using computerized tomography (CT) and magnetic resonance imaging (MRI).

(1) More than 50% of new cases are found incidentally. Kidney cancer is the most common tumor and now accounts for 3% of all cancers. Any solid mass larger than 3 cm should be considered malignant.

(2) The Bosniak classification of cystic renal masses is based on appearance on CT and presents the foundation for management of these masses based on risk of malignancy (Gkougkousis et al., 2010).

b. Many patients with kidney masses are asymptomatic, and masses remain nonpalable until the later stages of the disease.

(1) Most kidney cancers (e.g., renal cell carcinomas) are discovered incidentally by imaging studies for unrelated symptoms.

(2) Clinical signs, such as flank pain, gross hematuria, and palpable abdominal mass, may occur late in the disease along with metastatic symptoms such as bone pain.

(3) The aim of renal tumor biopsy is to determine malignancy and grade the renal mass (Ljungberg et al., 2010).

(4) Treatment options for renal cell cancers have expanded over the years. The most traditional approach has been to perform radical nephrectomy which predisposes the patient to CKD with attendant-associated risks.

(5) More recently, nephron-sparing procedures, such as partial nephrectomy, thermal ablation, and active surveillance, have become viable options (Campbell et al., 2009).

(6) Following surgery for renal cell cancer, the patient is at risk for sequelae such as proteinuria, glomerulosclerosis, and progression of kidney failure. Careful monitoring is warranted (Gkougkousis et al., 2010).

c. Wilms' tumor is a rare form of kidney cancer primarily seen in children, peaking at 3 to 4 years of age.

(1) It is one of the most common cancers of the kidney in this population and usually occurs unilaterally.

(2) Risk factors include female sex, African-American race, and positive family history.

(3) Treatment includes surgical resection followed by adjuvant chemotherapy and occasionally radiotherapy. Prognosis is quite good because of improvements in surgical treatment and chemotherapy (Carmichael et al., 2013).

5. Urinary tract infections (UTIs).

a. UTIs are the most common healthcare-associated infections. In the outpatient setting in the United States, UTIs account for 8.6 million visits to healthcare providers, 84% by women (Hooten, 2010). There are two main types of UTIs in adults: uncomplicated and complicated.

b. Uncomplicated UTIs.

(1) Acute uncomplicated cystitis in young women presents acutely with symptoms of dysuria, frequency, urgency, and occasionally suprapubic pain. Bacteriuria is also present.

(a) Most uncomplicated UTIs are caused by uropathogens – usually *Escherichia coli* (*E. coli*) – which are present in rectal flora and gain access to the bladder through the urethra.

(b) Treatment consists of a 3-day regimen of sulfonamides or fluoroquinalones. However, antimicrobial resistance has increased in the past few years, and new studies are underway to determine optimal treatment.

(c) Consideration of the adverse effects of this therapy, along with some newer agents, has resulted in updates to the guidelines (Gupta et al., 2011).

(2) Recurrent acute uncomplicated cystitis in women is often due to recurring infections and the persistence of the initial causative agent. Antimicrobial prophylaxis, behavioral modification strategies, and ingestion of cranberry products may be indicated.

(3) Acute uncomplicated pyelonephritis in women results from an ascending UTI that has infected the kidney.

(a) Symptoms can vary from a mild illness to a type of septic syndrome and can include fever, chills, flank pain, nausea, costrovertebral angle tenderness, and pyuria.

(b) Treatment with oral antimicrobials for 7 days is indicated for mild forms of the disease or parenteral therapy for hospitalized patients (Hooten, 2010).

(4) Acute cystitis in adults occurs in individuals with conditions with possible occult renal or prostate involvement.

(a) Contributing factors.
i. Male sex.
ii. Older adults.
iii. Pregnancy.
iv. Diabetes mellitus.
v. Recent urinary tract instrumentation.

vi. UTIs in childhood.
vii. Symptoms for more than 7 days.
      (b) Symptoms are the same as for
            uncomplicated UTIs.
      (c) A urine culture should be obtained, and
            it is important to assure that therapy is
            adequate because more serious
            complications can occur, especially in
            pregnant women or in individuals with
            diabetes (Hooten, 2010).
c. Complicated UTI may start with classic
    symptoms of cystitis, but may also include
    vague signs such as fatigue, nausea, abdominal
    discomfort, headache, or back pain for several
    weeks duration.
    (1) A cardinal sign is pyuria or bacteriuria.
          Diagnosis requires a urine culture.
    (2) Several underlying conditions can
          predispose patients to the development of
          complicated UTI. These include obstruction
          or other structural abnormalities; foreign
          bodies, such as catheters, stents, and tubes;
          and any condition that compromises
          immunity, such as with patients who have
          received a transplant (Hooten, 2010).
d. Catheter-associated infections are one of the
    most common infections worldwide due to the
    frequent use of urinary catheterization in
    hospitals and long-term care facilities (Hooten
    et al., 2010).
    (1) There is a high incidence of bacteriuria
          related to indwelling catheterization.
          Incidence approximates 3% to 10% per day.
    (2) The Infectious Disease Society of American
          has convened an expert panel to update the
          diagnosis and treatment of catheter-
          associated UTIs. Efforts are also geared to
          prevention of infection with alternative
          strategies to prevent the need for
          catheterization (Hooten et al., 2010).
    (3) Spinal cord injury changes the mechanisms
          of voiding and often necessitates catheter
          placement in the bladder making the
          treatment of UTI problematic.
          Fluoroquinilones are the agent of choice
          for treatment, but many pathogens have
          developed resistance (Hooten, 2010).
e. Prostatitis is related to reflux of infected urine
    from the urethra into the prostatic ducts and
    occurs at a rate of 2% to 10% in men during
    their lifetime. Symptoms vary widely, but
    recurrent UTIs with the same pathogen are a
    cardinal sign. Prostatitis is usually caused by
    gram negative bacteria, and duration of
    treatment should be continued for at least 30
    days (Hooten, 2010).
f. Papilliary necrosis occurs because the renal
    papillae are susceptible to ischemia, and any
    insults may cause necrosis.
    (1) In patients with diabetes, more than half
          will develop this condition after a UTI.
    (2) Cytoscopic surgery to remove obstructing
          papillae and administration of broad-
          spectrum antibiotics are recommended for
          treatment (Hooten, 2010).
g. Treatment of infectious diseases of the kidney is
    complex due to the changing number of
    antimicrobials, development of resistant
    strains, differing durations of therapy, and
    ongoing trials of various interventions. It is
    beyond the scope of this book to list all the
    various therapies in current use for specific
    infections.
h. Patient teaching should incorporate preventive
    measures such as urination after coitus and
    voiding when the urge occurs.
    (1) Review signs and symptoms of infection,
          including when to contact their healthcare
          provider.
    (2) Discuss with patients and family members
          the importance of completing all
          prescribed therapies and keeping all
          follow-up appointments (Hooten, 2010).
i. Tuberculosis of the urinary tract usually surfaces
    5 to 10 years after the primary tubercular
    infection is diagnosed. Many patients have no
    clinical symptoms, and some have persistent
    pyuria or hematuria with *Mycobacterium
    tuberculosis* isolated in urine cultures.
    (1) Imaging studies are used to evaluate the
          level of severity.
    (2) Treatment with antituberculosis drugs for 9
          months to 2 years may be indicated
          (Visweswaran & Bhat, 2010).
j. Fungal infections of the urinary tract are
    caused by Candida species which inhabit the
    perineum but are usually not found in the
    urine. *Candiduria* is the term used to denote
    candida infection in the urine.
    (1) Infection occurs when the fungus grows in
          the urine and infects the bladder wall and
          upper urinary tract.
    (2) Risk factors for candiduria include older
          age, female sex, use of antibiotics, urinary
          drainage devices, diabetes mellitus, and
          prior surgical procedures.
    (3) Imaging studies and complex urine
          cultures are used to diagnose candiduria.
    (4) Treatment with systemic antifungal agents
          may be warranted in some cases, and
          continuous bladder infusion of ampho-
          tericin may be indicated (Kauffman, 2010).
k. Glomerulonephritis (GN) related to infection is
    unusual but occurs primarily in patients with

diabetes, malignant neoplasm, acquired immunodeficiency syndrome (AIDS), and alcoholism.

l. Poststreptococcal glomerulonephritis (PSGN) has an effect on children ages 2 to 14 years and has a greater incidence in males.

   (1) Throat infection with *Streptococcus pyogenes* can result in PSGN along with ingestion of unpasteurized contaminated milk.

   (2) This infection is decreasing in industrialized countries and is altering from primarily affecting children to debilitated adults. It is common in developing countries within communities with poor socioeconomic circumstances.

     (a) Clinical presentation almost always includes a history of previous streptococcal infection in the skin or throat. Hypertension, edema, hematuria, and positive culture for the strep species are common findings.

     (b) Early antibiotic treatment with penicillin is indicated. Cephalosporins are indicated in those allergic to penicillin. Most children recover from PSGN, but treated adults may have mild proteinuria and microscopic hematuria.

     (c) Long-term monitoring of kidney function is warranted (Rodriguez-Iturbo et al., 2010).

m. Endocarditis-associated glomerulonephritis is community acquired, and 15,000 cases of infective endocarditis are seen in the United States each year.

   (1) The incidence rate has remained stable over the past few decades, but changes have been seen in the epidemiology.

   (2) There is a decrease in cases caused by rheumatic fever and a rise in cases linked to health care.

   (3) The incidence of endocarditis-associated GN in patients on hemodialysis is 20 to 60 times higher than in the general population.

     (a) The use of synthetic grafts and dialysis catheters increases their risks.

     (b) Treatment with antibiotics for 4 to 6 weeks can eliminate endocarditis but is associated with an increase in serum creatinine, along with hematuria and proteinuria (Rodriguez-Iturbe et al., 2010).

n. Viral infections resulting in GN cause deposition or formation of viral immune complexes, autoantibody formation, and virus-induced release of proinflammatory factors.

   (1) The most common causative viruses include human immunodeficiency virus (HIV) and hepatitis A, B, and C.

   (2) The cytomegalovirus can be found in recipients of a kidney transplant.

   (3) Treatment is directed to the specific causative agent (Rodriguez-Iturbe et al., 2010).

6. Glomerular diseases of the kidney. The glomerulus is the main functioning unit in the kidney, and disease in this area can affect overall kidney function.

a. Glomerular diseases lead to injury to the glomerular filtration barrier, which allows plasma proteins (proteinuria) and red blood cells (hematuria) to pass through the membrane into the urine.

b. These diseases are complex and can occur from direct insult to the kidney such as with infection or exposure to a nephrotoxic drug or as a result of secondary systemic diseases, such as diabetes or lupus nephritis (Floege & Feehally, 2010).

c. General mechanisms of glomerular injury.

   (1) Proteinuria is one of the main characteristics of glomerular disease and occurs because of damage to the glomerular basement membrane (GBM) and the podocytes.

   (2) Normal urine protein excretion is less than 150 mg in one 24-hour period.

     (a) Protein excretion less than 3.5 g per 24 hours is considered nonnephrotic.

     (b) Over 3.5 grams of protein excretion is considered nephrotic range.

     (c) It must be understood that nephrotic syndrome refers to a constellation of symptoms including heavy proteinuria (over 3.5 grams), hypoalbuminemia (serum albumin less than 3.0 g/dL), and peripheral edema (Floege & Feehally, 2010).

   (3) Immune mechanisms develop with glomerular disease. Antigen-antibody complexes arise within the circulation and localize in the glomerulus, causing dense deposition.

   (4) The complement system is activated, contributing to development of an inflammatory response and/or direct tissue injury.

   (5) Inflammation is caused by infiltration of inflammatory cells and proliferation of mesangial, epithelial, or endothelial cells (Schira, 2008).

d. Clinical presentation can vary according to the etiology and extent of disease.

(1) Hypertension, dependent, and periorbital edema are usually present.
(2) Laboratory studies include quantification of proteinuria and examination of urine for red blood cells or casts.
  (a) Certain serological studies, such as antinuclear and anti-DNA antibodies, cryoglobulins, rheumatoid factor, and anti-GBM antibodies, are also used to assist with diagnosis.
  (b) Urine electrophoresis detects the presence of monoclonal light or heavy chains (Floege & Feehally, 2010).

e. Classification of glomerulopathies is complex, but takes into account the etiology, onset and duration, clinical symptoms, serologic and morphologic findings, and pathophysiology.
(1) Kidney biopsy histopathology is assessed using variable methods that can discover the presence or absence of immune deposits, degree of cellular proliferation in various areas of renal parenchyma, and the presence of cellular or fibrous crescents (Floege & Feehally, 2010).
(2) Terms used to classify glomerular diseases.
  (a) *Diffuse* involves all glomeruli.
  (b) *Focal* involves some glomeruli.
  (c) *Segmental* involves portions of individual glomeruli.
  (d) *Membranous* involves glomerular wall thickening.
  (e) *Proliferative* indicates that the number of glomerular cells increases.
  (f) *Rapidly progressive* indicates that there is the expectation of continued loss of kidney function with minimal recovery potential.
  (g) *Primary* indicates disease that primarily occurs in the glomeruli without involvement of extra-renal sites.
  (h) *Secondary* indicates glomerular disease occurring as a result of a systemic process.
  (i) *Idiopathic* indicates that the cause is unknown.
  (j) *Acute pathologic* changes occur over days or weeks.
  (k) *Chronic* is slower and progressive denoting pathologic changes that develop over months or years (Schira, 2008).
(3) Treatment of glomerular disease is aimed at halting the inflammatory process and is geared to the specific etiology, control of symptoms, and effectiveness of various therapies, such as corticosteroids and immunosuppressive agents, in specific clinical situations (Appel & D'Agati, 2010).

f. Nephrotic syndrome is a clinical syndrome with characteristic symptoms of proteinuria (> 3.5 g/day), hypoalbuminemia (< 3.5 g/dL) edema, hypercholesterolemia, hypercoagulability, hyperlipidemia, and lipiduria. The metabolic effects of the syndrome can greatly influence the general health of the patient.
(1) Most episodes of nephrotic syndrome are self-limiting and respond to specific therapy. But in some patients, the condition can become chronic and lead to kidney failure.
(2) Patients with nephrotic syndrome are at increased risk for infection; thus, monitoring for signs and symptoms of infection is warranted. Many diseases present as nephrotic syndrome (Floege & Feehally, 2010).
(3) Nephritic syndrome is a condition that involves glomerular inflammation, leading to a decrease in GFR, nonnephrotic range proteinuria (< 3.5 g/day), edema, hypertension, and hematuria featuring red cell casts, resulting in brown-colored urine. Diseases associated with nephritic syndrome include:
  (a) Poststreptococcal GN.
  (b) IGA nephropathy.
  (c) Systemic lupus.
  (d) Postinfectious diseases such as endocarditis, abscesses, and access infections.

g. Rapidly progressive glomerulonephritis (RPGN) is a clinical scenario that presents acutely with a severity that causes kidney function to decrease over days or weeks. The patient may have clinical signs of nephritic syndrome that do not result in self-limitations. The following glomerular diseases can have a clinical presentation similar to RPGN:
(1) Goodpasture's disease (anti-GBM) is due to an autoantibody in the GBM and is associated with lung hemorrhages. Infiltration of the inflammatory cells causes local capillary wall damage in the lungs and kidneys.
(2) Vasculitis is associated with crescent formation and circulating antibodies to certain substances such as neutrophil cytoplasmic antigens (ANCA) seen with Wegener's granulomatosis.
(3) Immune complex diseases, such as systemic lupus erythematosus, poststreptococcal GN, and Pauci-immune crescentic GN, can

commonly present with clinical signs similar to what occurs with RPGN (Floege & Feehally, 2010).

7. Obstructive disorders of the kidney.
   a. Nephrolithiasis involves stone formation (calculus) (see Figure 1.38) within the renal tubules and collecting system; however, renal calculi are sometimes found within the ureters or bladder. It is prevalent in industrialized nations and has been increasing steadily over the last decade.

   (1) Recent studies have found an association between uric acid nephrolithiasis, metabolic syndrome, obesity, and type 2 diabetes (Sakhaee & Maalouf, 2008).

   (2) Risk factors that encourage formation of kidney stones include decreased urine volumes, saturation of urine with calcium, oxalate, phosphate, uric acid and cystine, acidic urine, and infections from bacteria.

   (3) The urine includes many ions and molecules that can form soluble complexes with the ionic parts of a stone. Crystals form and grow into a calculus that anchors to the renal epithelium (Monk & Bushinsky, 2010).

   (4) Pain and hematuria are the most common complaints of patients with kidney stones. The pain usually has an abrupt onset, appears to increase in severity over time, and occurs in the flank or loin area.
       (a) Macroscopic hematuria is common and occurs with large calculi. Passing of clots from hematuria can cause a colicky type pain.
       (b) Urine examination can disclose urine pH, characteristic crystals, and red blood cell count.
       (c) In the United States, the majority of kidney stones are made of calcium oxalate and calcium phosphate (37%), calcium oxalate (26%), and struvite (22%), with the remainder from uric acid and cystine.

   (5) Imaging studies such as a plain film of the abdomen, unenhanced CT, and renal ultrasound can uncover opacities in the kidneys and ureters. Analysis of retrieved stones will help in analyzing their chemical makeup, aid in identifying the underlying metabolic defects, and help to focus therapy (Monk & Bushinsky, 2010).

   (6) Nonpharmacologic treatment for kidney stones includes increased fluid intake to 2 to 2.5 L/day, restriction of salt intake, decreased intake of animal protein, and ingestion of age- and gender-appropriate

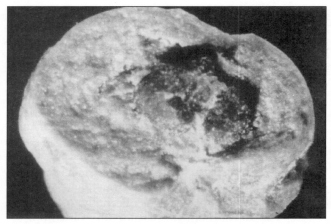

Figure 1.38. Renal calculus. Large kidney stone composed of calcium oxalate and uric acid core.

amounts of calcium. Multicomponent dietary changes depending on stone makeup are usually indicated.

   (7) Pharmacologic treatment with thiazides, citrate, or allopurinol may also decrease the risk for recurrent stones (Fink et al., 2013).

   (8) If the kidney stone does not pass spontaneously, surgical procedures may be necessary.

   (9) Newer techniques, such as extracorporeal shock wave lithotripsy, have changed the surgical management of larger obstructions (Gkougkousis et al., 2010).

   (10) Recurrence is a problem, and monitoring of kidney function along with assessment for bleeding and infection from stones are important components of care.

   b. Nephrocalcinosis involves augmented calcium content within the kidney. It can occur in the area of the renal pyramids (medullary) or can be localized in the renal cortex (cortical).
      (1) These disorders can be caused by a variety of conditions from altered calcium metabolism to tubular and anatomic diseases of the kidney.
      (2) Treatment is aimed at therapy for the underlying disease and preventive measures to prevent additional deposits of calcium (Monk & Bushinsky, 2010).

   c. Urinary tract obstruction results from structural or functional disorders that hamper normal urine flow and can result in significantly impaired kidney function.
      (1) Hydronephrosis is the dilatation of the urinary tract that may or may not result in urinary obstruction.
      (2) The peak incidence for this type of obstruction is during the second and third

decade of life. Outflow obstruction due to prostatic hypertrophy tends to occur in men over 60 years old with approximately 80% developing symptoms.

(3) Decline in GFR and renal handling of electrolytes and water excretion may be seen and can vary greatly depending on the duration of the obstruction and the hydration state of the patient.

(4) Clinical symptoms can vary but usually include pain and alterations in urine volume.

(5) Treatment is aimed at relief of the obstruction to decrease further kidney damage (Harris & Hughes, 2010).

d. Retroperitoneal fibrosis is a rare fibro-inflammatory disorder, but in the past decade many clinical reports have been appearing in the literature.

(1) This syndrome involves formation of fibrosclerotic tissue in the retroperitoneum, resulting in a periaortic mass that can encase the ureters (Pipitone et al., 2012).

(2) The cause is unknown, but the syndrome appears to be related to an autoimmune process with no specific immunologic markers.

(3) Nonspecific inflammatory markers, such as sedimentation rate and C-reactive protein, may indicate disease activity and can be used to judge response to treatment.

(4) Retroperitoneal fibrosis (see Figure 1.39) can also develop secondary to inflammation, infection, or malignant disease (Swartz, 2009).

(5) Clinical symptoms are dull pain in the abdomen, lower back, or flank area, but colicky pain can occur if the ureters are encased.

(6) If there is venous or lymphatic involvement, edema of the lower limbs may occur.

(7) Imaging procedures such as ultrasound, MRI, and CT are essential for diagnosis and to evaluate response to therapeutic interventions.

(8) The goal of treatment of retroperitoneal fibrosis is to ease the symptoms, reduce the size of the mass, relieve the obstruction, and avoid relapses. The initial approach to treatment is surgical or urologic intervention.

(9) Medical treatment with corticosteroid therapy can produce a short-term response that will decrease the pain and constitutional symptoms. Several steroid-sparing agents have also been used to achieve a longer-term response (Pipitone et al., 2012).

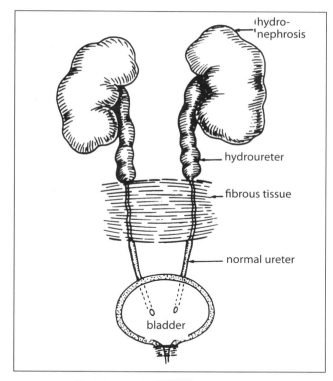

Figure 1.39. Retroperitoneal fibrosis. Fibrotic tissue develops in the retroperitoneal abdominal cavity and grows around and compresses the ureters. The compression creates a retrograde pressure up the urinary tract, causing the ureters to enlarge (hydroureter) and the kidneys to enlarge (hydronephrosis).

Source: Richard, C.J. (1986). *Comprehensive nephrology nursing.* Boston: Little, Brown. Used with permission.

(10) Mycophenolate or tamoxifen have a relatively safe profile and have been used successfully. Agents with a higher risk profile such as cyclophosphamide, azathioprine, and methotrexate can be used if necessary (Swartz, 2009).

M. Kidney problems caused by systemic diseases.
   1. Diabetes mellitus.
      a. Diabetes mellitus is a modification in the metabolism of carbohydrates, proteins, and fats.
         (1) It affects multiple systems, including the kidneys, and is associated with a reduction in insulin production and/or insulin use.
         (2) It is the leading cause of kidney failure in the United States (Ritz & Wolf, 2010).
         (3) Type 1 diabetes is an autoimmune disease and is typified by destruction of pancreatic islet cells leading to insulin deficiency. Although it can occur at any age, typically symptoms occur before the age of 30 years.
         (4) Type 2 diabetes is characterized by insulin resistance as well as insulin deficiency.

Type 2 diabetes is often preceded by metabolic syndrome consisting of visceral obesity, hypertension, insulin resistance, and dyslipidemia.

    (a) Initially, pancreatic beta cells counteract the insulin resistance, but eventually hyperglycemia occurs.

    (b) Although considered a disease of older adults, recently it has been occurring in adolescents and children (Ritz & Wolf, 2010).

b. The pathogenesis of diabetic nephropathy (DN) is a well-known microvascular complication of diabetes and is the leading cause of CKD stage 5 in the United States as well as other Western countries.

    (1) It is associated with both type 1 and type 2 diabetes. DN occurs in 20% to 40% of patients with diabetes (ADA, 2013b).

    (2) Hyperglycemia occurs initially and induces dysfunction in various cell types that result in progressive diabetic nephropathy (Kanwar et al., 2011).

    (3) Genetic factors play a large role in the development of nephropathy. Familial clusters have been found in both types 1 and 2 diabetes. Prevalence is increased in African Americans, Native Americans, Hispanic Americans, and Polynesians compared to Caucasians.

    (4) Hemodynamic changes occur early in the course of DN in the form of hyperfiltration. This occurs because of multiple factors, including glucose dependent effects that cause afferent arteriolar dilatation.

    (5) Hypertrophy is an early occurrence in DN and is associated with glomerular enlargement, resulting in an increase in the filtration surface area and an overall increase in kidney size.

    (6) Mesangial expansion is one of the characteristic changes noted in DN. It occurs because mesangial cells increase in number and size resulting in deposition of an extracellular matrix and development of glomerulosclerosis. Studies have shown that tight glucose control can help to mediate these changes.

    (7) Inflammation occurs as a result of infiltration by monocytes-macrophages and activated T lymphocytes in the glomerulus and interstitium.

    (8) Proteinuria is associated with a widening of the glomerular basement membrane (GBM) and the dysfunction occurring in the podocytes. These mechanisms allow serum proteins to escape across damaged basal membranes (Ritz & Wolf, 2010).

c. Diagnosis and clinical manifestations.

    (1) Recommendations for screening for DN by the American Diabetes Association suggest assessment of urine albumin excretion in type 1 patients with disease duration of 5 years or more and in patients with type 2 at the time of diagnosis (ADA, 2013b).

    (2) Serum creatinine should be measured annually to estimate GFR with an equation.

    (3) Albumin concentration can easily be measured in a spot urine sample that measures albumin to creatinine ratio. The advantage of measuring albumin levels is that uncovering microalbumuria detects DN early and can predict cardiovascular and renal risk.

        (a) Normal albumin excretion is less than 30 mg/day, and levels greater than 30 mg/day are considered increased.

        (b) From a historical standpoint, ratios between 30 and 299 mg/day were said to have *microalbuminuria*. Levels greater than 300 mg/day were referred to as *macroalbuminuria* (ADA, 2013b). These terms are no longer used.

    (4) In individuals with a body mass index greater than 30, albuminuria over 30 mg/day may be detected even without the presence of hypertension.

        (a) Patients with features of metabolic syndrome are at increased risk for kidney disease and cardiovascular disease.

        (b) Hypertension can develop prior to the onset of DN in patients with type 2 diabetes. Approximately 80% of patients are found to have an abnormal blood pressure at the time of diagnosis with type 2 disease (Ritz & Wolf, 2010).

    (5) Some important microvascular complications can occur in other organ systems due to diabetes. These include sensory polyneuropathy that results in paresthesias and impaired perception of pain that can ultimately result in foot problems.

        (a) Autonomic neuropathy can result in gastroparesis and diarrhea alternating with constipation. It can also affect cardiac innervations, resulting in a decreased ability to perceive pain during myocardial infarction or ischemic event.

        (b) Retinopathy is quite common and can be treated with improved ophthalmic techniques.

(c) Macrovascular complications include stroke, coronary disease, and peripheral arterial disease (Ritz & Wolf, 2010).

(6) The role that hyperglycemia plays in the development of DN has been studied over the last two decades. Two large controlled trials have demonstrated that A1C levels should be no greater than 7% to reduce the risk for developing microvascular complications such as DN.

(a) The Diabetes Control and Complications Trial (DCCT) demonstrated that intensive treatment of type 1 diabetes decreased the incidence of microalbuminuria by 39%.

(b) Results from the United Kingdom Diabetes Prospective Study (UKPDS) in type 2 diabetes indicated a 30% risk reduction for microvascular complications in those who had intensive glycemic control (Gross et al., 2005).

(c) Recent studies have examined the effect of glycemic control and risk of cardiovascular disease in individuals with type 2 diabetes.

d. Prevention and early detection of DN can lead to better patient outcomes by providing strategies that protect the kidneys and the cardiovascular system.

(1) Glycemic control should be individualized and take into account the duration of diabetes, cardiovascular disease, and ability to recognize hypoglycemia. Kidney Disease Outcomes Quality Initiative (KDOQI) recommends targeting the glycated hemoglobin (HbA1c) level to 7% regardless of the presence or absence of CKD (NKF, 2007).

(2) Control of blood pressure through the use of ACE inhibitors or ARBs is effective and provides some renoprotection.

(3) Appropriate treatment of dyslipidemia to lower CVD risk is an important component of care. Use of appropriate lipid-lowering agents is an integral part of patient management.

(4) Nutritional counseling on salt, potassium, and phosphate restriction is advised (NKF, 2007).

(5) Lifestyle modifications such as weight reduction, diet modification that includes less fat and salt intake, smoking cessation, and exercise have been shown to be effective (Ritz & Wolf, 2010).

e. Patient education strategies should be geared toward teaching the patient about the connection between optimal glycemic control and development of DN.

(1) Empowering patients to include lifestyle modifications needs to be encouraged.

(2) Stress the importance of keeping appointments to maintain ongoing assessment of kidney function (Gomez, 2011).

2. Hypertensive nephropathy is a chronic disease that is growing in prevalence worldwide, spanning racial and gender lines; it is usually asymptomatic and is the second most common cause of CKD stage 5. The damage occurring in the kidneys is called hypertensive sclerosis (Udani et al., 2011).

a. Definition. In 2003, the Seventh Joint National Committee on Prevention, Detection, Evaluation and Treatment of High Blood Pressure (JNC 7) provided guidelines for classification of blood pressure in adults and was reaffirmed by JNC 8.

b. The JNC 8 blood pressure classification system is the same as what was recommended in the JNC 7 report, although BP treatment targets are less stringent in JNC 8.

(1) For patients under 60 years, the recommendation is to initiate or intensify antihypertensive therapy when BP is 140/90 mmHg.

(2) For patients over 60 years, a less aggressive approach is recommended, with the target BP of 150/90 mmHg.

(3) In patients over 18 years of age with CKD, the target BP is 140/90 mmHg. The initial or supplemental treatment continues to advocate for the use of an angiotensin-converting enzyme inhibitor (ACE inhibitor) or angiotensin-receptor blocker (ARB), regardless of race or diabetes status.

(4) In the nonblack population, including those with diabetes, recommendations for initial therapy include use of a thiazide-based diuretic, calcium channel blocker, ACE inhibitors, or ARB.

(5) In the black population, it is recommended that initial therapy begin with a thiazide type diuretic or calcium channel blocker (James et al., 2014).

c. Recent clinical data and epidemiologic studies demonstrate the connection between blood pressure and the risk for cardiovascular disease, so a modification in how hypertension is defined and classified has occurred.

(1) The Hypertension Writing Group, a national assembly of hypertension specialists, proposed a new definition.

(2) It is not based on blood pressure reading alone, but takes into account target organ

damage, cardiovascular disease risk factors, and early disease markers (Giles, 2009).

d. Cardiovascular risk factors include older age, elevated BP, increased heart rate, obesity, dyslipidemia, diabetes mellitus, insulin resistance, smoking, family history of premature CVD, sedentary lifestyle, and psychosocial stressors.

   (1) CVD is the main long-term risk of hypertension and can be classified into pressure-related conditions such as stroke and heart failure.

   (2) Additionally, it can be classified into atherosclerotic conditions such as myocardial infarction.

e. Target organ damage can be apparent early in the process and includes cardiac signs such as left ventricular hypertrophy, symptomatic heart failure, angina pectoris, and ischemic heart disease.

   (1) Vascular damage results in peripheral artery disease, carotid disease, and aortic aneurysm.

   (2) Cerebrovascular damage is manifested in stroke, transient ischemic attacks, dementia, and loss of vision.

   (3) Kidney damage leads to albuminuria and CKD (Giles, 2009).

f. When causes of hypertension remain unknown, this type is considered primary or essential hypertension (Lawton et al., 2010). Pathology involved in hypertensive nephrosclerosis remains muddled, but two distinct initial injuries involve changes in the renal vasculature and lead to progressive injury.

   (1) Elastic fibers in the arterial circulation of the kidney are replaced by thickening in the intima and narrowing of the lumen resulting in decreased blood flow.

   (2) The afferent arterioles lose their ability to autoregulate because of dilatation. Eventually the glomeruli are damaged and are unable to autoregulate (Udani et al., 2011).

g. Causes of secondary hypertension.

   (1) Renal causes include renal parenchymal disease, acute and chronic GN, and renovascular disease, such as renal artery stenosis or arteritis.

   (2) Endocrine disorders such as primary aldosteronism, Cushing's syndrome, pheochromocytoma, and thyroid disease.

   (3) Oral contraceptives, mineralcortoids, glucocortoids, NSAIDs, amphetamines, cocaine, and other illicit drugs have been implicated.

   (4) Other factors involved include obstructive sleep apnea, obesity, and coarctation of the aorta. Pregnancy complications, such as preeclampsia or ecclampsia, can contribute to secondary hypertension (Lawton et al., 2010).

h. Diagnosis of primary hypertension should start with eliminating secondary sources listed above and accurate measurement of blood pressure. Arterial blood pressure is measured in the brachial artery by using a cuff-based sphygmomanometer and detecting sounds (auscultation) or recording vascular pulsations (oscillometric). Some tips for accuracy include:

   (1) Proper cuff size: the bladder of the cuff should encircle at least 80% of the arm.

   (2) Patient should be seated comfortably with the bared arm supported and the cuff at the level of the heart. 30 seconds should elapse between readings. The BP can be checked after 2 minutes in the standing position.

   (3) Ambulatory BP monitoring is beneficial. Home blood pressure monitoring is recommended because BP varies greatly during the day. It is recommended for patients with white coat and borderline hypertension. It is also useful in determining response to therapy including episodes of hypotension (Lawton et al., 2010).

i. Nonpharmacologic interventions.

   (1) These interventions are geared to management and prevention of HTN. Effective lifestyle changes include smoking cessation, weight reduction, physical exercise, reduction of salt intake, increase in fruit and vegetable intake, decrease in fat intake, and moderation of alcohol/caffeine intake and stress modulation.

   (2) Adoption and adherence to lifestyle modifications are difficult and remain problematic, but counseling might be effective for long-term management goals (Rayner et al., 2010).

j. Pharmacologic treatment of hypertension is complex and requires lifelong treatment with more than one drug. Many large randomized clinical studies have compared classes of drugs with placebo and different treatment strategies with regard to cardiovascular events. The recommendations are subject to change as new evidence surfaces (Williams, 2010). General classes of antihypertensive medications include:

   (1) Diuretics that may be thiazide type, loop type, or potassium-sparing diuretics.

   (2) Beta blockers that reduce cardiac output and differ in their duration of action and selectivity for beta-receptors (e.g., atenolol,

metoprolol, inderal, carvedilol, and others).
(3) Calcium channel blockers (CCBs), which are divided into two main groups.
    (a) Dihydropyridines block calcium channels inducing peripheral vascular relaxation with a corresponding decrease in BP (e.g., amlodipine, nefedipine).
    (b) Nondihydropyridines block calcium channels in cardiac muscle and decrease cardiac output (e.g., diltiazem, verapamil).
(4) Angiotensin-converting enzyme inhibitors (ACE inhibitors) work by blocking the conversion of angiotensin I to angiotensin II. The result leads to vasodilatation and a decrease in BP. In patients with impaired kidney function, it is important to monitor serum potassium levels (e.g., captopril, enalapril, lisinopril, and others).
(5) Angiotensin II receptor blockers (ARBs) are a newer class of drugs and work by blocking angiotensin II receptors, which inhibit vasoconstriction (e.g., losartan, valsartan, and others).
(6) It is important to note that both ACE inhibitors and ARBs are equally effective at decreasing albuminuria and preserving GFR (e.g., renoprotective properties).
(7) Centrally acting sympatholytic drugs target the activation of the sympathetic nervous system to decrease BP (e.g., clonidine, methydopa).
(8) Direct vasodilators work by relaxing smooth muscle and lowering vascular resistance (e.g., hydralazine, minoxidil).
(9) Alpha-receptor blockers block norepinephrine in the arteries and decrease vasoconstriction (e.g., doxazosin, prozosin, and others) (Schonder, 2006; Williams, 2010).
(10) Special populations require careful thought regarding choice of antihypertensive agents.
    (a) There is a high prevalence of hypertension in African Americans with more target organ damage. As a group, they tend to respond better to diuretics, CCBs, and decreased intake of salt.
    (b) For a variety of reasons such as arterial wall stiffening, decline in GFR due to aging, and decrease in drug clearance, hypertension is problematic in people 60 years or older. Because of these factors, dosages should be increased

gradually and medication regimens kept simple.
    (c) Patients with CKD should be started on ACE inhibitors and ARBs for their protective effect on the kidney (Williams, 2010).
k. Hypertensive emergency or urgency formerly known as "malignant" hypertension refers to marked elevations in BP with readings greater than 180/120 mmHg.
    (1) The onset is very rapid, resulting in severe target organ damage and may result in acute kidney injury.
    (2) Various pharmacologic agents can be used to gradually reduce the BP to prevent additional damage (Sarafides & Bakris, 2010).
l. Renovascular hypertension is a syndrome of increased BP related to clinical conditions that interfere with arterial circulation to the kidneys.
    (1) Patients with significant renal artery stenosis will have a decrease in renal perfusion leading to overstimulation of the renin-angiotensin-aldosterone system (RAS), resulting in hypertension.
    (2) Fibromuscular dysplasia involves the large and medium-sized renal arteries with lesions disrupting the vascular wall with deposition of collagen.
        (a) It is more common in young females and presents as early-onset hypertension.
        (b) It is commonly asymptomatic and may be found incidentally during angiography (Textor & Greco, 2010).
    (3) Atherosclerotic renovascular disease involves the narrowing of the renal arteries and is more common in patients older than 50 years; it is seen with systemic atherosclerosis.
        (a) Plaque and vascular calcification are present.
        (b) Associated with coronary, cerebro-vascular, peripheral vascular, and aortic disease (Textor & Greco, 2010).
    (4) Treatment of renovascular hypertension involves medical treatment with antihypertensives, examining modifiable cardiac risk factors such as smoking cessation and weight reduction, low dose aspirin, and control of hyperlipidemia with appropriate therapies.
        (a) Renal revascularization techniques, such as percutaneous transluminal renal angioplasty and stenting, have also been successful.

(b) Surgical revascularization is reserved for those patients not responsive to other therapies (Textor & Greco, 2010).

3. Systemic lupus erythematosus (SLE) is an inflammatory autoimmune disease that affects many organ systems including the kidney.

a. It is more common in African Americans, Afro-Carribeans, Asian Americans, and Hispanic Americans with peak incidence between 15 and 45 years and greater in females.

b. Risk factors for kidney involvement include lupus nephritis, low socioeconomic status, family history, younger age, and hypertension.

c. The pathology involved in SLE is related to autoantibodies combining with antigen, resulting in immune complexes that are not cleared adequately and deposit in various organs that result in an inflammatory response.

   (1) The localization of these immune complexes in the glomerulus activates complement and procoagulant factors.

   (2) Injures the capillaries and adjacent structures (Appel & Jayne, 2010).

d. Clinical symptoms of SLE vary, and the disease is characterized by episodic flares followed by periods of remission.

   (1) Renal symptoms include proteinuria, microhematuria, dysmorphic red blood cells and casts, and hypertension. Involvement of the kidneys occurs in 60% of young adults.

   (2) Extrarenal symptoms may include malaise, lack of appetite, weight loss, and low grade fever. Dermal findings include a classic "butterfly" rash on the face.

   (3) Additional symptoms include photo-sensitivity, arthralgias, Raynaud phenomenon, pleurisy, pericarditis, and pulmonary hypertension (Appel & Jayne, 2010).

e. Classification of SLE is multifaceted and is based on light microscopy, immunofluorescence, and electron microscope findings. The World Health Organization (WHO) developed a system in 1995; the International Society of Nephrology (ISN/Renal Pathology Society (RPS) updated the very complex classifications in 2004.

f. Treatment of SLE is geared to preservation of kidney function and treatment of systemic symptoms. It involves corticosteroids in high doses given intravenously (IV) followed by oral preparations.

   (1) Due to an increased risk of infectious complications and side effects, prolonged courses of these drugs are usually limited.

   (2) Cytotoxic agents such as cyclophos-phamide, which inhibits B cells, has been given orally and IV with some success.

   (3) Azathioprine and cyclosporine have been used successfully along with corticosteroids (Appel & Jayne, 2010).

g. Cosmetic side effects causing body image problems are common along with altered emotional status. Recognition of body image issues needs to be acknowledged (not overlooked) and appropriate counseling needs to be instituted.

4. Renal amyloidosis results from the deposition of abnormal glycoproteins in the kidneys and other organs.

a. These proteins cause fibril formation, which are produced by immunoglobulin light chains that deposit in the blood vessels, glomeruli, and tubules of the kidney.

b. The amyloid deposits can also affect the kidney, specifically the glomerular basement membrane (GBM), and result in noninflammatory glomerulopathy with notable enlargement of the kidney.

c. Immunoglobulin-associated amyloidosis (AL) involves free immunoglobulin subunits such as light chains.

   (1) The main clinical symptoms are weight loss and weakness along with nephrotic syndrome, orthostatic hypotension, and peripheral neuropathy. Bone pain may be present in those with multiple myeloma.

   (2) Cardiomyopathy and motility disturbances in the GI tract are seen.

   (3) Treatment may include a course of chemotherapy or treatment with melphalan and prednisone.

d. AA amyloidosis is due to prolonged elevation of serum amyloid A protein (SAA). Patients who have long-standing inflammatory disease are at increased risk.

   (1) The kidney is the main organ targeted; results in development of proteinuria and a subsequent rise in the serum creatinine level along with hepatomegaly and GI disturbances such as diarrhea and constipation.

   (2) Treatment of the underlying inflammatory disease is the aim of treatment (Ronco et al., 2010).

Section D

Assessment of Kidney Structure and Function

Sheila J. Doss-McQuitty

I. History and physical assessment. Table 1.11 provides a detailed outline for a history and physical assessment format for patients experiencing kidney problems. A basic understanding of interviewing and familiarity with physical assessment skills are prerequisites (Bickley, 2012; Seidel et al., 2011).

II. Physical assessment of the kidneys.

A. Patient preparation.
1. Before beginning the physical assessment, tell the patient what will happen, address questions and concerns, provide privacy, and help the patient relax.
2. The environment should be at a comfortable temperature with adequate lighting. The nurse needs to warm his or her hands and any equipment that will be used (such as a stethoscope).

B. Inspection.
1. Place the patient in a supine position with examiner on right side.
2. Inspect right and left upper quadrants at the midclavicular line, from a standing position and at eye level.
3. Inspect for raised areas, masses, or unusual pulsations (Bickley & Szilagyi, 2012; Seidel et al., 2011).
   a. Raised masses may be a large polycystic kidney or hypernephroma.
   b. Unusual pulsations may be an arterial aneurysm.
4. Inspect lower quadrant at midline. A distended bladder may be visible midline across the lower quadrants.

C. Auscultation.
1. Bell of the stethoscope is held lightly against the abdomen slightly to the right and left of the midline in both upper quadrants.
2. With the patient in a supine position, listen for a renal or aortic bruit (a low pitched murmur), indicating renal arterial stenosis or aortic aneurysm.
3. With the patient in a prone or sitting position, auscultate the entire costovertebral angle (area where the twelfth rib and vertebral column intersect) for bruits (Bickley, 2012; Seidel et al., 2011).

D. Palpation.
1. The kidneys.
   a. Normally, in an adult, the kidneys are not palpable, except on occasion the inferior pole of the right kidney. The left kidney is rarely palpable.
      (1) A clinician's success in palpating the right kidney is usually enhanced when examining a thin person or child.
      (2) In someone with easily palpable kidneys, it is important to determine if the kidneys are felt bilaterally (e.g., polycystic kidneys) or unilaterally (e.g., cyst, tumor). This will help determine likely pathologies.
      (3) Tenderness suggests additional pathology considerations such as infection (pyelonephritis) or enlargement (hydronephrosis).
   b. The kidneys are located deep in the abdomen and, as noted, are difficult to palpate.
      (1) Moderate to deep palpation is required.
      (2) Place one hand posteriorly under the flank and place the other hand anteriorly over the lower aspect of the upper quadrant on the same side of the body. Posteriorly elevate the kidney by pushing up, and ask the patient to breathe deeply. During exhalation, anteriorly palpate deeply for the kidney.
   c. Occasionally, the lower pole of a normal-sized right kidney is palpated as a solid, firm, but elastic mass that moves with inspiration (polycystic kidneys usually feel bumpy).
   d. Enlarged kidneys may indicate hydronephrosis, neoplasms, or polycystic disease.
2. Urinary bladder.
   a. Palpate bladder at midline 1 cm above symphysis pubis.
   b. A distended bladder feels smooth, round, and tense, and can extend above the umbilicus.
   c. The patient may feel pressure or the urge to void if the bladder is distended (Bickley, 2012; Seidel et al., 2011).

E. Percussion.
1. Kidneys are difficult to percuss anteriorly because they are located deep and posterior in the abdominal cavity.
2. Posteriorly percuss both sides of the costovertebral angle (CVA) for kidney tenderness or pain.
   a. Place the palm of one hand against the skin and gently strike the top of this hand with the ulnar surface of the other hand that has been made into a fist.
   b. CVA tenderness may indicate pyelonephritis, neoplasms, inflamed or bleeding cysts, calculi, or intermittent hydronephrosis.

Table 1.11

Health History and Physical Assessment Guide
for the Nephrology Nurse Caring for a Patient with Kidney Diseases

Patient's Name: **Date:**

Nurse's Name:

I. COMPREHENSIVE HEALTH HISTORY

A. Identifying data
   1. Age
   2. Birth date
   3. Sex
   4. Race
   5. Place of birth
   6. Marital status
   7. Occupation
   8. Religious preference and spiritual practices and beliefs

B. Source of history (i.e., patient, relative, friend, medical record) and nurse's judgment about the validity of the information

C. Chief complaint(s): stated in the patient's own words, if possible.

D. History of the present illness: the patient's chronologic explanation of the health problems for which he/she is seeking care
   1. The account should include:
      a, Onset of the problem
      b. The setting in which it developed
      c. Its manifestations
      d. Its treatments
      e. Its impact on the patient's life
      f. Its meaning to the patient
   2. The symptoms of the problems should be described in terms of seven dimensions:
      a. Body location
      b. Quality
      c. Quantity (severity)
      d. Timing (i.e., onset, duration, and frequency)
      e. Setting in which they occur
      f. Factors that aggravate or relieve the symptoms
      g. Associated manifestations

E. Past health history
   1. General state of health
   2. Childhood illnesses (i.e., measles, rubella, mumps, whooping cough, chicken pox, rheumatic fever, scarlet fever, polio, frequent "strep" throat)
   3. Immunizations and dates (i.e., tetanus, pertussis, diphtheria, polio (Salk and/or Sabin), measles, rubella, mumps, hepatitis)
   4. Adult illnesses: describe nature of each illness, date, treatment, and outcome in patient's own words if possible
   5. Psychiatric illnesses: describe nature of each illness, date, treatment, and outcome in patient's own words, if possible
   6. Operations: describe type of operation(s), date(s), and outcome(s), including organ/tissue transplants
   7. Other hospitalizations: reason(s), date(s), and outcome(s)
   8. Allergies: state substance(s) to which allergic; how each allergy manifests itself (signs and symptoms); prophylactic treatment, if any; date of past allergic response
   9. Current medications: state all prescription, over-the-counter, home remedy nonprescription, herbal drugs/teas, dietary/nutritional supplements, vitamins, minerals, and flower essences that the patient uses. Give dosage, frequency, and length of time taking. Elicit patient's understanding of reason(s) for each, its desired effects, and its side effects.
   10. Diet history
      a. ask for a 24-hour recall of all food and fluids consumed and dietary supplements, including amount of each and time of day
      b. ascertain any special dietary restrictions or requirements
      c. determine patient's understanding of reasons for dietary restrictions
      d. determine patient's ability to purchase and prepare necessary foods
   11. Sleep patterns
      a. usual bedtime and time of awakening
      b. difficulty falling asleep or staying asleep and associated reasons; aids to sleep
      c. daytime naps: how many and how long for each
      d. any recent changes in any of the above
   12. Habits
      a. describe exercise schedule
      b. coffee/tea: daily amount
      c. alcohol: type and usual daily consumption
      d. tobacco: type (cigarettes, cigars, pipe, chewing) and usual daily number
      e. recreational drugs: name drug and describe its use (Note: the patient may be reluctant to give this information about illegal drug use.)
   13. Environmental hazards
      a. recent recipient of x-ray contrast media
      b. ingestion of lead
      c. exposure or ingestion of mercury
      d. prolonged use of NSAIDs
      e. prolonged sulfonamide use
      f. prolonged aminoglycoside use

Table 1.11

Health History and Physical Assessment Guide
for the Nephrology Nurse Caring for a Patient with Kidney Diseases (page 2 of 9)

    g. "moonshine" ingestion
    h. exposure to radiation
    i. exposure to sprays, herbicides, pesticides, fumes (e.g., farmers, ranchers, loggers)
    j. others
  14. Ask patient to describe work and neighborhood where he/she lives; look for evidence of new industrial park or nuclear waste site, fumes, air pollution, water pollution.

F. Family History
    1. Give age and state of health or cause and age at death for each of the following family members:
       a. paternal and maternal grandparents
       b. parents
       c. siblings
       d. spouse
       e. children
    2. Question about the occurrence of the following conditions in any family member:
       a. diabetes mellitus
       b. tuberculosis
       c. heart disease
       d. high blood pressure
       e. stroke
       f. kidney disease
       g. cancer
       h. arthritis
       i. anemia
       j. headaches
       k. mental illness
       l. symptoms similar to those the patient is experiencing

	Typical Findings in Patients with Kidney Failure

G. Psychosocial history: Have the patient describe in his/her own words:
  1. His lifestyle, home situation, significant people in his life and any recent changes in each
  2. A typical day and recent changes
  3. The most important events in his life
  4. Spiritual/cultural/religious beliefs that influence his health or therapeutic regimen
  5. Educational background
  6. Current occupation
  7. Professional and personal goals
  8. Financial status and effect of illness on it; ability to manage cost of illness
  9. Travel in last year
	changes in lifestyle because of illness
	often changes in occupation or unemployed because of illness
	major financial problems because of cost of kidney failure treatment

H. Review of systems (from the patient's *subjective* point of view)
Note: As abnormalities arise, ask what the person does to treat them.
  1. General state of health
    a. usual weight
    b. recent decrease or increase in weight
    c. fever
    d. unusual weakness, fatigue, malaise
    e. pain
	losses in weight if anorexic or has nausea and vomiting
	gains in weight with fluid retention
	
	weakness, fatigue, malaise

2. Skin
    a. rashes
    b. bumps
    c. itching or dryness and how managed
    d. color changes
    e. changes in hair or nails
	dry, scaly skin
	severe itching
	
	grayish-bronze color with underlying pallor
	easy bruising, poor healing of cuts and scratches
	dry, brittle hair
	brittle split nails

3. Head
    a. headache: location, frequency, and treatment
    b. head injuries
  4. Eyes
    a. visual
    b. glasses or contact lenses: reason and length of time
    c. last eye examination
    d. pain
    e. excessive tearing
    f. double vision
    g. glaucoma
    h. cataracts
	frequent headaches
	
	decreased visual acuity
	redness
	pain
	double vision
	cataracts

Table 1.11

Health History and Physical Assessment Guide
for the Nephrology Nurse Caring for a Patient with Kidney Diseases (page 3 of 9)

	Typical Findings in Patients with Kidney Failure
5. Ears a. hearing acuity b. tinnitus c. vertigo d. earaches e. infection f. discharge	
6. Nose and sinuses a. frequent colds b. nasal stuffiness c. hay fever/allergies/sneezing d. nosebleeds e. sinus problems	nose bleeds
7. Mouth and throat a. condition of teeth and gums b. bleeding gums or mucous membranes c. last dental examination d. history of cavities e. sore, bleeding tongue f. history of sore throat (especially "strep" throat) g. hoarseness h. unusual taste in mouth i. unusual odor on breath	bleeding ammonia or urine smell to breath metallic taste in mouth sore, cracked, bleeding tongue and mucous membranes frequent "strep" throat may be precursor to some types of glomerulonephritis
8. Neck a. lumps b. "swollen glands" c. goiter d. pain	
9. Breasts a. lumps b. pain c. discharge from nipples d. self-examination knowledge and practice e. recent enlargement of breasts, especially for men	enlargement of breast tissue (for men)
10. Respiratory a. cough b. sputum (color, quantity, consistency) c. hemoptysis d. wheezing e. asthma f. bronchitis g. emphysema h. pneumonia i. tuberculosis j. pleurisy k. last tuberculin skin test and results l. last chest x-ray and results	tenacious sputum pneumonia
11. Cardiac a. heart trouble b. high blood pressure c. rheumatic fever d. heart murmurs e. dyspnea f. orthopnea g. paroxysmal nocturnal dyspnea h. edema i. chest pains j. palpitations k. last EKG or other cardiac evaluations and results	high blood pressure dyspnea orthopnea paroxysmal nocturnal dyspnea edema of feet and legs, and around eyes palpitations chest pain
12. Gastrointestinal a. dysphagia b. heartburn and treatment c. change in appetite d. nausea e. vomiting (have patient describe emesis) f. indigestion g. frequency and description of bowel movements h. change in bowel habits i. rectal bleeding	heartburn anorexia nausea, especially in the early morning vomiting indigestion constipation and/or diarrhea blood in vomitus and/or stools difficulty swallowing

Table 1.11

Health History and Physical Assessment Guide
for the Nephrology Nurse Caring for a Patient with Kidney Diseases (page 4 of 9)

	Typical Findings in Patients with Kidney Failure
j. constipation and treatment	
k. diarrhea and treatment	
l. abdominal pain	
m. food intolerances	
n. excessive flatus	
o. hemorrhoids	
p. jaundice	
q. liver or gall bladder problems	
r. hepatitis	
13. Urinary	
a. frequency of urination	polyuria in early kidney failure and
b. amount of each urination	in polycystic kidney disease
c. number of times gets up at night to urinate (nocturia)	nocturia in early kidney failure
d. recent increase or decrease in amount of each urination	decreased amount of urine in late kidney failure
e. pain during urination (dysuria)	blood in urine
f. difficulty starting urination (hesitancy)	depending on cause of renal problem,
g. urgency	patient may report history of:
h. dribbling at end of urination	dysuria
i. starting and stopping of stream during urination	hesitancy
j. blood in urine (hematuria)	urgency
k. color of urine	dribbling
l. burning during urination	burning during urination
m. incontinence or enuresis	incontinence or enuresis
n. history of urinary tract infections and treatment	history of frequent urinary tract infections
o. history of urinary tract stones and treatment	history of urinary tract stones
p. surgeries, such as kidney donation, kidney transplant recipient, bladder surgery, or stents.	
If patient on dialysis:	
a. date of initiation	
b. type of dialysis	
c. date of last dialysis	
d. where treated (home, in-center)	
e. complications	
14. Genito-reproductive	
a. males	problem achieving and/or maintaining erection
(1) discharge from penis or sores on penis	
(2) history of sexually transmitted disease(s) and treatment	decreased libido
(3) hernias	infertility
(4) pain or masses in testicles	
(5) recent decrease in size of testicles	
(6) ability to achieve and maintain an erection	
(7) recent change in interest in sex	
(8) frequency of intercourse	
(9) contraceptive measures	
b. females	failure to menarche (children)
(1) age at menarche	infertility
(2) regularity, frequency, and duration of menstrual periods	amenorrhea or irregular menstrual periods
(3) amount of bleeding during menstrual periods	decreased libido
(4) bleeding between periods or after intercourse	
(5) recent changes in frequency or duration of periods	
(6) frequency of intercourse; recent changes in interest in sex	
(7) ability to achieve orgasm	
(8) number of pregnancies; number of live births; number of spontaneous, therapeutic, or induced abortions	
(9) date of last menstrual period	
(10) dysmenorrhea	
(11) age of menopause	
(12) last Pap smear and results	
(13) contraceptive measures, use of hormones, creams	
15. Musculoskeletal	
a. joint pains or stiffness	joint pain
b. arthritis	gout
c. gout	arthritis
d. backache	stiff joints
e. if any of above are present, describe location and symptoms (i.e., swelling, redness, pain, stiffness, weakness, limitation of motion or activity)	muscle pains
	leg cramps
	restlessness
f. muscle pains, cramps, or spasms	

Table 1.11

Health History and Physical Assessment Guide
for the Nephrology Nurse Caring for a Patient with Kidney Diseases (page 5 of 9)

	Typical Findings in Patients with Kidney Failure

16. Peripheral vascular
    a. pain on walking
    b. leg cramps
    c. varicose veins
    d. thrombophlebitis
    e. recent hair loss from extremities
	leg cramps
	pain on walking

17. Neurologic
    a. fainting
    b. seizures
    c. localized weakness
    d. numbness
    e. tingling or burning sensations
    f. tremors
    g. paralysis
    h. memory loss
    i. alteration in state of mental acuity
	fainting
	seizures
	muscle weakness
	numbness, tingling, burning of soles of feet
	
	footdrop
	decreased interest in environment
	decreased ability to do abstract reasoning

18. Psychiatric
    a. unusual nervousness, anxiety
    b. mood changes
    c. depression
    d. loss of interest in usual recreation activities
    e. depression
	mood swings
	depression
	anger
	hostility

19. Endocrine
    a. thyroid problems
    b. heat or cold intolerance
    c. excessive sweating
    d. excessive thirst, hunger, or urination
    e. diabetes mellitus
    f. problems with conception
	heat and/or cold intolerance
	excessive thirst, hunger (diabetic nephropathy)
	infertility

20. Hematologic
    a. anemia
    b. easy bruising or bleeding
    c. history of blood transfusion: dates, reasons, and reactions
    d. fatigue, malaise
	anemia
	easy bruising and bleeding
	fatigue
	malaise

II. SYSTEMATIC PHYSICAL EXAMINATION (from the examiner's objective point of view)
Note: As abnormalities arise, ask what the person does to treat them.
 	
A. General survey
  1. Observe the patient's apparent state of health and signs of distress
  2. Height
  3. Weight
  4. Correlate height and weight to determine appropriateness for each patient.
  5. Observe posture, activity, gait, dress, grooming, personal hygiene, odors to breath or body, facial expressions, manner, affect, reaction to other people, state of awareness.
	low weight for height if patient anorexic
	high weight for height if patient has fluid overload
	appears chronically or acutely ill, often emaciated, apathetic, poorly groomed, low energy level, halitosis, body odor, uses defense mechanisms.

B. Vital signs
  1. Blood pressure: lying, sitting, and standing
  2. Oral or rectal temperature; observe for hypothermia or hyperthermia
  3. Count radial pulse rate
  4. Count respiratory rate
	usually hypertensive
	possible orthostatic hypotension
	hyperthermic (due to infection)
	abnormal pulse rate and rhythm

C. Skin
  1. Inspect color, evidence of bleeding, bruising, excoriation
  2. Palpate
    a. moisture: dryness, sweating, oiliness
    b. temperature (with backs of examiner's fingers)
    c. mobility and turgor: lift a fold of skin and note ease with which it moves (mobility) and speed with which it returns into place (turgor)
  3. Observe skin lesions and describe their anatomic locations, distribution, arrangement, type of lesion (macules, papules, vesticles, bulla, erosion, etc.), and color
  4. Inspect and palpate fingernails and toenails for color, shape, and lesions
  5. Inspect and palpate the head and body hair for quantity, distribution, and texture
	pale, grayish-bronze color
	ecchymoses
	purpura
	excoriated and reddened areas
	dry
	delayed wound healing
	poor turgor and mobility
	
	brittle, split nails
	red, brown, or white bands
	scant (do not confuse with normal male balding), dry, brittle hair

Table 1.11

Health History and Physical Assessment Guide
for the Nephrology Nurse Caring for a Patient with Kidney Diseases (page 6 of 9)

	Typical Findings in Patients with Kidney Failure
D. Eyes	
1. Test visual acuity using a Snellen eye chart, or have the patient read small newspaper or magazine print up close and then large print several feet away	decreased visual acuity double vision
2. Inspect eyebrows for quantity and distribution of hair and scaliness of skin	dry, scaly skin under eyebrows
3. Inspect eyelids for edema, color, lesions, adequacy with which the eyelids close to cover the corneas	edema of eyelids which may prevent their closing completely
4. Inspect the conjunctivas and sclera for color, especially jaundice and pallor	pale or red, inflamed conjunctiva yellow sclera
5. Using oblique lighting, inspect the cornea and lens of each eye for opacities	opacities of cornea and lens
6. Inspect the size, shape, and equality of the pupils	
7. Test direct and consensual pupillary reaction to light (CN III)	
8. Test the pupillary reaction to accommodation	
9. Assess the extraocular movements through the six cardinal fields of gaze (CN III, IV, VI)	nystagmus
10. Using the ophthalmoscope, examine the fundus of each eye; note the outline and color of the optic disc; inspect for nicking of junctions of arterioles and veins	retinopathy outline of optic disc blurred hemorrhages nicking at arteriovenous crossings papilledema
E. Ears	
1. Inspect the auricles for deformities and lesions	hard nodules or lumps in auricles
2. Using an otoscope, inspect the ear canal and drum; note discharge, redness, swelling of the drum	decreased hearing acuity
3. Test auditory acuity by asking the patient to repeat numbers whispered by the examiner (CN VIII).	
F. Nose	
1. Inspect for deformity and inflammation	pale mucous membranes
2. Using a nasal speculum and light source, inspect the nasal mucosa for color, swelling, exudate, and bleeding	bleeding
G. Mouth and pharynx	
1. Inspect the lips for color, moisture, lumps, ulcerations, cracking, and bleeding	dry, cracked lips with bleeding
2. Using a light source, inspect the buccal mucosa for color, pigmentation, ulcerations, nodules, and bleeding	pale, ulcerated, bleeding mucous membranes inflamed, bleeding gums
3. Inspect the gums and teeth for inflammation, swelling, retraction, bleeding, caries, and loose or missing teeth	dry, cracked, bleeding tongue
4. Inspect the tongue for color, ulcerations, bleeding	
5. Inspect under the surface of the tongue and floor of the mouth for redness, nodules, and ulcerations	
6. Note and describe the smell of the breath	smell of ammonia and urine to breath
7. Using a tongue blade and light source, inspect the pharynx; describe color, exudate, edema, ulcerations, tonsillar enlargement	
H. Neck	
1. Palpate lymph nodes, using pads of index and middle fingers, and note enlargement	
2. Inspect and palpate trachea for deviation from midline	
3. Palpate the lobes of the thyroid; note size, shape, symmetry, tenderness, and nodules	
I. Thorax and lungs	
1. Inspect the posterior and anterior chest for rate, rhythm, and effort of breathing; deformities of the thorax; shape of chest; bulging interspaces during expiration	rapid, deep respirations in acidosis crackles pleural rubs
2. Auscultate the anterior and posterior lung fields for normal vesicular breath sounds and adventitious sounds (crackles, rhonchi, rubs)	
J. The heart	
1. Inspect and palpate each of the following areas for pulsations, lifts, heaves, and thrills	
a. aortic area (2nd intercostal space, right sternal border)	
b. pulmonic area (2nd intercostal space, left sternal border)	
c. 3rd left intercostal space (Erb's point)	
d. right ventricular area (lower half of sternum and parasternal area on the left)	
e. apical (left ventricular) area (5th intercostal space, just medial to the left midclavicular line)	
f. epigastric area (lower sternum and xiphoid process)	

Table 1.11

Health History and Physical Assessment Guide
for the Nephrology Nurse Caring for a Patient with Kidney Diseases (page 7 of 9)

	Typical Findings in Patients with Kidney Failure

2. Using the stethoscope, auscultate each of the following areas:
  a. aortic area (2nd intercostal space, right sternal border)
  b. pulmonic area (2nd intercostal space, left sternal border)
  c. Erb's point (3rd intercostal space, left sternal border)
  d. tricuspid area (5th intercostal space, left sternal border)
  e. mitral area (5th intercostal space, just medial to left midclavicular line)
  f. listen with bell and then diaphragm of stethoscope in each area
  g. assess the following:
    (1) first heart sound for intensity and splitting
    (2) second heart sound for intensity and splitting
    (3) systolic and diastolic murmurs
    (4) pericardial friction rub
3. Assess the rate and rhythm of the radial and carotid pulses
4. Using a stethoscope and sphygmomanometer, measure the arterial blood pressure
5. With the patient's upper torso at a 15°–30° angle, assess the internal and external jugular veins for level of distension
	
	murmurs
	pericardial friction rub
	
	irregular pulse rate
	hypertension
	paradoxical pulse (in pericardial effusion)
	distended jugular veins

K. Peripheral vascular system
1. Inspect arms, noting size and symmetry, color and texture of skin, nail beds, venous pattern, and edema
2. Inspect the legs, noting size and symmetry; color and texture of skin; nail beds; hair distribution on the lower legs, feet, and toes; rashes, scars, ulcers, venous enlargement, and edema.
3. Palpate each peripheral pulse:
  a. radial
  b. ulnar
  c. brachial
  d. femoral
  e. popliteal
  f. dorsalis pedis
  g. posterior tibial
4. Grade peripheral pulses based on a 4-point scale:
  0 – completely absent
  1 – barely palpable
  2 – expected, normal
  3 – full, increased
  4 – bounding
5. Perform an Allen test to assess patency of radial and ulnar arteries (especially important in patients who will have an artery in the forearm used for an AV shunt or fistula formation)
6. Assess external arteriovenous shunt or fistula or graft for patency and for adequate circulation to extremity distal to the shunt or fistula. Inspect exit site of external AV shunt for signs of inflammation. Inspect internal AV fistula or graft for scar tissue, redness, infection, presence of pulsation
	edema
	pale, cyanotic nail beds
	
	weak or absent peripheral pulses

L. Breasts and axillae 1. Inspect the female breasts for size and symmetry, masses, dimpling, flattening, color, edema, venous pattern, size and shape of nipples, direction in which nipples point, discharge from nipples 2. Palpate the female breasts for induration, tenderness, nodules 3. Inspect the male breasts for nodules, swelling, ulcerations 4. Palpate the male breasts for nodules, glandular enlargement (gynecomastia) 5. Inspect the axillae for rash and infection 6. Palpate auxiliary lymph nodes for enlargement and tenderness	 gynecomastia
M. The abdomen 1. Inspect the skin for scars, striae, dilated veins, rashes, and lesions 2. Inspect the contour of the abdomen for masses, enlarged organs, peristalsis, pulsations 3. Using the diaphragm of the stethoscope, auscultate for bowel sounds 4. Auscultate for bruits over the aorta, iliac arteries, and femoral arteries 5. Lightly percuss in all four quadrants, checking for normal sound of tympany or dullness of ascitic fluid 6. Percuss the upper and lower liver borders, and measure the span at the right midclavicular line 7. Palpate in all four quadrants for masses and tenderness 8. Palpate the lower liver border for consistency, tenderness, enlargement 9. Palpate right and left kidneys, noting size, contour, and tenderness 10. Assess for kidney tenderness at left and right costovertebral angles	 distended abdomen bruits ascites enlarged liver kidney tenderness

Table 1.11

Health History and Physical Assessment Guide
for the Nephrology Nurse Caring for a Patient with Kidney Diseases (page 8 of 9)

	Typical Findings in Patients with Kidney Failure

N. Male Genitalia
  1. Assess sexual maturation
    a. size and shape of penis and testes
    b. color and texture of scrotal skin
    c. character and distribution of pubic hair
  2. Inspect foreskin, if present, for phimosis and paraphimosis
  3. Inspect the glans for ulcers, scars, nodules, and signs of inflammation
  4. Inspect the urethral meatus for size and discharge
  5. Palpate the penis, noting tenderness and induration
  6. Inspect the scrotum for lumps, swelling, excoriation, and signs of inflammation
  7. Palpate each testis and epididymis, noting size, consistency, nodules and swelling
  8. Inspect for scar of past kidney implant
	in pubescent boys, underdeveloped penis and testes and absence of pubic hair for age
	
	decreased size of testes

O. Female Genitalia
  1. Assess sexual maturation
    a. character and distribution of pubic hair
    b. breast development
  2. Inspect labia majora, labia minora, clitoris, urethral orifice, vaginal opening for inflammation, ulcerations, discharge, swelling, or nodules
  3. Inspect for scar of past kidney transplant
	in pubescent girls, absence of pubic hair and decreased breast development for age

P. Musculoskeletal
  1. Assess each joint for:
    a. limitation in range of motion
    b. swelling
    c. tenderness
    d. heat
    e. redness
    f. crepitation
    g. deformities
    h. symmetry
  2. For renal patients, especially important to assess the following joints:
    a. hands and wrists
    b. elbows
    c. shoulders
    d. ankles
    e. knees
    f. hips
    g. spine
	decreased range of motion of joints
	swelling
	tenderness
	skin warm to touch
	red skin over joints
	deformities

Q. Nervous system
  1. Cranial nerves assessment
    I. Olfactory: have patient identify familiar odors
    II. Optic: test visual acuity; using an ophthalmoscope, inspect the fundus
 	
    III. Oculomotor
    IV. Trochlear ⎰ Inspect shape and size of the pupils; test pupillary reaction to light; test extraocular movements through the six cardinal fields of gaze, noting loss of movement in any direction and nystagmus
    VI. Abducens ⎱
    V. Trigemial
       Motor: Assess strength of temporal and masseter muscles
       Sensory: Assess for pain and light touch on the forehead, cheek and chin, bilaterally
       Assess for corneal reflex
    VII. Facial
       Motor: Inspect symmetry of face; assess ability to raise eyebrows, frown, show teeth, smile, puff out cheeks
    VIII. Acoustic: Assess hearing acuity
    IX. Glossopharyneal ⎰ Listen for hoarseness of the voice;
    X. Vagus ⎱ assess gag reflex
    XI. Spinal Accessory: Assess strength of shoulder muscles (trapezial)
    XII. Hypoglossal: Assess ability of tongue to protrude in midline and to move side to side
	decreased ability to identify odors
	
	nystagmus
	
	decreased sensation
	
	facial weakness
	decreased hearing acuity

Table 1.11

Health History and Physical Assessment Guide
for the Nephrology Nurse Caring for a Patient with Kidney Diseases (page 9 of 9)

	Typical Findings in Patients with Kidney Failure
2. Screening motor examination	
a. assess posture and balance during walking and standing	poor posture
b. perform a Romberg test	weakness of extremities
3. Screening sensory examination	
a. assess patient's ability (with his/her eyes closed) to identify points of sharp and light touch by the examiner	decreased sensation
b. stereognosis	
4. Reflexes	
a. using a reflex hammer, assess each reflex:	decreased reflexes
(1) biceps	
(2) triceps	
(3) brachioradialis	
(4) knee	
(5) ankle	
(6) plantar response (Assess plantar flexion or dorsiflexion of foot in response to stroking sole of foot.)	
b. grade each reflex on a 5-point scale:	
4+: very brisk; hyperactive	
3+: brisker than average	
2+: average; normal	
1+: somewhat decreased	
0 : no response	
R. Mental Status	

3. A distended bladder is dull to percussion above the symphysis pubis (Bickley, 2012; Seidel et al., 2011).

III. Kidney pain.

A. Assessment.
1. Careful assessment of urinary tract pain aids in differential diagnosis of intrarenal, postrenal, and/or extrarenal disorders and provides information for the management of the pain.
2. Assess the location, intensity, onset, pattern(s), and description/characterization of pain.
   a. Identify aggravating (what worsens) and alleviating (what improves) factors.
   b. Positional factors change with body movement.
   c. Associated signs and symptoms that occur with the pain.
3. Clarify the location of the pain (Eaton, 2013; Taal et al., 2012).
   a. Kidney pain or nephralgia is generally felt in the flank(s) and along the costovertebral angle in the back and is not altered by position changes.
   b. Ureteral pain is felt in the groin or genital area.
   c. Bladder pain is felt in the suprapubic to upper thigh area.
   d. Urinary tract pain is often perceived slightly below the ribs to the upper thighs and can be bilateral or unilateral.

B. Pain pathway.
1. Nociceptors (pain receptors) are located throughout the renal capsule and urinary collecting system (i.e., renal pelvis to external urethral sphincter).
2. Most of the kidney lacks nociceptors. Therefore extensive damage and complete loss of kidney function can occur without nephralgia.
3. Renal nociceptors transmit information to afferent (sensory) neurons that enter the dorsal spinal cord between T10 and T12.
4. Anterolateral spinal tracts transmit all pain information to the brain.
5. Testicular pain may accompany kidney pain because nerves from the renal plexus communicate with the spermatic plexus (Eaton, 2013; Taal et al., 2012).

C. Nephralgia.
1. Kidney pain is classified primarily as nociceptive visceral pain, meaning it arises from an intact nervous system in the kidney. Neuropathic kidney pain occurs less frequently and generally indicates damage to the nervous system (e.g., loin pain–hematuria syndrome).
2. If the renal capsule is punctured, distended, or inflamed, nephralgia occurs.
   a. When the renal capsule is punctured (such as with a biopsy or trauma), dull deep pain or intense pressure is felt. True nephralgia is

evident with a closed renal biopsy. Because cutaneous nociceptors are anesthetized, the needle passes through the skin painlessly. As the needle penetrates the renal capsule, deep nephralgia is felt because the capsule nociceptors are stimulated.

   b. Distention or inflammation of the renal capsule causes a dull, constant pain (as seen with neoplastic growths, bleeding from trauma, inflammation with edema formation, pyelonephritis, and inflamed or bleeding cysts).

  3. Acute obstruction in the intrarenal collecting system can cause pain if the renal pelvis is distended. Slowly developing calculi in the renal pelvis, however, can be painless.

  4. Ischemia caused by occlusion of renal blood vessels (e.g., from an embolus, arteriosclerotic disease, or tumor) results in constant dull or sharp pain (Eaton, 2013; Taal et al., 2012).

D. Referred pain.
  1. Pain that originates in viscera and is felt on the skin is referred pain.
  2. Renal (visceral) and cutaneous sensory/afferent neurons enter the spinal cord adjacent to each other.
  3. When renal sensory neurons are stimulated, concurrent stimulation of cutaneous neurons occurs and the nephralgia feels as though it originates in the skin.
  4. Renal pain is felt in dermatomes T10–L1.

E. Flank pain is classic for the presence of renal calculi (e.g., kidney stone) in the absence of fever.
  1. It will be important for the clinician to differentiate the origination of the pain source.
  2. A classic presentation would be pain that occurs acutely, originates in the flank area, and radiates to the groin, urethra, or abdomen accompanied by hematuria.
  3. Even though rarely considered, nausea and vomiting occurs in about 50% of patients with acute renal colic due to nephrolithiasis (Litwin & Saigal, 2012).
  4. However, it must be understood that flank pain is also associated with other pathologies including pyelonephritis or hydronephrosis.

F. Renal colic.
  1. Colic refers to spasm in a tubular or hollow organ accompanied by pain.
  2. Renal colic is often associated with movement of a stone down the ureter.
  3. Renal colic is an excruciating pain that increases in intensity, plateaus, and then decreases. The pain may radiate from the flank into the genital area (testicle or labia).

  4. Renal colic is treated with analgesia and fluid support (Eaton, 2013; Taal et al., 2012).

IV. Urine collection for analysis.

A. Use clean catch or midstream method for bacterial and routine urine analysis.
  1. Cleanse external genitalia.
  2. Have patient urinate approximately 100 mL (if possible) to flush out urethral bacteria and leukocytes. Discard.
  3. Then collect urine in a sterile container.

B. Urine specimens can be collected by bladder catheterization or suprapubic aspiration of the bladder.
  1. These are both invasive procedures that may lead to urinary tract infection. Therefore, these are done when no alternative noninvasive method is available.
  2. When a bladder catheter is in place, using aseptic technique, collect freshly excreted urine from the drainage system according to the manufacturer's instructions.

C. To ensure accurate analysis, deliver urine to the laboratory immediately. The specimen may be refrigerated up to 1 hour. Urine that remains at room temperature for 1 hour undergoes the following changes:
  1. Crystals form.
  2. Red blood cells hemolyze.
  3. Leukocytes lyse and release leukocyte esterase.
  4. Nitrites degrade.
  5. Tubercle bacilli die.
  6. Bacteria grow, consume glucose, and decompose urea to ammonia.
  7. Ammonia increases the urine pH.
  8. Many casts disintegrate in an alkaline environment (Kee, 2013; Rabinovitch, 2009).

V. Macroscopic urinalysis (see Table 1.12).

A. Physical characteristics.
  1. Normal yellow color is due to the presence of urochrome and urobilin pigments.
  2. Concentration of urine affects color. Dilute urine is less colored and concentrated urine is more orange colored.
  3. Urine color may be changed by drug and dye excretion, pigments, type of foods eaten, and cellular substances (for example, leukocytes make urine white, bile pigments make urine yellow-brown or greenish, and beets make urine burgundy).
    a. Hematuria can be microscopic or macroscopic, resulting in a range of color from yellow to

Table 1.12

Urinalysis

Macroscopic Analysis		
	Normal	**Alteration**
Color	Clear Pale yellow or amber	Cloudy with infection Lighter if dilute; darker if concentrated Changed by foods, cellular debris
Specific gravity	1.005–1.030	Increased with volume deficit Decreased with volume excess
Omsolality	100–1200 mOsm/kg	Increased with volume deficit Decreased with volume excess
pH	4.5–8	Increased with Fanconi syndrome; renal tubular acidosis
Glucose	Negative	Diabetes mellitus
Ketones	Negative	Starvation, vomiting, ketoacidosis
Leukocyte esterase	Negative	Inflammation, infection
Nitrites	Negative	Infection
Red blood cells	Negative–few	Inflammation, trauma, calculi, neoplasm
Protein	Negative/trace or < 30 mg/day	Increase in glomerular disease, tubular disease
Microscopic Analysis/Sediment		
	Normal	**Alteration**
Crystals	Negative	Calculi – specific to type
Casts		
Hyaline	0–few	Stress, fever, volume deficit, renal parenchymal disease
Red cell	0	Glomerulonephritis
White cell	0	Inflammation, infection
Fatty	0	Nephrotic syndrome
Renal tubular epithelial	0	Interstitial nephritis, acute tubular necrosis, transplant rejection
Granular	0	Renal parenchymal disease
Waxy or broad	0	Advanced kidney disease

bright red. Hematuria can originate from anywhere along the urinary tract (see Sediment later in this chapter).

b. Normal urine is clear. Cloudiness results from phosphates, urates, pH changes, bacteria, cells, crystals, or lipids.

c. Normal urine foams slightly when shaken. Proteinuria causes increased foam and may indicate kidney disease, such as the nephrotic syndrome (see Protein and Related Substances).

4. Degradation of urea to ammonia causes the characteristic smell of urine. Bacteriuria can increase urea breakdown and cause urine to have a much stronger ammonia smell.

5. Unusual urine odor may also result from ketonuria, phenylketonuria, alkaptonuria, hypermethioninemia, maple syrup urine disease, and the ingestion of certain foods such as asparagus (Kee, 2013; Rabinovitch, 2009).

B. Volume.
   1. Nurses provide one of the most valuable bedside tests for hospitalized patients: assessment of urine output.
      a. They may ultimately be the first to recognize a reduction in urine output signifying the need for evaluation and treatment.
      b. Urine output is monitored closely within an acute care setting because a significant reduction (less than 0.5 mL/kg/hr for 6 hours) meets the criterion of acute kidney injury (AKI) (Valette & du Cheyron, 2013).
   2. A minimal daily urinary volume of approximately 500 mL (SI = 0.5 L) is required to excrete wastes.
   3. The maximum diuretic volume is approximately 20 L (SI = 20 L).
   4. Urine is formed at about 1 mL/min (SI = .001 L/min).
   5. Clinically, less than 30 mL/hr (SI = .03 L/hr) warrants investigation.
   6. Daily urine volume can vary and is influenced by multiple variables, such as fluid intake, hydration status, and adequacy of kidney function (Daugirdas, 2014; Raff, 2002).

C. Specific gravity and osmolality. Urine specific gravity normally ranges from 1.005 to 1.030. Osmolality ranges from 100 to 1200 mOsm/kg H_2O. The kidneys help to maintain normal plasma osmolality primarily because the kidneys are to excrete urine with an osmolality markedly different from that of plasma.
   1. Specific gravity measures the density of a solution compared to the density of water, which is one (1.000). Specific gravity is altered by the presence of proteins, cells, casts, and other substances, whereas osmolality is not altered by these substances.
   2. Osmolality measures the number of solute particles per kilogram of water.
   3. Osmolality is the most accurate measurement of the kidney's ability to concentrate or dilute urine.
   4. The more concentrated the urine, the higher the osmolality (as with fluid volume depletion). The more dilute the urine, the lower the osmolality (as with fluid volume excess or diabetes insipidus).
   5. Blood and urine osmolality are measured simultaneously to determine if the kidneys are responding correctly to the body's fluid status.
      a. Blood osmolality is approximately 280 to 300 mOsm/kg H_2O (SI = 280 to 300 mOsm/kg H_2O).
      b. Healthy kidneys maintain a constant plasma osmolality by excreting urine with an increased osmolality when the plasma osmolality increases, or excreting urine with a low osmolality when the plasma osmolality decreases.

   6. There are times when the urine specific gravity is falsely elevated, such as when measured after a patient has been administered radiographic dye. This can result in a specific gravity as high as 1.03, if measured close to the time of the procedure.
   7. On the other hand, a low-urine specific gravity may be caused by excessive fluid intake, diabetes insipidus, or from diuretics (Litwin & Saigal, 2012).

D. Urine pH.
   1. Normal range of urine pH is 4.5 to 8 (SI = pH 4.5 to 8).
   2. pH is influenced by many extrarenal factors, such as drugs, electrolyte imbalances, and systemic pH changes.
   3. A change in urine pH seldom indicates kidney disease, except with renal tubular acidosis and Fanconi syndrome (in these cases, the urine is alkaline).
   4. With pregnancy, urine pH is more alkaline, especially in the morning. This is normal and does not indicate kidney disease (Kee, 2013; Rabinovitch, 2009).

E. Glucose in the urine.
   1. Glycosuria with normally functioning kidneys is due to plasma glucose that exceeds the renal threshold for glucose reabsorption (e.g., diabetes mellitus, excessive carbohydrate intake, highly emotional states, pregnancy, and dysfunction of the pituitary gland).
   2. A plasma glucose level of 180 mg/dL must be generally exceeded in someone with normal kidney function for glycosuria to occur. With pregnancy, glycosuria can occur without hyperglycemia.
   3. Glycosuria without hyperglycemia occurs with kidney impairment (e.g., Fanconi syndrome and with exposure to nephrotoxins). Fanconi syndrome may result from disease processes (e.g., multiple myeloma), heavy metal exposure, and certain medications (e.g., cisplatin, aminoglycosides) (Haque et al., 2012).

F. Ketones.
   1. Ketones are an end product of fat metabolism.
   2. Ketonuria results from an increased catabolism of fatty acids due to starvation, vomiting, extreme temperature exposure, extreme overexertion/ physical exercise, alcoholic or diabetic ketoacidosis, and a large vitamin C intake.
   3. Ketonuria is a poor indicator of kidney disease.

G. Nitrites.
   1. Urine does not normally contain nitrites.
   2. In the bladder, many gram-negative and some gram-positive bacteria convert nitrates

(substances related to protein metabolism) to nitrites.
3. Bacterial conversion of nitrates to nitrites takes 4 hours or more. Therefore, the best time to test is the first urine specimen of the morning.
4. Presence of nitrites in urine is detected by a color change test and reported as positive or negative.
5. A positive nitrites test indicates bacterial infection in the urinary tract (greater than 10,000 organisms per mL).
6. Factors that interfere with accurate test results are high urine specific gravity, abundance of urinary ascorbic acid, low dietary intake of protein, urine pH less than 6, and prolonged storage of urine (nitrites will degrade) (Baumgarten & Gehr, 2011; Daugirdas, 2014; Raff, 2002).

H. Urinary electrolytes.
1. Many factors affect the quantity of electrolytes excreted in the urine.
   a. Their daily range is quite variable.
   b. It is beneficial to analyze urinary electrolyte composition from a 24-hour specimen and correlate the results with plasma electrolyte levels.
2. Certain electrolytes are altered with kidney disease (e.g., sodium and potassium).
   a. Recent evidence reflects less favorable diagnostic capacity than once appreciated.
      (1) Historically, the fractional excretion of sodium (FENa) was used to assist in differentiating prerenal acute kidney injury (AKI) from acute tubular necrosis (ATN).
      (2) Over time, it has been realized that this once simple diagnostic parameter (e.g., FENa) has too many exceptions.
   b. Now there are promising new urinary biomarkers (e.g., neutrophil gelatinase-associated lipocalin, NGAL) for diagnosing AKI that offer better diagnostic utility (Macedo & Mehta, 2009).
3. The most important parameter to clarify the presence of prerenal failure is fluid replacement.
   a. If kidney function returns to the previous baseline within 1 to 3 days after optimization of volume status, then this would be consistent with a diagnosis of a prerenal origin.
   b. Persistent kidney failure would be suggestive of ATN.
4. An examination of urinary sediment for renal tubular epithelial cells and casts has improved prognostic utility more than the evaluation of the urinary excretion of urea or sodium (Perazella & Coca, 2012).
5. Urine chemistries have a fairly limited role in providing reliable information to differentiate between prerenal AKI and ATN.

6. The ability to concentrate urine is at times impaired with AKI resulting in electrolyte and/or water wasting (e.g., ATN). At times, the urine remains essentially unchanged from the glomerular filtrate produced as early as the proximal tubule (Perazella & Coca, 2012).

I. Urinary protein.
1. Overview.
   a. Normally, individuals excrete small quantities of protein in the urine.
   b. Proteinuria is often the first evidence of progressive kidney disease and thus an important tool for diagnosing early kidney disease.
   c. Urinary protein excretion in excess of 150 mg/day is often associated with kidney disease.
   d. The type of protein in the urine has heightened significance.
      (1) Albumin can signify chronic kidney disease related to diabetes, glomerular disease, and hypertension.
      (2) Low-molecular-weight globulins are suggestive of tubulointerstitial disease (KDIGO, 2013a).
2. Normal urinary excretion of albumin is approximately 30 mg/day (SI = 0.73 μmol/day).
   a. Microalbuminuria is defined as urine excretion of albumin between 30 and 150 mg/day (SI = 0.73–2.2 μmol/day).
   b. The presence of microalbuminuria helps to diagnose, plan, and evaluate treatment, and monitor disease progression of diabetic nephropathy.
   c. The reagent on most dipstick tests is sensitive to albumin with 99% sensitivity and specificity.
   d. Follow-up analysis of significant proteinuria should be done by sending a urine specimen to the laboratory.
   e. Table 1.13 describes how dipstick results correspond with laboratory values of proteinuria.
   f. With increasing amounts of protein in the urine, foaming occurs (like whisking an egg white).
3. Proteinuria greater than 150 mg/24 hour (SI = 2.2 μmol/24 hr) is significant and should be evaluated thoroughly. Proteinuria may indicate glomerular capillary disease, such as nephrotic syndrome or glomerulonephritis.
4. With pregnancy, proteinuria up to 300 mg/day (SI = 4.4 μmol/day) is considered within normal limits.
5. Proteinuria may be transient or persistent.
   a. Transient proteinuria reflects a temporary change in the glomerulus and is generally benign and self-limited; e.g., as can be seen in

Significant proteinuria may be missed in dilute urine & may be overdiagnosed in conc. urine.

Table 1.13

Proteinuria – Correlation of Dipstick and Amount of Protein

Dipstick Result	Amount of Protein
Trace	5–10 mg/dL
1+	30 mg/dL
2+	100 mg/dL
3+	300 mg/dL
4+	1000 mg/dL

congestive heart failure, with exercise, or fever.
   b. Persistent proteinuria reflects malfunction of the glomerulus or tubules and requires additional investigation. Patients who have evidence of persistent proteinuria on two or more tests spaced 1 to 2 weeks apart should be diagnosed with chronic kidney disease and undergo further evaluation (KDIGO, 2013a).
6. Proteinuria can be estimated from a random "spot" urine sample, preferably obtained in the morning, first-voided specimen.
   a. Collect a minimum of 10 mL and measure the protein and creatinine in the urine.
   b. Calculate the ratio of urinary protein in mg/urinary creatinine in mg. Normally, the ratio in an adult is approximately 0.2 or 200 mg/day (SI = 2.92 μmol/day); in a child 0.5 or 500 mg/day (SI = 7.3 μmol/day).
   c. As proteinuria increases, the ratio increases (e.g., ratio of 3.5 = 3.5 gm/day [SI = 51.3 μmol/day] proteinuria).
   d. Obtaining a spot urine sample for the purposes of detection and monitoring proteinuria in both children and adults has been shown to have the diagnostic equivalence to that of a 24-hour urine total protein sample (Methven et al., 2010).
7. Significant aminoaciduria occurs with elevated plasma amino acid levels (hepatic disorders), high protein intake, and renal tubular disorders (e.g., cystinuria and Hartnup disease) (Baumgarten & Gehr, 2011; Daugirdas, 2014).

J. Additional substances.
   1. Urinary excretion of uric acid. Most of uric acid (70%) is removed from the body in urine. A small amount of uric acid is removed in stool. However, if the kidneys are no longer able to remove adequately, uric acid will increase in the blood and form crystals that can deposit into joints causing gout. It must be understood that not everyone with an elevated uric acid level in the blood will

develop gout. People may have a diet rich in purine-rich foods or have chronic kidney disease. Patients with kidney disease have a reduced capacity for elimination.
   a. Daily urinary excretion is variable and influenced by diet and protein metabolism.
   b. Hyperuricosuria is associated with malignant neoplasms, antineoplastic agents, and gout.
      (1) May result in calculi formation and renal impairment.
      (2) The correlation of an elevated uric acid level and the development of kidney disease or the role uric acid plays in having a causal relationship with hypertension or vascular disease requires additional research (Feig, 2009).
   c. Some hyperuricosuria is normal in pregnancy due to the increased glomerular filtration rate.
   2. Urinary excretion of urea.
      a. Variable amount is excreted daily depending on diet, fluid balance, and kidney function.
      b. Altered urinary urea levels suggest kidney disease and need to be correlated with blood urea nitrogen levels. Urine urea levels usually decrease with kidney failure.
   3. Urinary excretion of myoglobin.
      a. Myoglobin is a protein found in muscle cells where it accepts oxygen from hemoglobin and stores oxygen for use by the mitochondria.
      b. Filtered by the nephron and excreted in the urine.
      c. Myoglobinuria occurs with excessive skeletal muscular trauma (called rhabdomyolysis) and does not necessarily indicate kidney disease.
      d. Excessive myoglobinemia may cause kidney impairment because one of myoglobin's metabolites is potentially nephrotoxic (Baumgarten & Gehr, 2011; Daugirdas, 2014).

VI. Examination of urinary sediment.

A. To complete the evaluation of a urine specimen, microscopic examination of the urine sediment is essential.
   1. To perform an examination of urinary sediment, at least 10 mL of urine must be centrifuged for 5 minutes.
   2. The top layer of supernatant is discarded while the bottom pellet is retained for examination under a microscope (see Figure 1.40).

B. Determining the significance of urinary cells.
   1. Squamous epithelial cells represent normal desquamation from the lower urinary tract, and a few are normal.
   2. Transitional cells, renal tubular cells, and oval fat bodies originate from the upper urinary tract with

disorders such as acute tubular necrosis, acute glomerulonephritis, pyelonephritis, and nephrotic syndrome.

3. Erythrocytes (red blood cells [RBCs]).
   a. RBCs are not normally found in the urine. However, presence of a few RBCs does not always represent pathology. If one or more can be seen in every high-power field and contamination (e.g., menstruation) is ruled out, then this is abnormal.
   b. An increased number indicates disruption of the genitourinary tract vasculature, e.g., inflammation, lesions, trauma, neoplasms, moving calculi, and cystic disease.
   c. Erythrocytes that originate from the kidney are usually broken and accompanied by red cell casts. Red blood cell casts are consistent with glomerulonephritis.

4. Leukocytes and bacteria in the urine. Pyuria, the abnormal presence of leukocytes in the urine, appears with infection. The location of the infection cannot be known with certainty. It could be in the upper or lower urinary tract, or the cells could represent glomerulonephritis.
   a. A few leukocytes and bacteria are normally present in urine.
   b. An increased number of leukocytes, bacteria, or both nitrites and leukocyte esterase indicate inflammation in the urinary tract, e.g., infection.
      (1) Leukocyte esterase is an enzyme found in azurophilic or primary neutrophil granules and released with inflammation.
         (a) Leukocyte esterase is reported as negative or positive and may be quantified as trace, small (+), moderate (++), or large (+++).
         (b) A false positive result may occur if urine has vaginal secretions or cells.
         (c) An erroneous high positive result occurs when urine remains at room temperature. Over time, more leukocytes lyse, and more leukocyte esterase is released.
         (d) Substances that can affect test accuracy are the presence of ascorbic acid, glucose, albumin, cephalexin, tetracycline, cephalothin, and large quantities of oxalic acid in the urine.
      (2) Casts usually accompany leukocytes and bacteria that originate in the kidney.
      (3) Bacteria are surrounded by an antibody when they originate in the kidney.
         (a) A full inflammatory reaction may take about a week, and that is when the antibody-coated bacteria will be visible in the urine.

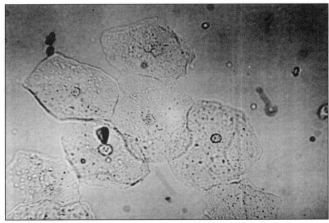

A. Squamous epithelial cells from lower urinary tract.

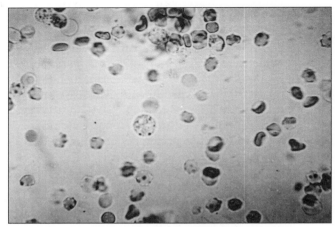

B. Numerous red blood cells and occasional white blood cells.

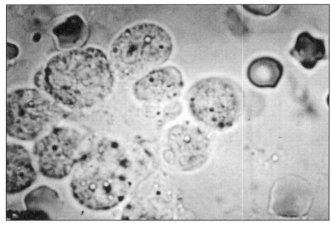

C. Clusters of white blood cells.

Figure 1.40. Urinary sediment.

orthostatic proteinurea – excretion varies diurnally & c posture – lowest values c night & then c supine

transient benign proteinurea – may develop in response to stress – fever, exercise, cardiac failure

(b) With repeated infections, the antibody-coated bacteria will appear more quickly.

(4) Persistent leukocyturia without bacteriuria may indicate the presence of fungi, yeast, or tubercule bacilli.

d. Eosinophils in the urine.

(1) Eosinophiluria indicates a hypersensitivity reaction intrarenally, such as acute interstitial nephritis, urinary tract infection, and renal transplant rejection.

(2) Eosinophiluria is affirmed by Wright stain when urine pH is greater than 7 (SI = pH 7), or by Hansel stain when the urine pH is less than 7 (Baumgarten & Gehr, 2011; Daugirdas, 2014).

C. Urine microscopy and evaluation of crystals.

1. Crystalluria is an abnormal urinary finding and may or may not be related to kidney disease.

2. Crystal formation is pH dependent, can develop any place along the urinary tract, is enhanced by fluid volume depletion, and can result in calculi (see Figure 1.41).

a. Crystals found in acid urine are uric acid, calcium oxalate, calcium sulfate, amorphous urate, cystine, leucine, or tyrosine.

b. Crystals found in alkaline urine are phosphates, calcium carbonate, or ammonium biuret.

c. Drugs and dyes can also crystallize.

D. Urine microscopy and evaluation of casts.

1. Casts are formed or molded in the tubular lumen of the kidney. They are called casts (cylindruria) because of the molding process. Urinary casts are either formed in the distal convoluted tubule (DCT) or the collecting duct (distal nephron). Casts are not formed in the proximal convoluted tubule (PCT) or loop of Henle.

2. Casts are composed of Tamm-Horsfall protein and other substances associated with inflammation such as cellular debris, immunoglobulins, and pigments. Tamm-Horsfall protein is a mucoprotein that forms the base of casts and is formed and secreted by cells of the ascending loop of Henle, distal tubule, and collecting duct.

3. Casts are important indicators of kidney disease and aid in identifying the type of disease.

a. Decreased tubular fluid flow or stasis, increased acidity, and increased solute concentration favor cast formation.

b. Casts generally form in the favorable environments of the distal tubule and collecting duct.

c. Casts can dissolve in alkaline urine.

d. Although casts vary in length, size, and width, they are cylindrical because the tubular lumen is cylindrical.

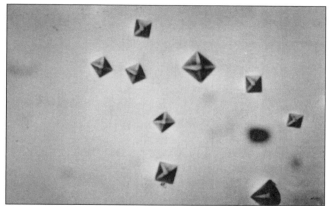

A. Calcium oxalate crystals.

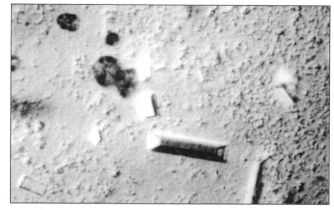

B. Triple phosphate crystals.

Figure 1.41. Urinary crystals.

e. Casts are classified by their appearance and composition.

4. Types of casts (see Figure 1.42).

a. Hyaline casts are acellular and a few in the urine are normal.

(1) A transient increase in urinary hyaline casts can occur with stress, strenuous exercise, fever, and fluid loss.

(2) A persistent increase may indicate renal parenchymal disease.

b. Red cell casts contain fragments of erythrocytes and are associated with glomerular disruption and bleeding as in glomerulonephritis, Goodpasture syndrome, renal trauma, and lupus nephritis.

c. White cell casts contain leukocyte fragments and are associated with inflammation as in pyelonephritis and interstitial nephritis.

d. Fatty casts contain lipoid material, are present with fatty degeneration of tubular epithelium, and are associated with nephrotic syndrome, diabetic glomerulosclerosis, and lupus erythematosus.

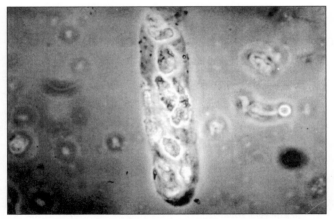

A. Tubular epithelial cell cast.

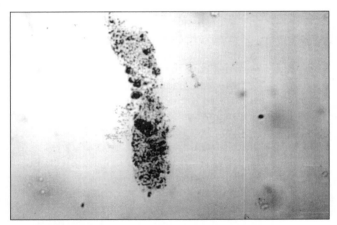

B. Coarse granular cast.

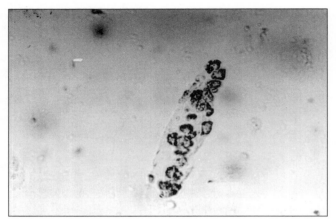

C. White blood cell cast.

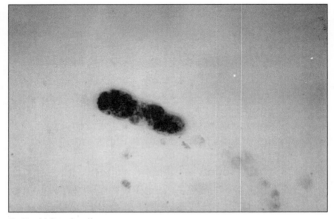

D. Red blood cell cast.

Figure 1.42. Urinary casts.

e. Renal tubular epithelial cell casts are composed of sloughed tubular epithelium and associated with acute tubular necrosis and transplant rejection.

f. Broad casts contain epithelium and are large because they form in the collecting duct. The presence of broad casts indicates significant damage to the tubules of the nephron and suggests advanced kidney disease.

g. Granular casts indicate kidney disease and represent final degeneration of cellular casts and/or aggregation of serum protein with Tamm-Horsfall protein.

   (1) Granular casts are described as fine or coarse. There is no clinical difference between them.

   (2) Pigmented granular casts contain portions of heme pigments, myoglobin, hemoglobin, or a combination, and may be named for the pigment (e.g., hemoglobin cast).

   (3) Heavily pigmented granular casts may be called muddy brown casts and are one of

the casts associated with acute tubular necrosis.

h. Waxy casts are the final degeneration of granular casts.

   (1) Indicate advanced kidney disease, and are sometimes called kidney failure casts.

   (2) Associated with diabetic nephropathy, renal amyloidosis, and CKD stage 5 (Baumgarten & Gehr, 2011; Daugirdas, 2014).

VII. **Blood analysis in evaluation of kidney function.**

A. Serum creatinine is a biochemical marker used by clinicians to evaluate kidney function in acute and chronic conditions. It is a poor marker of CKD because it does not become elevated until over 50% of kidney function is lost. It is also influenced by diet, muscle mass, age, and medications. As an index for AKI, it increases too late following injury. For these reasons, other markers are under investigation. For now, serum creatinine is routinely measured, standardized, and inexpensive to obtain.

1. Normal 1 mg ± 0.3 mg/dL (SI = 88 mmol/dL) and pregnant woman 0.46 mg ± 0.3 mg/dL (SI = 37 mmol/dL).
2. An end product of phosphocreatine, a high energy substance used to form ATP to be used as energy by muscles.
3. Slightly higher in men than women because of larger muscle mass in men.
4. Fluctuates minimally throughout the day and from day to day.
5. Regulated and excreted by the kidneys.
6. Rises with kidney failure, severe muscle breakdown, or both.
7. An elevated creatinine is a fair indicator of kidney function when the person is considered to be in a steady metabolic state (not acutely ill) and there is no evidence of muscle breakdown.
   a. Plasma creatinine of 2 mg/dL (SI = 176 mmol) indicates an approximate 50% loss of kidney function. A plasma creatinine of 8 to 9 mg/dL (SI = 704 to 792 mmol/dL) indicates an approximate 90% loss of kidney function.
   b. The plasma creatinine rises when over 50% of kidney function is lost.
8. As the ability of the kidneys to remove creatinine decreases, the plasma creatinine increases. As the plasma creatinine doubles, the creatinine clearance decreases. Creatinine clearance is the same as glomerular filtration rate.
9. Because plasma creatinine varies from person to person related to muscle mass, it is important to obtain a baseline for each person and calculate a glomerular filtration.
10. Plasma creatinine is less reliable as an indicator of kidney failure with malnourishment, liver failure, and heart failure. In these situations, creatinine clearance is more accurate.
11. In pregnancy, plasma creatinine is lower because of increased clearance of creatinine. Therefore, a slight rise in plasma creatinine (> 0.9 mg/dL [SI = 78 mmol/dL]) should be investigated.

B. Blood urea nitrogen (BUN).
1. Normal 10 to 20 mg/dL (SI = 3.6 to 7.1 mmol/L); in pregnant woman 8.7 mg ± 1.5 mg/dL.
2. An end product of endogenous or exogenous (dietary) protein metabolism.
3. Influenced by fluid volume changes, dietary protein intake, and catabolism.
4. 75% is excreted by the kidney and 25% by the bowel.
5. The BUN rises with kidney failure, increased protein breakdown (e.g., gastrointestinal bleeding and fever), and fluid volume depletion.
   a. With kidney failure, the kidney does not excrete urea effectively, and blood levels rise over time.
   b. With bleeding in the GI tract, the blood is digested (including plasma protein), and as with any protein, urea is an end product and absorbed into the blood.
   c. With fluid volume depletion, although the number of urea molecules stays constant, they appear increased in proportion to the low number of water molecules.
6. Changes in BUN must be correlated with changes in plasma creatinine to assess kidney failure.
7. In pregnancy, the BUN is lower because of increased renal clearance. As with plasma creatinine, a slight rise should be investigated.
8. The BUN and plasma creatinine rise simultaneously in kidney failure (Daugirdas, 2014; Kee, 2013).

C. Cystatin C role in evaluation of kidney function.
1. Cystatin C is a cysteine protease inhibitor produced by the body's cells at a constant rate.
2. Filtered by the glomerulus and reabsorbed completely by the tubules.
3. May be used as an alternative to serum creatinine or creatinine clearance for screening and monitoring.
4. Elevated levels indicate decreased kidney function (decreased glomerular filtration rate).
5. May be more useful in monitoring kidney function in critically ill patients; tends to rise more quickly than creatinine.
6. May be useful in predicting higher risk of CKD among older adults without known kidney disease.
7. Not affected by diet, inflammation, gender, age, or race.

D. Although many electrolytes, pH, and nonelectrolytes are regulated and excreted by the kidney, numerous extrarenal factors influence their plasma levels and must be considered in assessing kidney function.
1. As an example, plasma potassium is regulated and excreted by the kidneys, but its movement into and out of cells is influenced by insulin, aldosterone, cellular damage, and pH changes.
2. After disorders of these extrarenal factors are excluded, a rise in serum potassium along with a rise in creatinine and BUN is an indicator of worsening kidney failure.

E. Erythropoiesis is regulated by renal erythropoietin. With chronic kidney disease, anemia occurs, and the hematocrit, hemoglobin, and the erythrocyte counts are decreased.

F. Substances that the kidney secretes can be measured, such as plasma renin.

1. Renin is elevated in some forms of hypertension and renal artery stenosis.
2. Renin is normally elevated in pregnancy.
3. Plasma renin concentration is obtained with a blood sample drawn when the patient is in an upright position (stimulates renin release).
4. Concentration values.
   a. Normal sodium diet.
      (1) The normal adult living in the United States consumes about 4 to 6 grams of sodium daily. The kidneys excrete sodium at a rate of 2.9 to 24.0 ng/mL/hr in ages 20 to 39.
      (2) In an adult 40 years of age, the kidneys will excrete sodium at a rate of 2.9 to 10.8 ng/mL/hr.
   b. Low-sodium diet.
      (1) A low-sodium diet is considered to be 2 grams or less per day. This would translate into a urinary sodium excretion rate of 0.1 to 4.3 ng/mL/hr for someone 20 to 39 years old.
      (2) For someone 40 years of age on a sodium restricted diet, sodium excretion would be somewhat less, around 0.1 to 3.0 ng/mL/hr.

G. Plasma substances that are altered with specific kidney diseases can be measured, including antibodies, complement, and autoantibodies.
   1. Antibodies are composed of globulin proteins and termed *immunoglobulins* (Ig).
      a. The classes of these antibodies and typical values are:
         (1) IgG 565 to 1765 mg/dL (SI = 5.65 to 17.65g/L).
         (2) IgA 85 to 385 mg/dL (SI = 0.85 to 3.85 g/L).
         (3) IgM 55 to 375 mg/dL (SI = 0.55 to 3.75 g/L).
         (4) IgD Minimal.
         (5) IgE Minimal.
      b. A rise in IgG and IgM is associated with nephropathy, such as SLE or Sjögren's syndrome.
      c. IgA rises with Berger's disease (glomerular pathology) and pregnancy hypertension.
      d. IgE rises with allergic reactions.
   2. Normal complement values are:
      a. Total complement: 75 to 160 U/mL (SI = 75 to 160 U/L).
      b. C3 55 to 120 mg/dL (SI = 0.55 to 1.20 g/L).
      c. C4 20 to 50 mg/dL (SI = 0.20 to 0.50 g/L).
      d. Complement decreases with inflammatory kidney diseases.
   3. Autoantibodies are normally absent. Therefore their presence indicates pathology. Autoantibodies and kidney diseases associated with them include:

      a. Anti-DNA: systemic lupus erythematosus (SLE) and scleroderma.
      b. Antiglomerular basement membrane: Goodpasture syndrome.
      c. Antinuclear: SLE, scleroderma, and Sjögren's syndrome.
      d. Anti-sm-B: SLE (sm = smooth muscle).
      e. Anti-ss-A and Anti-ss-C (ss = Sjögren's syndrome).

[handwritten annotation: creatinine excretion rate varies with muscle mass. In particular women, elderly have lower creatinine generation rate thus artificially inflates ratio of protein to albumin to creatinine]

VIII. **Creatinine clearance.**
A. Creatinine clearance.
   1. Overview.
      a. Creatinine clearance to assess kidney function is an imperfect test if measured directly with a 24-hour urine sample or estimated by calculation of the glomerular filtration rate.
      b. Measurement of inulin excretion is considered the gold standard, but this requires intravenous infusion and timed blood samples that must be done over several hours. This makes inulin infusions a less than optimal tool for measuring kidney function.
      c. Creatinine is freely filtered by the glomerulus, but is also secreted by the proximal tubules.
      d. A 24-hour urine collection is also difficult to accurately obtain and is no longer routinely used for determining creatinine clearance.
      e. Serum creatinine based equations for GFR are more accurate (Cirillo, 2010).
   2. Creatinine clearance is the amount of blood cleared of creatinine in 1 minute by the glomerular capillaries.
   3. After creatinine is filtered through the glomerular capillaries, it passes through the nephron with minimal change and is excreted. Creatinine clearance is a measure of the GFR.
   4. Creatinine clearance is a good clinical indicator of kidney function. As kidney function decreases, creatinine clearance decreases.
   5. Normal creatinine clearance for a young adult is about 110 to 120 mL/min.

B. Procedure. Collect a 24-hour urine specimen and one blood specimen drawn at the midpoint of the urine collection.
   1. The volume of urine and quantity of creatinine in the blood and urine are measured.
   2. These values are inserted into formulas that calculate creatinine clearance (Daugirdas, 2014; Kee, 2013).

C. Formulas for creatinine clearance (CrCl).
   1. Basic formula:

$$CrCl = \frac{U_{Cr} \times U_{Vol}}{P_{Cr} \times T_{min}} \qquad Corrected\ CrCl = \frac{CrCl \times 1.73}{BSA}$$

   U_{Cr} =   Urine creatinine   BSA = Body surface area
   U_{Vol} =   Urine volume
   P_{Cr} =   Plasma creatinine
   T_{min} =   Time in minutes

   2. Approximately 10% of urinary creatinine is secreted into the tubular lumen. Therefore, the above formula overestimates GFR by about 10%. Thus, a more accurate GFR is obtained by multiplying the results by 90% (0.90).
   3. Creatinine clearance can be estimated by the following formula:
      Cr Cl = [(140 – age) x TBW] / (SCr x 72)
      TBW = weight in kg
      SCr in mg/dL
      a. For females, the above result is multiplied by 85% (0.85).
      b. This calculation does not require a 24-hour urine collection and is an estimate rather than direct measure of the creatinine clearance.
   4. Another formula for creatinine clearance is the MDRD (Modification of Diet in Renal Disease) formula:
      a. 186 x (plasma creatinine) – 1.154 x (age in years) – 0.203.
      b. For females, the above result is multiplied by 0.742.
      c. For African Americans, the above result is multiplied by 1.210.
      d. The MDRD formula is complex due to the negative log algebra functions. As a result, a calculator is needed to compute the creatinine clearance.
      e. The MDRD formula is generally considered a more accurate estimate of creatinine clearance than the Cockcroft-Gault formula. However, many clinicians and reference books use the Cockcroft-Gault equation due to ease of calculation.
   5. For children (1 week to 18 years), the Schwartz equation is often used:
      a. (length [cm] x k) / serum creatinine.
      b. k = 0.45 for infants 1 to 52 weeks old.
      c. k = 0.55 for children 1 to 13 years old.
      d. k = 0.55 for adolescent females 13 to 18 years old.
      e. k = 0.7 for adolescent males 13 to 18 years old (Daugirdas, 2014; Kee, 2013).

IX. Imaging studies.

A. Overview.
   1. Imaging studies are crucial to the diagnosis and successful management of patients with kidney disease.
   2. Frequently, imaging studies are obtained in an effort to determine the etiology for kidney injury or kidney disease.
   3. Most commonly, studies are obtained in an effort to evaluate for the presence of vascular diseases, vesicoureteral reflux, urinary tract obstruction, kidney stones, renal cyst, or mass.
   4. Kidney ultrasound is by far the most common imaging study obtained.

B. Radionuclide tests.
   1. Involve administration of a radionuclide tracer agent (e.g., 99mTc dimercaptosuccinic acid [DMSA]). The kidneys uptake and excrete the tracer allowing measurement of kidney function in each kidney.
   2. A renal scan is frequently obtained to evaluate renal perfusion. This includes evaluation for renal artery stenosis and thrombosis. A more specific type of scan called a radionuclide cystography is the best choice for detection of vesicoureteral reflux, especially in children (Dyer et al., 2001).
      a. A radionuclide (low-dose radioactive substance) is injected intravenously. The radioactive substance circulates through the kidneys and is excreted in the urine.
      b. Renal scans depict accumulation of the radionuclide by the kidneys and primarily provide information related to anatomy. For example, in renovascular disease hypoperfused areas are poorly visualized (Michota, 2001; Snyder, 2005).
      c. A renal scan is a diagnostic tool used to detect renal artery stenosis. An evaluation for the presence of artery stenosis might be invoked in patients who have resistant hypertension despite appropriate management and a history of atherosclerotic disease (O'Neill et al., 2011).
   3. Renogram.
      a. Procedure is same as the renal scan.
      b. As the radionuclide circulates through the kidneys, scintillators count the agent's activity, and curves are generated that describe blood flow, glomerular filtration, and tubular secretion (Michota, 2001; Snyder, 2005).
   4. Patient preparation for above tests.
      a. Explanation of the procedure, which is painless and noninvasive (except for the venipuncture). There is a slight amount of radiation from the radioisotope. Most of this radiation exposure occurs to the kidneys and bladder. Almost all

radiation is gone from the body in 24 hours. Caution is advised if the patient is pregnant or breastfeeding.
   b. Required to sit or lie quietly during the test.
   c. No special posttest care (Michota, 2001). The patient may be asked to drink plenty of fluids and urinate frequently to help remove the radioactive material from the body.

C. Renal arteriogram.
   1. Outlines renal arterial vasculature and differentiates the type of renovascular disorder. For example, it can identify the high vascularity of a malignant neoplasm; or, differentiate between stenosed or misplaced vessels (see Figure 1.43).
   2. Indications for an arteriogram include persistent hematuria, blunt trauma, hypertension, renal arterial disease, renal mass, and preparation for kidney surgery.
   3. Procedure.
      a. A radiopaque dye is injected intravenously (IV) or through a catheter.
      b. Numerous roentgenograms are taken.
      c. The IV catheter is removed and a pressure dressing applied to the catheter insertion site.
   4. The iodine-based radiopaque dye is potentially nephrotoxic and allergenic.
      a. Should be used with caution, and in the lowest dose possible in patients with diabetes mellitus,

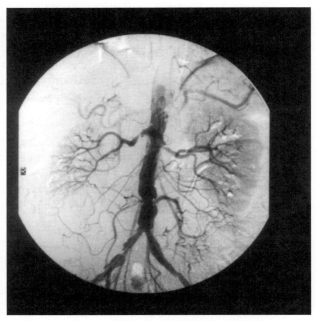

Figure 1.43. Abdominal aortogram and renal arteriogram. Bilaterally, renal arteries are narrowed near their exit from the aorta. The right kidney is small and the left kidney is normal size. The distal aorta and right common iliac artery have moderate to high-grade stenosis.

diabetic nephropathy, preexisting kidney disease, vascular disease, multiple myeloma, older adults, and in the presence of fluid volume depletion (Niell et al., 2013).
      b. Individuals with an allergy to iodine or seafood may be unable to receive an iodine-based dye.
   5. Patient care before the arteriogram.
      a. Description of the test.
      b. Assessment for allergy to the dye.
      c. Explanation that as the dye is being injected, an unusual taste may be sensed in the mouth.
      d. Explanation of posttest care and vital signs monitoring.
   6. Patient care after a renal arteriogram:
      a. Bed rest for 4 to 12 hours (variable; may be shorter or longer depending on the patient and length/difficulty of the procedure).
      b. Frequent assessment of vital signs and pedal pulses for peripheral circulation.
      c. Assessment for bleeding or hematoma formation at the catheter insertion site.
      d. Maintenance of the pressure dressing for 24 hours.
      e. Adequate hydration.
      f. Observation for nephrotoxic and/or allergic reactions to the dye.
   7. Complications associated with a renal arteriogram include inflammation, hematoma, thrombus, embolus, arteriovenous fistula formation, atheroma dislodgement, acute decrease in kidney function (nephrotoxic reaction), and anaphylactic reaction to dye (Revell et al., 2010).

D. Renal venogram.
   1. Outlines the renal venous vessels.
   2. The procedure and patient care are same as for the renal arteriogram.

E. Magnetic resonance angiography (MRA).
   1. Arteries can be visualized with increasing accuracy.
   2. Can be an alternative to traditional renal angiography for people at risk for complications associated with contrast media.
   3. See MRI for additional discussion regarding patient care and procedure (Michota, 2001).

X. Roentgenogram's utility in evaluating kidney disease.

A. Plain roentgenogram (x-ray) of the kidneys, ureters, and bladder (KUB).
   1. Visualizes the size, shape, position, and number of kidneys, ureteral, and bladder structures.
   2. Identifies radiopaque objects, foreign bodies, calculi, neoplasms, or air.

B. Significance of findings.
   1. Size and shape.
      a. Large or irregular shaped kidneys may indicate hydronephrosis, cysts, or neoplasms.
      b. Small kidneys may indicate chronic glomerulonephritis or nonfunctioning kidneys.
      c. The kidneys lengthen a few centimeters with pregnancy.
   2. Air around or inside the kidney may indicate severe infection.
   3. A nebulous or indistinct kidney border may indicate neoplasm or inflammation.

C. Patient teaching.
   1. A KUB is noninvasive, painless, requires no dyes, and can be done in an upright or lying position.
   2. No special patient preparation or posttest care is required.

XI. Ultrasound studies are used to evaluate kidney disease routinely.

A. Overview.
   1. A majority of kidney cancers are found by routine surveillance imaging studies like ultrasound (American Cancer Society, 2013).
   2. Kidney ultrasound is recommended for evaluation of kidney failure of unknown etiology.
   3. However, the benefit of obtaining a kidney ultrasound when evaluating AKI is not entirely clear.
   4. Other risk stratification criteria may provide more diagnostic significance than information obtained for a kidney ultrasound in specific patient population groups (Licurse et al., 2010).

B. During the renal ultrasound, inaudible, nonharmful sound waves are reflected off the kidneys. Photographs are made that identify renal anatomy and true kidney depth.

C. Patient teaching.
   1. Procedure is noninvasive and painless.
   2. Requires that the patient remain in the prone or sitting position for about 30 minutes.
   3. No special care before or after the procedure is required.

D. Limitations.
   1. Ribs, adipose tissue, and gas in the bowel can interfere with sound wave reflections.
   2. Interpretation is difficult in obese individuals.
   3. Interpretation is difficult if the kidneys are high under the ribs and/or behind a gas-filled gastrointestinal tract.

E. Significance of findings.
   1. Outlines hydronephrosis.

   2. Differentiates between a cyst that is fluid-filled and a tumor that is solid.
   3. During pregnancy, the kidneys will be larger.

XII. Computerized axial tomography (CAT/CT).

A. Dual energy CT allows better visualization and differentiation of the genitourinary structures (e.g., determining chemical composition of renal calculi) (Dalrymple et al., 2007).

B. Numerous roentgenograms are taken, each about 10 degrees apart, and transmitted into a computer that creates an image of the kidney and calculates its density.

C. Significance of findings.
   1. CAT is more sensitive than an ultrasound. A renal lesion that does not enhance is not a neoplasm.
   2. Detects and characterizes renal masses. Kidneys are a common site for extra-renal malignancy, such as non-Hodgkins lymphoma.
   3. Visualizes renal vascular disorders and inferior vena cava tumors.
   4. Identifies filling defects of the collecting system and regional lymph nodes.

D. CT can be performed with or without intravenous dye. The patient is observed for an allergic response to the dye during and after the test.

E. Patient teaching.
   1. Test is painless.
   2. A supine position for 10 to 15 minutes is required.
   3. May have to hold breath for short periods of time during the test.
   4. Machine makes some noise.
   5. After the test, no special care is required.

XIII. Magnetic resonance imaging (MRI).

A. The advantages of obtaining an MRI is that it does not require ionizing radiation and it has better contrast resolution compared to a computerized tomography (CT) scan.

B. MRI is a painless, noninvasive procedure that provides visual information about soft tissue.

C. The MRI scanner applies a strong magnetic field that causes protons to align themselves with the magnetic field. Emission of radio waves causes the magnetic field to rotate or resonate.

D. The rotating fields generate electric signals that a computer analyzes, creating an image on a screen. Images are available in all planes.

E. Significance of findings.
   1. Visualizes renal vessels, possible extension of neoplasm in the renal vein and/or inferior vena cava.
   2. Visualizes retroperitoneal structures.
   3. Identifies renal masses. MRI does not differentiate benign from malignant tumors.

F. Patient teaching.
   1. Test is painless.
   2. Need to lie still in a horizontal position on a table.
   3. The table is moved into a tube-like structure that may create a feeling of claustrophobia. An "open" MRI is available that does not require a closed structure.
   4. In general, anyone wearing removable metal objects will be asked to remove them before the test (e.g., rings). Individuals with pacemakers and aneurysm clips should not undergo an MRI. Individuals with other types of implanted metal will need to undergo an individualized risk assessment.
   5. Takes about 40 to 90 minutes.
   6. The room may feel cool, and it is warmer inside the magnet.
   7. The magnet makes noise like a jack hammer so ear plugs or covering are worn.
   8. Sedation is available based on the patient's need.
   9. Individuals with CKD stages 4 and 5 should undergo MRI only if necessary.
      a. In about 2.5% of these individuals, an adverse reaction to gadolinium (the contrast agent used in MRI) may cause nephrogenic systemic fibrosis (NSF).
      b. NSF is characterized by thickening and hardening of the skin (most commonly in the extremities) that progresses to joint immobility and may present 2 weeks to 18 months after receiving gadolinium.

G. Posttest care is determined by the use or absence of sedation during the test (Michota, 2001; Rydahl et al., 2008).

XIV. Excretory urograms.

A. Intravenous pyelography (IVP).
   1. Provides information about the size, shape, and position of the urinary tract structures, and renal excretory function, such as twisted ureters, misplaced kidneys, and obstructed calyces.
   2. A radiopaque dye is injected intravenously, circulates through the kidneys, and is excreted in the urine. Roentgenograms are taken as the dye circulates through the urinary tract.
   3. The iodine-based dye used for the IVP is potentially nephrotoxic and allergenic.
      a. Should be used with caution, and in the lowest

dose possible in patients with diabetes mellitus, diabetic nephropathy, preexisting kidney disease, vascular disease, multiple myeloma, older adults, and in the presence of fluid volume depletion.
      b. Individuals with an allergy to iodine or seafood may be unable to receive an iodine-based dye.
   4. Patient preparation for an IVP.
      a. Explanation of the procedure.
      b. A clear, empty gastrointestinal tract.
      c. Good hydration.
      d. Assessment of kidney function (creatinine clearance).
      e. Assessment of allergy to the dye, iodine, or seafood.
   5. Posttest care.
      a. Maintaining good hydration.
      b. Watching for allergic reaction.
      c. Evaluating kidney function for nephrotoxicity to the dye.

B. Retrograde pyelogram.
   1. Provides anatomic information about the collecting system of the urinary tract, such as the position of a ureteral calculus.
   2. Procedure.
      a. Patient preparation is similar to an IVP.
      b. The procedure may be uncomfortable – pressure and an urge to void are felt.
      c. Bladder and ureteral catheterizations are performed.
      d. A radiopaque dye is injected through the catheters into the urinary tract and roentgenograms are taken.
         (1) As the catheters are removed, more dye is injected and x-ray is taken.
         (2) About 5 minutes after the catheters are removed, another x-ray is taken.
         (3) If a ureteral obstruction is identified, a stent may be left so urine can drain (Michota, 2001; Steggall & Omara, 2008).
   3. Potential complications.
      a. Urinary tract infection.
      b. Perforation of the bladder or ureter.
      c. Ureteral edema with possible obstruction.
      d. Hematuria.
      e. Discomfort from the dye (unusual taste).
   4. Postprocedure care.
      a. Assess for and treat complications.
      b. Assess for bleeding, infection, characteristics of the urine, and ability to void to completely empty the bladder (using a bladder scanner may be helpful to determine bladder volume).
      c. Assess for pain and/or ureteral, bladder, or urethral spasms. Administer analgesics.
      d. Provide and encourage hydration.

C. Antegrade pyelogram (nephrostomogram).
  1. Provides anatomic visualization of the urinary collecting system.
     a. May include the renal pelvis.
     b. Will include the ureter.
     c. May include the bladder.
  2. Indicated with a ureteral, ureteropelvic, or ureterovesical obstruction when an intravenous or retrograde pyelography cannot be done.
  3. Procedure.
     a. Contrast material is injected into the renal pelvis via a percutaneous needle or a nephrostomy tube (if present), and x-rays are taken (Michota, 2001; Snyder, 2005; Steggall & Omara, 2008).
     b. Patient preparation and postcare are similar to a kidney biopsy (following section) and retrograde pyelogram.
        (1) Pain occurs with this procedure as with a kidney biopsy because a needle punctures the kidney.
        (2) No pain is felt if a nephrostomy tube is in place.
     c. Potential complications.
        (1) Allergic reaction to the dye.
        (2) Urinary tract bleeding.
        (3) Urinary tract infection.
     d. Generally, minimal concern about potential nephrotoxicity of the contrast material unless it refluxes through the calyces and into the papillae.

XV. Kidney biopsy.

A. Purpose, indications, and contraindications.
  1. A kidney biopsy determines the nature and extent of kidney disease for diagnosis, treatment, and prognosis.
     a. It is a relatively safe procedure with a complication rate of less than 0.1%.
     b. Consideration must be given as to whether the biopsy results will change the course of management.
  2. Indications.
     a. Unexplained acute kidney injury (AKI) with two normal size kidneys, no evidence of obstruction, and no obvious cause for dysfunction.
        (1) Most of the time, AKI is explained by prerenal disease, acute tubular necrosis, and urinary tract obstruction.
        (2) These conditions are usually diagnosed clinically without need for biopsy.
     b. Significant and persistent proteinuria with two normal-sized kidneys, no evidence of obstruction, and no obvious cause for dysfunction.

c. Kidney biopsy is usually not indicated in the case where the cause of the glomerulonephropathy can almost be pinpointed to a prior infectious event (e.g., streptococcal pharyngitis).
     d. Suspected kidney involvement in systemic disease (e.g., active lupus nephritis).
     e. Kidney transplant dysfunction of unknown etiology.
  3. Contraindications.
     a. Hemorrhagic tendencies.
     b. Uncontrolled hypertension (blood pressures exceeding 160/95 mmHg).
     c. Sepsis.
     d. Solitary kidney is a relative contraindication.
     e. Small shrunken kidneys measuring less than 9 cm.
     f. Large polycystic kidneys.
     g. Hydronephrosis.
     h. Documented kidney neoplasm.
     i. Urinary tract infection.
     j. Frequent coughing, sneezing, or both.
     k. Uncooperative patient.
     l. According to a study focusing on the benefit of a biopsy in persons age 80 or more years, there appears to be some clinical benefit. The study reported that kidney biopsy in the elderly modified treatment in 67% of cases, particularly in those with AKI. Age is not a contraindication for kidney biopsy (Moutzouris et al., 2009).

B. Procedure.
  1. A biopsy is an invasive procedure requiring strict aseptic technique.
  2. Small section of cortical tissue is obtained by a needle and examined histologically (by a pathologist with experience in kidney biopsy tissue analysis) by light, immunofluorescence, and/or electron microscopy.
     a. Light microscopy magnifies tissue approximately 750 times and electron microscopy 54,999 times.
     b. Immunofluorescence is a staining technique used to study immunopathologic processes and can identify complement and antibodies.
  3. A kidney biopsy can be done by the open or closed/percutaneous method. The percutaneous method is done more frequently (see Figure 1.44).
  4. Open method.
     a. Surgical procedure.
        (1) The kidney is exposed.
        (2) Biopsy needle is inserted into the kidney under direct visualization.
     b. Indicated when percutaneous biopsy is hazardous (e.g., with an obese or restless patient).

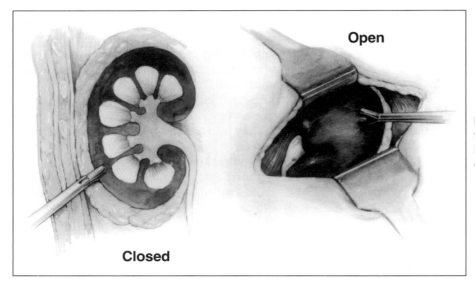

Figure 1.44. Kidney biopsy. Technique for closed/percutaneous and open kidney biopsy. The biopsy needle is enlarged for illustrative purposes.

c. Patient preparation is similar to any major abdominal operation and includes the preparation for a closed or percutaneous kidney biopsy (explained below).
d. Advantages include direct visualization of kidney and better control of bleeding, and can be done with other abdominal surgeries.
e. Disadvantages include the risks of surgery, e.g., risk of anesthesia, an operation, lengthened recovery, and infection.
5. Closed or percutaneous method.
a. Procedure.
   (1) Can be done at the bedside if patient is unable to go to medical imaging department. The kidney position is sometimes marked on the skin with ultrasound if biopsy is performed at a different time or location.
   (2) Patient is prone with pillows under abdomen to elevate kidney.
   (3) Patient with a transplanted kidney will be supine because of the position of the allograft in the iliac fossa.
   (4) Skin is cleansed and anesthetized.
   (5) With the patient holding his or her breath, the biopsy needle is inserted with aid of ultrasound. Breathing would cause the needle to move slightly because the kidneys are in contact with the diaphragm.
   (6) Patient may complain of pain and/or intense pressure as the needle enters the innervated renal capsule.
   (7) Tissue samples are taken and prepared, needle removed, pressure dressing applied to puncture site.
   (8) Patient remains in position for 20 to 30 minutes.
   (9) An ultrasound may be completed after the

biopsy to identify any immediate postprocedure bleeding (Walso et al., 2009).
b. Patient preparation.
   (1) Explanation of the procedure and postprocedure care.
   (2) Signed informed consent.
   (3) Pain will be felt when needle enters kidney (this is an example of visceral pain).
   (4) Patient responsibilities (e.g., position and holding breath).
   (5) Hematologic and kidney function assessment.
   (6) Determination of kidney position and depth (usually by CT or ultrasound).
   (7) Vital sign monitoring.
   (8) Mild sedation.
   (9) Urinate before procedure.
   (10) NPO 8 to 12 hours before (variable).
6. Postprocedure care for percutaneous and open kidney biopsy.
a. Monitor vital signs frequently for first 24 to 48 hours to detect intrarenal and/or extrarenal bleeding and infection.
b. Assess for other signs and symptoms of bleeding including pallor, dizziness, lightheadedness, decrease in erythrocytes, hematocrit, and/or hemoglobin, backache, and/or flank pain.
c. Collect serial urine specimens to evaluate hematuria (redness should decrease with each sample).
d. Maintain bed rest and pressure dressings to prevent bleeding.
e. Assess puncture site for bleeding and/or signs and symptoms of inflammation.
f. Assess pain with administration of analgesics (opioids often indicated). Cold therapy and therapeutic touch may also be beneficial.

g. Educate and assist with splinting puncture site to decrease discomfort with coughing and deep breathing.

h. Instruct patient to drink liberal amounts of fluids to maintain dilute urine and prevent intrarenal clot formation.

i. Give emotional and psychological support.

j. Limit strenuous activity, heavy lifting for 1 to 2 weeks.

7. Complications.
   a. Persistent hematuria.
   b. Infection.
   c. Perirenal and/or intrarenal arteriovenous fistula.
   d. Aneurysm.
   e. Laceration of organs and/or blood vessels adjacent to the biopsied kidney (Michota, 2001; Taal et al., 2012).

SECTION E
Chronic Kidney Disease
Joni Walton

I. Prevalence of CKD.

A. Overview.
1. Millions of people in the United States have chronic kidney disease (CKD).
   a. Two different sources, the Centers for Disease Control and Prevention (CDC) and the National Kidney Foundation (NKF), estimate there are around 20 to 26 million with CKD (CDC, 2014; NKF, 2013b).
   b. The statistics become even more alarming when you consider the global impact; 10% to 16% of people worldwide have CKD (NKF, 2013b).
2. While CKD is highly prevalent, most are unaware that they have it and remain undiagnosed.
   a. As a consequence of this lack of awareness, CKD has been labeled the "silent epidemic" by the NKF (NKF, 2013b).
   b. Approximately 9 out of 10 people with CKD stage 3 do not know they have the disease.
3. CKD continues to be the major cause of physician visits, hospitalizations, and lost productivity.
4. In the United States, CKD is the 8th leading cause of death.
5. Unfortunately, the preferred treatment of CKD stage 5 with kidney transplantation is remarkably low.
   a. In 2011, fewer than 15,000 people received a kidney transplant.

b. In September 2014, 109,184 people were on the waiting list in hopes of receiving a kidney.
   c. Considering these numbers, it is easy to understand why so many die while waiting for a transplant (Organ Procurement and Transplant Network, 2014).

B. The demographics of CKD.
1. The incidence of CKD is higher in females and adults over age 70.
2. CKD progression to stage 5 is more likely to occur in males (CDC, 2010).
3. Geographic destiny seems to matter in the determining the prevalence of CKD.
   a. The south has more adults with CKD than other regions of the United States.
   b. The majority of adults living with kidney disease are married with an annual income less than $35,000.
   c. Adults under the age of 65 years living with CKD usually have insurance.
   d. Still, many with CKD are uninsured (Schiller et al., 2012).
4. The majority of Americans with CKD are Caucasian.
5. However, a disproportionate number of African Americans, Native Hawaiians, Asian Americans, and American Indians have CKD (Schiller et al., 2012).
   a. Mexican Americans are 1.5 times more likely to develop CKD.
   b. African Americans are four times more likely than whites to develop CKD (CDC, 2010).
      (1) African Americans with hypertension may have a genetic variant that increases their likelihood for CKD.
      (2) The nonmuscle myosin heavy chain 9 gene (MYH9) has been implicated in the progression of CKD in this population (KDIGO, 2012c).

C. The relevance of age and CKD.
1. Children achieve an adult level of GFR by the age of 3 years.
2. Kidney function peaks by the third decade of life, usually denoting a GFR of around 120 mL/min/1.73 m^2.
3. After the age of 30, GFR tends to decline by 0.8 to 1 mL/min/1.73 m^2 per year.
4. Older adults tend to develop CKD at a higher rate than younger adults.
   a. Kidney sclerosis occurs with age.
   b. Functioning renal mass declines; decrease in the number of functioning nephrons.
   c. Kidney weight decreases.
   d. Age-related loss of kidney function might not

always have implications for an individual's health (Arora, 2013).

D. Genetics and CKD.
1. Table 1.14 provides a list of some of the inherited diseases related to the kidneys.
2. Research in CKD genetics is in its infancy and full of promise for new developments.
3. Pharmacogenomics is an exciting field that provides individualized genetic data that allows healthcare providers to identify medications that may cause nephrotoxicity, drug interactions, and harmful side effects. This individualized data can help enhance and optimize pharmacologic treatment (Luttropp et al., 2009).
4. Nephrotic syndrome, such as in Alport syndrome or progressive tubulointerstitial disease, is a genetic disease.
5. Atypical hemolytic uremic syndromes and kidney damage may develop secondary to inherited diseases such as metabolic or systemic disorders (Vehaskari, 2011).
6. The apolipoprotein L-1 (APOL1) located near the MYHY gene may play a role in focal glomerulosclerosis in African Americans (Friedman et al., 2011).
7. Albuminuria is also linked to a single-nucleotide polymorphism in the SHROOM3 gene (Ellis et al. 2012).

E. Social or environmental risk factors.
1. Epidemiologists have reported that high fluoride content in ground water, exposure to fertilizers, and pesticides in farming communities caused a significant increase in kidney disease in Sri Lanka (IRIN, 2008).
   a. Approximately 50% of fluoride that is ingested is filtered by the kidneys. In the United States, doses of fluoride contained in drinking water are far below what would be considered toxic levels (Xiong et al., 2007).
      (1) Exposure to environmental toxins as a cause for kidney disease is not routinely considered in the United States.
      (2) However, it needs to be considered when there is no apparent etiology.
   b. In 2012, Sri Lanka had a high prevalence of CKD among male farmers.
      (1) Over 2 years, health officials in Sri Lanka documented a 25% increase in CKD.
      (2) Dehydration and contaminated water may be a factor causing CKD in this population.
   c. The Chinese herb aristolochic acid is nephrotoxic.
      (1) People living in rural Croatia, Romania, Serbia, Bosnia, and Bulgaria experienced an endemic of a noninherited condition called Balkan nephropathy.
      (2) Caused by the toxin aristolochic acid that causes kidney failure and bladder cancer (NIH, 2011).

Table 1.14

Inherited Kidney Diseases

Cystic Kidney Diseases	Inherited Metabolic Diseases	Other Inherited Diseases	Other with Genetic Influence
Autosomal dominant polycystic kidney disease	Diabetes mellitus	Alport syndrome and variants	Reflux nephropathy
Autosomal recessive polycystic kidney disease	Genetic amyloidosis	Bartter syndrome	Hemolytic uremic syndrome
Nephronophthisis	Anderson-Fabry disease	Congenital nephrotic syndrome	
Medullary sponge kidney	Renal Fanconi syndrome	Primary immune glomerulonephritis	
Associated with tuberous sclerosis, Lowe's syndrome, Von Hippel-Lindau diseases and other syndromes	Hyperoxaluria	Primary immune glomerulonephritis	

Based on Devuyst et al. (2014)

2. Industrial chemicals and heavy metals can cause CKD (Soderland et al., 2010).
   a. Young men working as manual laborers in the Northwestern region of Nicaragua have an increased prevalence of CKD and urinary tract infections called *chisata*, a syndrome of dysuria among sugarcane workers.
   b. The higher prevalence of CKD has been attributed to the more frequent antibiotics, NSAIDs, diuretics, dehydration, and resultant volume depletion (Ramirez-Rubio et al., 2013).
3. Up to 5% of NSAIDs users experience adverse renal events, and older adults are at significant risk (Luciano & Peraxella, 2012).
4. Iodinated contrast mediums have been implicated in contrast-induced acute kidney injury (CI-AKI) in people with comorbidities, e.g., hypertension and adult-onset diabetes (Bansal, 2012; Solomon & Dauerman, 2010).
   a. Damage results from iodinated contrast media that remains stagnant in the kidneys and causes direct renal tubular cellular damage.
   b. Cytotoxicity is impacted by a decrease in renal blood flow that ultimately leads to medullary ischemia.

F. Physiologic risk factors.
1. Hypertension (HTN) and diabetes are the most common causes for CKD.
   a. Diabetes is the leading cause of CKD worldwide.
   b. It has been estimated that about 40% of patients with diabetes have diabetic-associated nephropathy (KDIGO, 2012c).
2. The National Kidney Disease Education Program (NKDEP, 2012) reported that 44% of new patients starting dialysis have diabetes-induced nephropathy.
3. Age-related loss of kidney mass is a key factor in the development of CKD.
4. Obesity, elevated lipids, cardiovascular disease, and acute kidney injury from drugs, toxins, and infections compounds the risks for CKD.
5. In the United States, longevity, obesity, and type 2 diabetes perpetuate the development of kidney disease (Hajhosseiny et al., 2013).
6. During the past decade, clinicians have diagnosed and treated glomerulonephritis earlier than in the past, which has resulted in a reduced incidence (CDC, 2014).

II. Etiology and pathophysiology of CKD.

A. Overview.
1. It is important for nephrology nurses to understand that the pathogenesis of CKD is multifactorial and complex; it impacts almost all body systems.
2. Systemic diseases, if present prior to CKD, can accelerate the progression of both the disease and CKD (KDIGO, 2013a).
3. The human body has an impressive ability to compensate for decreased kidney function.
4. The kidneys are able to maintain homeostasis up to a 25% loss in glomerular filtration rate (GFR) allowing for preservation of solute clearance.

B. Loss of nephrons.
1. The pathophysiology of CKD is dependent upon the specific underlying etiology; however, there are several mechanisms that occur following the loss of nephron mass that are common to the overall pathogenesis.
   a. Increased intrarenal activity of the renin-angiotensin system.
   b. Adaptive hyperfiltration.
   c. Glomerular capillary pressure and flow increase, causing glomerular hypertension leading to systemic HTN.
   d. Vasoactive molecules, cytokines, and growth factor cause structural and functional hypertrophy of nephrons.
   e. Glomerulosclerosis.
   f. Tubulointerstitial inflammation leading to fibrosis and scarring (Heuther & Forshee, 2010).
2. Intact nephron theory.
   a. In progressive nephropathy, the "intact nephron theory" hypothesizes that normal kidney function is temporarily sustained by surviving nephrons.
   b. Heuther and Forshee (2010) explain that "nephrons are capable of a compensatory hypertrophy and expansion or hyperfunction in their rates of filtration, reabsorption, and secretion and can maintain a constant rate of excretion in the presence of overall declining GFR" (p. 1390).
   c. This process of progressive renal dysfunction with compensatory hyperfiltration and hypertrophy is the primary pathophysiology of CKD.
   d. This is compounded by nephrotoxins (e.g., NSAIDs, aminoglycosides, and heavy metals), hypertension, dyslipidemia, smoking, diabetes, and acute kidney injury.
   e. With a loss of approximately 50% of the nephrons, the serum creatinine will double in value and the GFR will decrease by 50% (Arora, 2013). With this realization, it is understandable why so many people have undiagnosed CKD, as early stages are asymptomatic with powerful physiologic compensatory mechanisms in place.

C. Creatinine, GFR, and albuminuria.
1. Creatinine is affected by race and ethnicity, muscle

mass, diet, nutrition (high protein diets and supplements), and muscle-wasting disorders.

2. Creatinine is released by muscle tissue and excreted through glomerular filtration.

3. As the GFR decreases, serum creatinine increases in an inverse relationship.
   a. Serum creatinine alone is not an accurate measure of CKD because creatinine is impacted by age, gender, race, body muscle mass and fat, metabolic state, pharmacologic agents, and lab analytical procedures.
   b. However, it continues to be used as a surrogate marker in GFR estimating equations.

4. The best indicator of kidney function is a calculated plasma GFR. GFR provides an estimate of the filtering capacity and rate of which an ultrafiltrate of plasma is produced by the glomeruli per unit of time.

5. Normally, proteins are reabsorbed in the proximal convoluted tubules, and due to molecular size and charge, are restricted from entering Bowman's space and the renal interstitium. It is thought protective mechanisms in the glomerular wall prevent the transmural passage of proteins.
   a. Glomerular endothelium pores.
   b. Network of hydrated collagen.
   c. Interdigitations network of podocytes in a slit diaphragm.

6. In proteinuria, damaged epithelial cells allow proteins to pass through these protective barriers, and damage is compounded by the proteins themselves.

7. Fibrosis and sclerosis occurs as a result of protein-mediated toxicity on the cells (Lerma, 2013). It is not entirely clear whether albumin or nonalbumin proteins are responsible for nephrotoxicity.

8. Albuminuria is an early marker of kidney dysfunction.
   a. Defective glomerular basement membrane.
   b. Overproduction of proteins.
   c. Systemic disease impacts the kidneys' ability to reabsorb proteins.

9. The extent of proteinuria is widely recognized as a marker of the severity of CKD and as a predictor of future decline in GFR.
   a. More important, a reduction in proteinuria translates into a protection from further decline in patients with diabetic and nondiabetic kidney disease.
   b. Progression of kidney disease with proteinuria.
      (1) Consistent experimental evidence supports the crucial role of proteinuria in accelerating kidney disease.
      (2) Multiple pathways are involved.
         (a) Increased glomerular permeability, resulting in proteinuria.

      (b) Leads to excessive proximal tubular reabsorption of protein.
      (c) Increase in inflammatory mediators within the renal tubules.
      (d) Vasoactive and inflammatory genes are activated.
      (e) Resulting in interstitial inflammatory changes and fibroblast proliferation.
      (f) Ultimately causing renal scarring (Cravedi & Remuzzi, 2013).

10. Urinary albumin is the most frequently assessed measure of kidney damage in clinical practice, reflecting endothelial damage caused by either systemic diseases or kidney disease (Levey & Kinker, 2013).

D. Fluid, electrolytes, and acid-base.
   1. CKD impacts the kidneys' ability to balance salt, water, and acid-base balance.
   2. Highly adaptive remaining nephrons are able to maintain fluid balance until the GFR drops to 20 mL/min, and then compensatory mechanisms begin to fail.
   3. When the GFR reaches about 20 mL/min, there is a decrease in sodium and free-water elimination, resulting in extracellular volume expansion causing signs of fluid overload, most notably peripheral edema.
   4. The kidneys also lose the ability to eliminate potassium when aldosterone secretion and distal blood flow decline (Arora, 2013).
   5. Potassium shifts from intracellular space to extracellular space with evolving acidosis, resulting in development of hyperkalemia.
   6. In CKD, the proximal tubules are unable to produce adequate amounts of ammonia to eliminate endogenous acids, causing metabolic acidosis.
      a. Metabolic acidosis in CKD leads to protein imbalance, negative nitrogen balance, increased protein degradation, increased essential amino acid oxidation, reduced albumin synthesis, and lack of adaptation to a low protein diet causing protein-energy malnutrition (Arora, 2013).
      b. The bones suffer because calcium is a buffer for acidosis resulting in the depletion of minerals and renal osteodystrophy (Arora, 2013).
      c. In the early stages of CKD, acid is eliminated by excretion of hydrogen ions by the kidneys in the form of acid and ammonium.
      d. Each nephron increases excretion of ammonium, which activates the renin-angiotensin and complement systems, producing endothelium-1, known to cause inflammation and damage the kidneys.

e. Bicarbonate from bone, tissue, and extracellular fluid buffers the retained acid in the body.

f. The level of ammonium excretion decreases when GFR is less than 40 mL/min and metabolic acidosis develops.

g. There are severe consequences of chronic metabolic acidosis leading to complex health problems, worsening endocrine disorders, and aggravating systemic inflammation leading to increased mortality (Kovesdy, 2013).

E. Calcium, vitamin D, phosphate, and bone.
1. Alterations in mineral and bone metabolism begins in the early stages of CKD and progresses over time with further loss of kidney function.
2. Hypocalcemia occurs in response to acidosis and is further impacted by vitamin D3 due to impaired synthesis in the kidneys, thus decreasing absorption of calcium in the intestines (Arora, 2013).
3. Phosphate retention further disrupts production of vitamin D3.
4. In the later stages of CKD, phosphate is not adequately filtered from the kidneys, leading to development of hyperphosphatemia.
5. Excessive phosphates are known to bind to calcium in the soft tissues and deposit in tissues leading to soft tissue calcification and vascular calcifications (Shanahan et al., 2011). This adaptive mechanism does not allow serum phosphate to increase until the later stages of CKD.
6. Pathogenesis of secondary hyperparathyroidism in CKD is thought to be caused by the down regulation of parathyroid receptors on the parathyroid gland. Both vitamin D and calcium receptors are down regulated, causing elevation in parathyroid hormone, reduction in serum calcium, and low vitamin D levels.
   a. This down regulation affects fibroblast growth factor that has been implicated in hyperplasia of the parathyroid glands and vascular calcification (Cunningham et al., 2011).
   b. Secondary hyperparathyroidism has been linked to the development of bone and mineral defects, vascular and soft tissue calcification, and cardiovascular disease.

III. Systemic impact of CKD.

A. Metabolism.
1. Insulin sensitivity is diminished with hyperparathyroidism, resulting in glucose intolerance.
2. Individuals with diabetes, metabolic syndrome, and nondiabetes are impacted by insulin resistance and oxidative stress. This has a plausible association with development of vascular and renal injury (Heuther & Forshee, 2010).
3. In addition to altered bone and mineral metabolism, a negative nitrogen balance occurs from changes in protein, fat, and carbohydrate metabolism. When glomeruli are diseased, protein will leak into the urine, causing proteinuria and indicating kidney damage.
4. Proteinuria in itself can cause damage to the kidneys and increase the progression of CKD through the inflammatory process described earlier.
5. Inflammatory cell infiltration can accelerate damage to the kidneys by causing tubular inflammation and fibrogenesis that further decrease GFR and increase cardiovascular risk (Cravedo & Remuzzi, 2013).
6. Renal excretion of medications. The kidneys play a vital role in pharmacokinetics.
   a. Individuals with CKD do not have normal renal metabolism or clearance of many medications (Arora, 2013).
   b. The individual patient and GFR need to be taken into account, as well as the pharmacokinetic principles of the drug.
      (1) Calculating doses and dosing intervals based on GFR.
      (2) Many drugs require renal adjustment (reduced dose).
   c. In CKD, drug metabolites can cause serious side effects and toxicities from accumulation that can lead to life-threatening complications.
   d. There are three primary effects in individuals with CKD described by Doogue and Polasek (2011).
      (1) Drugs have higher steady-state concentrations.
      (2) Increased vulnerability to the drug effect.
      (3) Drug effect may be exaggerated.
   e. A general principle to remember is "decreased drug clearance results in higher drug concentrations and hence greater drug effects" (p. 1).
   f. Nurses realize the valuable role the clinical pharmacist plays in medication consultation and dosing in CKD.

B. Cardiovascular.
1. Metabolic abnormalities, oxidative stress, and proinflammatory mediators are known to accelerate the progression of cardiovascular disease in CKD (Heuther & Forshee, 2010).
2. CKD is an independent risk factor for development of cardiovascular disease and more important than smoking or dyslipidemia. There is a body of evidence that supports the relationship between decreased GFR and increased cardiovascular disease (Herzog et al., 2011).
3. Proteinuria is also an independent predictor of cardiovascular disease and mortality (Hajhosseiny et al., 2013).

a. Hajhosseiny and colleagues (2013) came to the conclusion that proteinuria is the single strongest predictor of cardiovascular disease in CKD.

b. Proteinuria has also been implicated in development of arrthymias such as atrial fibrillation, complete heart block, asystole, and ventricular tachycardia and ventricular fibrillation.

c. The strong association with proteinuria and cardiovascular disease specifically includes development of coronary heart disease, myocardial infarction, stroke, acute mitral regurgitation, and cardiogenic shock (Hajhosseiny et al., 2013).

4. The pathophysiologic mechanisms of endothelial dysfunction in CKD are not clearly defined. Oxidative stress and the inflammatory process have been known to play a powerful role in the acceleration of vascular aging (Cozzolino, 2013).

a. Endothelial nitric oxide synthesis, availability, and function play a key role in prevention of cardiovascular disease by antiinflammatory, antiadhesive, antiplatelet, and vasodilating functions.

b. Proteins broken down into dimethylarinines cause a dysfunction in nitric oxide synthesis and endothelial function (Hajhosseiny et al., 2013).

c. Cardiac remodeling is induced with myocyte hypertrophy and dysfunction, increase in interstitial fibrosis, and a decrease in capillary density with a resultant increased left ventricular hypertrophy (LVH).

d. Concentric LVH is seen in up to 42% of individuals with CKD and an even higher incidence in patients receiving dialysis.

e. Cardiac autonomic dysfunction can occur, resulting in arrhythmias such as tachycardia, potentiating development of orthostatic hypotension, activity intolerance, and impaired heart rate.

5. In addition to endothelial dysfunction, extraosseous vascular deposition of calcium has been known to occur within the coronary arteries, secondary to complex bone and mineral disorders.

6. Vascular calcification is a significant cause of mortality in CKD and leads to stroke, peripheral arterial disease, coronary artery disease, and congestive heart failure.

a. Vascular calcification inhibits normal vasodilatation of vasculature due to the stiffness in the vessels caused by calcium deposits in the media of the vessel.

b. This tends to be more common in patients receiving dialysis and is thought to be related to administration of vitamin D and oral calcium containing phosphate binders.

c. Coronary perfusion decreases, pulse pressure increases, and atherosclerotic plaques form (Afzali & Goldsmith, 2012).

7. Atherogenesis is accelerated by dyslipidemia as CKD causes a decrease in high-density lipoprotein (HDL), the "good" cholesterol, and an increase in low-density lipoprotein, the "bad" cholesterol (LDL), and triglycerides. In uremic states, there is a further decline in HDL.

8. Pericarditis may occur with worsening uremia and cause cardiac tamponade.

C. Pulmonary.
1. Fluid retention tends to occur, resulting in development of heart failure and pulmonary edema.
2. Dyspnea and activity intolerance are manifested by tachypnea and shortness of breath.
3. Metabolic acidosis may cause hyperventilation as seen in Kussmaul breathing, protein-energy malnutrition, weakness of muscles, and fatigue (Arora, 2013).
4. Hyperventilation with increased tidal volume or respiratory rate is common, causing compensatory metabolic acidosis (Heuther & Forshee, 2010).

D. Hematologic.
1. Hypercoagulation, anemia, and platelet dysfunction are the primary hematologic disorders in CKD.
2. Clotting factors, thrombin, fibrin, and fibrinolysis contribute to hypercoagulation as well as thrombosis.
3. Anemia is usually categorized as normocytic nomochromic due to a decrease in production of erythropoietin as well as a decrease in red blood cell (RBC) life span.
a. The kidney produces approximately 90% of erythropoietin, while the liver and other organs produce only 10%.
b. Kidney dysfunction impacts RBC development and availability.
c. Other factors may contribute to anemia in CKD including vitamin B12, iron, and folate deficiencies.
d. Bleeding tendency and malnutrition may also occur in CKD.
e. Refractory anemia, not responsive to erythropoietin replacement, has been known to occur with hyperparathyroidism, chronic inflammation, and shortened RBC survival.
f. Eosinophilia and prolonged bleeding time are common in CKD.
g. Iron deficiency anemia tends to have a significantly high prevalence in patients with CKD (KDIGO, 2012b).

E. Immune.
   1. The pathogenesis surrounding immune dysfunction in CKD is not clearly understood.
   2. People with CKD do not fully respond to vaccinations. For example, it has been reported that patients who are on dialysis and receive the hepatitis B vaccine develop less of a protective response as compared to those persons not on dialysis.
   3. The inflammatory response in itself is immunosuppressive. Theoretically, chronic inflammation, as well as oxidative stress, leads to accelerated tissue degeneration (Cozzolino, 2013), similar to an accelerated aging process.
   4. There is a suppressed cell-mediated immune response, antibody production, and phagocytosis in CKD (Heuther & Forshee, 2010).

F. Gastrointestinal.
   1. As people with CKD develop high levels of urea, erosive esophagitis, gastritis, and duodenitis can develop.
   2. Symptoms of gastrointestinal distress tend to occur in the later stages (e.g., nausea/vomiting).
   3. Hypotension during dialysis can cause ischemic colitis (Thomas et al., 2013).
   4. Halitosis may be experienced in uremia due to salivary enzymes breaking down urea.
   5. Malnutrition in the form of protein energy wasting (PEW) is seen in up to 75% of people with CKD on kidney replacement therapy and is associated with poor outcomes (Jadeja & Kher, 2012).
      a. Alterations in protein synthesis and degradation occur in PEW and are manifested by unintentional weight loss, malnutrition, and a decrease in body mass index (BMI), body fat, serum cholesterol, and albumin.
      b. The kidneys are responsible for amino acid oxidation as well as protein metabolism (Bonanni et al., 2011).
      c. PEW can be impacted by alterations in hormones.

G. Endocrine.
   1. CKD alters the concentration of growth hormone, insulin, thyroid and parathyroid hormone, and prostaglandins.
   2. There is a higher incidence of hypothyroidism and goiter in CKD (Palmer & Henrick, 2013). Iodine is cleared by the kidney through glomerular filtration, which can interfere with thyroid production. In individuals who are uremic, decreased levels of T3 are related to an increase in mortality from cardiovascular event (Palmer & Henrich, 2013).
   3. Nitric oxide synthesis, resistance to growth

hormone, low testosterone, insulin resistance, or altered insulin signaling all play a key role in protein energy wasting (Bonanni et al., 2011).
   4. Both women and men with CKD experience sexual dysfunction. Men may experience a decreased libido, impotence, oligospermia, and infertility.
      a. Levels of free and total testosterone are lower in men with CKD.
      b. As CKD progresses, women experience decreased estrogen, amenorrhea, and decreased libido.
      c. Guglielmi (2013) reports that only 7% of women with CKD stage 5 who are childbearing age receiving dialysis become pregnant due to anovulation, early menopause, and hormonal abnormalities.
      d. Pregnancy can accelerate progression of CKD, and fetal outcomes are impacted, especially in advanced CKD. Of those receiving dialysis, there is significant intrauterine growth restriction of the fetus, prematurity, and preeclampsia.
   5. Children with CKD have impaired growth due to disturbances in growth hormone metabolism and insulin-like growth factor-l. Short stature is also attributed to malnutrition, decreased taste, appetite, anorexia, and increased water intake (Tönshoff, 2013).

H. Neurologic.
   1. Individuals progressing to CKD stage 5 are at increased risk for stroke, cognitive dysfunction, both autonomic and peripheral neuropathies, restless legs, dysesthesias, and myopathy.
   2. Peripheral neuropathies are common in individuals with advancing CKD and often lead to weakness and decreased functional capacity (Krishnan & Kiernan, 2009).
   3. With progression in CKD, neurophysiologic alterations occur, sometimes resulting in an altered mental status and, in extreme cases, encephalopathy. These toxin-mediated symptoms resolve quickly following kidney transplant and diminish somewhat with initiation of dialysis.
   4. Uremic toxicity and hyperkalemia cause axonal membrane dysfunction, impeding nerve conduction; potassium should be considered a uremic neurotoxin.
   5. Impotence is a sign of autonomic dysfunction in men with CKD.
   6. Carpal tunnel syndrome is common in individuals on dialysis.
      a. Attributed to deposits of amyloid in the tissues.
      b. Due to a decrease in clearance of β-microglobulin.
      c. Results in median nerve entrapment.

7. CKD is a risk factor for cognitive impairment.
   a. Memory, verbal, and executive functioning are impacted by uremia.
   b. Cognitive function improves with kidney transplant (Krishnan & Kiernan, 2009).

I. Integumentary.
   1. Bruising, bleeding, hematomas, and ecchymosis are commonly seen from alterations in platelet and bleeding times.
   2. Pallor may be seen from anemia.
   3. Pruritus of the limbs, thorax, and head can occur and is often more severe at night.
      a. Uremic pruritus may occur with or without uremia.
      b. The etiology of uremic pruritus is thought to be multifactorial.
      c. One theoretical cause is related to the heightened inflammatory response seen in advanced stages of CKD as evidenced by increases in C-reactive protein, a biomarker for inflammation (Kuypers, 2009).
   4. Individuals with CKD stage 5 and calciphylaxis develop benign fatty lesions on the abdomen.

J. Alterations in bones and mineral metabolism in CKD.
   1. There is a dysfunction of the homeostasis of minerals altering levels of growth factor, parathyroid hormone (PTH), and vitamin D.
      a. This imbalance is thought to contribute to development of vascular endothelial changes within the walls of the coronary arteries and systemic blood vessels.
      b. As phosphates are retained in the body, free calcium binds with phosphate and decreases the level of calcium.
      c. Secondary hyperparathyroidism results from retained phosphorus, low levels of vitamin D, and a reduction in serum calcium.
      d. Ultimately, alterations in bone and mineral biochemical parameters cause a state of high turnover of bone disease or osteitis fibrosa cystica. However, with treatment and in certain patients, the opposite can occur (low-turnover bone disease).
   2. The parathyroid glands have calcium-sensing receptors that respond to a negative feedback from calcium.
      a. Hypertrophied parathyroid glands are less responsive to calcium, and an autonomic state develops (unable to decrease the levels of PTH), creating tertiary hyperparathyroidism (Chauhan et al., 2012).
      b. PTH receptors are downregulated on the bone.
      c. Calcium salts tend to deposit in the medial layer of arteries, producing a stiff, noncompliant vessel.
   3. Investigative efforts have suggested that the process includes an accelerated death of vascular smooth muscle (London et al., 2013).
      a. Individuals with CKD not yet receiving dialysis develop muscle wasting, which tends to be reversible once they begin dialysis.
      b. The wasting progression is not fully understood.
   4. Mineral and bone disease and the influence of secondary hyperparathyroidism in CKD lead to early skeletal changes, bone loss, low bone mineral density, and risk for fractures (Akkupalli et al., 2013).
   5. Vitamin D3 deficiency occurs and leads to osteomalacia (John et al., 2013).
      a. CKD progression results in a higher risk of fractures and secondary mortality (Miller, 2013).
      b. Children with CKD with short stature will also have delayed bone maturation (Tönshoff, 2013).

IV. Definition, classification, and staging of CKD.

A. Overview.
   1. Most of the information presented focuses on definition, classification, and staging of CKD and is based on evidence-based recommendations from Kidney Disease Improving Global Outcomes (KDIGO, 2013a).
   2. The goal of KDIGO is to improve care of individuals with CKD.
   3. Recommendations were rated by KDIGO International Work Group for strength as 1 (recommend), 2 (suggest), or NG (not graded).
   4. The supporting evidence was graded as A (high), B (moderate), C (low), and D (very low) based on strength of the evidence.
   5. The evidence review team was from Tufts Center for Kidney Disease in Boston.

B. Kidney Disease: Improving Global Outcomes (KDIGO).
   1. Primarily, there were two significant changes to the new KDIGO guidelines that included:
      a. Adding the etiology/cause of CKD.
      b. Staging of albuminuria to the classification system.
   2. KDIGO also lists abbreviations, acronyms, and other nomenclature.
      a. The term *CKD* is used for any stage of CKD.
      b. *CKD-ND* implies CKD without a kidney transplant and nondialysis.
      c. *CKD-T* implies nondialysis with a kidney transplant.
   3. The stage of kidney disease is listed following CKD as CKD 1, 2, 3, 4, or 5, with CKD 5HD

referring to stage 5 hemodialysis dependent, and CKD 5PD referring to stage 5 peritoneal dialysis-dependent (KDIGO, 2012d).

C. Definition of CKD.
1. CKD is defined by the workgroup as "abnormalities of the kidney structure or function, present for > 3 months, with implications for health. CKD is classified based on cause, GFR category, and albuminuria category" (KDIGO, 2013a).
2. The 3-month time period is important to distinguish CKD from acute kidney disease (Levey & Inker, 2013).

D. Classification of CKD.
1. In addition to the GFR and albuminuria category, KDIGO work group recommends that CKD be classified on etiology or cause of CKD.
2. CKD can be caused by a large group of disorders or diseases that alter the kidney function and structure (KDIGO, 2013a).
3. Genetic conditions may also lead to CKD.

E. Staging of CKD.
1. CKD stages are based upon the GFR (mL/min/1.73 m^2).
2. Age, gender, and body size are the primary variables used when estimating the GFR with normal ranges estimated at 120–130 mL/min/1.73 m^2.
3. There is variability in the GFR estimates by predication equations due to errors in measurement, variability of lab methods, and difficulty in obtaining accuracy at ranges of the GFR (> 60 mL/min/1.73 m^2).
4. The GFR may vary in response to age, body mass, meals, exercise, posture, changes in blood pressure, amount of protein in the diet, glucose control, extracellular fluid volume, and high salt intake.
5. KDIGO (2013a) recommends that the initial assessment of CKD be made using serum creatinine and the GFR estimating equation (eGFR) [1A evidence grade].
   a. GFR estimating equation that is calculated from serum creatinine to obtain the GFR is labeled as "eGFRcreat" (KDIGO, 2013, p. 6).
   b. See the National Kidney Foundation (2013) at http://www.kidney.org/professionals for the following GFR calculators:
      (1) CKD-EPI equation.
      (2) CKD-EPI cystatin C equation.
      (3) CKD-EPI creatinine-cystatin C equation.

F. eGFRcreat equation.
1. Researchers continue to identify improved precision in the GFR estimation.

   a. Newer equations have assisted in optimal classification of CKD.
   b. Currently, the CKD-EPI equation seems to provide the best overall estimation with minimal misclassifications (Levey et al., 2009) and is recommended by KDIGO (2013a).
2. The CKD-EPI equation may not be optimal for individuals at the low and high end of GFR ranges and in all population groups (e.g., very young and very old).
3. From a public health perspective and in clinical practice, the CKD-EPI equation is currently the most precise (Earley et al., 2012).
   a. Labs must follow specific calibration requirements.
   b. Round serum creatinine to the nearest whole number when using µmol/l (international units) and nearest 100th when using mg/dL (conventional units).
   c. Understand what situations would cause eGFRcreat to be less than accurate (e.g., acutely ill).
   d. When reporting eGFRcreat using the 2009 CKD-EPI creatinine equation, may use other GFR estimates if it is proven to be more accurate (KDIGO, 2013a).
   e. Measurement and use of cystatin C as a biomarker for estimating GFR is considered to be more accurate than creatinine. But, at present, there is no standardization in laboratory measurement of cystatin C.

G. eGFRcys. Cystatin C is a low-molecular-weight protein found in the body and abundant in immune cells; when elevated, it is a marker of kidney dysfunction, cardiovascular risk, and stroke.
1. It is not dependent upon gender, muscle mass, or diet.
2. Normal urinary cystatin C level in healthy people is 100 µg/l.
3. Elevated levels of cystatin C are also related to increased mortality and are predictors of clinical outcomes in CKD (Peralta et al., 2010).
4. KDIGO recommends measuring cystatin C when eGFR measured from serum creatinine is less than accurate [2B evidence grade].
5. Cystatin C may detect early kidney disease, allograft rejection, and acute kidney injury that is not evident with measures of eGFRcreat.
6. Cystatin C is used in monitoring medication nephrotoxicity and predicting cardiovascular mortality.
7. Cystatin C might provide a better marker for diagnosing CKD in people with higher levels of GFR. It is most often used to measure GFR in adults with an estimated GFR of 45 to 59 mL/min/1.73m^2. It is thought to be most useful in

circumstances where it is needed to confirm the diagnosis of CKD (e.g., older kidney donor).
8. Cystatin C generation may be affected by thyroid dysfunction, heterophilic antibodies, race/ethnicity other than U.S./European Black and White, and use of corticosteroids (KDIGO, 2013a).

H. Albuminuria.
1. In relation to kidney function, mortality, and morbidity, albuminuria is a key predictor of prognosis (KDIGO, 2013).
2. Albuminuria is associated with a higher risk of cardiovascular disease, cardiovascular events, and cardiovascular mortality (Tonelli, Muntner, & Lloyd, 2012).
3. Normally, less than 30 mg of albumin is lost in the urine over a 24-hour period, and it is a more accurate measure than total urinary protein that is found in earlier stages of CKD.
4. Nephrology nurses can play an important role in maintaining the accuracy of urinary albumin testing by educating the patients on the timing of collection. First voided sample in the morning is best [2B level of evidence].
5. The KDIGO work group prefers using the albumin-to-creatinine ratio (ACR) for the most accurate measurement followed by:
   a. Urine protein-to-creatinine ratio (PCR).
   b. Reagent strip urinalysis for total protein with automated reading.
   c. Reagent strip urinalysis for total protein with manual reading.
      (1) Reagent strips have been used in primary care for years and are considered less accurate than ACR measurement.
      (2) These strips are operator and manufacturer dependent with many false positives. They are affected by colored compounds such as bilirubin or drugs such as ciprofloxacin, quinine, and chloroquine (KDIGO, 2013a).
6. The KDIGO work group strongly encourages clinicians to understand that the clinical setting may impact the measurement and interpretation of albuminuria and that repeat testing using quantitative lab measurements using ACR may be indicated to confirm findings.
7. The term *microalbuminuria* is outdated and should not be used by labs or clinicians (KDIGO, 2013a).
8. There may be individual variations of albuminuria.
   a. Menstrual blood, urinary tract infection, and exercise may cause transient elevations in albuminuria (KDIGO, 2013a).
   b. Individuals who have paraplegia, muscular dystrophy, and amputations may have variability in creatinine excretion due to lower muscle mass.

c. For children, gender, race, age, high BMI, and puberty status must be considered when evaluating urinary excretion of protein or albumin.
d. Proteinuria may be used in place of albuminuria for children with CKD of any age; a total urinary protein excretion of > 40 mg/m^2/hr or > 3grams/1.83 m^2/day is considered nephritic in origin (KDIGO, 2013a).

I. 24-hour urine collection.
1. Is not routinely obtained now that spot urines provide accurate estimation of protein loss in 24 hours calculating a urine albumin-to-creatinine ratio (UACR).
2. However, when a 24-hour urine sample is ordered for creatinine and blood urea nitrogen clearance, it must be done properly to be accurate.
   a. The patient is given a plastic container for collection of all urine over a 24-hour period as an outpatient.
   b. This can also be done with inpatients in the hospital.
   c. The urine collection jug is placed in a bucket of ice or in the refrigerator.
   d. The patient is given a urinal or a specimen collection pan to collect every drop of urine. Men may urinate directly into the jug.
   e. A lid to the jug is secured tightly, and the jug is placed in a bag and put into the refrigerator.
   f. A 24-hour urine is started in the morning and timed exactly after the patient's first voiding (for example, 7:20 a.m.).
   g. The first morning voiding is not included in the 24-hour urine and is flushed.
   h. Time the collection following the first voiding after the patient empties his or her bladder.
      (1) On day 2, the patient is asked to urinate upon waking (as in the example, 7:20 a.m.) and save the urine in the collection jug.
      (2) If the patient urinates upon rising at 6:30 a.m. (example) the patient is asked to try to empty his or her bladder again for the final time at 7:20 a.m. (example).
   i. The patient can drink water 1 hour before the final voiding time to help with urination.
2. This test should not be done within 3 days of the patient receiving radiocontrast media (Dugdale, 2013).
3. A UACR of greater than 30 mg/g (30 mg albumin for each gram of creatinine) is considered elevated and should be retested in 2 weeks. If the second test is high, this is persistent proteinuria (NKUDIC, 2010).

V. Evaluation and progression of CKD.

A. The prevalence of CKD may vary by specific ethnic groups related to a prevalence of risk indigenous to that region.
1. Risks might include a higher incidence of comorbid, environmental, and social conditions evident in particular regions of the world.
2. Nephrotoxic medications, urinary tract obstruction, and volume depletion are common to all countries; however, other risk factors may vary by country of origin.
3. The majority of research on progression of CKD has been done on North American Whites and African Americans.
4. Because of the importance to document true deterioration in kidney function, KDIGO (2013) has defined progression as a "change of category of eGFR or albuminuria or both, as well as a numeric change over an established period of time" (p. 69).
5. Progression of CKD is related to several factors including (KDIGO, 2013a):
   a. The cause of CKD.
   b. Level of GFR.
   c. Level of albuminuria.
   d. Age.
   e. Sex.
   f. Race/ethnicity.
   g. Elevation in BP.
   h. Hyperglycemia.
   i. Dyslipidemia.
   j. Smoking.
   k. Obesity.
   l. History of cardiovascular disease.
   m. Ongoing exposure to nephrotoxic agents.

B. Deterioration in kidney function.
1. A 23% or greater decrease in eGFR from baseline is considered an aggressive decline, and a sustained decline of more than 5 mL/min/1.73 m^2/year is considered a rapid progression (KDIGO, 2013a).
2. There are many factors that predict progression of CKD that are modifiable or preventable, such as blood pressure, hyperglycemia, dyslipidemia, smoking, obesity, and exposure to nephrotoxic agents.
3. Prediction tools are recommended for use to evaluate progression of CKD.
4. It would be important to refer individuals to a nephrologist who need kidney replacement therapy (KRT) in the next 12 months as evidenced by a prediction tool for education, vascular access, and transplantation [1B grade evidence].
   a. There is no clear evidence of the relationship between the timing for nephrology referral and improved patient outcomes.
   b. An objective of Healthy People 2020 is to increase care by a nephrologist at least 1 year prior to KRT in those with CKD (Healthy People, 2013). KDIGO (2013) Work Group recommends referral to a nephrologist after potentially reversible or modifiable factors are corrected or with a rapidly declining GFR.
5. KDIGO (2013a) identified consequences and benefits of early and late referral to a nephrologist (see Table 1.15).

VI. Management of complications of CKD.

A. Overview.
1. The KDIGO (2013a) Work Group promotes optimum healthy lifestyle for individuals with CKD with the goal of delaying the progression of CKD.
2. A team approach can support kidney-specific strategies with implementation of interventions to control modifiable factors.
3. Lowering blood pressure and individualizing BP targets according to age decreases morbidity and progression of CKD.
4. A nurse can play a valuable role as a team member, empowering lifestyle modifications in individuals and their families.

B. Lifestyle and blood pressure control.
1. Individuals with CKD are encouraged to achieve a healthy weight ranging from a BMI of 20 to 25 and be committed to a daily exercise program for optimum cardiovascular fitness and tolerance of 30 minutes five times per week [1D grade of evidence].
2. Adiposity (obesity) is a strong risk factor for diabetes.
3. Weight reduction has been demonstrated to lower blood pressure in those who are overweight.
4. Alcohol intake should be limited to less than one standard size drink a day for women and two for men with attention to size of glass or ounces of alcohol [2D grade of evidence].
5. Exposure to secondhand smoke and cigarette smoking itself are clearly modifiable risk factors that have a direct effect on blood pressure and cardiovascular health.

C. Blood pressure and interruption of RAAS.
1. Vital to the delay of progression of CKD (not graded):
   a. Control of blood pressure.
   b. Interruption or blockage of the renal-angiotension-aldosterone system (RAAS) that accelerates BP response.
2. KDIGO Blood Pressure Guidelines (2012c) call for individualized BP targets based on age, cardiovascular disease, progression of CKD,

Table 1.15

Early Versus Late Referral: Consequences and Benefits

Consequences of late referral	Benefits of early referral
Anemia and bone disease	Delay needed to initiate RRT
Severe hypertension and fluid overload	Increased proportion with permanent access
Low prevalence of permanent access	Greater choice of treatment options
Delayed referral for transplant	Reduced need for urgent dialysis
Higher initial hospitalization rate	Reduced hospital length of stay and cost
Higher 1-year mortality rate	Improved nutritional status
Less patient choice of RRT modality	Better management of CVD and comorbid conditions
Worse psychosocial adjustment	Improved patient survival

Abbreviations: CVD – cardiovascular disease; RRT – renal replacement therapy.

Source: Kidney Disease: Improving Global Outcomes (KDIGO) CKD Work Group. KDIGO 2012 Clinical Practice Guideline for the Evaluation and Management of Chronic Kidney Disease. *Kidney International Supplements 2013*; 3: 1–150 (originally table 35 on page 114). Used with permission.

retinopathy, other preexisting diseases or disorders, and tolerance to treatment.

3. Adults with urine albumin levels of ≤ 30 mg/24 hours whose blood pressure is > 140 mmHg systolic or > 90 mmHg diastolic need to be treated with antihypertensives [1B grade evidence].

4. If there is evidence of albuminuria ≥ 30 mg/24 hours and blood pressure is > 130 mmHg systolic or > 80 mmHg diastolic, treat with an antihypertensive [2D grade evidence].

5. In older adults it is important to assess for orthostatic hypotension and postural dizziness in individuals with CKD who are taking antihypertensives and then tailor treatment to monitor for adverse events [not graded].

6. For children, antihypertensives are recommended when blood pressure is consistently above the 90th percentile for height, gender, and age [1C grade evidence] with a target goal of blood pressure in the 50th percentile [2D grade evidence].

D. Blood pressure lowering agents.
1. The process of individualizing BP treatment takes into account comorbidities, modification of lifestyle, age, and adverse effects of blood pressure lowering agents.

2. KDIGO BP guidelines (2012c) recommend tailoring treatment to the individual with CKD. Renin-angiotensin-aldosterone system blockers (RAAS), such as ACE-I and ARBs, are an important part of regulation of blood pressure and albuminuria.

3. Aldosterone antagonists, such as spirolactone, have been used since the 1950s to lower blood pressure with an increased risk of hyperkalemia. (NEPRON D study refutes this claim, higher risk

for AKI and hyperkalemia.)

4. Direct renin inhibitors (DRIs), such as aliskiren, prevent angiotension I from converting to angiotension II by binding to renin. Aliskiren has a black-box warning and should not be used in combination ACE-I and ARBs in people who have diabetes or CKD with GFR less than 60 mL/min/1.73 m^2 due to the risk for stroke, hyperkalemia, hypotension, and renal complications.

5. Diuretics, beta blockers, calcium channel blockers, centrally acting alpha-adrenergic agonist, direct vasodilators, and alpha-blockers continue to be used in lowering blood pressure (KDIGO, 2012c).

E. ACE-I and ARBs.
1. In adults who have diabetes, KDIGO recommends an angiotensin-receptor blocker (ARB) or angiotensin-converting enzyme inhibitor (ACE-I) to provide antihypertensive effect as well as renal protection [2D grade evidence].

2. These classes of drugs have demonstrated a capacity to slow the progression of nephropathy in patients with diabetes and hypertension and are considered the preferred drug of choice.

3. They cause a generalized arterial vasodilatation both systemically and in the afferent and efferent arterioles of the glomeruli; result in an increasing GFR and albuminuria (KDIGO, 2012c).

4. In individuals with albuminuria, these medications provide renal protection by decreasing albuminuria, resulting in increasing GFR. There is also a reduction in aldosterone.

5. A possible secondary benefit includes the suppression of the development of fibrosis as well as improved cardiac and vascular remodeling (KDIGO, 2012c).

6. At this time, all drugs in the ACE-I and ARB class

appear to be similar with no one drug demonstrating superiority.

   a. They can also be administered with calcium-channel or beta blockers and diuretics for treatment of high blood pressure.

   b. KDIGO suggests that an ACE-I or an ARB be used in children [2D grade evidence] for additional renal protection.

   c. Increasing the blockade of the RAAS with dietary sodium restriction, an ACE-I, or an ARB also decreases albuminuria – a target for therapy.

   d. Adherence to ACE-I may be difficult for individuals due to the side effect of a dry persistent cough, which is attributed to the accumulation of bradykinin that occurs with the conversion of angiotension I to angiotensin II in up to 20% of individuals.

   e. ACE-I and ARB may be contraindicated with individuals with renal artery stenosis and dehydration (vomiting, fever, diarrhea, sepsis) due to a significant decrease in GFR in these clinical situations.

   f. These medications have teratogenic effects in pregnancy, and caution must be taken in women of childbearing age by implementing birth control strategies (KDIGO, 2012c).

F. Adherence to treatment.

   1. Researchers have identified that there is poor adherence to medication regimens in individuals with CKD as well as less than optimal control of blood pressure.

   2. The individual patient's perception of the cost vs. benefits of treatment has been identified to play a key role in adherence.

   3. It is recommended that providers avoid prescribing medications that are costly and inconvenient to take (KDIGO, 2012c).

G. Salt intake. KDIGO (2012c) guidelines for blood pressure management state that salt intake be limited to less than 90 mmol or 2 grams of sodium per day [1C graded evidence].

   1. Increased salt intake impacts fluid volume, retention of fluid, and peripheral edema in individuals with elevated blood pressure and CKD.

   2. Nurses can encourage ways to decrease salt intake and avoid added salt. It is recommended that salt be eliminated in cooking and replaced with other spices such as onions, lemon, rosemary, or garlic.

   3. Teach individuals with CKD not to use salt substitutes due to potassium content and risk of hyperkalemia. Advise them to avoid table salt, bouillon cubes, packaged seasoning mixes, monosodium glutamate, soy sauce, barbecue sauce, and meat tenderizers.

   4. Pasta, rice, and potato dinner mixes are very high in sodium as well as smoked, spiced, and cured meat, fish, poultry, bacon, ham, sausage, hot dogs, lunch meat, and frozen pizzas.

   5. Processed cheeses, buttermilk, salad dressings, and most cottage cheeses are high in sodium. Salted popcorn, chips, pretzels, nuts, and other packaged snacks should be eliminated from the diet.

   6. Teach patients how to read nutrition labels and to estimate daily salt intake to stay within the 2 gram sodium limit. Avoid drinking softened water due to the added sodium (Kaplan & Olendzkki, 2013).

H. Protection from acute kidney injury in CKD.

   1. Individuals with CKD are at increased risk for acute kidney injury (AKI).

   2. Social, environmental, and pharmacologic factors that would cause AKI must be controlled or avoided. These include dehydration, radiocontrast media, over-the-counter medications (NSAIDs), nephrotoxic medications, and chronic disease (diabetes, gout, heart failure).

   3. Nephrotoxic medications increase risk for AKI.

     a. Education provided by nurses has proven valuable in empowering the individuals with CKD to protect their kidneys from further damage.

     b. Screen all patients with CKD if scheduled for procedures using contrast media to see if they are taking metformin. Taking metformin with CKD has the potential risk of developing lactic acidosis when placed at risk for states of dehydration, infection, NPO status, or requiring IV administration of iodinated contrast media.

     c. Nephrology nurses need to be aware of the dangers for patients when metformin is administered. It is important to educate not only the patient, but also his/her family and other nurses on withholding metformin until kidney function is at baseline and the patient can return to drinking fluids normally (Vallerand et al., 2013).

     d. KDIGO has identified specific cautionary measures related to pharmacotherapy in patients with CKD (e.g., dose ranges that are known to be nephrotoxic).

     e. Oral phosphate-containing preps for colonoscopy need to be avoided in individuals with CKD as it can induce phosphate nephropathy.

I. Nutrition therapy.

   1. The American Dietetic Association (2010) recommends guidance from a registered dietitian for all people with CKD to prevent malnutrition,

electrolyte problems, and mineral disorders, and to halt rapid progression of CKD.

2. Initial assessment.
   a. Interview to determine intake of nutrients and food selection.
   b. Any use of supplements, herbals, botanicals, and medications.
   c. An individual's beliefs, attitudes, lifestyle, and behaviors related to foods.
   d. Their readiness to make lifestyle changes.
   e. Their access to food, nutrition, and supplies (ADA, 2010).

3. The primary goal is to treat protein-energy malnutrition in CKD.
   a. When dietary protein intake is excessive or severely restricted, problems develop in adults with CKD.
   b. With excessive food intake, there is an accumulation of metabolic wastes and uremic toxins that may result in a decrease in kidney function.
   c. KDIGO (2013a) supports avoiding protein intake of greater than 1.3 g/kg/day [2C graded evidence]. In adults with diabetes [2C grade of evidence] or those without diabetes who have CKD G4 or G5 GFR categories [2B grade of evidence], it is recommended that protein be decreased to 0.8 g/kg/day.
   d. For individuals with CKD and diabetes, the ADA (2010) also prescribes limiting protein in the diet to 0.8 g of protein per kg of body weight per day.
   e. Dietary protein restriction is not recommended in:
      (1) Children, due to growth and development problems.
      (2) Adults with malnutrition.

J. Control of blood glucose.
   1. In those with type 2 diabetes, poor glycemic control is a key predictor of mortality.
   2. Individuals with diabetes and CKD must implement a multifactorial plan that addresses glycemic control. They must also address control of blood pressure, and when indicated, management with ACE-I or ARBs, statins, and antiplatelet therapy [not graded].
      a. With the goal of preventing or delaying the progression of CKD, hemoglobin A1C (Hgb A1C) target of 7.0% in nonpregnant adults will decrease the microvascular problems associated with diabetes such as retinopathy, neuropathy, nephropathy, and macrovascular disease [1A grade of evidence].
      b. For those with decreased life expectancy or who have a higher risk of developing hypoglycemia, it is not recommended to treat Hgb A1C to less than 7.0%.

K. Anemia in CKD.
   1. Fatigue, weakness, headache, and irritability are commonly seen in people with anemia (Schrier & Auerbach, 2013). KDIGO anemia clinical practice guidelines (2012b) identify iron deficiency as the most commonly encountered anemia in CKD.
   2. Hemoglobin (Hgb) measurement is the gold standard for assessment of the severity of anemia.
   3. Hgb is measured in grams per 100 mL in the United States, and each gram carries 1.34 mL of oxygen. KDIGO (2012b) identified Hgb levels for diagnosing anemia in adults and children (see Table 1.16).
      a. In children with CKD:
         (1) Aged 0.5 to 5 years is < 11.0g/dL or 110g/L.
         (2) Aged 5 to 12 years is < 11.5 g/dL or 115 g/L.
         (3) Aged 12 to 15 years is < 12.0 g/dL or 120 g/L.
      b. In adults with CKD.
         (1) For females aged 15 years or older, anemia is diagnosed with a level of < 12.0 g/dL or 120 g/L.
         (2) For men, Hgb level of < 13.0 g/dL or 130 g/L is diagnostic of anemia [not graded].
   4. Diagnostic Hgb levels require further anemia evaluation to identify other potential causes other than assuming the cause is related to a reduction in endogenous erythropoietin.
   5. Evaluating red blood cells (RBC) indices assists the provider with identifying the morphologic type of anemia. Here are the most frequently used RBC indices:
      a. Mean corpuscular hemoglobin (MCH) evaluates amount (weight, mass) of Hgb in the cell and reflects the color. MCH is the mass of Hgb per RBC and described as normochromic, hypochromic, or hyperchromic.
      b. Mean corpuscular volume (MCV) evaluates size. The MCV evaluates cell size which identifies if the RBCs are normocytic, microcytic, or macrocytic.
      c. Mean corpuscular hemoglobin concentration (MCHC) evaluates the concentration of Hgb (average weight) in the cell. The MCHC is the ratio of Hgb mass to Hgb volume and reflects concentration. The RBC indices identify the morphologic characteristics of the RBC (Curry, 2012).
      d. The red cell distribution width (RDW) is also assessed to evaluate if the RBC are the same size or if they vary from each other in size and shape.
      e. In CKD, anemia is generally normochromic (normal MCH) and normocytic (normal MCV). Long-standing iron deficiency anemia is both microcytic (decreased MCV) and hypochromic (decreased MCH).
   6. Folate and vitamin B12 deficiencies are unlikely in CKD but are routine in a workup for anemia.

Table 1.16

Hemoglobin Thresholds Used to Define Anemia

Age or gender group	Hemoglobin threshold: g/dL (g/L)
Children	
6 mo-5 yr	11.0 (110)
5-12 yr	11.5 (115)
12-15 yr	12.0 (120)
Non-pregnant females > 15 yr	12.0 (120)
Pregnant females > 15 yr	11.0 (110)
Men > 15 yr	13.0 (130)

Abbreviations: mo – month; yr – year.

Reproduced with permission from World Health Organization. Worldwide prevalence of anaemia 1993-2005: WHO global database on anaemia.368 In: de Benoist B, McLean E, Egli I and Cogswell M (eds), 2008; accessed: http://whqlibdoc.who.int/publications/2008/9789241596657_eng.pdf

Source: Kidney Disease: Improving Global Outcomes (KDIGO) CKD Work Group. KDIGO 2012 Clinical Practice Guideline for the Evaluation and Management of Chronic Kidney Disease. *Kidney International Supplements 2013*; 3: 1–150 (originally table 28 on page 81). Used with permission.

Folate and vitamin B12 would show a macrocytic RBC (elevated MCV).

7. Inherited thalassemia disorders often cause microcytic RBCs (decreased MCV).

8. When evaluating for iron, it is important to assess both the availability of iron to support erythropoiesis as well as the patient's iron stores (KDIGO, 2012b).
   a. Transferrin saturation (TSAT) measures the availability of iron.
   b. Iron stores are commonly evaluated by serum ferritin levels, but in CKD the inflammatory process can increase serum ferritin levels.
   c. Bone marrow aspiration remains the gold standard for evaluation of iron storage but is costly and inconvenient.
   d. In addition to the TSAT and ferritin levels, iron status can also be evaluated by the reticulocytes Hgb content and by the percentage of RBCs that are hypochromic (decreased MCH).
   e. Most people with CKD have normal storage of iron in the bone marrow (KDIGO).

9. Treatment of iron deficiency.
   a. Both the risks and benefits of iron therapy must be assessed by the clinician [not graded] (KDIGO, 2012b).
   b. Nurses recall that oral iron is not absorbed in the stomach, but in the duodenum and in the proximal jejunum as well.
   c. Oral iron is inexpensive and must be taken with some precaution to obtain the best absorption.
   d. Food decreases absorption; oral iron should be administered 2 hours before meals.
   e. Antacids interfere with absorption and should not be taken within 4 hours of taking oral iron (Schrier & Auerbach, 2013).
   f. Oral iron can cause nausea, vomiting, constipation, or diarrhea, and seems to be dose dependent.
   g. Sustained release or enteric coated medications are usually inadequate for treatment of iron deficiency (Schrier & Auerbach, 2013).
   h. People who have gastrointestinal intolerance to oral iron tablets may experience fewer side effects with ferrous sulfate elixir.
   i. Daily dosing of oral iron in adults with iron deficiency is 150 to 200 mg a day of elemental iron in divided doses.
   j. Elemental iron in various iron preparations.
      (1) A 325 mg tablet of ferrous sulfate contains 65 mg of elemental iron.
      (2) A 325 mg tablet of ferrous gluconate has 36 mg of elemental iron.
      (3) A 325 mg tablet of ferrous fumarate has 98 mg of elemental iron (Schrier & Auerbach, 2013).
   k. Iron administration must be guided by the clinical status, response to iron therapy, recent blood losses, treatment with erythropoiesis-stimulating agents (ESA), and outcomes of ferritin, TSAT, and Hgb levels [not graded] (KDIGO, 2012b).
   l. For those who do not tolerate oral iron, parenteral iron can be given, but this route of administration carries a risk of anaphylactic-type reactions (Schrier & Auerbach, 2013).
      (1) The manufacturer recommends that a test dose of iron salt (Infed® or Dexferrum®) be given at weekly intervals of 1, 2, and 3 weeks. A test dose is recommended: 25 mg over 5 minutes while observing the patient for reactions.
      (2) If no reactions occur by 60 minutes after a test dose, then the remaining dose is administered at 75 mg at a rate of less than 50 mg/minute diluted in 250 to 1000 mL of normal saline.
      (3) The 60-minute monitoring period is a KDIGO anemia guideline for IV iron dextran [1B level of evidence] and for IV nondextran iron [2C level of evidence]. Parenteral iron should always be administered by trained personnel who can provide resuscitative measures and treat adverse reactions.
      (4) During week 4, dosing 100 mg given intravenously over 5 minutes at less than 50 mg/minute can be initiated. This can be

Table 1.17

**Potentially Correctable Versus Noncorrectable Factors
Involved in the Anemia of CKD, in Addition to ESA Deficiency**

Easily correctable	Potentially correctable	Impossible to correct
Absolute iron deficiency Vitamin B12/folate deficiency Hypothyroidism ACEi/ARB Nonadherence	Infection/ inflammation Underdialysis Hemolysis Bleeding Hyperparathyroidism PRCA Malignancy Malnutrition	Hemoglobinopathies Bone marrow disorders

ACEi– angiotensin-converting enzyme inhibitor; ARB – angiotensin-receptor blocker; PRCA – pure red cell aplasia.

Source: Kidney Disease: Improving Global Outcomes (KDIGO) Anemia Work Group. KDIGO Clinical Practice Guideline for Anemia in Chronic Kidney Disease. *Kidney International Supplements 2012*; 2: 279–335 (originally table 3 on page 307). Used with permission.

repeated until the prescribed dose and lab values are reached (Lexicomp, 2013).

(5) Patients with systemic infections should avoid receiving parenteral iron [not graded].

(6) See specific dosing recommended by manufacturer for infants and children.

m. Ferritin and TSAT must be evaluated every 3 months during:

(1) ESA treatment or change in ESA dose.

(2) The point where there is a decision to stop or continue iron therapy.

(3) Periods of blood loss [not graded] (KDIGO, 2012b).

n. Optimizations of erythropoiesis with ESA therapy. Iron and ESA therapies are used to treat anemia and to decrease red cell transfusions and their risks [1B].

(1) ESA is used to treat anemia by stimulating the erythroid progenitor cells to form and then release reticulocytes in bone marrow to mature into erythrocytes.

(2) Increases in Hgb are seen with ESA approximately 10 days after initiation of treatment. ESA increases the risk of stroke by increasing peripheral vascular resistance, blood pressure, and blood viscosity.

(3) In 2011, the FDA issued a black box warning that ESAs carry greater risks for "death, serious adverse cardiovascular reactions, and stroke" (FDA, 2011, p. 1) when Hgb targets exceed 11 g/dL.

(4) The FDA recommends that ESAs are initiated when Hgb falls below 10 g/dL to decrease the need for an RBC transfusion. Berns (2011), a nephrologist, has questioned this recommendation because it was based on a limited number of trials and patient populations and applied to the whole population with CKD.

(5) KDIGO Anemia Clinical Practice Guidelines (2012b) note that therapy needs to be individualized. Individuals who suffer a decreased quality of life may have improvement in symptoms when receiving ESA therapy and target Hgb over10.0 g/dL (< 100 g/L) [not graded].

6) Before treatment of anemia with ESA, individuals with CKD must have all correctable causes of anemia addressed [not graded] while balancing the risks and benefits of treatment [1B level of evidence] considering hypertension, stroke, and risk for loss of vascular access that occur with higher Hgb levels (see Table 1.17).

(7) ESA therapy is recommended with a high level of caution in individuals who have acute malignancy that can be cured and CKD [1B level of evidence], a history of stroke [1B level of evidence], or a history of malignancy [2C level of evidence].

(8) ESA therapy is not supported by KDIGO Anemia Clinical Practice Guidelines (2012b) for adults with CKD ND with Hgb over10 g/dL (100g/L) [2D level of evidence].

o. If the Hgb is less than10 g/dL (100 g/L) in adults with CKD ND, the decision should be

individualized and based on these criteria.
(1) Need for a blood transfusion.
(2) Rate of decline of Hgb.
(3) Previous response to iron therapy.
(4) Symptoms related to anemia [2C level of evidence].

p. Adults with CKD 5D should be started on ESAs to prevent drops in Hgb below 9.0 g/dL (900 g/L) [2B level of evidence].

q. KDIGO suggests that the decision to initiate ESA in children with CKD be based on several factors, such as potential harm vs. quality of life, performance in school, and need for transfusion. If treated, goal for Hgb is 11.0 to 12.0 g/dL (110 to 120 g/L) [2D grade of evidence].

r. Dosing of ESA is based on body weight, clinical evaluation, and Hgb levels [2D level of evidence]. Dose adjustments are made on the same criteria including current ESA dose [1B level of evidence].
(1) Withholding ESA doses is not recommended during therapy, and lowering the dose is preferred when the Hgb has increased too rapidly or exceeded target [2C level of evidence].
(2) A subcutaneous or intravenous route of administration of ESA therapy is used for CKD 5HD and subcutaneous route for individuals with CKD ND and CKD 5PD [2C level of evidence].
(3) Frequency is based on the patient's tolerance, CKD stage, treatment settings, type of ESA and preference [2C level of evidence].

s. During ESA therapy:
(1) Hgb levels should be assessed every month during the initiation of ESA therapy, monthly for individuals with CKD stage 5D, and every 3 months during the maintenance phase for individuals with CKD ND [not graded].
(2) In those patients who demonstrate minimal or no response in Hgb with ESA therapy, KDIGO suggests individualizing therapy and discourages against escalating dose beyond "double the initial weight-based dose" (2012b, p. 286) [2D level of evidence].

10. Androgens are not recommended as an adjunct treatment to ESA [1B level of evidence] and KDIGO suggests against using vitamins C, D, E, folic acid, L-carnitine, and pentoxifylline as adjuvant to treatment [2D level of evidence].

11. If a patient develops antibody-mediated pure red cell aplasia (PRCA), it is recommended to stop ESA therapy [1A level of evidence]. Treatment for PRCA begins with peginesatide [1B level of evidence]. Evaluate for PRCA.
a. A rapid or sudden drop in Hgb with the coinciding onset of pancytopenia (reduction WBC and platelets) might create suspicion for the possibility of PRCA.
b. If the patient is requiring transfusions every week or more [not graded].

12. RBC transfusions for chronic anemia.
a. To avoid allosensitization, RBC transfusions are to be avoided in those individuals who are eligible for organ transplantation [1C].
b. Transfusions may be indicated in those with ESA resistance, bone marrow failure, stroke, malignancies, or other hemoglobinopathies where ESA is not recommended or ineffective [2C].
c. The decision to transfuse is not based on one isolated Hgb value but on individual symptoms, stabilization of hemorrhagic condition, and preoperative correction where the benefits outweigh the risks [2C].
d. In those patients who are receiving frequent transfusions, it is important to monitor ferritin levels.

L. Mineral and bone disorders: A newer term is *CKD-MBD* (see Table 1.18).
1. CKD-MBD is a complex group of disorders that involves bone, minerals, and hormones as well as significant abnormalities in the cardiovascular system and coronary arteries caused by a process of calcification (Chauhan et al., 2012).
2. CKD-MBD increases the patient's risk of mortality due to the damages caused to the cardiovascular system. Chauhan and colleges recommend that clinicians must "think beyond the bones," as the bone's disease is contributing to blood vessel calcification.
3. Renal osteodystrophy.
a. The systemic impact of CKD occurs with the onset of CKD prior to diagnosis.
b. Dysfunction in mineral and bone metabolism in CKD can lead to systemic abnormalities in the metabolism of vitamin D, calcium, phosphorus, and PTH early in the disease.
(1) This results in problems with linear growth, strength, bone growth, mineralization, and causes calcification of soft tissue and vessels (KDIGO, 2009).
(2) In CKD, there are changes in the pathologic structure and morphology of the osseous structures; known as renal osteodystrophy and includes osteomalacia, osteoporosis, and secondary hyperparathyroidism.
(3) The term *CKD-MBD* includes the spectrum

Table 1.18

KDIGO Classification of CKD-MBD and Renal Osteodystrophy

Definition of CKD–MBD
A systematic disorder of mineral and bone metabolism due to CKD manifested by either one or a combination of the following: • Abnormalities of calcium, phosphorus, PTH, or vitamin D metabolism. • Abnormalities in bone turnover, mineralization, volume, linear growth, or strength. • Vascular or other soft-tissue calcification.
Definition of renal osteodystrophy
• Renal osteodystrophy is an alteration of bone morphology in patients with CKD. • It is one measure of the skeletal component of the systemic disorder of CKD-MBD that is quantifiable by histomorphometry of bone biopsy.

CKD – chronic kidney disease; CKD-MBD – chronic kidney disease-mineral and bone disorder; KDIGO – Kidney disease: Improving Global Outcomes; PTH – parathyroid hormone.

Source: Kidney Disease: Improving Global Outcomes (KDIGO) CKD–MBD Work Group. KDIGO Clinical Practice Guideline for the Diagnosis, Evaluation, Prevention, and Treatment of Chronic Kidney Disease–Mineral and Bone Disorder (CKD–MBD). *Kidney International 2009*; (Suppl. 113): 76: S1–S130 (originally table 1 on page S4). Used with permission.

of not only bone disorders but also systemic mineral, cardiovascular diseases associated with alterations in bone and mineral metabolism.

(4) Patients will complain of generalized bone pain, as well as pain with ambulation and activity. A primary concern with renal osteodystrophy is the increased incidence of fractures (Kline, 2013).

c. In renal osteodystrophy, there is bone reabsorption common in the proximal femur and tibia, humerus and distal clavicle, and phalanges due to the hyperphosphatemia, decreasing serum ionized calcium, which in turn, causes hyperparathyroidism.

d. Osteomalacia occurs when there is reduced bone turnover (forming process) that causes softening of the bones. This process is accelerated by a decrease in calcium levels that is a response to hyperphosphatemia and vitamin D deficiency (Kline, 2013).

e. Infants with CKD stages 2 to 5D must have close monitoring of growth with quarterly measurements of length, and children must have height assessed at least every year [1B]. Deformities of the legs and arms are seen in younger children with delays in growth, and they have an increased risk for scoliosis and slipped capital femoral epiphysis (Kline, 2013).

f. Serum lab tests measuring calcium, phosphorus, alkaline phosphate, and PTH need to be obtained. Monitoring begins in adults every 6 to 12 months with CKD stage 3 [IC], and in children testing begins at CKD stage 2 [2D].

g. KDIGO suggests that calcidiol 25 (OH) D levels

be evaluated in CKD stages 3 to 5D and that vitamin D deficiency is treated [2C].

h. Treatment of CKD-MBD should be treated based on trends in laboratory values, not a single isolated lab value [1C].

(1) Clinicians.

(a) Should evaluate serum phosphorus and calcium together to guide clinical practice [2D] with consistent laboratory techniques.

(b) Should be notified if the lab changes methods or assays to optimize the interpretation of the data [1B].

(2) For CKD stages 2 to 5 not on dialysis, phosphate is maintained in the normal range. However, there are no identified optimal levels or normal range for phosphate.

(3) Quarles (2013) recommends maintaining serum phosphate levels between 3.5 and 5.5 mg/dL for individuals receiving dialysis (1.13 to 1.78 mmol/L).

4. Bone testing and biopsy.

a. Bone density testing is not accurate in CKD stages 3b to 5, and KDIGO does not recommend bone mineral density screening [2B].

b. Bone biopsy, although invasive, is still the best method for obtaining an accurate diagnosis for patients with CKD stages 3 to 5D who have unexplained bone fractures, chronic bone pain, or suspicion of aluminum toxicity [NG].

c. In general, for these CKD stages, bone biopsy is not a routine suggestion because in this population it does not have predictive value of fractures as it does in the normal population [2B].

d. KDIGO suggests that prediction of bone turnover can be done using the PTH or alkaline phosphatase (bones specific) [2B].

e. Specific bone tests that look at collagen synthesis and breakdown, such as procollagen type I C terminal propeptide, deoxypyridinoline, pyridinoline, or cross-laps, can be done to assess bone disease [2B], but KDIGO suggests "not" doing these tests routinely in CKD stages 3 to 5D [2C].

5. Vascular calcification.
   a. Calcium is commonly deposited within the intima and media layers in artherosclerosis. For individuals receiving dialysis, it more commonly occurs in the medial layer, causing stiffness of the vessels, i.e., noncompliance (Afzali & Goldsmith, 2012).
   b. Afzali & Goldsmith (2012) report there has been an acceleration of vascular calcification with the use of oral phosphate binders containing calcium and the use of oral vitamin D among people on dialysis.
   c. Blood vessel stiffness is caused by progressive calcification and is associated with sudden cardiac death. Calcification is also increased with diet and the type of dialysate (Afzali & Goldsmith, 2012).
   d. Individuals with vascular and valvular calcifications who have CKD stages 3 to 5D are considered to be at highest cardiovascular risk [2A].
   e. Echocardiogram, CT scan, and plain lateral abdominal films can be obtained to assess for the presence of valvular or vascular calcifications in CKD stages 3 to 5D [2C] (KDIGO, 2009).

6. Treatment.
   a. The treatment of CKD-MBD involves evaluation of serum calcium, serum phosphorus, serum iPTH (intact PTH), and vitamin D levels in addition to assessing for the presence of vascular calcification.
   b. When initiating treatment, it is important to individualize and take into consideration the stage of CKD, side effects of the medications, drug interactions, and the presence of other bone and mineral disorders and treatments.
   c. For those with CKD, KDIGO suggests to not routinely prescribe vitamin D supplements or analogs, without documented deficiency, for the purpose of suppressing increased levels of PTH in those who are not on dialysis.
   d. KDIGO suggests treatment of hyperphosphatemia for specific CKD stages (see Table 1.19) and for hyperparathyroidism.
   e. Historically, each oral phosphate binder has had its own problems. Long-term

administration of aluminum hydroxide resulted in toxicity as tissues accumulated and absorbed aluminum.

f. After abandoning aluminum-containing binders, calcium salts were used for management of hyperphosphatemia. Calcium carbonate dissolves in an acid pH and has diminished effectiveness when taking H2 blockers. Calcium acetate is more efficient because it can be taken with H2 blockers (acid blockers) at a lower dose than calcium carbonate (Quarles, 2013).

g. Debate continues on which oral phosphate binder is the best for treatment. With the development of noncalcium binders such as sevelamer, an ion binder, and lanthanum, an earth element, comes expense and new side effects. Sevelamer hydrochloride (Renagel®) increases the risk of metabolic acidosis in CKD; thus sevelamer carbonate (Renvela®) was developed.

h. All binders are more effective when taken with meals because less calcium is absorbed. Calcium intake must not exceed 2000 mg/day or 1.5 g of elemental calcium per day.

i. The area of controversy in CKD is appropriate dose, target range, and formulation of vitamin D (KDIGO, 2012b).

j. There is not adequate research to support the use of bisphosphonates in CKD stage 4.

7. Low phosphorus diet.
   a. Foods rich in protein are major sources of phosphorus. Packaged foods, fast foods, and thickeners also have higher added phosphorus (processed).
   b. Reading labels can help identify phosphorus in food, as it may be in the form of disodium dihydrogen pyrophosphate.
   c. Nephrology nurses and dietitians can teach patients by using the handout from the National Kidney Disease Education Program (NKDEP) (2010).
   d. Carbonated beverages may also contain phosphorus (e.g., dark sodas). Nuts, lentils, beans, oatmeal, bran cereals, dairy, meat, poultry, and fish contain increased levels of phosphates.
   e. Foods with no or little phosphorus additives are ideal (Noori et al., 2010).
   f. For adults with CKD, phosphorus is limited to 800 to 1000 mg per day (Castle, 2012).
   g. Diet alone is usually not adequate in reducing phosphorus levels to a normal range, and oral phosphate binders are needed.
   h. Nutrition is not compromised by restricting phosphorus, but nutritional supplements may be indicated in some people (Quarles, 2013).

Table 1.19

Phosphate-Binding Compounds

Binder source	Rx	Forms	Content (mineral/metal/element)	Potential advantages	Potential disadvantages
Aluminum hydroxide	No	Liquid, tablet, capsule	Aluminum content varies from 100 to > 200 mg (per tablet)	Very effective phosphate-binding capacity; variety of forms.	Potential for aluminum toxicity; altered bone mineralization, dementia; GI side effects
Calcium acetate	Yes/no	Capsule, tablet	Contains 25% elemental Ca^{2+} (169 mg elemental Ca^{2+} per 667 mg cap)	Effective phosphate-binding, potentially for enhanced phosphate-binding capability over $CaCO_3$ potentially less calcium absorption	Potential for hypercalcemia-associated risks including extraskeletal calcification and PTH suppression; GI side effects
Calcium carbonate	No	Liquid, tablet, chewable, capsule, gum	Contains 40% elemental Ca^{2+} (200 mg elemental Ca^{2+} per 500 mg $CaCO_3$)	Effective, inexpensive, readily available	Potential for hypercalcemia-associated risks including extraskeletal calcification and PTH suppression; GI side effects
Calcium citrate	No	Tablet, liquid, capsule	Contains 22% elemental Ca^{2+}	Not recommended in CKD	Enhancement of aluminum absorption; GI side effects
Calcium ketoglutarate					Similar to other calcium salts, costly, GI side effects, potentially less hypercalcemic than calcium carbonate or acetate, not well studied
Calcium gluconate		Tablet, powder			Similar to other calcium salts, not well studied
Ferric citrate					GI side effects, not well studied
Magnesium/calcium carbonate	No	Tablet	Approx 28% Mg^{2+} (85 mg) per total mg carbonate and 25% elemental Ca^{2+} (100 mg) per total $CaCO_3$	Effective; potential for lower calcium load than pure calcium-based binders	GI side effects, potential for hypermagnesemia, not well studied
Magnesium carbonate/ calcium acetate	Yes	Tablet			Lack of availability worldwide, assumed to have similar effects of its components
Sevelamer-HCl	Yes	Caplet	None	Effective; no calcium/metal; not absorbed; potential for reduced coronary/aortic calcification when compared with calcium-based binders in some studies; reduces plasma concentration of LDL-C	Cost; potential for decreased bicarbonate levels; may require calcium supplement in presence of hypocalcemia; GI side effects
Sevelamer carbonate	Yes	Caplet, powder	None	Effective; no calcium/metal; not absorbed; assumed to have similar advantages as sevelamer-HCl; potentially improved acid-base balance	Cost; may require calcium supplement in the presence of hypocalcemia; GI side effects
Lanthanum carbonate	Yes	Wafer, chewable	Contains 250, 500, or 1000 mg elemental lanthanum per wafer	Effective; no calcium; chewable	Cost; potential for accumulation of lanthanum due to GI absorption, although long-term clinical consequences unknown; GI side effects

CKD – chronic kidney disease; GI – gastrointestinal; LDL-C – low-density lipoprotein cholesterol; PTH – parathyroid hormone.

Source: Kidney Disease: Improving Global Outcomes (KDIGO) CKD–MBD Work Group. KDIGO Clinical Practice Guideline for the Diagnosis, Evaluation, Prevention, and Treatment of Chronic Kidney Disease–Mineral and Bone Disorder (CKD–MBD). *Kidney International 2009*; (Suppl. 113): 76: S1–S130 (originally table 19 on page S53). Used with permission.

8. Chronic metabolic acidosis in CKD.
   a. In chronic metabolic acidosis, there are some compensatory effects that adjust the blood pH. The adjustment is the result of the bicarbonate buffers in the bone, extracellular fluid, tissue, and respiratory system (hyperventilation) that compensate for the acidosis.
   b. This occurs at the expense of other systems, and chronic metabolic acidosis compounds complex health problems.
   c. Catabolism of muscle protein, bone resorption, osteopenia, systemic inflammation, hypotension, malaise, resistance to growth hormone and insulin, hypertriglyceridemia, impaired cardiac functioning, worsening of secondary hyperparathyroidism, and increased mortality result from chronic metabolic acidosis (KDIGO, 2013a; Kovesdy, 2013).
   d. The acidosis is associated with a GFR < 40 mL/minute. Low serum bicarbonate levels in CKD are related to an increased risk for loss of kidney function.
   e. There is a decrease in the acidosis when kidney replacement therapy is initiated due to the buffers added to the dialysate.
   f. In children, chronic metabolic acidosis stunts growth; treatment with bicarbonate slows the progression of CKD.
   g. In adults, treatment is not initiated routinely due to the added sodium and the risk of increase fluid volume.
   h. KDIGO (2013a) suggests that serum bicarbonate levels less than 22 mmol/L should be treated with supplementation of oral bicarbonate [2B].
   i. Throughout the world, bicarbonate treatment is cost effective, easy to obtain, and affordable for those with CKD (KDIGO, 2013a).

VII. Management of comorbidities associated with CKD.

A. CKD is a complex systemic disease that requires individualized management using a team approach while empowering the individual as an agent of self-care.
   1. Lifestyle modifications are important to slow the progression of CKD. Therapeutic lifestyle modifications discussed previously must be a priority for individuals with CKD.
   2. CKD accelerates many pathologic conditions in the body, and aging brings with it a high prevalence of comorbidities.
   3. Individuals with CKD may have other interrelated comorbidities that increase mortality and morbidity and accelerate CKD. There is an increased cardiovascular disease risk for all individuals with CKD [1A].
      a. It appears that CKD and its comorbidities are a pathologic cycle of disease processes that leads to atherosclerosis, arteriosclerosis, and cardiovascular events.
      b. Hypertension is a primary risk factor for CKD, and CKD-MBD has increased risk for vascular calcification.
   4. Anemia has to be addressed; proteinuria reduced; and blood pressure, blood glucose, and lipid targets achieved (KDIGO, 2013a).
   5. It is common to see normal or low cholesterol levels in patients with CKD due to malnutrition and muscle wasting.
   6. Lower levels of high-density lipoprotein (HDL), the good cardioprotective cholesterol, and high levels of the bad low-density lipoprotein (LDL) add additional risks for cardiovascular disease.
      a. Up to 50% of individuals with CKD have hypertriglyceridemia due to defects in triglyceride removal (Appel, 2013).
      b. The national guidelines for detection, evaluation, and treatment of adults with high blood cholesterol are set by the Adult Treatment Panel (ATP).
      c. With a diagnosis of CKD, fasting lipid profiles need to be obtained [1C].
      d. Physical activity, weight loss, abstinence from alcohol, and modification of diet can decrease triglyceride levels.
   7. Statin therapy or statin/ezetimibe combination is recommended by KDIGO (2013b) for treatment of lipid disorders in those with the following:
      a. CKD GFR < 60 mL/min/1.73 m^2.
      b. Younger than 50 years of age.
      c. Not receiving dialysis.
      d. Do not have kidney transplant [1A] (KDIGO, 2013b).
      e. Ages 18 to 49 years, with the above criteria, should also receive statin therapy if they have diabetes, coronary artery disease, prior stroke, or < 10% 10-year risk of having a myocardial infarction [2A].
      f. Statins are lipid-lowering agents that inhibit an enzyme (HMG-CoA) responsible for the synthesis of cholesterol and are contraindicated in pregnancy. Pharmaceutical companies have categorized statins as category X, meaning they are contraindicated. Category A provides reassurance as the safest category, while category X strictly denotes that a drug is contraindicated.
      g. Statin therapy is first-line treatment for hypertriglyceridemia as they lower both triglycerides and LDL, and raise HDL, resulting in reduced atherosclerotic events.

h. Grapefruit juice increases levels of statins and the risk for muscle breakdown and rhabdomyolysis (Vallerand et al., 2013).

B. Coronary artery disease.
1. The pathophysiologic process in CKD-MBD leads to vascular calcification of the coronary arteries.
2. There is a lack of research that includes people with CKD and coronary syndrome.
   a. Until there is research data that proves otherwise, treatment of acute coronary syndromes in CKD should be similar to those without CKD using aspirin, beta blockers, ACE/ARBs, clopidogrel, and immediate reperfusion (Hurzog et al., 2011).
   b. KDIGO CVD work group reports there is evidence of increased mortality in those with CKD who have surgical coronary revascularization with significant operative complications.
   c. Percutaneous angioplasty may be an option; however, it adds an additional risk of contrast-induced nephropathy. When percutaneous interventions are required, this often necessitates administration of additional contrast dye, thus increasing the risk to the kidneys.
   d. Individuals with CKD who are at risk for CVD without increased risk for bleeding should be prescribed antiplatelet medications to prevent CVD [2B].

C. Heart failure.
1. The incidence of heart failure is correlated with worsening CKD.
2. Diastolic heart failure (DHF) has slightly higher mortality than systolic heart failure (SHF) leading to pump failure and sudden cardiac death (Herzog, 2011).
   a. In SHF, the ejection fraction (ventricular contraction) is impaired; thus the heart does not pump blood adequately. The ventricular wall thickness is decreased.
   b. In DHF, the ejection fraction of the ventricle is normal; however, the ventricles do not have normal filling/relaxation during diastole and the patient presents with symptoms of heart failure.
      (1) The ventricular wall thickness is increased.
      (2) Changes in the myocardium, pressure overload from chronic uncontrolled hypertension, and volume overload add to ventricular dysfunction and heart failure.
      (3) Diastolic dysfunction can occur early in CKD prior to the development of left ventricular hypertrophy (LVH).

c. Individuals with heart failure experience significant fatigue, activity intolerance, and fluid retention.
d. Echocardiogram remains the gold standard for diagnosis of LVH and heart failure. LVH can be related to anemia in people with early CKD (KDIGO, 2013a).
e. Education and counseling are necessary to control heart failure and prevent hospital admissions.
f. Salt restriction, diuresis, and escalation in pharmacologic therapy are necessary to treat heart failure.
g. Beta blockers are recommended for use in heart failure, and bisoprolol or carvedilol is standard therapy for systolic heart failure.

D. Peripheral arterial disease.
1. There is a relationship between CKD and peripheral arterial disease (PAD).
2. To assess for peripheral arterial disease, KDIGO (2013a) recommends listening for bruits, checking for pulses, palpating skin temperature and capillary refill, looking for skin ulcers or nonhealing wounds, and measuring ankle-brachial index [1B].
3. A symptom analysis must assess ischemic leg pain with rest, claudication, and walking.
4. Antiplatelet therapy is recommended to reduce ischemic events (ACCF/AHA, 2013).

E. Diabetes.
1. Throughout the world, diabetes is the primary cause of CKD, and people with diabetes often have poor kidney function.
2. The incidence of diabetes is quickly rising in developing nations (KDIGO, 2013a). People with CKD and diabetes have significant reductions in GFR and progress more rapidly.
   a. They also have higher rates of adverse events, including hospitalization, risk for AKI, diastolic heart failure, infection, peripheral arterial disease (PAD), and foot ulcers.
   b. The risk for foot amputation increases as GFR decreases (KDIGO, 2013a).
   c. People with diabetes and CKD have more in-hospital AKI. It is vital that nurses monitor for dehydration and nephrotoxic medications, and that they follow guidelines for temporarily discontinuing metformin and also preventing radiocontrast-induced kidney injury.
3. A1C or glycohemoglobin is a serum blood measurement of the average blood glucose over a 3-month period or life of the red blood cell (NIDDK, 2012b).
   a. This test does not require fasting and is measured in percentage.

(1) Normal is less than 5.7%.
(2) Prediabetes is 5.7% to 6.4%.
(3) Diabetes is over 6.5%.
(4) Optimal Hgb A1C is less than 7% (53 mmol/mol) to prevent progression of vascular complications [1A].

b. Hgb A1C less than 6.5% does not seem to improve mortality and may cause hypoglycemia (Aronow, 2013). KDIGO (2013a) states: "In people with CKD and diabetes, glycemic control should be part of a multifactorial interventions strategy addressing blood pressure control and cardiovascular risk, promoting the use of angiotensin-converting enzyme inhibition or angiotensin-receptor blockade, statins, and antiplatelet therapy where clinical indication" (p. 76).

4. Albuminuria in people with diabetes increases the risk of CVD, and lifestyle changes to control risk factors that are modifiable will reduce the progression of CKD.

5. Smoking cessation is of utmost importance in those with diabetes and CKD, as smoking increases kidney damage in those with diabetes (KDIGO, 2013a).

6. Nerve damage or neuropathies are related to the duration of diabetes and the long-term exposure of the nerves to high glucose.
   a. Nurses are aware of peripheral neuropathies; however, people with diabetes can get neuropathy of the peripheral nerves, autonomic, proximal, and focal nerves.
      (1) The autonomic nerves affect the heart and blood vessels, lungs, urinary tract, sex organs, eyes, and the digestive system (NIDDK, 2012b).
      (2) Disruptions in the autonomic nervous system can lead to alterations in sensory and motor pathways that might result in patient specific complaints such as asymptomatic hypoglycemia (patient is unaware of a low blood glucose), orthostatic hypotension, gastroparesis, dysphagia, urinary retention, sexual dysfunction, and problems with thermoregulation.
      (3) The best treatment is prevention with maintaining therapeutic blood glucose with daily monitoring.
      (4) Pharmacologic treatment for painful neuropathies is tricyclic antidepressants, other antidepressants, and anticonvulsants (NIDDK, 2012b).
   b. Podiatric assessment should be done on a regular basis for those with diabetes [2A] (ACCF/AHA, 2013).
      (1) Daily foot inspection must be routine for those with diabetes.

(2) Patients with diabetes should be instructed regarding proper footwear, cleaning, and moisturizers.

7. Oral care is also important to decrease risk for infection.

8. Annual eye exams by a professional are recommended to assess for retinopathy (NIDDK, 2013).

9. Recommendations for immunizations are listed in Figure 1.45.

10. Diabetes educators, clinics, nurse educators, and dietary educators can assist people with diabetes.
    a. It is recommended that adults with diabetes and CKD limit dietary protein to 0.8 g/kg/day [2C].
    b. KDIGO recommends following the American Diabetes Association guidelines in children.

11. Termininology appropriateness.
    a. Using "ic" at the end of the disease (diabetic, asthmatic) is considered inappropriate and dehumanizing and must be avoided by healthcare providers.
    b. Put the person first, the disease second, as in "people with diabetes."
    c. Individuals with CKD struggle with the lack of respect they perceive from the healthcare system. Demonstrating compassion and respect improves the therapeutic nurse–patient relationship.

VIII. Living with CKD.

A. Overview.
   1. CKD is a long-term complex disease with many coexisting and comorbid conditions.
   2. It impacts all aspects of life from the time of diagnosis until death.
   3. As CKD progresses, it comes with additional physical, emotional, social, and financial burdens that can restrict lifestyle (Finnegan-John & Thomas, 2013).
   4. The complexity and healthcare demands of CKD can make many individuals and families feel helpless and powerless (Muhammad et al., 2012).
   5. Nephrology nurses understand that the physical and emotional burdens of living with CKD are real, and the stresses and frustrations are difficult to manage (NKF, 2009).
   6. Bragazzi (2013) reported that CKD brings a significant psychological burden that is often overlooked in daily clinical practice.

B. Coping with diagnosis and daily life with CKD.
   1. The initial diagnosis of CKD is often difficult to accept for the majority of people. In a focus group study of people living with CKD, many expressed initial shock, confusion, vulnerability, and felt overwhelmed (Tong et al., 2009).

2. As CKD progresses, four primary themes emerge in the research.
   a. Confronting mortality.
   b. Lack of choice.
   c. Gaining information.
   d. Weighing alternatives.
3. Nephrology nurses can assist patients in gaining information and allow them to weigh alternatives and give them choices to avoid a sense of powerlessness.
4. Within the therapeutic nurse–patient relationship, nurses can encourage conversations with patients allowing for the sharing of frustrations and challenges.
5. Regarding treatment choices and decision making, patients report that the experiences of other patients with CKD were influential, in addition to the opinions of their family (Morton et al., 2010). Often, family influences are based upon the convenience of treatment options on the family itself and not necessarily the choice of the patient.

C. Normalcy.
1. It is important to stay involved in activities, sports, hobbies, play, recreation, and the responsibilities of daily living.

2. Life satisfaction is increased when individuals with CKD and their families return to their normal routine such as school, work, and other activities (NKF, 2009).
3. The Americans with Disabilities Act (ADA) protects those with CKD from discrimination when they need to take time away from work for treatment or therapies.
4. Individuals with CKD are encouraged to talk about emotions, fears, and concerns with family members as a healthy coping mechanism.
   a. Self-reports of dissatisfaction with family support, feeling like a burden on family and friends, feelings of isolation, and the inability to participate in social activities due to health problems were related factors that increase mortality in those with CKD stage 5D (Untas et al., 2011).
   b. Strong family relationships with a sense of warmth, caring, and support can decrease stress.
5. Normalcy for young women often includes pregnancy and childbearing. These normal life situations are not promoted in women of child-bearing age with CKD due to the poor pregnancy outcomes.

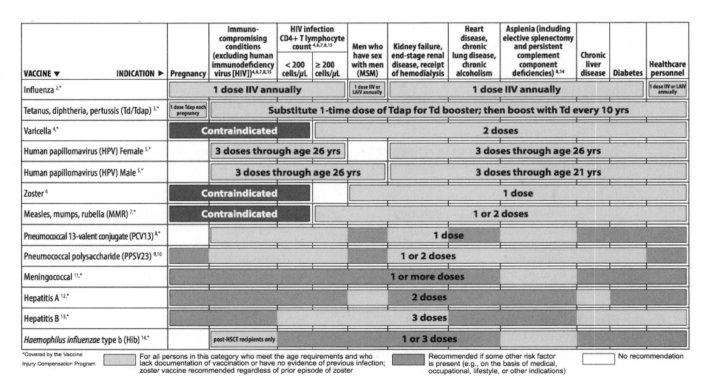

Figure 1.45. Vaccines that might be indicated for adults based on medical and other indications.

Source: Centers for Disease Control and Prevention (CDC). (2011). Immunization Practices. MMWR, 60(RR-2), 40-41. (Available from http://www.cdc.gov/vaccines/schedules/downloads/adult/adult-combined-schedule.pdf).

a. Women who seek fertility and pregnancy, successful kidney transplantation is the optimal way to restore fertility.
b. Women with CKD who do become pregnant need to be managed by a team including a perinatologist and nephrologist.
c. Nurses can help facilitate grieving in women of childbearing age who are unable to conceive by allowing time for patients to share their feelings of loss.

D. Fatigue.
1. Overview.
   a. Energy levels, activities and exertion, fitness, and fatigue are problems that impact the daily lives of people with CKD.
   b. Bonner and associates (2010) reported that individuals with CKD experience significant levels of fatigue and are unable to participate in many activities.
   c. This is more common in females and older adults.
2. Researchers identified that parents of children with CKD reported low energy levels, weakness, and increased frequency of falling asleep during the day with GFR < 50 mL/min/1.73 m^2.
3. Decreased quality of life was related to low energy, weakness, and sleepiness during the day as well as trouble sleeping (Roumelioti et al., 2010).
4. Tong and researchers (2013) identified that fatigue and increased need for sleep affected both work and social activities. Many study participants felt guilty and helpless from "wasting" time sleeping (p. 691).

E. Stressors.
1. Stress is similar for men and women.
2. Coping strategies are used more often in women (Harwood et al., 2011).
3. Most commonly reported stressors:
   a. Sleep problems.
   b. Fatigue
   c. Peripheral neuropathy.
4. Optimism is a powerful effective coping strategy to use with stress and was reported as commonly used (Harwood et al., 2009).
5. Reframing is a technique that has been effective in dealing with negativity and stressful situations. It works by looking at the situation in a positive light and identifying possible good in the situation.
6. As CKD progresses, the demands and stressors change.
7. Decisions for kidney transplantation or initiation of dialysis are additional stressors. Kidney transplant represents hope. Researchers identified that a failed transplant causes grief, loss, and dread of returning to dialysis.

a. Finnegan-John and Thomas (2013) examined the impact of CKD stage 5 on the quality of life and reported that study participants often spoke of dialysis as suffering "fatigue, infertility, low energy, mood and physical changes to the body, for example, catheter, weight gain, and scarring."
b. One study participant called her fistula an "internal grub." Makaroff and Molzahn (2012) identified three challenges of individuals with CKD-D that caused study participants to contemplate withdrawal from dialysis
   (1) The "unpredictability" of CKD.
   (2) The relentless nature of the "work."
   (3) Quality of life.
c. Nephrology nurses must be aware that from the patient's perspective, CKD is a burden that causes suffering and decreases quality of life (Finnegan-John & Thomas, 2013).

F. Spirituality.
1. Research shows that a high level of spirituality in individuals with CKD stage 5D helps "focus on themselves in order to face their problems related to the disease" and plays a positive role in mental health (Theofilou, 2012, p. 3).
2. Depression, social dysfunction, somatic symptoms, anxiety, and insomnia are also decreased with increases in spirituality. Health locus of control increases as spirituality increases. (Theofilou, 2011).
3. Interconnections to a deity, inner self, friends, family, community, and nature are components of spirituality.
   a. Development of connectedness within each realm enhances spirituality and inner strength.
   b. Spirituality may include religion for many people, and for most it involves praying and a relationship with a deity.
   c. As nurses, there is an acknowledgment that all people are spiritual in nature, and this is unique for each individual person.
   d. Nurses can also be advocates for spiritual interventions such as prayer, meditation, finding meaning and purpose, and helping the patient increase awareness of spiritual resources (Bragazzi & Del Puente, 2013).

G. Depression.
1. Decreased quality of life, increased mortality and morbidity, and hospitalization are related to depression in those with CKD (Finkelstein et al., 2010; Hedayati et al., 2010).
2. There is an increase in cardiovascular events in those with CKD and depression; this widespread problem is underdiagnosed and treated (Hedayati et al., 2012).

3. Of psychiatric disorders, depression is most common in CKD. Major depression in individuals with diabetes and CKD-G5 is associated with a greater risk of mortality (Young et al., 2010).
4. Depression co-occurs with anxiety, which leads to increased somatic symptoms, decreased social life, decreased sexual functioning, and insomnia (Theofilou, 2011).
   a. Research participants reported feeling trapped because while their appearance seemed normal, inside they felt ill and exhausted (Tong et al., 2009).
   b. Nephrology nurses can screen patients and monitor for depression and take an active role in facilitating treatment with both medication and cognitive behavioral therapy (Hedayati et al., 2012).
5. Sexual dysfunction is related to depression in women with CKD (Guglielmi, 2013).

H. Sexuality.
1. Self-esteem, fatigue, anemia, cardiovascular disease, weakness, insomnia, depression, and decreased quality of life can all cause sexual dysfunction. Sexual desire, arousal, orgasm, distress, and painful intercourse can play a role in sexual dysfunction (Prescott et al., 2013).
2. In women with CKD, 55% report lack of sexual arousal (Vecchio et al., 2010).
   a. In woman with CKD on hemodialysis, sexual dysfunction is associated with menopause, diabetes, diuretics, low serum albumin, depression, less education, and age (Strippoli & CDS Group, 2012).
   b. This multifactorial problem causes women with CKD G4 to 5 to have two times more sexual dysfunction than gender and age-matched healthy controls (Prescott et al., 2013). These same problems are related to decreased quality of life (Guglielmi, 2013).
   c. Women with CKD experience early menopause.
   d. Treatment of menopausal symptoms with hormone replacement therapy must be individualized due to the additional cardiovascular risk of blood clots and stroke.
   e. Topical lubricants can be helpful to decrease vaginal dryness and pain with intercourse.
3. In men with CKD, erectile dysfunction and lack of orgasm are reported in up to 80% of men (Vecchio et al., 2010).
4. Physiologic changes add to the complexity of sources causing sexual dysfunction. These include low testosterone, vascular calcification, nerve damage from hypertryglceridemia, diabetes, other neuropathies, and medications (antihypertensives, antidepressants).

5. Sexual dysfunction in men with CKD can be treated with erectile dysfunction medications as recommended by a healthcare practitioner. They are contraindicated for those on nitrates.
6. For both men and women with sexual dysfunction, it is important to address physiologic and psychological factors involved.
   a. Correction of anemia, blood pressure, albuminuria, hyperlipidemia, and hormonal imbalances may improve sexual function; however, in men, pharmacologic therapy is often needed.
   b. For women, there is currently no pharmacologic therapy for sexual dysfunction. Treatment of vaginal dryness with oils and lubricants can decrease painful intercourse.
7. Cognitive behavior therapy, support groups, social support, reframing, optimism, and treatment of depression can help strengthen coping skills.

IX. Empowerment strategies to delay progression of CKD.

A. Overview.
1. The primary outcome in empowering individuals with CKD with self-care management is to:
   a. Delay the progression of CKD.
   b. Prevent and manage comorbid conditions.
2. This must be done by minimizing the impact of CKD upon someone's lifestyle and supporting a full, rich, active lifestyle.
3. Many individuals in CKD G1 to G2 do not have symptoms, and it can be a challenge to motivate them to modify lifestyle.
4. It is important to assess the individual's confidence in his/her ability to make lifestyle changes, set realistic goals, and carry out tasks.
5. There are many tools available for nurses to assess the learning styles and individualize teaching for the complex patient (Inott & Kennedy, 2011). Both time and frustration can be spared if the teaching is tailored to the correct learning style (auditory, kinesthetic, and visual).
6. Cultural factors must also be taken under consideration. Materials must be appropriate for the age, gender, and ethnicity of the individual.

B. Enhancing self-care and management.
1. Self-care and management in CKD can be complex and initially overwhelming, especially if hypertension and diabetes are involved.
2. It can be time-consuming and a challenge to follow a restricted diet and to maintain a blood pressure log, blood glucose log, and medication administration log.
3. Many educators believe that patients must master

one task before a new one is added. Nurses can guide patients with their self-care in a gentle, compassionate manor.
   a. Miller and Rollnick (2012) describe compassion as promoting the welfare of another with a commitment to pursue their best interest and "to benevolently seek and value the well-being of others" (p. 20).
   b. Enhancing self-care and management improves management of symptoms, quality of life, and coping; it also decreases healthcare utilization and cost (Novak et al., 2013).
4. People with CKD want to be treated with respect and holism.
   a. Tong and researchers (2013) reported that study participants with CKD feel like they are treated as a disease entity without emotional or psychological support from the healthcare team.
   b. Individuals with CKD want to be at the center of the healthcare team and participate in decision making.
   c. Members of the health team can be patient-centered and form mutually agreed-upon plans of care.
   d. Referral to social workers, counselors, chaplains, or talking to other individuals with CKD can enhance coping strategies (NKF, 2009). Miller and Rollnick (2012) describe necessary components to promote change within the nurse–patient relationships.
      (1) Demonstrating affirmation of the person's efforts and strengths.
      (2) Respecting autonomy.
      (3) Demonstrating value of the patient's absolute worth.
      (4) Understanding the patient's internal perspective or demonstrating accurate empathy.
5. Building a therapeutic relationship is a key factor in promoting self-care and healthy behavior changes.

C. Transtheoretical model of intentional change.
   1. Successful change often occurs in stages.
   2. Failure for self-change is most likely to be due to a lack of guidance.
   3. Prochaska and colleagues (2007) are clinical psychologists and researchers with over 50 research studies refining the Transtheoretical Model of Intentional Change (TTM) model for successful change.
      a. These experts recommend that healthcare professionals understand the six stages of change and identify which stage their patient is in for appropriate facilitation of behavior change.
      b. The purpose of this model is to promote and maintain healthy lifestyle change. This is one of the leading models used for successful behavior change in health care.

D. Motivational interviewing.
   1. Another successful strategy for promoting and maintaining healthy behavioral change is motivational interviewing.
      a. The purpose of this technique is to create a safe and supportive environment and to facilitate contemplation of one's behavior and to:
         (1) Help explore the behavior.
         (2) Make a cost-benefit analysis of the status quo.
         (3) Decrease potential resistance to change.
         (4) Clarify goals.
         (5) Assist developing realistic strategies to facilitate realistic behavioral changes (Miller & Rollnick, 2012).
      b. The authors identify a common problem with the helping professions, called the "righting reflex" (p. 5).
         (1) This entails persuading a person to change and attempting to fix behaviors by directing others to change often in a confrontational, authoritarian style.
         (2) These approaches tend to evoke defensiveness, anger, shame, powerlessness, and resistance to change.
      c. Confrontation, expert opinion, lecturing, labeling, blaming, and preaching do not have a role in motivational interviewing.
      d. People are more likely to be persuaded to change by their own voice than that of another.
   2. Miller and Rollnick (2012) have developed the following questions to inspire personal reflection and guide change while making the person feel empowered, understood, respected, and engaged.
      a. Why would you want to make this change?
      b. How might you go about it in order to succeed?
      c. What are the three best reasons for you to do it?
      d. How important is it for you to make this change and why?
      e. So what do you think you will do?
   3. With ongoing research, nurses can learn conversational techniques that empower patients with CKD, enhance their well-being, and promote healthy lifestyles.
      a. A nurse can print these five questions on an index card to use as a resource when the righting reflex occurs. This will help guide the discussion and allow patients to persuade themselves to change.
      b. It is imperative that the patient and the healthcare team have adequate administrative support, both financial and within the system structure. Time and scheduling for patient

education and self-care management should be given.

   c. Nurses need to move away from "a paternalistic model to a partnership" that is truly patient-centered (Novak et al., 2013, p. 193).

4. The administration must support empowerment of patient self-care and management by scheduling time for staff education and development of their expertise in CKD (Novak et al., 2013).

   a. Nurses can do a comprehensive assessment of the patient's learning style, readiness to learn, stage of change, resources, family support, impedance to change, behaviors, and ability to carry out self-care and management.

   b. Novak and colleagues (2013) recommend that patients are also screened for anxiety, depression, emotional distress, and social support.

   c. If systems are in place within organizations to center on the patient, in order to educate and empower them, the program would include preparation for the progression of CKD and patient choices of kidney replacement therapy.

E. Preparation for kidney replacement therapy (KRT).

1. A number of motivational interviewing techniques can be used to introduce KRT using an unbiased and objective approach.

2. Denial is a healthy coping mechanism for most people and it is often difficult to visualize future progression of CKD.

3. The individual with CKD may prefer a referral to a nurse educator for formal education on KRT modalities.

4. Speaking with other patients on KRT is often helpful.

5. Many organizations provide tours of the dialysis unit or visitation with a patient on home hemodialysis.

   a. For those who are visual learners, The National Kidney and Urological Diseases Information Clearinghouse (NKUDIC) has many resources available for patients and families.

   b. There may be patients who opt out of KRT and prefer palliative or hospice care.

   c. As previously discussed, individualized patient-centered education includes optimum under-standing, and it takes time to change ways of thinking and behavior.

F. CKD is a dynamic and complex systemic disease that impacts all aspects of the individual's physiologic and psychological being.

1. Kidney disease is difficult, and its complexities are challenging to understand – for the nurse and more so for the individual and family.

2. Motivational interviewing can be implemented to persuade the patient to make healthy lifestyle changes to decrease the progression of CKD and to manage symptoms.

3. Self-care and management are of primary importance in maintaining therapeutic control of blood pressure, blood glucose, lipid levels, and CKD-MBD. Individuals with CKD must care for their nutrition and follow daily diet restrictions to prevent malnutrition and albuminuria.

4. Nephrology nurses can prepare individuals with CKD for kidney replacement therapies or kidney transplant through education, counseling, and discussion.

5. Teaching can be tailored to the learning type and individualized to meet the needs of the patient.

References

Afzali, B., & Goldsmith, D.J.A. (2012). Vascular calcification in chronic kidney disease. *UpToDate*. Retrieved from www.uptodate.com

Aitken, E., Carruthers, C., Gall, L., Kerr, L., Geddes, C., & Kingsmore, D. (2013). Acute kidney injury: Outcomes and quality of care. *QJM An International Journal of Medicine, 106*(4), 323-332

Akkupalli, L., Paravathi, G., Somasundaram, M., & Muni Radha, J. (2013). Bone mineral density in chronic kidney disease patients. *International Journal of Biological & Medical Research, 4*(1), 2870-2874.

American Cancer Society (2013). *Cancer facts and figures 2013*. Atlanta, Georgia. Retrieved from http://www.cancer.org/acs/groups/cid/documents/webcontent/003107-pdf.pdf

American College of Cardiology Foundation/American Heart Association (ACCF/AHA). (2013). ACCF/AHA practice guidelines: Management of patients with peripheral artery disease. *Circulation, 127*, 1-19.

American Diabetes Association (ADA). (2013a). *Genetics of diabetes*. Retrieved from http://www.diabetes.org/diabetes-basics/genetics-of-diabetes.html

American Diabetes Association (ADA). (2013b). Standards of medical care in diabetes – 2013. *Diabetes Care, 36*(Suppl. 1). doi:10:2337/dc13-SO11

American Dietetic Association. (2010). *Chronic kidney disease evidence-based nutrition practice guideline*. Chicago: American Dietetic Association. Retrieved from http://www.guideline.gov/content.aspx?id=23924&search=ckd

American Kidney Fund (AKF). (2012). *Kidney disease statistics*. Retrieved from https://www.kidney.org/news/newsroom/factsheets/FastFacts

American Nurses Association (ANA) and International Society of Nurses in Genetics (ISONG). (2007). *Genetics/genomics nursing: Scope and standards of practice*. Silver Spring, MD: Nursesbooks.org

American Nurses Credentialing Center (ANCC). (2014*). Advanced genetics nursing certification eligibility criteria*. Retrieved from http://www.nursecredentialing.org/Certification/ExamResources/Eligibility/ECategory/Advanced-Genetics-Eligibilty.html

American Society of Human Genetics (ASHG). (1998). Professional disclosure of familial genetic information. *American Journal of Human Genetics, 62*, 474-483.

Appel, G., & D'Agati, V. (2010). Primary and secondary (non-genetic) causes of focal and segmental glomerulosclerosis. In J.

Floege, R. Johnson, & J. Feehally, (Eds.), *Comprehensive clinical nephrology* (4th ed., pp 228-240). St. Louis, MO: Elsevier/Saunders.

Appel, G. & Jayne, D. (2010). Lupus nephritis. In J. Floege, R. Johnson, & J. Feehally (Eds.), *Comprehensive clinical nephrology* (4th ed., pp. 308-321). St. Louis: Elsevier/Saunders.

Aronow, W.S. (2013). Hemoglobin A1c, blood pressure, and serum low-density lipoprotein cholesterol goals in diabetics. *World Journal of Cardiology, 5*(5), 119-123.

Arora, P. (2013). Chronic kidney disease. *Medscape*. Received from emedicine.medscape.com

Aslam, A., & Coulson, I.H. (2013). Cowden syndrome (multiple hamartoma syndrome). *Clinical and Experimental Dermatology*, n/a-n/a. doi: 10.1111/ced.12140

Bansal, R. (2012). Contrast-induced nephropathy. *Medscape*. Retrieved from http://emedicine.medscape.com/article/246751-overview

Baumgarten, M., & Gehr, T. (2011) Chronic kidney disease: Detection and evaluation. *American Family Physician, 84*(10), 1138-1148.

Baylis, C., & Davison, J. (2010). Renal physiology in normal pregnancy. In J. Floege, R. Johnson, & J. Feehally, *Comprehensive clinical nephrology* (4th ed., pp. 497-515). St. Louis: Elsevier/Saunders.

Becker, M. (2013a, October). *Clinical manifestations and diagnosis of gout.* From UpToDate: http://www.uptodate.com

Becker, M. (2013b, March). *Diuretic-induced hyperuricemia and gout.* From UpToDate: http://www.uptodate.com

Bello, A., Kawar, B., El Kossi, M., & El Nahas, M. (2010). Epidemiology and pathophysiology of chronic kidney disease. In J. Floege, R. Johnson, & J. Feehally (Eds.), *Comprehensive clinical nephrology* (4th ed., pp. 907-918). St. Louis: Elsevier/Saunders.

Berns, J.S. (2011). ESA therapy for kidney patients: Is it ever safe? *Medscape nephrology*. Retrieved from www.medscape.com

Berns, J.S. (2013). Anemia and left ventricular hypertrophy in chronic kidney disease. *UpToDate*. Retrieved from www.uptodate.com

Bickley, L.S., & Szilagyi, P.G. (2012). *Bates' guide to physical examination and history taking* (11th ed.). Philadelphia: Lippincott Williams & Wilkins.

Bonanni, A., Mannucci, I., Verzola, D., Sofia, A., Saffioti, S., Gianetta, E., & Gaibotto, G. (2011). Protein-energy wasting and mortality in chronic kidney disease. *International Journal of Environmental of Research and Public Health, 8*(5), 1631-1654. doi:10.3390/ijerph8051631

Bonner, A., Wellard, S., & Caltabiano, M. (2010). The impact of fatigue on daily activity in people with chronic kidney disease. *Journal of Clinical Nursing, 19*(21-22), 3006-3015.

Bragazzi, N.L. (2013). c. *Health Psychology Research, 1*, e26.

Brown, S.M. (2009). *Essentials of medical genetics* (2nd ed.). Hoboken, NJ: John Wiley & Sons.

Campbell. S., Novick, A., Belldegrun, A., Blute, M., Chow, G., Derweesh, I., … Uzzo, R. (2009). Guideline for management of the clinical T1 renal mass. *The Journal of Urology*, 182, 1271-1279. doi:10.1016/j.juro.2009.07.004

Carmichael, S., Pulliam, J., & D'Orazio, J. (2013). Delayed tumor resection in a 5-year-old child with bilateral Wilms tumor. *Journal of Surgical Case Reports*, 3. doi:10.1093/jscr/rjt012

Castle, E.P. (2012). Low-phosphorus diet: Best for kidney disease? *Mayo Clinic Health.* Retrieved from www.mayoclinic.com/health/food-and-nutrition/HQ01212

Centers for Disease Control and Prevention (CDC). (2014). *National chronic kidney disease fact sheet: General information and national estimates on chronic kidney disease in the United States, 2010.* Atlanta, GA: U. S. Department of Health and Humans Services.

Chand, S., McKnight, A.J., & Borrows, R. (2014). Genetic polymorphisms and kidney transplant outcomes. *Current Opinion in Nephrology and Hypertension.* Retrieved from http://www.ncbi.nlm.nih.gov/pubmed/25188274

Chan-Smutko, G. (2012). Genetic testing by cancer site: Urinary tract. *The Cancer Journal, 18*(4), 343-349. doi:10.1097/PPO.0b013e31826246ac

Chertow, G.M., Burdick, E., Honour, M., Bonventre, J.V., & Bates, D.W. (2005). Acute kidney injury, mortality, length of stay, and costs in hospitalized patients. *Journal of American Society of Nephrology, 16*(11), 3365-3370. doi:10.1681/ASN.2004090740

Cirillo, M. (2010). Evaluation of glomerular filtration rate and of albuminuria/proteinuria. *Journal of Nephrology, 23*(2), 125-132.

Coca, S., Yalavarthy, R., Concato, J., & Parikh, C. (2008). Biomarkers for the diagnosis and risk stratification of acute kidney injury: A systemic review. *Kidney International, 73*(9) 1008-1016.

Coleman, J.A. (2008). Familial and hereditary renal cancer syndromes. *The Urologic Clinics of North America, 35*(4), 563-572.

Connolly, J., & Neild, G. (2010). Congenital anomalies of the kidney and urinary tract. In J. Floege, R. Johnson, & J. Feehally (Eds.), *Comprehensive clinical nephrology* (4th ed., pp. 609-626). St. Louis: Elsevier/Saunders.

Consensus Panel on Genetic/Genomic Nursing. (2009). *Essentials of genetic and genomic nursing: Competencies, curricula guidelines, and outcome indicators* (2nd ed) Silver Spring, MD: American Nurses Association.

Corrigan, R.M. (2001). The experience of the older adult with end-stage renal disease on hemodialysis. *Queen's University Masters Thesis.* Kingston, Ontario Canada.

Cozzi, F., Marson, P., Cardareli, S., Favaro, M., Tison, T., Tonello, M., … Doria, A. (2012). Prognosis of scleroderma renal crisis: A long-term observational study. *Nephrology Dialysis Transplantation, 27*(12), 4398-4403.

Cozzolino, M. (2013). Prevention and treatment of CKD-MBD. *Nephro-Urology Monthly, 5*(2), 773-774. doi:10.5812/humonthly.9372

Cravedi, P., & Remuzzi, G. (2013). Pathophysiology of proteinuria and its value as an outcome measure in CKD. *British Journal of Clinical Pharmacology, 76*(4), 516-523. doi:10.1111/bcp.12104

Cunningham, J., Locatelli, F., & Rodriguez, M. (2011). Secondary hyperparathyroidism: Pathogenesis, disease progression, and therapeutic options. *Clinical Journal of the American Society of Nephrology, 6*(4), 913-921. doi:10.2215/CJN.06040710

Cupples, W. (2007). Interactions contributing to kidney blood flow autoregulation. *Current Opinion in Nephrology and Hypertension, 16*(1), 39-45.

Curry, C.V. (2012). Mean corpuscular volume (MCV). *Medscape.* Retrieved from http://emedicine.medscape.com/article/2085770-overview#aw2aab6b2

Dalrymple, N., Prasad, S., El-Merhi, F., & Chintapalli, K. (2007). Price of isotropy in multidetector CT. *Radiographics, 27*(1), 49-62.

Daniels, M.S. (2012). Genetic testing by cancer site: Uterus. *The Cancer Journal, 18*(4), 338-342. doi:10.1097/PPO.1090b1013e3182610cc3182612

Daugirdas, J.T., Blake. P.G., & Ing, T.S. (2014). *Handbook of dialysis* (5th ed.). Philadelphia, PA: Lippincott Williams & Wilkins.

Devuyst, O., Knowers, N., Remuszzi, G., & Schaefer, F. (2014). Rare inherited kidney diseases: Challenges, opportunities and perspectives, *Lancet, 24*(383), 1844-1859.

Dixon, B., Hulbert, J., & Bissler, J. (2010). Tuberous sclerosis complex renal disease. *Nephron Experimental Nephrology, 118*(1), 15-20. doi:10.1159/000320891

Doogue, M.P., & Polasek, T.M. (2011). Drug dosing in renal disease. *Clinical Biochemist Review, 32*(2), 69-73.

Dugdale, D.C. (2013). Protein urine test. *MedlinePlus.* Retrieved from http://www.nlm.nih.gov/medlineplus/ency/article/003580.htm

Dyer, R., Chen, M., & Zagoria, R. (2001). Intravenous urography: Technique and interpretation. *Radiographics, 21*(4), 799-821.

Earley, A., Miskulin, D., Lamb, E.J., Levely, A.S., & Uhlig, K. (2012). Estimating equations for glomerular filtration rate in the era of creatinine standardization: A systemic review. *Annals of Internal Medicines, 156*(11), 785-795. doi:10.7326/0003-4819-156-6-201203200-00391

Eaton, D.C., & Pooler, J. (2013). *Vander's renal physiology* (8th ed.). St. Louis: McGraw-Hill.

Eitner, F. (2010). Acquired cystic kidney disease and malignant neoplasms. In J. Floege, R. Johnson, & J. Feehally (Eds.), *Comprehensive clinical nephrology* (4th ed., pp. 1010-1015). St. Louis: Elsevier/Saunders.

Ellis, J.W., Chen, M.H., Foster, M.C., Liu, C.T., Larson, M.G., de Boer, I., ... CARe Renal Consortium. (2012). Validated SNPs for eGFR and their associations with albuminuria. *Human Molecular Genetics, 21*(14), 3293-3298.

Eng, C. (2012). PTEN Hamartoma tumor syndrome (PHTS). *Gene Reviews*. Retrieved from http://www.ncbi.nlm.nih.gov/books/NBK1488/

Feig, D. (2009). Uric acid: A novel mediator and marker of risk in chronic kidney disease? *Current Opinion in Nephrology and Hypertension, 18*(6), 526-530.

Fink, H., Ishani, A., Taylor, B., Greer, N., MacDonald, R., Sadiq, S., ... Wilt, T. (2012). *Chronic kidney disease stages 1-3: Screening, monitoring and treatment comparative effectiveness*, No. 37, Agency for Healthcare Research and Quality, Report No. 11(12)-EHC0. Retrieved from http://www.ncbi.nlm.nih.gov/books/NBK84564/

Fink, H., Wilt, T., Eidman, K. Garimella, P., MacDonald, R., ... Monga, M. (2013). Medical management to prevent recurrent nephrolithiasis in adults: A systemic review for an American College of Physicians clinical guideline. *Annals of Internal Medicine, 158*, 535-543.

Finkelstein, F.O., Wuerth, D., & Finkelstein, S.H. (2010). An approach to addressing depression in patients with chronic kidney disease. *Blood Purification, 29*(2), 121-124.

Finnegan-John, J., & Thomas, V.J. (2013). The psychosocial experience of patients with end-stage renal disease and its impact on quality of life: Findings from a needs assessment to shape service. *ISRN Nephrology*. doi:10.5402/2013/308986

Floege, J. & Feehally, J. (2010). Introduction to glomerular disease: Clinical presentations. In J. Floege, R. Johnson, & J. Feehally (Eds.), *Comprehensive clinical nephrology* (4th ed., pp. 193-207). St. Louis: Elsevier/Saunders.

Food and Drug Administration (FDA). (2011). FDA drug safety communication: Modified dosing recommendations to improve the safe use of erythropoiesis-stimulating agents (ESAs) in chronic kidney disease. *FDA Drugs*. Retrieved from http://www.fda.gov

Foreman, J. (2010). Fanconi syndrome and other proximal tubule disorders. In J. Floege, R. Johnson, & J. Feehally (Eds.), *Comprehensive clinical nephrology* (4th ed., pp. 584-595). St. Louis: Elsevier/Saunders.

Frantzen, C., Links T.P., & Giles R.H. (2012). Von Hippel-Lindau disease. *Gene Reviews*. Retrieved from http://www.ncbi.nlm.nih.gov/books/NBK1463/

Friedman, D.J., Kozlitina, J., Genovese, G., Jog, P., & Pollak, M.R. (2011). Population-based risk assessment for APOL1 on renal disease. *Journal of American Society Nephrology, 22*(11), 2098-2105.

Gabree, M., & Seidel, M. (2012). Genetic testing by cancer site: Skin. *The Cancer Journal, 18*(4), 372-380 doi:10.1097/PPO.1090b1013e3182624664.

Gaff, C.L., & Bylund, C.L. (2011). *Family communication about genetics*. New York: Oxford University Press.

Garg, A., & Herts, B.R. (2012). Birt-Hogg-Dube syndrome. *The Journal of Urology, 188*(4), 1343-1344. doi:1016/j.juro.2012.06.125

Giles, T. (2009). Rethinking hypertension in the 21st century: An overview of the expanded definition and classification of hypertension. *CME Medscape,* Retrieved from http://www.medscape.org/viewarticle/708548

Gkougkousis, E., Jain, S., & Mellon, J.K. (2010). Urologic issues for the nephrologist. In J. Floege, R. Johnson, & J. Feehally (Eds.), *Comprehensive clinical nephrology* (4th ed., pp. 716-725). St. Louis: Elsevier/Saunders.

Glassock, R. (2010). Other glomerular disorders and antiphosholipid syndrome. In J. Floege, R. Johnson, & J. Feehally (Eds.), *Comprehensive clinical nephrology* (4th ed., pp. 335-343). St. Louis: Elsevier/Saunders.

Gomez, N. (Ed.). (2011). *Nephrology nursing scope and standards of practice* (7th ed.). Pitman, NJ: American Nephrology Nurses' Association.

Greco, K.E. (2003). Nursing in the genomic era: Nurturing our genetic nature. *MEDSURG Nursing, 12*(5), 307-312.

Greco, K.E., & Mahon, S.M. (2003). Genetics nursing practice enters a new era with credentialing. *Internet Journal of Advanced Nursing Practice, 5*(2).

Greco, K.E., Tinley, S., & Seibert, D. (2012). Essential genetic and genomic competencies for nurses with graduate degrees. Silver Spring, MD: American Nurses Association and the International Society of Nurses in Genetics. Retrieved from http://www.nursingworld.org/genetics

Gross, J., DeAzevedo, S., Silverado, S., Canani, L., Caramori, M., & Zelmanovitz, T. (2005). Diabetic nephropathy: Diagnosis, prevention and treatment. *Diabetes Care, 28*(1), 164-176.

Guay-Woodford, L. (2010). Other cystic disorders. In J. Floege, R. Johnson, & J. Feehally (Eds.), *Comprehensive clinical nephrology* (4th ed., pp. 543-559). St. Louis: Elsevier/Saunders.

Guglielmi, K.L. (2013). Women and ESRD: Modalities, survival, unique considerations. *Advances in Chronic Kidney Disease, 20*(5), 411-418.

Guillevin, L., Bérezné, A., Seror, R., Teixeira, L., Pourrat, J., Mahr, A., ... Mouthon, L. (2012). Scleroderma renal crisis: A retrospective multicentre study on 91 patients and 427 controls. *Rheumatology, 51*(3), 460-467.

Gunder, L.M., & Martin, S.A. (2011). *Essentials of medical genetics for health professionals*. Sudbury, MA: Jones & Bartlett Learning.

Gupta, K., Hooten, T., Naber, K., Wult, B., Colgan, R., ... Soper, D. (2011). International clinical practice guidelines for the treatment of acute uncomplicated cystitis and pyelonephritis in women: A 2010 update by the Infectious Diseases Society of America and the European Society for Microbiology and Infectious Diseases. *Clinical Infectious Diseases, 52*(5) e103-e120. doi:10.1093/cid/ciq257

Gupta, N., Seyama, K., & McCormack, F.X. (2013). Pulmonary manifestations of Birt-Hogg-Dubé syndrome. *Familial Cancer,* 1-10. doi:10.1007/s10689-013-9660-9

Hajhosseiny, R., Khavandi, K., & Gondsmith, D.J. (2013). Cardio-vascular disease in chronic kidney disease: Untying the Gordian knot. *International Journal of Clinical Practice, 67*(1), 14-31.

Hall, J. (2011). Guyton and Hall textbook of medical physiology (12th ed.). Philadelphia: Saunders.

Hall, J.E., Abdollahian, D.J., & Sinard, R.J. (2013). Thyroid disease associated with cowden syndrome: A meta-analysis. *Head & Neck, 35*(8), 1189-1194. doi:10.1002/hed.22971

Hallan, S., & Orth, S. (2010). The KDOQI 2002 classification of chronic kidney disease: For whom the bell tolls. *Nephrology Dialysis Transplantation, 25*, 2832-2836. doi:10.1093/ndt/gfq370

Happé, H., & Peters, D.J. (2014). Translational research in ADPKD: Lessons from animal models. *Nature Reviews Nephrology*. doi:10.1038/nrneph.2014.137

Harris, K., & Hughes, J. (2010). Urinary tract obstruction. In J. Floege, R. Johnson, & J. Feehally (Eds.), *Comprehensive clinical nephrology* (4th ed., pp. 702-715). St. Louis: Elsevier/Saunders.

Harwood, L., Wilson, B., & Sonrop, J. (2011). Sociodemographic differences in stressful experiences and coping amongst adults with chronic kidney disease. *Journal of Advanced Nursing, 67*(8), 1779-1789.

Harwood, L., Wilson, B., Locking-Cusolito, H., Sontrop, J., & Spittal, J. (2009). Stressors and coping in individuals with chronic kidney disease. *Nephrology Nursing Journal, 36*(3), 265-276, 301.

Haskari, V.M. (2011). Genetics and CKD. *Advances in Chronic Kidney Disease, 18*(5), 317-323.

Haque, S., Arieta, G., & Batlle, D. (2012). Proximal renal tubular acidosis: A not so rare disorder of multiple etiologies. *Nephrology Dialysis Transplantation, 27*(12), 4273-4287.

Healthy People 2020. (2013). Chronic kidney disease. Retrieved from http://www.healthypeople.gov

Hedayati, S.S., Minhajuddin, A.T., Afshar, M., Toto, R.D., Trivedi, M.H., & Rush, A.J. (2010). Association between major depressive episodes in patients with chronic kidney disease and initiation of dialysis, hospitalization, or death. *Journal of the American Medical Association, 303*(19), 1946-1953.

Hedayati, S.S., Yalamanchili, V., & Finkelstein, F.O. (2012). A practical approach to the treatment of depression in patients with chronic kidney disease and end-stage renal disease. *Kidney International, 81*, 247-255.

Herzog, C.A., Asinger, R.W., Berger, A.K., Charytan, D.M., Díez, J., Hart, R.G., … Ritz, E. (2011). Cardiovascular disease in chronic kidney disease. A clinical update from Kidney Disease: Improving Global Outcomes (KDIGO). *Kidney International, 80*(6), 572-586. doi:10.1038/ki.2011.223.

Hooten, T., Bradley, S., Cardenos, D., Colgen, R., … Nicolle, L. (2010). Diagnosis, prevention, and treatment of catheter-associated urinary tract infection in adults: 2009 international clinical practice guidelines from the Infectious Disease Society of America. *Clinical Infectious Diseases, 50*(5), 625-663. doi:10.1086/650482

Hooten, T. (2010). Urinary tract infections in adults. In J. Floege, R. Johnson, & J. Feehally (Eds.), *Comprehensive clinical nephrology* (4th ed., pp. 629-640). St. Louis: Elsevier/Saunders.

Huether, S.E., & Forshee, B.A. (2010). In K.L. McCance, S.E. Huether, V.L. Brasher, & N.S. Rote (Eds.), *Pathophysiology: The biologic basis for disease in adults and children* (6th ed.). Maryland Heights, MO: Elsevier/Mosby.

Inglese, M. (2007). Von Hippel-Lindau disease: An overview. *Nephrology Nursing Journal, 34*(4), 390-394.

Inott, T., & Kennedy, B.B. (2011). Assessing learning styles: Practical tips for patient education. *Nursing Clinics of North America, 46*(3), 313-320.

Integrated Regional Information Networks (IRIN). (2008, July 15). Sri Lanka: Rising kidney disease among farmers puzzles researchers. *IRIN: Humanitarian News and Analysis.*

Integrated Regional Information Networks (IRIN). (2012, August 12). Sri Lanka: Drought link with kidney disease risk. *IRIN: Humanitarian News and Analysis.*

Isakova, T., Xie, H., Yang, W., Xie, D., Anderson, A.H., Scialla, J., … Chronic Renal Insufficiency Cohort (CRIC) Study Group. (2011). Fibroblast growth factor 23 and risks of mortality and end-stage renal disease in patients with chronic kidney disease. *Journal of American Medical Association, 305*(23), 2432-2439.

Jadeja, Y.P., & Kher, V. (2012). Protein energy wasting in chronic kidney disease: An update with focus on nutritional interventions to improve outcomes. *Indian Journal of Endocrinology & Metabolism, 16*(2), 246-251. doi:10.4103/2230-8210.93743

James, P., Oparil, S.,Carter, B., Cushman, W., Dennison-Himmelfarb, C. Handler, C., … Ortiz, E. (2014). Evidence-based guidelines for the management of high blood pressure in adults: Report from the panel members appointed to the Eighth Joint National Committee (JNC 8). *The Journal of the American Medical Association, 311*(5), 507-520. doi:10.1001/jama.2013.284427

Jefferson, J., Thurman, J., & Schrier, R. (2010). Pathophysiology and etiology of acute kidney injury. In J. Floege, R. Johnson, & J. Feehally (Eds.), *Comprehensive clinical nephrology* (pp. 797-812). St. Louis: Elsevier/Saunders.

Joannidis, M., Metnitz, B., Bauer, P., Schusterschitz, N., Moreno, R., Druml, W., & Metnitz, P.G. (2009). Acute kidney injury in critically ill patients classified by AKIN versus RIFLE using SAPS 3 database. *Intensive Care Medicine*, 1692-1702.

John, S.G., Siqrist, M.K., Taal, M.W., & McIntyre, C. W. (2013). Natural history of skeletal muscle mass changes in chronic kidney disease stage 4 and 5 patients: An observational study. *PLoS One, 8*(5) e65372. doi:10.1371/journal.pone.0065372

Jorde, L., Care, J., Bamshad, J., & White, R. (2000). *Medical genetics.* St. Louis: Mosby.

Kaefer, M., Zurakowski, D., Bauer, S., Retik, A., Peters, C., Atala, A., & Treves, S. (1997). Estimating normal bladder capacity in children. *Journal of Urology, 158*(6), 2261-2264.

Kanwar, Y. Sun, L., Xie, P., Lui, F., & Chen, S. (2011). A glimpse of various pathogenic mechanisms of diabetic nephropathy. *The Annual Review of Pahologic Mechanisms of Disease, 6*, 395-423. doi:10.1146/annrev.pathol.4.119807.0922150

Kaplan, N.M., Bakris, G.L., & Forman, J.P. (2013, June 16). Genetic factors in the pathogenesis of primary (essential) hypertension. Retrieved from http://www.uptodate.com/contents/genetic-factors-in-the-pathogenesis-of-primary-essential-hypertension

Kauffman, C. (2010). Fungal infections of the urinary tract. In J. Floege, R. Johnson, & J. Feehally (Eds.), *Comprehensive clinical nephrology* (4th ed., pp. 649-653). St. Louis: Elsevier/Saunders.

Kee, J.L. (2013). *Laboratory and diagnostic tests with nursing implications* (9th ed.). Upper Saddle River, NJ: Prentice Hall.

Kestenbaum, B., & Drueke, T. (2010). Disorders of calcium, phosphate, and magnesium metabolism. In J. Floege, R. Johnson, & J. Feehally (Eds.), *Comprehensive clinical nephrology* (4th ed., pp. 130-147). St. Louis: Elsevier/Saunders.

Kidney Disease: Improving Global Outcomes (KDIGO). (2009). Clinical practice guideline for the diagnosis, evaluation, prevention, and treatment of chronic kidney disease-mineral and bone disorder. *Kidney International Supplement, 113*, S1-130. doi:10.1038/ki.2009.188. Retrieved from http://www.ncbi.nlm.nih.gov/pubmed/19644521

Kidney Disease: Improving Global Outcomes (KDIGO). (2012a). Acute Kidney Injury Work Group. Clinical practice guideline for acute kidney injury. *Kidney International Supplements, 2*(1), 1-138. Retrieved from http://www.kdigo.org/clinical_practice_guidelines/pdf/KDIGO%20AKI%20Guideline.pdf

Kidney Disease: Improving Global Outcomes (KDIGO). (2012b). Anemia Work Group. KDIGO clinical practice guidelines for anemia in chronic kidney disease. *Kidney International Supplements, 2*(4), 279-335. Retrieved from http://www.guideline.gov/content.aspx?id=38245

Kidney Disease: Improving Global Outcomes (KDIGO). (2012c). Blood Pressure Work Group. KDIGO clinical practice guideline for the management of blood pressure in chronic kidney disease. *Kidney International Supplements, 2*(5), 337-414. Retrieved from http://www.kdigo.org/clinical_practice_guidelines/pdf/KDIGO_BP_GL.pdf

Kidney Disease Improving Global Outcomes (KDIGO. (2013a). CKD Work Group. Clinical practice guideline for the evaluation and management of chronic kidney disease. *Kidney International*

Supplements, 3(1). Retrieved from http://www.kdigo.org/clinical _practice_guidelines/pdf/CKD/KDIGO_2012_CKD_GL.pdf

Kidney Disease: Improving Global Outcomes (KDIGO). (2013b). Lipid Work Group. Clinical practice guideline for lipid management in chronic kidney disease. *Kidney International, Suppl. 3*, 259-305.

Kline, M.J. (2013). Imaging in osteomalacia and renal osteodystrophy. *Medscape*. Retrieved from http://emedicine.medscape.com/article/392997-overview

Kopp, J., Fabian, J., & Naicker, S. (2010). Human immunodeficiency virus infection and the kidney. In J. Floege, R. Johnson, & J. Feehally (Eds.), *Comprehensive clinical nephrology* (4th ed., pp. 675-683). St. Louis: Elsevier/Saunders.

Krishnan, A.V., & Kiernan, M.C. (2009). Neurological complications of chronic kidney disease. *Nature Reviews Neurology, 5*, 542-551. doi:10.1038/nrneurol.2009.138

Kuypers, D.R. (2009). Skin problems in chronic kidney disease. *Nature Clinical Practice Nephrology, 5*, 157-170. doi:10.1038/ncpneph1040

Lawton, W., Luft, F. & DiBonna, G. (2010). Normal blood pressure control and the evaluation of hypertension. In J. Floege, R. Johnson, & J. Feehally (Eds.), *Comprehensive clinical nephrology* (4th ed., pp. 395-410). St. Louis: Elsevier/Saunders.

Lewington, A., Cerdá, J., & Mehta, R. (2013). Raising awareness of acute kidney injury. *Kidney International, 84*(3), 457-467.

Lea, D.H., Williams, J., & Donahue, M.P. (2005). Ethical issues in genetic testing. *Journal of Midwifery Women's Health, 50*(3), 234-240. http://www.medscape.com/viewarticle/505222_4

Lerma, E.V. (2013). Proteinuria. *Medscape*. Retrieved from emedicine.medscape. com/article/238158-overview

Levey, A., & Coresh, J. (2012). Chronic kidney disease. *Lancet, 379*, 165-180. doi:10.1016/50140-6736(11)60178-5

Levey, A., de Jong, P., El Nahas, M., Astor, C., Matsuhita, K., ... Eckardt, K.U. (2010). The definition, classification and prognosis of chronic kidney disease: A KGIGO Controversies Conference Report. *Kidney International, 80*(1), 17-28. doi:10.1038/ki.2010.483

Levey, A.S., & Inker, L.A. (2013). Definition and staging of chronic kidney disease in adults. *UpToDate*. Retrieved from http://www.uptodate.com

Levey, A.S., Stevens, L.A., Schmid, C.H., Zhang, Y.L., Castro, A.F., Feldman, H.I., ... CKD-EPI (Chronic Kidney Disease Epidemiology Collaboration). (2009). A new equation to estimate glomerular filtration rate. *Annals of Internal Medicines, 150*(9), 604-612.

Lexicomp. (2013). Iron dextran: Drug information. *UpToDate*. Retrieved from http://www.uptodate.com

Licurse, A., Kim, M., Dziura, J., Forman, H., Formica, R., Makarov, D., ... Gross, C. (2010). Renal ultrasonography in the evaluation of acute kidney injury: Developing a risk stratification framework. *Archives of Internal Medicine, 170*(21), 1900-1907.

Lindor, N.M., McMaster, M.L., Lindor, C.J., & Greene, M.H. (2008). Concise handbook of familial cancer susceptibility syndromes (2nd ed.). *Journal of the National Cancer Institute Monographs,* (38), 1-93. doi:10.1093/jncimonographs/lgn001

Lines, S., & Lewington, A. (2009). Acute kidney injury. *Clinical Medicine, 9*(3), 273-277.

Little, M., Georgas, K., Pennisi, D., & Wilkinson, L. (2010). Kidney development: Two tales of tubulogenesis. *Current Topics in Developmental Biology, 90*, 193-229. doi:10.1016/S0070-2153(10)90005-7

Litwin, M., & Saigal, C. (2012). Kidney stones in adults. National Kidney and Urologic Diseases Information Clearinghouse, National Institutes of Health, National Institute of Diabetes and Digestive and Kidney Diseases. Washington, D.C. Retrieved from http://kidney.niddk.nih.gov/kudiseases/pubs/stonesadults/Kidney StonesAdults_508.pdf

Ljungberg, B., Cowan, N., Hanbury, D., Hora, M.,Kuczyk, M., ... Sinescu, I. (2010). EAU guidelines on renal cell carcinoma: The 2010 update. *European Urology, 58*, 398-406. doi:10.1016/j.eururo.2010.06.032

London, G.M., Pannier, B., & Marchais, S.J. (2013).Vascular calcifications, arterial aging and arterial remodeling in ESRD. *Blood Purification, 35*, 1-3.

Luciano, R., & Perazella, M.A. (2012). NSAIDS: Acute kidney injury. *UpToDate*. Retrieved from uptodate.com

Luyckx, V., & Brenner, B. (2010). The clinical importance of nephron mass. *Journal of the American Society of Nephrology, 21*(6), 898-910.

Luttropp, K., Lindholm, B., Carrero, J.J., Glorieux, G., Schepers, E., Vanholder, R., ... Nordfors, L. (2009). Genetics/genomics in chronic kidney disease –Towards personalized medicine? *Progress in Uremic Toxin Research Seminars in Dialysis, 22*(4), 417-422. doi:10.1111/j.1525-139X.2009.00592.x

Macedo, E., & Mehta, R. (2009). Prerenal failure: From old concepts to new paradigms. *Current Opinion in Critical Care, 15*(6), 467-473.

Macedo, E.B. (2010). Prevention and nondialytic management of acute kidney injury. In J. Floege, R. Johnson, & J. Feehally (Eds.), *Comprehensive clinical nephrology* (4th ed., pp. 830-841). St. Louis: Elsevier/Saunders.

Mahon, S. (2013). Allocation of work activities in a comprehensive cancer genetics program. *Clinical Journal of Oncology Nursing, 17*(4), 397-404. doi:10.1188/13.cjon.397-404

Mahon, S.M., & Crecelius, M.E. (2013). Practice considerations in providing cancer risk assessment and genetic testing in women's health. *Journal of Obstetric, Gynecologic, & Neonatal Nursing*, n/a-n/a. doi:10.1111/1552-6909.12033

Makaroff, K.S., & Molzahn, A. (2012). Living with dying in chronic kidney disease. *University of Alberta*. Retrieved from http://www.uvic.ca/hsd/illnessnarratives/assets/docs/videos/anna _May_2012.pdf

Menko, F.H., van Steensel, M.A., Giraud, S., Friis-Hansen, L., Richard, S., Ungari, S., ... European BHD Corsortium. (2009). Birt-Hogg-Dubé syndrome: Diagnosis and management. *The Lancet Oncology, 10*(12), 1199-1206.

Methven, S., MacGregor, M., Traynor, J., O'Reilly, D., & Deighan, C. (2010). Assessing proteinuria in chronic kidney disease: Protein-creatinine ratio versus albumin-creatinine ratio. *Nephrology Dialysis Transplantation, 25*(9), 2991-2996.

Michota, F.A. (2001). *Diagnostic procedures handbook* (2nd ed.). Hudson, OH: Lexi-Comp.

Miller, P.D. (2013). Osteoporosis in patients with chronic kidney disease: Diagnosis, evaluation, and management. *UpToDate*. Retrieved from http://www.uptodate.com

Miller, W.R., & Rollnick, S. (2012). Motivational interviewing: *Helping people change* (3rd ed.). New York: Guilford Press.

Monk, R., & Bushinsky, D. (2010). Nephrolithiasis and nephrocalcinosis. In J. Floege, R. Johnson, & J. Feehally (Eds.), *Comprehensive clinical nephrology* (4th ed., pp. 687-701). St. Louis: Elsevier/Saunders.

Monsen, R.B. (2005). *Genetics nursing portfolios: A new model for credentialing*. Silver Spring, MD: American Nurses Association.

Morrison, P.J., Donnelly, D.E., Atkinson, A.B., & Maxwell, A.P. (2010). Advances in the genetics of familial renal cancer. *Oncologist, 15*(6), 532-538.

Morton, R.L., Tong, A., & Webster, A.C. (2010). The views of patients and carers in treatment decision making for chronic kidney disease: Systematic review and thematic synthesis of qualitative studies. *British Medical Journal, 340*, c112.

Moutzouris, D., Herlitz, L., Appel, G., Markowitz, G., Freudenthal, B., Radhakrishnan, J., & D'Agati, V. (2009). Renal biopsy in the very elderly. *Clinical Journal of the American Society of Nephrology, 4*(6), 1073-1082.

Muhammad, S., Noble, H., Banks, P., Carson, A., & Martin, C.R. (2012). How young people cope with chronic kidney disease: Literature review. *Journal of Renal Care, 38*(4), 182-190.

National Coalition for Health Professional Education in Genetics (NCHPEG). (2014). Interpreting the results of a genetic or genomic test. Retrieved from http://www.nchpeg.org/index.php?option=com_content&view=article&id=172&Itemid=64

National Comprehensive Cancer Network (NCCN). (2013). Genetic/familial high risk assessment: Breast and ovarian, version 1.2013. Retrieved from most current guideline available at http://www.nccn.org

National Institute of Diabetes and Digestive and Kidney Diseases (NIDDK). (2012a). The A1C test and diabetes. *National Diabetes Information Clearinghouse (NDIC).* Retrieved from http://diabetes.niddk.nih.gov/dm/pubs/A1CTest/

National Institute of Diabetes and Digestive and Kidney Diseases (NIDDK). (2012b). Diabetic neuropathies: The nerve damage of diabetes. *National Diabetes Information Clearinghouse (NDIC).* Retrieved from http://diabetes.niddk.nih.gov/dm/pubs/neuropathies/index.aspx

National Institute of Diabetes and Digestive and Kidney Diseases (NIDDK). (2013). Prevent diabetes problems: Keep your eyes healthy. *National Diabetes Information Clearinghouse (NDIC).* Retrieved from http://diabetes.niddk.nih.gov/dm/pubs/complications_eyes/index.aspx

National Institutes of Health (NIH). (2011). Balkan endemic nephropathy. *Genetic and Rare Diseases Information Center (GARD).* Retrieved from http://rarediseases.info.nih.gov/gard/8576/disease/resources/1

National Kidney Disease Education Program (NKDEP). (2010). Phosphorus: Tips for people with chronic kidney disease (CKD). Retrieved from http://nkdep.nih.gov/resources/nutrition-phosphorus.shtml

National Kidney Disease Education Program (NKDEP). (2012). At risk for kidney disease? *National Kidney Disease Education Program.* Retrieved from http://nkdep.nih.gov/learn/are-you-at-risk.shtml

National Kidney Foundation (NKF). (2009). Coping effectively: A guide to living well with kidney failure. Retrieved from http://www.kidney.org/sites/default/files/docs/coping.pdf

National Kidney Foundation (NKF). (2013a). Calculators for health professionals. Retrieved from http://www.kidney.org/professionals/KDOQI/gfr_calculator

National Kidney Foundation (NKF) (2013b). Chronic kidney disease – A growing problem. Retrieved from http://www.kidney.org/news/newsroom/factsheets/CKD-A-Growing-Problem.cfm

National Kidney and Urologic Diseases Information Clearinhouse (NKUDIC). (2010). Proteinuria. Retrieved from http://kidney.niddk.nih.gov/kudiseases/pubs/proteinuria/

Niell, B., Vartanians, V., & Halpern, E. (2013). Improving education for the management of contrast reactions: An online didactic model. *Journal of the American College of Radiology, 30*(13), S1546-1440.

Noori, N., Sims, J.J., Kopple, J.D., Shah, A., Colman, S., Shinaberger, C.S., … Kalantar-Zadeh, K. (2010). Organic and inorganic dietary phosphorus and its management in chronic kidney disease. *Iran Journal of Kidney Disease, 4*(2), 89-100.

Novak, M., Costantini, L., Schneider, S., & Beanlands, H. (2013). Approaches to self-management in chronic illness. *Seminars in Dialysis, 26*(2), 188-194.

Okusa, M., & Rosner, M. (2013). *Overview of the management of acute kidney injury (acute renal failure).* UpToDate. Retrieved from http://www.uptodate.com

O'Neill, W., Bardelli, M. & Yevzlin, A. (2011). Imaging for renovascular disease. *Seminars in Nephrology, 31*(3), 272-282.

Oncology Nursing Society. (2009). Cancer predisposition genetic testing and risk assessment counseling [Position statement]. Retrieved from http://www.ons.org/Publications/Positions/Predisposition

Organ Procurement and Transplant Network (OPTN). (2014). Health resources and service administration. *Transplant information database.* Retrieved from http://optn.transplant.hrsa.gov/data/

Palmer, B., & Alpern, R. (2010). Metabolic acidosis. In J. Floege, R. Johnson, & J. Feehally (Eds.), *Comprehensive clinical nephrology* (4th ed., pp. 155-166). St. Louis: Elsevier/Saunders.

Palmer, B.F., & Henrich, W.L. (2013). Thyroid function in chronic kidney disease. *UpToDate.* Retrieved from http://www.uptodate.com

Paparo, L., Rossi, G., Delrio, P., Rega, D., Duraturo, F., Liccardo, R., … De Rosa, M. (2013). Differential expression of PTEN gene correlates with phenotypic heterogeneity in three cases of patients showing clinical manifestations of PTEN hamartoma tumour syndrome. *Hereditary Cancer in Clinical Practice, 11*(1), 8.

Peralta, C.A., Katz, R., Sarnak, M.J., Ix, J., Fried, L.F., De Boer, I., … Schlipak, M.G. (2010). Cystantin C identifies chronic kidney disease patients at higher risk for complications. *Journal of the American Society of Nephrology, 22*(1), 147-155.

Perazella, M., & Coca, S. (2012). Traditional urinary biomarkers in the assessment of hospital acquired AKI. *Clinical Journal of the American Society of Nephrology, 7*(1), 167-174.

Pichler, R., Hugo, C., & Johnson, R. (2010). Geriatric nephrology. In J. Floege, R. Johnson, & J. Feehally (Eds.), *Comprehensive Clinical Nephrology* (4th ed., pp. 785-794). St. Louis: Elsevier/Saunders.

Pilarski, R., & Nagy, R.. (2012). Genetic testing by cancer site: Endocrine system. *The Cancer Journal, 18*(4), 364-371. doi:10.1097/PPO.1090b1013e3182609458

Pipitone, N., Vaglio, A., & Salvari, C. (2012). Retroperitoneal fibrosis. *Best Practice & Research Clinical Rheumatology, 26*(4), 439-449.

Pollak, M., Genovese, G., & Friedman, D. (2012). APOL1 and kidney disease. *Current Opinion in Nephrology & Hypertension, 21*(2), 179-182.

Pope, J. (2007). The diagnosis and treatment of Raynaud's phenomenon: A practical approach. *Drugs, 67*(4), 517-525.

Post, T., & Burton, R. (2013, July). *Diagnostic approach to the patient with acute kidney injury (acute renal failure) or chronic kidney disease.* UpToDate. Retrieved from http://www.uptodate.com

Prakash, J., Brojen Singh, T., Ghosh, B., Malhotra, V, Rathore, A., Vohra, R., … Usha, P. (2013). Changing epidemiology of community-acquired acute kidney injury in developing countries: Analysis of 2405 cases in 26 years from eastern India. *Clinical Kidney Journal, 6*(2), 150-155.

Prescott, L., Eidemak, I., Harrison, A.P., & Molsted, S. (2013). Sexual dysfunction is more than twice as frequent in Danish female predialysis patients compared to age- and gender-matched healthy controls. *International Urology and Nephrology, 46*(5), 979-984. doi:10.1007/s11255-013-0566-0

Prochaska, J.O., Norcross, J.C., & DiClemente, C.C. (2007). *Changing for good: A revolutionary six-stage program for overcoming bad habits and moving your life positively forward.* New York: William Morrow/HarperCollins.

Quarles, L.D. (2013). Treatment for hyperphosphatemia in chronic kidney disease. *UpToDate.* Retrieved from http://www.uptodate.com

Rabinovitch, A. (2001). *Urinalysis and collection, transportation, and preservation of urine specimens: Approved guideline* (2nd ed.). Wayne, PA: National Committee for Clinical Laboratory Standards.

Raff, H. (2002). *Physiology secrets* (2nd ed.). Philadelphia: Belfus & Hanley.

Ramirez-Rubio, O., Brooks, D.R., Amador, J.J., Kaufman, J.S., Weiner, D.E., & Scammell, M.K. (2013). Chronic kidney disease in Nicaragua: A qualitative analysis of semi-structured interviews with physicians and pharmacists. *BMC Public Health, 13*, 350. doi:10.1186/1471-2458-13-350

Rayner, B., Charlton, K., Lambert, E., & Derman, W. (2010). Nonpharmacologic prevention and treatment of hypertension. In J. Floege, R. Johnson, & J. Feehally (Eds.), *Comprehensive clinical nephrology* (4th ed., pp. 421-429). St. Louis: Elsevier/Saunders.

Reidy, K., & Rosenblum, N. (2009). Cell and molecular biology of kidney development. *Seminars in Nephrology, 29*(4), 321-337.

Revell, M., Pugh, M., Smith, & Mclnnis, L. (2010). Radiologic studies in the critical care environment. *Critical Care Nursing Clinics of North America, 22*(1), 41-50.

Riche, D.M. (2012). ATP IV: Predicting guideline updates. UMC. Retrieved from http://www.umc.edu/uploadedFiles/UMCedu/Content/Education/Academic_Affairs/Continuing_Health_Professional_Education/Fam%20Med%20Riche.pdf

Riley, B., Culver, J., Skrzynia, C., Senter, L., Peters, J., Costalas, J., … Trepanier, A. (2012). Essential Elements of genetic cancer risk assessment, counseling, and testing: Updated recommendations of the National Society of Genetic Counselors. *Journal of Genetic Counseling, 21*(2), 151-161. doi:10.1007/s10897-011-9462-x

Ritz, E., & Wolf, G. (2010). Pathogenesis, clinical manifestations and natural history of diabetic nephropathy. In J. Floege, R. Johnson, & J. Feehally (Eds.), *Comprehensive clinical nephrology* (4th ed., pp. 359-376). St. Louis: Elsevier/Saunders.

Rodriguez-Iturbe, B., Burdmann, E., & Barsoum, R. (2010). Glomerular diseases associated with infection. In J. Floege, R. Johnson, & J. Feehally (Eds.), *Comprehensive clinical nephrology* (4th ed., pp. 662-674). St. Louis: Elsevier/Saunders.

Ronco, P., Aucouturier, P., & Moulin, B. (2010). Renal amyloidosis and glomerular diseases with monoclonal immunoglobulin deposition. In J. Floege, R. Johnson, & J. Feehally (Eds.), *Comprehensive clinical nephrology* (4th ed., pp. 322-334). St. Louis: Elsevier/Saunders.

Rossert, J., & Fischer, E. (2010). Acute interstitial nephritis. In J. Floege, R. Johnson, & J. Feehally (Eds.), *Comprehensive clinical nephrology* (4th ed., pp. 729-737). St. Louis: Elsevier/Saunders.

Roumelioti, M.E., Wentz, A., Schneider, M.F., Gerson, A.C., Hooper, S., Benfield, M., … Unruh, M.L. (2010). Sleep and fatigue symptoms in children and adolescents with CKD: A cross-sectional analysis from the chronic kidney disease in children (CKiD) study. *American Journal of Kidney Diseases, 55*(2), 269-280.

Runyon, B. (2013, February). Hepatorenal syndrome. *UpToDate*. Retrieved from www.uptodate.com

Rydahl, C., Thomsen, H., & Marckmann, P. (2008). High prevalence of nephrgenic systemic fibrosis in chronic renal failure patients exposed to gadodiamide, a gadolinium-containing magnetic resonance contrast agent. *Investigative Radiology, 43*(2), 141-144.

Sakhaee, K., & Maalouf, N. (2008). Metabolic syndrome and uric acid nephrolithiasis. *Seminars in Nephrology, 28*(2), 174-180.

Sarafides, P., & Bakris, G. (2010). Evaluation and treatment of hypertensive urgencies and emergencies. In J. Floege, R. Johnson, & J. Feehally (Eds.), *Comprehensive clinical nephrology* (4th ed., pp. 445-450). St. Louis: Elsevier/Saunders.

Schiller, J.S., Lucas, J.W., & Peregoy, J.A. (2012). Summary health statistics for U.S. adults: A national health interview survey, 2011. *National Center for Health Statistics. Vital Health Stat, 10*(256) Retrieved from http://www.cdc.gov/nchs/data/series/sr_10/sr10_256.pdf

Schira, M. (2008). Pathophysiology. In C. Counts (Ed.), *Core curriculum for nephrology nurses* (5th ed., pp. 33-62). Pitman, NJ: American Nephrology Nurses' Association.

Schonder, K. (2006). Pharmacology of renal disease. In Molzahn, A., & Butera, E. (Eds.), *Contemporary nephrology nursing: Principles and practice* (2nd ed., pp 395-415). Pitman, NJ: American Nephrology Nurses' Association.

Schrier, R., Coffman, T., Falk, R., Molitoris, B., & Neilson, E. (2012). *Schrier's diseases of the kidney* (9th ed.). Philadelphia: Lippincottt Williams & Wilkins.

Schrier, S.L., & Auerbach, M. (2013). Treatment of iron deficiency anemia. *UpToDate*. Retrieved from www.uptodate.com

Schwartz, G., Brion, L., & Spitzer, A. (1987). The use of plasma creatinine concentration for estimating glomerular filtration rate in infants, children, and adolescents. *Pediatric Clinics of North America, 34*(3), 571-590.

Seidel, H.M., Ball, J.W., Dains, J.E., Flynn, J.A., Solomon, B.S., & Stewart, R.W. (2011). *Mosby's guide to physical examination* (7th ed.). St. Louis: Mosby.

Seller-Pérez, G., Herrera-Gutiérrez, M.E., Maynar-Moliner, J., Sánchez-Izquierdo-Riera, J.A., Marinho, A., & Luis do Pico, J. (2013). Estimating kidney function in the critically ill patients. *Critical Care Research and Practice. 2013*(ID 721810). doi:10.1155/2013/721810

Shanahan, C.M., Crouthamel, M.H., Kapustin, A., & Giachelli, C.M. (2011). Arterial calcification in chronic kidney disease: Key roles for calcium and phosphate. *Circulation Research, 109*(6), 697-711.

Shehata, B.M., Stockwell, C.A., Castellano-Sanchez, A.A., Setzer, S., Schmotzer, C.L., & Robinson, H.. (2008). von Hippel-Lindau (VHL) Disease: An update on the clinico-pathologic and genetic aspects. *Advances in Anatomic Pathology, 15*(3), 165-171. doi: 10.1097/PAP.0b013e31816f852e

Slickers, J., Olshan, A., Siega-Riz, A., Honein, M., Aylsworth, A. (2008). Maternal body mass index and lifestyle exposures and the risk of bilateral renal agenesis or hypoplasia: The National Birth Defects Prevention Study. *American Journal of Epidemiology, 168*(11), 1259-1267.

Soderland, P., Lovekar, S., Weiner, D.E., Brooks, D.R., & Kaufman, J.S. (2010). Chronic kidney disease associated with environmental toxin and exposures. *Advances in Chronic Kidney Disease, 17*(3), 254-264. doi:10.1053/j.ackd2010.03.011

Solomon, R., & Dauerman, H.L. (2010). Clinician update: Contrast induced acute kidney injury. *Circulation, 122*, 2451-2455. doi:10.1161/CIRCULATIONAHA.110.953851

Song, R., & Yosypiv, I. (2011). Genetics of congenital anomalies of the kidney and urinary tract. *Pediatric Nephrology, 26*(3), 353-364. doi:10.1007/s00467-010-1629-4

Stamatakis, L., Metwalli, A.R., Middelton, L.A., & Marston Linehan, W. (2013). Diagnosis and management of BHD-associated kidney cancer. *Familial Cancer, 1-6.* doi:10.1007/s10689-013-9657-4

Steggall, M., & Omara, M. (2008). Urinary tract stones: Types, nursing care and treatment options. *British Journal of Nursing, 17*(9), S20-S30.

Stevens, L., Shastri, S., & Levey, A. (2010). Assessment of renal function. In J. Floege, R. Johnson, & J. Feehally (Eds.), *Comprehensive clinical nephrology* (4th ed., pp. 31-38). St. Louis: Elsevier/Saunders.

Strippoli, G.F.M., & Collaborative Depression and Sexual Dysfunction (CDS) in Hemodialysis Working Group. (2012). Sexual dysfunction in woman with ERD requiring hemodialysis. *Clinical Journal of the American Society of Nephrology, 7*(6), 974-981.

Susantitaphong P., Cruz, D.N., Cerda, J., Abulfaraj, M., Alqahtani, F., Koulouridis, I., Jaber, B.L., & the Acute Kidney Injury Advisory Group of the American Society of Nephrology. (2013). World incidence of AKI: A meta-analysis. *Cinical Journal of the American Society of Nephrology, 8*(9), 1482-1493. doi: 10.2215/CJN.00710113

Swartz, R. (2009). Idiopathic retroperitoneal fibrosis: A review of the pathogenesis and approaches to treatment. *American Journal of Kidney Diseases, 54*(3), 546-553. doi:10.1053/j.ajkd.2009.04.019

Taal, M., Chertow, G., Marsden, P., Skorecki, K., Yu, A., & Brenner, B. (2012). *Brenner and Rector's the kidney* (9th ed.). Philadelphia: Elsevier Saunders.

Teplick, A., Kowalski, M., Biegel, J., & Nichols, K. (2011). Screening in cancer predisposition syndromes: Guidelines for the general pediatrician. *European Journal of Pediatrics, 170*(3), 285-294. doi:10.1007/s00431-010-1377-2

Textor, S., & Greco, B. (2010). Renovascular hypertension and ischemic renal disease. In J. Floege, R. Johnson, & J. Feehally (Eds.), *Comprehensive clinical nephrology* (4th ed., pp. 451-468). St. Louis: Elsevier/Saunders.

Theofilou, P.A. (2011). Sexual functioning in chronic kidney disease: The association with depression and anxiety. *Hemodialysis International, 16*(1), 76-81.

Theofilou, P. (2012). The relationship between religion/spirituality and mental health in patients on maintenance dialysis. *Journal of Woman's Health Care,* S2:001 doi:10.4172/2167-0420.S2-001

Thomas, P., Panackal, C., John, M., Joshi, H., Mathai, S., Kattickaran, J., & Igbal, M. (2013). Gastrointestinal complications in patients with chronic kidney disease – A 5-year retrospective study from a tertiary referral center. *Renal Failure, 35*(1), 49-55. doi:10.3109/0886022X.2012.731998

Tonelli, M., Muntner, P., Lloyd, A., Manns, B.J., Klarenbach, S., Pannu, N., … Hemmelgarn, B.R. (2012, June 19). Risk of coronary events in people with chronic kidney disease compared with those with diabetes: A population-level cohort study. *Lancet, 380.* doi:10.1016/S0140-6736(12)60572-8

Tönshoff, B. (2013). Pathogenesis, evaluation and diagnosis of growth impairment in children with chronic kidney disease. *UpToDate.* Retrieved from http://www.uptodate.com

Tong, A., Henning, P., Wong, G., McTaggart, S., Mackie, F., Carroll, R.P., & Craig, J.C. (2013). Experiences and perspectives of adolescents and young adults with advanced CKD. *American Journal of Kidney Diseases, 61*(3), 375-384.

Tong, A., Sainsbury, P., Chadban, S., Walker, R.G., Harris, D. C., Carter, S.M., … Craig, J.C. (2009). Patients' experiences and perspectives of living with CKD. *American Journal of Kidney Diseases, 53*(4), 689-700.

Toro, J.R. (2008). Birt-Hogg-Dubé syndrome. *Gene Reviews.* Retrieved from http://www.ncbi.nlm.nih.gov/books/NBK1522/

Torres, V., & Harris, P. (2010). Autosomal dominant polycystic kidney disease. In J. Floege, R. Johnson, & J. Feehally (Eds.), *Comprehensive clinical nephrology* (4th ed., pp. 529-542). St. Louis: Elsevier/Saunders.

Torres, V., & Harris, P. (2009). Autosomal dominant polycystic kidney disease: The last 3 years. *Kidney International, 76*(2), 149-168. doi:10.1038/ki2009.128

Triplitt, C. (2012). Understanding the kidneys' role in blood glucose regulation. *American Journal of Managed Care, 18*(Suppl. 1), S11-16.

Udani, S., Lazich, J., & Bakris, G. (2011). Epidemiology of hypertensive kidney disease. *Nature Reviews, 7,* 11-21 doi:10.1038/nrneph.2010.154

United States Renal Data System (USRDS). (2014). *Costs of chronic kidney disease.* Retrieved from http://www.usrds.org/2012/view/v1_07.aspx

Valette, X., & du Cheyron, D. (2013). A critical appraisal of the accuracy of the RIFLE and AKIN classifications in defining "acute kidney insufficiency" in critically ill patients. *Journal of Critical Care, 28*(2), 116-125.

Vallerand, A.H., Sanoski, C.A., & Deglin, H.H. (2013). Atorvastatin. *Davis's drug guide* (13th ed.). Philadelphia: F.A. Davis.

VanPutte, C., Regan, J., Seeley, R., Stephens, T., Tate, P., & Russo, A. (2013). Seeley's anatomy and physiology (10th ed.). Philadelphia: Science Engineering & Math/McGraw-Hill.

Varga, J. (2013). *Overview of the clinical manifestations of systemic sclerosis (scleroderma) in adults.* From uptodate.com: http://www.uptodate.com

Varga, J., & Fenves, A. (2013, October). *Scleroderma renal crisis. UpToDate.* Retrieved from http://www.uptodate.com

Vecchio, M., Navaneethan, S.D., Johnson, D.W., Lucisano, G., Graziano, G., Saglimbene, V., … Strippoli, G.F. (2010). Interventions for treating sexual dysfunction in patients with chronic kidney disease. *The Cochrane Library.*

Visweswaran, R.K., & Bhat, S. (2010). Tuberculosis of the kidney. In J. Floege, R. Johnson, & J. Feehally (Eds.), *Comprehensive clinical nephrology* (4th ed., pp. 641-648). St. Louis: Elsevier/Saunders.

Wasser, W., Tzur, S., Wolday, D., Adu, D., Baumstein, D., Rosset, S., … Skorecki, K. (2012). Population genetics of chronic kidney disease: The evolving story of APOL1. *Journal of Nephrology, 25*(5), 603-618.

Weitzel, J.N., Blazer, K.R., MacDonald, D.J., Culver, J.O., & Offit, K. (2011). Genetics, genomics, and cancer risk assessment. *CA: A Cancer Journal for Clinicians, 61*(5), 327-359. doi:10.3322/caac.20128

Whelan, A. J., Ball, S., Best, L., Best, R.G., Echiverri, S.C., Ganshow, P., … Stallworth, J. (2004). Genetic red flags: Clues to thinking genetically in primary care practice. *Primary Care, 31*(3), 497-508.

Wilding, A., Ingham, S.L., Lalloo, F., Clancy, T., Huson, S.M., Moran, A., & Evans, D.G. (2012). Life expectancy in hereditary cancer predisposing diseases: An observational study. *Journal of Medical Genetics, 49*(4), 264-269. doi:10.1136/jmedgenet-2011-100562

Williams, B. (2010). Pharmacologic treatment of hypertension. In J. Floege, R. Johnson, & J. Feehally (Eds.), *Comprehensive clinical nephrology* (4th ed., pp. 430-444). St. Louis: Elsevier/Saunders.

Woodward, C. (2009). United States government grows a family health tree, helping people trace hand-me-down genetic risks. *CMAJ Canadian Medical Association Journal, 180*(7), 707. doi:10.1503/cmaj.090368

Wyatt, C., & Klotman, P. (2013, November). Overview of kidney disease in HIV-positive patients. *UpToDate.* Retrieved from http://www.uptodate.com

Xiong, X., Liu, J., He, W., Xia, T., He, P., Chen, X., … Want, A. (2007). Dose-effect relationship between drinking water and fluoride levels and damage to liver and kidney function in children. *Environmental Research, 103*(1), 112-116.

Yang, L., & Bonventre, V. (2010). Diagnosis and clinical evaluation of acute kidney injury. In J. Floege, R. Johnson, & J. Feehally (Eds.), *Comprehensive clinical nephrology* (4th ed., pp. 821-829). St. Louis: Elsevier/Saunders.

Young, R.A., Von Korff, M., Heckbert, S.R., Ludman, E.J., Rutter, C., Lin, E.H.B., … Katon, W.J. (2010). Association of major depression and mortality in Stage 5 diabetic chronic kidney disease. *General Hospital Psychiatry, 32*(2), 119-124.

Zappitelli, M. (2008). Epidemiology and diagnosis of acute kidney injury. *Seminars in Nephrology, 28*(5), 436-446.

Exercise of Understanding
Label the internal structures of the kidney.

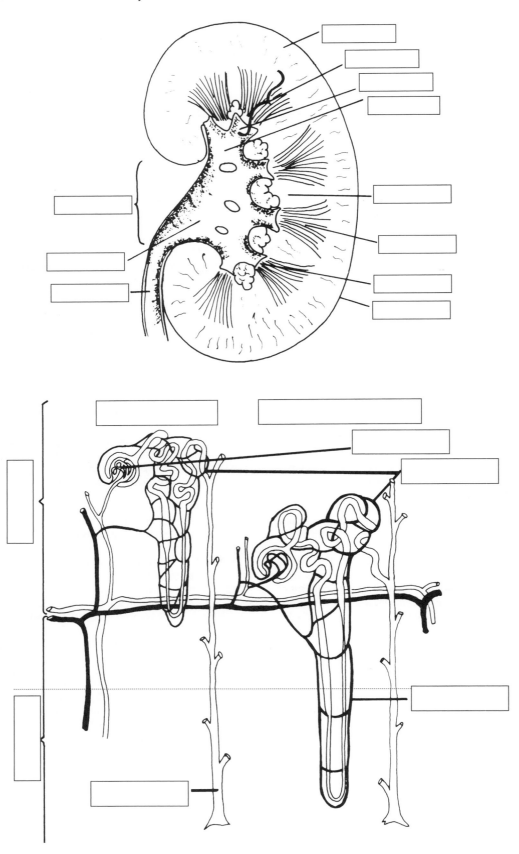

CHAPTER **2**
Chronic Kidney Disease

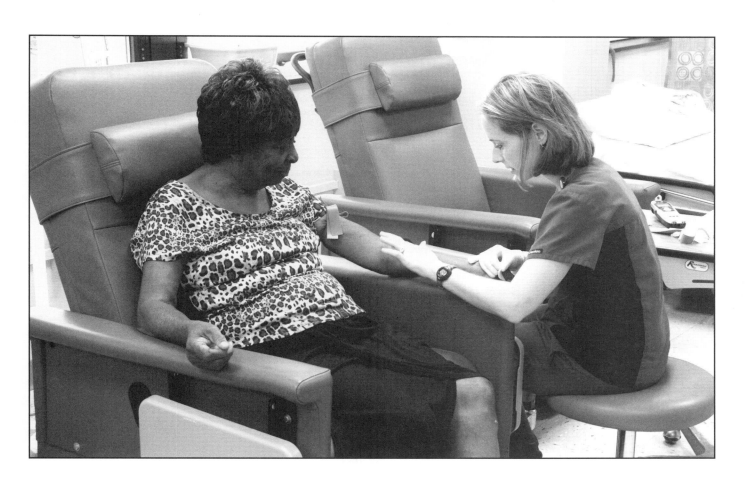

Chapter Editor
Debra J. Hain, PhD, ARNP, ANP-BC, GNP-BC, FAANP

Authors
Debra J. Hain, PhD, ARNP, ANP-BC, GNP-BC, FAANP
Mary S. Haras, PhD, MS, MBA, APN, NP-C, CNN

CHAPTER **2**

Chronic Kidney Disease

This offering for **1.7 contact hours with 1.0 contact hour of pharmacology content** is provided by the American Nephrology Nurses' Association (ANNA).

American Nephrology Nurses' Association is accredited as a provider of continuing nursing education by the American Nurses Credentialing Center Commission on Accreditation.

ANNA is a provider approved by the California Board of Registered Nursing, provider number CEP 00910.

This CNE offering meets the continuing nursing education requirements for certification and recertification by the Nephrology Nursing Certification Commission (NNCC).

To be awarded contact hours for this activity, read this chapter in its entirety. Then complete the CNE evaluation found at **www.annanurse.org/corecne** and submit it; or print it, complete it, and mail it in. Contact hours are not awarded until the evaluation for the activity is complete.

Example of reference for Chapter 2 in APA format. Two authors for entire chapter.

Hain, D.J., & Haras, M.S. (2015). Chronic kidney disease. In C.S. Counts (Ed.), *Core curriculum for nephrology nursing: Module 2. Physiologic and psychosocial basis for nephrology nursing practice* (6th ed., pp. 153-188). Pitman, NJ: American Nephrology Nurses' Association.

Interpreted: Chapter authors. (Date). Title of chapter. In ...

Cover photo by Counts/Morganello.

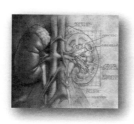

CHAPTER 2

Chronic Kidney Disease

Purpose

Chronic kidney disease (CKD) is a global health issue affecting about 8% to 16% of the world's population and is associated with poor health outcomes. These include increased all-cause mortality and cardiovascular mortality, progression of kidney disease to CKD stage 5 (formerly known as ESRD), cognitive impairment, anemia, mineral and bone disorders, increased risk for fractures, and acute kidney injury. Diabetes mellitus and hypertension are the most common causes of CKD in the United States. Early identification and intervention are essential to reduce mortality and morbidity and to slow the progression of CKD (Eckardt et al., 2013; Jha et al., 2013).

Nephrology nurses play a vital role as members of interprofessional teams focusing on health promotion, disease prevention, slowing the progression of CKD, and reducing cardiovascular mortality. This chapter will provide the best available evidence at the time of publication to support interventions aimed at improving health outcomes of patients with CKD.

Objectives

Upon completion of this section, the learner will be able to:
1. State the definition and classification of CKD.
2. Discuss epidemiology of CKD in the United States.
3. Identify screening measures for CKD.
4. Describe the interventions focused on reducing mortality, morbidity, and improving health outcomes in patients with CKD.
5. Summarize strategies for management of complications and comorbidities associated with CKD.
6. Discuss educational strategies for individuals with CKD.

SECTION A
Introduction to Chronic Kidney Disease

I. Definition and classification of chronic kidney disease.

A. Chronic kidney disease (CKD) has been defined as "either kidney damage or GFR < 60 mL/min/1.73 m² for ≥ 3 months. Kidney damage is defined as pathologic abnormalities or markers of damage, including abnormalities in blood or urine tests or imaging" (National Kidney Foundation [NKF], 2002a).

B. Kidney disease has been classified in 5 stages based on level of kidney function, progressing from stage 1 to stage 5 according to the Kidney Disease Outcomes Quality Improvement (KDOQI) CKD classifications (NKF, 2002a) (see Table 2.1).

Table 2.1

Stages of CKD

Stage	Description	GFR (mL/min/1.73 m²)
1	≥ 90	Kidney damage with normal or increased GFR
2	60–89	Kidney damage with mild decrease in GFR
3	30–59	Moderate decrease in GFR
4	15–29	Severe decrease in GFR
5	<15 (or dialysis)	Kidney failure

Adapted from National Kidney Foundation, Inc. (NKF). (2002). *KDOQI clinical practice guidelines for chronic kidney disease: Evaluation, classification, and stratification. Part 4. Definition and classification of stages of chronic kidney disease.* Used with permission.

C. Emerging evidence supports the need for a more global approach to definition and classification of CKD. In 2012, Kidney Disease Improving Global Outcomes (KDIGO) Clinical Practice Guideline for the Evaluation and Management of CKD provided updated definition, classification, and stratification from an international perspective.

D. CKD is now defined as "abnormalities of kidney structure or function, present for > 3 months, with implications for health and CKD is classified based on cause, GFR category, and albuminuria category (CGA)." The KDIGO classification is similar to the KDOQI classification, but expands the stage 3 category to differentiate mild to moderate and moderate to severe decrease in GFR (see Table 2.2).

II. Global epidemic of CKD.

A. There are global risk factors contributing to the development of CKD. Deaths in the United States and worldwide related to the risk factors of hypertension (13%), elevated blood glucose (6%), physical inactivity (6%), and obesity (5%) have been identified (World Health Organization [WHO], 2012).

B. In the United States, the leading causes of CKD are diabetes and hypertension. In developing countries, 43% of persons with CKD did not have diabetes or hypertension, suggesting that glomerulopathies are a major contributor (Couser et al., 2011).

III. Epidemiology of CKD in the United States.

A. Incidence.
1. Incidence is defined as the "rate of occurrence of new cases of a CKD in the population being studied" (Centers for Disease Control [CDC], 2011).
2. Although CKD affects all racial and ethnic groups, there is a higher incidence in African Americans (3.6 times higher) and Asians (1.4 times higher) as compared with European Whites; and Hispanics (1.5 times higher) compared to non-Hispanics (Stevens et al., 2011).
3. Age-adjusted and sex-adjusted incidence of kidney failure in the black race was 2.6 times higher than in non-Blacks (Derose et al., 2009).

B. Prevalence. Defined as "the number of CKD cases existing in a given population at a given period of time" (CDC, 2011).
1. According to the United States Renal Data System (USRDS, 2013), the prevalence of CKD has increased from 12.3% to 14% in the period 1988–1994 to 2005–2010. From 1999 to 2010, 15%

Table 2.2

GFR Categories in CKD

GFR category	GFR (ml/min/1.73m²)	Terms
G1	≥ 90	Normal or high
G2	60–89	Mildly decreased *
G3a	45–59	Mildly to moderately decreased
G3b	30–44	Moderately to severely decreased
G4	15–29	Severely decreased
G5	< 15	Kidney failure

Abbreviations: CKD – chronic kidney disease; GFR – glomerular filtration rate
*Relative to young adult level
In absence of evidence of kidney damage, neither GFR category G1 nor G2 fulfill the criteria for CKD.

Source: Kidney Disease: Improving Global Outcomes (KDIGO) CKD Work Group. KDIGO 2012 Clinical Practice Guideline for the Evaluation and Management of Chronic Kidney Disease. *Kidney International Supplements 2013*; 3: 1–150 (originally table 5 on page 27). Used with permission.

to 16% of adults over the age of 20 had evidence of CKD stages 1 to 4 (CDC, 2011).
2. Estimated point prevalence of all nonkidney failure Medicare population was 2.72 million in 2011 (USRDS, 2013). In the Medicare population for those over the age of 65, the prevalence of CKD was 10% (USRDS, 2013).

C. Risk factors.
1. Older age, diabetes, hypertension, cardiovascular disease, hyperlipidemia, obesity, and a family history of CKD have been associated with CKD (CDC, 2010; USRDS, 2013). Low socioeconomic status has been linked to increased risk for CKD (Couser et al., 2011).
2. In children.
   a. Genetic conditions, congenital anomalies of the kidney and urinary tract, and glomerulo-nephritis can lead to CKD (Kennedy et al., 2012) and contribute to approximately 67% of CKD in developed countries (Harambat et al., 2012).
   b. Rare causes of CKD in children include adenine phosphoribosyltransferase (APRT) deficiency, cystinuria, Dent disease, familial hypomagnesemia with hypercalciuria and nephrocalcinosis (FHHNC), and primary hyperoxaluria (PH) (Edvardsson et al., 2013).

D. Predicting prognosis.
1. Several variables should be considered when attempting to predict prognosis (KDIGO, 2013a).

a. Cause of CKD.
b. GFR category.
c. Albuminuria category.
d. Other risk factors and comorbid conditions.

2. Predicting the prognosis can aid in decision making regarding the best treatment for individuals (see Table 2.3).

3. The Kidney Failure Risk Equation (Tangri et al., 2011) can be used to predict the probability of treated kidney failure (dialysis or transplantation) for patients with CKD stage 3 to 5. Determining the probability of kidney failure may be helpful as providers engage in shared decision making with patients about nephrology referrals, timing of dialysis access placement, and living related kidney transplant. It is available at http://www.qxmd.com/calculate-online/nephrology/kidney-failure-risk-equation

IV. Screening.

A. Who should be screened? Anyone at high risk for developing CKD should be screened for kidney disease.

1. Individuals with diabetes, hypertension, and cardiovascular disease or those with metabolic syndrome or persons with a family history of these diseases should be screened.

a. Metabolic syndrome is a constellation of metabolic factors that increase a person's risk for cardiovascular disease. Metabolic syndrome is present when an individual has three or more of the following:
   (1) Abdominal waist circumference (men ≥ 40 inches and women ≥ 35 inches).
   (2) Triglycerides ≥ 150 mg/dL.
   (3) HDL < 40 mg/dL in men and 50 mg/dL in women.
   (4) Systolic BP ≥ 130 mmHg and diastolic ≥ 85 mmHg.
   (5) Fasting glucose ≥ 100 mg/dL (www.heart.org).

b. The U.S. Preventive Services Task Force (USPSTF, 2012) identified that approximately 11% of adults in the United States have CKD, and that those with the above conditions should be screened.

Table 2.3 **Prognosis of CKD by GFR and Albuminuria Categories: KDIGO 2012**				**Persistent albuminuria categories** **Description and range**		
				A1	A2	A3
				Normal to mildly increased	Moderately increased	Severely increased
				< 30 mg/g < 3 mg/mmol	30–300 mg/g 3–30 mg/mmol	> 300 mg/g > 30 mg/mmol
GFR categories (mL/min/1.73m²) Description and range	G1	Normal or high	≥ 90			
	G2	Mildly decreased	60–89			
	G3a	Mildly to moderately decreased	45–59			
	G3b	Moderately to severely decreased	30–44			
	G4	Severely decreased	15–29			
	G5	Kidney failure	< 15			

Dark gray, low risk (if no other markers of kidney disease, no CKD); Light blue, moderately increased risk; Light gray, high risk; Dark blue, very high risk.

Abbreviations: CKD – chronic kidney disease; GFR – glomerular filtration rate; KDIGO – Kidney Disease: Improving Global Outcomes.

Source: Kidney Disease: Improving Global Outcomes (KDIGO) CKD Work Group. KDIGO 2012 Clinical Practice Guideline for the Evaluation and Management of Chronic Kidney Disease. *Kidney International Supplements 2013*; 3: 1–150 (originally figure 9 on page 34). Used with permission.

c. The USRDS (2013) identified that "having both diabetes and hypertension greatly increases the odds of developing CKD" (p. 56). Individuals with diabetes, hypertension, or cardiovascular disease are two to four times more likely to develop CKD than persons without those conditions (USRDS, 2013).

2. Ethnic groups of African Americans, Asians, and Hispanics, as well as those from lower socioeconomic groups. In a study by Cho and colleagues (2013), healthy Koreans with metabolic syndrome were 1.5 times more likely to develop CKD than those without metabolic syndrome.

3. Children. The American Academy of Pediatrics (1993) recommends urine screening at infancy, early childhood, late childhood, and adolescence.

4. Asymptomatic adults.
   a. The USPSTF (2012) does not recommend routine screening for CKD in asymptomatic adults without diagnosed CKD.
      (1) Testing and monitoring for CKD for the purpose of chronic disease management (including monitoring patients with diabetes or hypertension) is not covered by this recommendation.
      (2) Although there is lack of evidence regarding routine screening in primary care settings, screening for urine protein (microalbuminuria or macroalbuminuria) and obtaining serum creatinine to estimate eGFR are feasible, especially for those at risk.
      (3) The American Diabetes Association recommends screening all individuals with diabetes.
      (4) The NIH Joint National Committee on Prevention, Detection, Evaluation and Treatment of High Blood Pressure recommends screening individuals with hypertension.
      (5) Considering these recommendations, the USPSTF suggests there is minimal to no harm in screening people at risk (i.e., older adults and people with diabetes and hypertension).
   b. The American College of Physicians (ACP) (2013) also recommends against screening in asymptomatic adults without risk factors.
   c. Since 2000, the National Kidney Foundation's Kidney Early Evaluation Program (KEEP) has been performing community screenings for at-risk population 18 years and older. Several publications describing KEEP have shown the benefits of early identification and referral. Information about KEEP can be found at http://www.kidney.org

B. Evaluation.
   1. Laboratory studies can assist with diagnosis.
      a. Urine protein for microalbuminuria or macroalbuminuria and urine creatinine can help detect early signs of kidney damage.
      b. Urinary loss of albumin and protein. Commonly referred to as albumin excretion rate (AER) and protein excretion rate (PER). Urinary AER ≥ 30 mg/24 hours sustained for 3 months or greater indicates CKD. This value is considered approximately equivalent to an albumin-to-creatinine ratio (ACR) in a random untimed urine sample of ≥ 30 mg/grams or ≥ 3 mg/mmol (KDIGO, 2013a, p. 22).
         (1) This should be correlated with other clinical findings when diagnosing CKD (KDIGO, 2013a).
         (2) Evidence indicates that there is a high prevalence of older adults with decreased eGFR who may also have an increased ACR that does not represent CKD but rather normal aging (see Module 5, Chapter 2) (see Table 2.4).
      c. Urine sediment or urine dipstick should be examined for the presence of red blood cells, white blood cells, and casts in persons at increased risk for developing CKD (NFK, 2002b).
      d. Serum creatinine can be used to estimate GFR. "Criteria for CKD include markers of kidney damage (albuminuria, as indicated by an albumin excretion rate of 30 mg/24 hours or greater and an albumin-creatinine ratio of 3 mg/mmol or greater [≥ 30 mg/g]); urine

Table 2.4

Albuminuria Categories in CKD

Category	AER (mg/24 hr)	ACR (mg/mmol)	ACR (mg/g)	Terms
A1	< 30	< 3	< 30	Normal to mildly increased
A2	30–300	3–30	30–300	Moderately increased *
A3	30–300	> 30	> 300	Severely increased **

Abbreviations: AER – albumin excretion rate; ACR – albumin-to-creatinine ratio.
 * Relative to young adult.
** Including nephrotic syndrome (usually > 2200/24 hours [ACR 42220 mg/g; 4220 mg/mmol]).

Source: Kidney Disease: Improving Global Outcomes (KDIGO) CKD Work Group. KDIGO 2012 Clinical Practice Guideline for the Evaluation and Management of Chronic Kidney Disease. *Kidney International Supplements* 2013; 3: 1–150 (from page 5). Used with permission.

sediment abnormalities; electrolyte and other abnormalities due to tubular disorders" (ACP, 2013).

2. Imaging studies. The decision to have a patient undergo imaging studies must be weighed against the risks. Recommendations do not endorse screening individuals who are not at risk for CKD (NFK, 2002b).

a. Ultrasound provides a general appearance of the kidney, the size of the kidneys, and whether there is increased echogenicity.
   (1) Renal ultrasound mass screening for congenital anomalies in infants was not supported in a large, longitudinal study in Italy (Caiulo et al., 2012).
   (2) An ultrasound can detect hydronephrosis from urinary obstruction or ureteral reflux. It may also detect the presence of cysts suggestive of polycystic kidney disease.

b. Intravenous pyelography (IVP) may be useful to identify renal asymmetry or abnormalities within the kidney, such as stones, tumors, or scars.

c. Computed tomography (CT) scan is the gold standard for detecting kidney stones, but may also reveal renal artery stenosis in addition to obstruction or tumors.
   (1) Precautions. Consider those at risk for contrast-induced acute kidney injury (CIAKI), which has been linked to increased risk of mortality and morbidity (Weisbord et al., 2008). It is important to implement strategies to reduce the risk of AKI (see Module 4).
   (2) Individuals at risk.
       (a) Patients with CKD, particularly those with CKD and DM.
       (b) Older adults (≥ 65 years).
       (c) People with metabolic syndrome, prediabetes, hyperuricemia, hypertriglyceridemia, and impaired fasting glucose who undergo coronary intervention may be at risk (Laville & Juillard, 2010).

d. Magnetic resonance imaging (MRI) is beneficial to detect renal vein thrombosis, lesions, cysts, etc. When MR angiography with gadolinium is used, it may help diagnose kidney disease.
   (1) Precautions with MRI with gadolinium.
       (a) For patients with impaired kidney function, administration of gadolinium-chelate based contrast agents (GBCA) has been associated with development of nephrogenic systemic fibrosis (NSF).
       (b) NSF was first recognized in 2006 as a skin disorder and later as a devastating systematic disorder.
       (2) Factors increasing the risk of NSF.
           (a) Exposure and underlying kidney disease.
           (b) Infection, inflammation, vascular disease, hypercoagulability, hypercalcemia, erythropoiesis-stimulating agents (ESAs), and iron therapy (Perazella & Shirali, 2014).
       (3) Prevention is the best approach.
           (a) Identify high risk patients; other options should be considered, such as non-GBCA if possible.
           (b) If GBCA has to be used, the lowest dose should be given. If a macrocyclic GBCA is used:
               i. ESA and iron are restricted immediately before and after the exam.
               ii. Kidney recovery from AKI should occur prior to GBCA.
               iii. Performing hemodialysis within hours of GBCA exposure is recommended if the person has ESRD (Perazella & Shirali, 2014).

e. Nuclear scans are beneficial to determine kidney size and function, problems with renal blood vessels, acute pyelonephritis, or scar tissue.

SECTION B

CKD Disease Management

I. Goals of therapies.

A. The goals of therapies are aimed at delaying the progression of CKD, reducing cardiovascular risks, treating uremic complications, and preparing patients for kidney replacement therapy.

B. An essential aspect of managing CKD is treating the specific cause of CKD, as well as other reversible conditions that may contribute to the progression of CKD or increase the risk for cardiovascular disease (CVD) (Stevens et al., 2009).
   1. All individuals with CKD should be considered at risk for cardiovascular disease; strategies to reduce this risk should be a key aspect in the plan of care.
   2. Nontraditional cardiovascular risk factors.
      a. Anemia.
      b. Hyperhomocysteinemia.
      c. Abnormal calcium and phosphorus metabolism.
      d. Oxidative injury.
      e. Inflammation (Schiffrin et al., 2007).

C. Role of inflammation.
1. Low-grade inflammation has been observed in patients with kidney failure and has been identified as a significant contributor to increased risk for cardiovascular mortality and morbidity (Stenvinkel et al., 2008).
2. In a population of adults with CKD stage 3 and 4, as compared to people with normal kidney function, there was evidence of low-grade inflammation that was associated with endothelial dysfunction and atherosclerosis. Although the endothelial dysfunction was less severe than those with kidney failure, cardiovascular damage begins before the person starts dialysis (Recio-Mayoral et al., 2011).

D. The plan of care should consider specific health conditions relative to the stage of CKD and take an interprofessional approach focusing on the array of factors known to be associated with progression of CKD and increased cardiovascular risk factors (KDIGO, 2013a).

E. Regardless of the stage of CKD, lifestyle interventions should be instituted for all patients with CKD as a way to reduce cardiovascular risk factors, including:
1. Smoking cessation.
2. Dietary sodium reduction.
3. Weight management.
4. Physical activities (Gansevoort et al., 2013).

II. Slow the progression of CKD.

A. Reduce proteinuria.
1. Definition of proteinuria. Proteinuria is a general term for the presence of protein in the urine and can be a reflection of abnormal loss of plasma proteins due to:
   a. Increased glomerular permeability to large molecular weight proteins (albuminuria or glomerular proteinuria).
   b. Incomplete tubular reabsorption of normally filtered low-molecular weight proteins (tubular proteinuria).
   c. Increased plasma concentration of low-molecular weight proteins (overproduction proteinuria, such as immunoglobulin light chains) (KDIGO, 2013a, p. 21).
2. Proteinuria can be the result of tubular damage as well as from the lower urinary tract.
   a. Evidence indicates that proteinuria has a pathogenesis role in the progression of CKD (Muntner et al., 2005).
   b. Proteinuria is associated with increased risk for all-cause mortality and cardiovascular

mortality in patients with CKD (Agrawal et al., 2009).
3. Clinical terminology generally refers to albuminuria (albumin is one type of plasma protein) instead of proteinuria.
   a. Albumin is the principal component of urinary protein in most kidney diseases (KDIGO, 2013a).
   b. Studies have shown that decreasing eGFR and increased albuminuria are strongly correlated with cardiovascular disease (Gansevoort et al., 2013).
4. Approaches to reducing proteinuria/albuminuria.
   a. An angiotensin receptor blocker (ARB) or ACE inhibitor (ACE-I) should be considered for adults with diabetes and CKD who have urine albumin excretion between 30 and 300 mg in 24 hours (KDIGO, 2013a).
   b. Individuals with CKD and urine excretion > 300 mg in 24 hours should be treated with an ARB or ACE-I regardless of diabetes status (present or not) (KDIGO, 2013a).
   c. In patients with diabetic kidney disease, treatment with an ACE-I titrated to normalization of albumin excretion should be considered when elevated ACR is confirmed with two different specimens on 2 different days.
      (1) This should be obtained over a 6-month interval following efforts to improve glycemic control and get BP to target (None et al., 2014).
      (2) Patients with diabetic kidney disease should have routine monitoring of urine albumin excretion to assess response to therapy and progression of disease (None et al., 2014).
      (3) There is a lack of sufficient evidence to support combining ARB or ACE-I to prevent progression of CKD (KDIGO, 2013a); however, some providers will prescribe off-label use of the combination as they attempt to achieve the best clinical outcomes possible.

B. Protein intake.
1. Too much protein intake can lead to accumulation of uremic toxins while not enough protein in the diet can result in loss of lean body mass and malnutrition.
2. Controversy exists regarding protein restriction as a way to slow the progression of CKD. Restricting protein can reduce uremic toxins that are linked to suppression of appetite and incite muscle wasting, which can lead to higher mortality and morbidity risks (KDIGO, 2013a).
3. When making a decision regarding protein restriction, nephrology professionals should

individualize their approach to care by considering residual kidney function and age of the person. Older adults are at risk for nutritional deficits, and restricting protein in a pediatric population may be detrimental to their growth (KDIGO, 2013a).

4. KDIGO Clinical Practice Guideline (2012a) recommendations.
   a. In adults with CKD who are at risk for progression.
      (1) Lowering protein intake to 0.8 g/kg/day in adults, with or without diabetes, and GFR < 30 mL/min/1.73 m².
      (2) Avoid high protein intake (> 1.3 g/kg/day).
   b. For patients with diabetic kidney disease, reducing the amount of dietary protein below usual intake is not recommended. Evidence has not shown that this intervention:
      (1) Alters glycemic control.
      (2) Reduces CVD risks.
      (3) Alters the course of GFR decline (None et al., 2014).

5. Consultation with a renal dietitian can be extremely helpful to determine the best protein sources, to educate the patient, and to monitor nutritional status (see Module 2, Chapter 6).
   a. Medicare beneficiaries are eligible for Medical Nutritional Therapy (MNT) (http://www.medicare.gov/coverage/nutrition-therapy-services.html), which is described later in the chapter.
   b. Diabetes Self-Management Training (DSMT) is another available service for individuals with diabetes. Information regarding this benefit can be found at http://www.diabeteseducator.org/

C. Glycemic control.
   1. The National Kidney Foundation (NKF) KDOQI Clinical Practice Guideline for Diabetes and CKD (2012) recommends a target hemoglobin A1C (Hgb A1c) of ~7.0% to prevent or delay the progression of the microvascular complications of diabetes, including diabetic kidney disease.
      a. It is not recommended to treat to an A1C < 7.0% for those at risk for hypoglycemia.
         (1) Consider A1C > 7.0% in patients with comorbidities or limited life expectancy and risk of hypoglycemia.
         (2) A1C > 8% may be appropriate for some individuals (None et al., 2014).
      b. In patients with CKD and diabetes, an interprofessional approach to glycemic control should be taken. It is important to address BP control and implement strategies aimed at reducing CVD risks and promoting the use of ACE-I or ARB, and statins when clinically indicated.
   2. Research has shown the importance of good glycemic control, especially the longer a p has diabetes (None et al., 2014).
   3. An A1C should be drawn at least twice a year in individuals who are meeting treatment goals, and quarterly in those with treatment changes and or not meeting goals (None et al., 2014).
   4. Lowering the A1C below or around 7% has been shown to reduce microvascular complications associated with diabetes.
   5. More stringent A1C < 7% (< 6.5) for selected individuals is recommended if done without significant hypoglycemia or other adverse events (None et al., 2014).

D. Blood pressure control.
   1. Hypertension (HTN) is a leading cause of cardiovascular mortality and morbidity (i.e., kidney disease, heart disease, and stroke).
   2. Patients with a history of hypertension are at risk for CKD (Inker & Levey, 2014).
      a. Hypertension is one of the most common causes for CKD.
      b. HTN can be a consequence of CKD (Mahmoodi et al., 2012).
   3. If the BP ≥ 115/75, there is an increased risk for cardiovascular mortality for every increase in 20 mmHg systolic blood pressure (SBP) and 10 mmHg diastolic blood pressure (DBP) (Chobanian et al., 2003).
   4. Measuring BP correctly is essential for appropriate classification, which can help determine the best treatment strategies. It is important to use the proper technique for taking the blood pressure. Katakam et al. (2008) propose these guidelines.
      a. Have person relax for at least 5 minutes before taking the blood pressure.
      b. The person's arm should be supported for the measurement.
      c. The stethoscope bell should be used (not the diaphragm).
      d. Blood pressure should be checked in both arms; the arm with the higher reading should be used for other readings (lying, standing).
      e. All measurements should be separated by at least 2 minutes.
      f. Measure the blood pressure in the sitting, standing, and lying positions if possible.
      g. Use the correct cuff size and note if a larger or smaller than normal cuff size is used.
   5. Cuff size, recommended by the American Heart Association (Pickering et al., 2005).
      a. Arm circumference of 27 to 34 cm; cuff should be "adult" size or 16 x 30 cm.
      b. Arm circumference of 35 to 44 cm; cuff should be "large adult" size or 16 x 36 cm.
      c. Arm circumference of 45 to 52 cm; cuff should be an "adult thigh" size or 16 x 42 cm.

6. Decisions to treat are based on repeated measurements.
   a. Readings can vary from day to day, and due to physiologic and environmental changes can vary at different times of the day. Multiple BP readings during the day may provide beneficial information that can guide treatment, with the goal of reducing end-organ damage. Evidence supports that home blood pressure monitoring (HBPM), if done correctly, can provide a more accurate picture of BP than office blood pressure monitoring (OBPM) (Sanghavi & Vassalotti, 2014).
      (1) Advantages of OBPM: commonly used in RCTs and reimbursed with office visit.
      (2) Disadvantages of OBPM: can be highly variable, observer bias may be present, and can be inaccurate due to white coat hypertension.
      (3) Advantages of HBPM: can be a stronger predictor of hypertensive end-organ damage, can improve adherence to BP medication when combined with other supportive interventions, can detect white coat hypertension, and is low cost.
      (4) Disadvantages of HBPM: requires training and device calibration, may be out-of-pocket expense, unreliable in atrial fibrillation, and can exacerbate anxiety disorder and obsessive-compulsive behavior (Sanghavi, p. 116).
   b. KDIGO guidelines emphasize this by using the term "consistently" when recommending BP goal (i.e., maintain BP that is consistently ≤ 140 mmHg) (KDIGO, 2012a, p. 344).
7. The Seventh Report of the Joint National Commission of Prevention, Detection, Evaluation, and Treatment of High Blood Pressure (JNC 7) classifies BP (see Table 2.5) and provides an evidence-based approach to prevention and management of hypertension (Chobanian et al., 2003). JNC-8 was recently published and will be discussed later in the chapter.
8. To slow the progression of CKD and reduce cardiovascular risks.
   a. It is critical to achieve optimal control of blood pressure, while assessing for symptoms such as postural dizziness.
   b. Individuals with diabetes and older adults have risks for autonomic neuropathy, placing them at risk for orthostatic hypotension (KDIGO, 2012a; Stokes, 2009).

Table 2.5

Blood Pressure Classification

BP Classification	Systolic BP (mm/Hg)	Diastolic BP (mm/Hg)
Normal	< 120	< 80
Prehypertension	120–139	80–89
Stage 1 hypertension	140–159	90–99
Stage 2 hypertension	≥ 160	≥ 100

Adapted from *The Seventh Report of the Joint National Committee on Prevention, Detection, Evaluation, and Treatment of High Blood Pressure*, page 11, NIH, National Heart, Lung, and Blood Institute, NIH Publication No. 04-5230, August 2004.

III. Decrease mortality and morbidity risk.

A. Cardiovascular disease is the leading cause of death in patients with CKD. The risk increases as the GFR declines and when microalbuminuria is present (Weiner & Sarnak, 2014).
   1. These patients have a higher mortality risk after an acute myocardial infarction (MI) with an increased risk for another MI, heart failure, and sudden cardiac death.
   2. A strong association exists between CKD with a lower eGFR and acute coronary syndrome, stroke, heart failure, and sudden cardiac death.
   3. Individuals with an eGFR below 15 mL/min/1.73 m^2 have the highest risk for CVD (KDIGO, 2013a).

B. Anemia has been linked with CVD and CKD.
   1. However, correction of hemoglobin to higher target levels can lead to worse cardiovascular outcomes (Eckardt et al., 2009).
   2. Two landmark studies, the Cardiovascular Risk Reduction by Early Anemia Treatment with Epoetin Beta (CREATE) and the Correction of Hemoglobin and Outcomes in Renal Insufficiency (CHOIR), led to the FDA's black box warning (covered later in the chapter) regarding higher risk for death and serious cardiovascular events when administering erythropoietin-stimulating agents (ESA) to target Hgb levels of 13.5 to 14.5 g/dL.

C. Left ventricular hypertrophy (LVH) commonly occurs as CKD progresses.
   1. LVH reflects target organ damage.
   2. LVH is associated with CVD (Shlipak et al., 2005).

D. It is essential that healthcare professionals implement interventions that address modifiable cardiovascular risk factors, control blood pressure and diabetes, and slow the progression of CKD (KDIGO, 2013a) as discussed in this chapter.

IV. Reduce the risk of hospitalization and improve health outcomes.

A. Care coordination.
1. Care coordination can be defined as "a function that helps ensure that the patient's needs and preferences are met over time with respect to health services and information sharing across people, functions, and sites and the deliberate organization of patient care activities between two or more participants (including the patient) involved in patient's care to facilitate the appropriate delivery of healthcare services … the best coordination model is one in which a patient experiences care that is patient centered, high quality, and cost-effective" (Camicia et al., 2013, pp. 491-492).
2. The best model is one that takes an integrated, interprofessional team approach to care and includes at least one care coordinator (often a nurse) (ANA, 2012).
   a. Although there are many models of care coordination involving registered nurses (RNs) and advanced practice registered nurses (APRNs), few have focused on nephrology practice.
   b. Barrett and colleagues (2011) conducted a randomized clinical trial exploring the impact of a nurse-coordinated model of care in patients with CKD stages 3 and 4.
      (1) Participants (40 to 74 years old) who had an eGFR between 25 and 60 mL/min/1.73 m^2 were randomized to one of two groups.
      (2) One group received usual care; the other group received usual care plus nurse-coordinated care that was focused on reducing CVD risk factors.
      (3) The nurse followed medical protocols in collaboration with a nephrologist.
      (4) The main outcome of the intervention was achievement of quality of life as measured by:
         (a) KDQOL-SF (Hays et al., 1997).
         (b) WHOQOL-BREF (Harper & Power, 1998).
         (c) The HUI Mark2 (Furlong et al., 2001).
         (d) Client Satisfaction Questionnaire 8 (Attkisson & Greenfield, 2004) measured satisfaction in care.
         (e) Decreased resource utilization.
         (f) Evaluation of clinical outcome measures such as CVD, mortality, amputation, and dialysis.
      (5) The results identified that many of th participants had nonprogressive kidney disease but continued to have high cardiovascular risks. and the intervention did not significantly affect rate of eGFR decline.
      (6) Limitations to this study.
         (a) Participant referral was obtained from a community laboratory and not from a nephrologist, and the participants were more likely to have nonprogressive kidney disease.
         (b) Recruitment bias may have been present.
      (7) Despite study limitations, the findings provide a foundation for future research.
3. There is a need for further research on care coordination in this complex population. In the current healthcare environment, effective care coordination models are essential as healthcare professionals, including nephrology nurses, strive to achieve optimal clinical outcomes, such as reducing potentially avoidable hospitalization.
   a. An important focus of care coordination is reducing potentially unnecessary hospitalizations.
      (1) There is a global effort aimed at achieving this goal.
      (2) Care coordination is an essential aspect of many initiatives.
   b. As nephrology nurses engage in care coordination activities, it is essential to consider the goals of the Triple Aim (Berwick et al., 2008).
      (1) Improve health of populations.
      (2) Improve quality of care and patient satisfaction.
      (3) Reduce healthcare costs.
4. A nurse practitioner (Hain) represented ANNA as a member of the American Nurses Association Congress on Nursing Practice and Economics health policy workgroup who developed a White Paper and Position Statement on the role of nurses in care coordination (ANA, 2012). These documents can serve as resources for nephrology nurses as they engage in care coordination (available to ANA members on the website http://www.nursingworld.org).

B. Collaborative practice with primary care providers.
1. Primary care providers and nephrology healthcare professionals should comanage patients with CKD by engaging collaborative practice through care coordination efforts (Stevens et al., 2009).
   a. Early screening and treatment may slow the progression of CKD and reduce CVD risks (Murphree & Thelen, 2010).

b. Collaboration between nephrology and primary care providers may also lead to appropriate and timely referrals.

2. Late referral to nephrology has been linked to less than optimal health outcomes. Some of the reasons for late referral include (Wauters et al., 2005):
   a. Disease-related issues (e.g., irreversible acute kidney injury or superimposed on CKD).
   b. Patient-related issues can occur when the patient either does not understand the potentially progressive nature of CKD or there are psychological factors (e.g., depression, denial) that impact the individual's willingness to follow recommendations for nephrology referral.
   c. Physician-related problems can either be associated to nephrology or primary care providers.
      (1) Primary care providers (PCPs) may feel they can take care of patients' health problems without consulting nephrology, and they may fear losing clinical responsibility if they refer to nephrology. In addition, there is evidence that PCPs do not feel they have received adequate training as to when to refer to nephrology.
      (2) Nephrology providers may not have the time necessary to educate the patient and family about CKD, and communication with the PCP may be limited or not occur at all. APRNs practicing in nephrology are uniquely positioned to lead initiatives related to interprofessional collaboration across healthcare settings.

3. There is controversy regarding when to refer to nephrology. Referral based on eGFR may lead to inappropriately labeling individuals with CKD, especially older adults with eGFR 45 to 59 mL/min/1.73 m² (see Module 5, Chapter 2).

4. Considering CVD risks associated with CKD, collaboration between primary care and nephrology providers may help reduce these risks and improve outcomes (Hemmelgarn et al., 2010).

5. The benefits of early identification and nephrology referral include:
   a. Provision of specific treatment based on diagnosis.
   b. Slowing/arresting CKD progression.
   c. Evaluation and management of CKD and comorbid conditions and/or complications (e.g., anemia, malnutrition, bone disease, acidosis).
   d. Planning and preparing for kidney replacement therapy.
   e. Psychological support.
   f. Provision of palliative care when appropriate (KDIGO, 2013).

6. Referral may be necessary (KDIGO, 2013a) when a patient exhibits:
   a. AKI or abrupt sustained fall in GFR.
   b. GFR < 30 mL/min/1.73m2 (GFR categories G4-G5).
   c. Consistent albuminuria (ACR ≥ 300 mg/g or AER ≥300 mg/24 hours).
   d. Progression of CKD (25% decline in eGFR from baseline; rapid progression sustains decline eGFR if more than 5 mL/min/1.73m²).
   e. Urinary red cell casts, RBC > 20 per high-power field sustained and not readily explained.
   f. CKD and hypertension refractory to treatment with four or more antihypertensive agents.
   g. Persistent abnormalities of serum potassium.
   h. Recurrent or extensive nephrolithiasis.
   i. Hereditary kidney disease.

C. Referral to other healthcare professionals.
   1. Nephrology nurses have historically collaborated with other healthcare professionals. When and who to refer patients with CKD is a decision that should be shared between healthcare professionals and patients and their family members.
   2. Social workers may address psychosocial issues and mental health problems that individuals with CKD can face.
   3. Dietitians are excellent resources for nutritional counseling and Medical Nutritional Therapy (MNT) (presented later in the chapter). Consideration should be given for a consultation with a dietitian to help patients with CKD engage in a healthy weight-loss program when appropriate.
   4. Older adults with risk of falls (Hain, 2012) or other physical problems may benefit from consultation with a physical therapist and/or occupational therapist (see Module 5, Chapter 2).
   5. Individuals often experience challenges coping with advancing disease and may benefit from support groups. Therefore, it is important to consider recommending that the person join a local support group. However, not all people want to be part of a support group, so it is essential to take a person-centered approach and determine the individual's preferences. In situations when patients refuse to attend a support group, counseling may be beneficial.

D. Reduce the risk of acute kidney injury (AKI).
   1. Evidence supports that there is a link between AKI and CKD.
      a. Areef and colleagues (2009) conducted a study to determine the incidence rates and hazard ratios for developing AKI in older adults.
      b. The researchers concluded that older adults

with preexisting CKD are at significant risk for AKI and that the occurrence of AKI may accelerate progression of CKD.
2. Assessment and treatment of AKI are beyond the scope of this chapter. It is important that nephrology nurses educate patients with CKD about the risk factors of AKI and discuss preventive strategies to reduce the risk. AKI is discussed in Chapter 1 of this module and in Module 4.

V. Management of complications associated with various stages of CKD.

A. Anemia is a decreased concentration of hemoglobin (Hgb) that leads to reduced oxygen-carrying capacity in the blood. Anemia is a common complication of CKD. The risk of anemia increases with decline in kidney function and is frequently seen in stages 3 to 5.
1. In people with stable kidney function, evaluation for other causes of anemia should be considered before assuming that anemia is related to CKD (KDIGO, 2012b). About 15% to 20% of individuals in CKD stages 1 to 3 and up to 70% in patients with kidney failure have anemia (McFarlane et al., 2008).
2. Causes of anemia related to CKD (Wish, 2014).
   a. Erythropoietin deficiency is the primary cause of anemia in CKD; declining GFR can result in erythropoietin deficiency (kidneys produce about 90% of erythropoietin).
   b. Iron deficiency.
   c. Acute and chronic inflammation.
   d. Severe hyperparathyroidism (occurs in later stages of CKD).
   e. Aluminum toxicity.
   f. Folate deficiency.
   g. Shortened RBC lifespan (from 120 days in people without CKD to 60 to 90 days in individuals with CKD).
   h. Loss of RBCs if undergoing hemodialysis due to inability to return all of the red blood cells.
3. Evaluation.
   a. The frequency of evaluation is based on KDIGO guidelines (2012c) for patients with CKD who are not receiving dialysis.
      (1) For adults with CKD and no anemia, measure the Hgb level:
         (a) When clinically indicated.
         (b) At least annually for adults with CKD stage 3.
         (c) At least twice per year for adults with CKD stages 4 to 5.
      (2) For adults with anemia and CKD stages 3 to 5 and not being treated with an erythropoiesis-stimulating agent (ESA), measure Hgb level at least every 3 months.

   b. Clinical manifestations (usually begin when the Hgb $\leq$ 10 g/dL).
      (1) Fatigue.
      (2) Cognitive deficits/difficulty with concentration.
      (3) Decrease overall feelings of well-being.
      (4) Loss of libido.
      (5) Cardiovascular complications.
         (a) May be asymptomatic and insidious.
         (b) Can increase CVD mortality and morbidity risks.
         (c) Those with CAD may experience increased episodes of angina.
         (d) Left ventricular hypertrophy (LVH).
            i. Linked to poor health outcomes, such as hospitalization and mortality in patients with CKD.
            ii. Decrease in Hgb of 0.5 g/dL below normal correlates with 32% increase for risk of LVH.
4. Diagnosis of anemia based on KDIGO guidelines (2012c) for patients with CKD who are not receiving dialysis. Initial evaluation should include the following tests.
   a. Complete blood count, which includes Hgb, red blood cell indices, white blood cell count and differential, and platelet count.
      (1) Hgb < 13.0 g/dL in males and 12.0 g/dL in women (WHO, 1968).
         (a) These criteria were based upon data from a population with individuals younger than 65 years of age; the criteria may or may not be applicable to the older adult (Beutler & Waalen, 2006; Mindell et al., 2013).
         (b) This definition may not be appropriate for some racial and ethnic groups, particularly African Americans (Beutler & West, 2005). There is a need for further research exploring how anemia is defined in these populations.
      (2) Normochromic (normal size red blood cells as indicated by normal mean corpuscular volume [MCV], normochromic (normal RBC, color as indicated by normal mean corpuscular Hgb concentration [MCHC]).
         (a) Low MCV suggests iron deficiency but can also be seen in thalassemia.
         (b) High MCV may indicate vitamin B12 or folate deficiency.
   b. Absolute reticulocyte count.
   c. Serum vitamin B12 and folate level.
   d. Depending on the clinical presentation stool for occult blood.
   e. Erythropoietin levels are not routinely used to

identify erythropoietin deficiency from other causes.

f. Iron stores.

(1) Serum ferritin level (≤ 30 μg/L indicate deficiency). Ferritin levels > 30 μg/L do not necessarily indicate adequate iron stores; ferritin is an acute phase reactant that increases in the setting of acute or chronic inflammation independent of iron stores.

(2) Serum transferrin saturation (TSAT).

(3) Iron deficiency.

(a) Absolute or functional iron deficiency is indicated when TSAT < 16% in person with CKD anemia. Absolute iron deficiency equates with decreased total body iron stores.

(b) Functional iron deficiency.

i. Pharmacologic stimulation of RBC production when using an ESA.

ii. Hepcidin, a peptide produced by the liver, interferes with RBC production by decreasing availability of iron in the setting of inflammation and infection (Wish, 2014).

5. Treating anemia based on KDIGO guidelines (2012c) for patients with CKD who are not undergoing dialysis. Erythropoiesis-stimulating agents (ESA) are used to treat anemia to reduce the need for packed red blood cell transfusion (PRBC).

a. Recombinant human erythropoietin (rHuEPO), first introduced in the 1980s, was a major breakthrough for treating anemia related to CKD. ESAs are recombinant human erythropoietin and bind to the erythropoietin receptor. There are three ESAs in use at this time.

(1) Epoetin alfa.

(2) Epoetin beta.

(3) Darbepoetin.

b. Evidence has emerged regarding the benefits of treating anemia with an ESA in this population; however, other clinical trials led to the 2011 FDA black box warning regarding the risk of death, myocardial infarction, stroke, venous thrombosis, thrombosis of vascular access, and tumor progression and recurrence.

c. Information and recommendations from the FDA.

(1) The risk of stroke or cardiovascular events is greater when administering an ESA to target Hgb ≥ 11 g/dL.

(2) The lowest dose that will maintain Hgb levels sufficient to reduce the need for PRBC transfusion should be used.

(3) The risks and benefits of ESA therapy should be weighed.

(4) The dose should not be increased more frequently than once every 4 weeks; decreases can occur more frequently, but frequent dose adjustments should be avoided as much as possible.

(5) If Hgb rises rapidly (i.e., > 1g/dL in any 2-week period) the dose should be reduced by 25% or more as needed.

(6) For those who do not respond adequately to a specific dose (Hgb increase < 1 g/dL in 4 weeks of therapy), it should be increased by 25%. Increasing the dose more than once a month is not recommended.

(7) For those who do not respond adequately over a 12-week escalation period, further increase to the ESA dose is unlikely to improve the response and may actually increase the risks for adverse events.

(8) Evaluate other causes of anemia. Discontinuation of the ESA should be considered if responsiveness does not improve (hyporesponsiveness is discussed later in the chapter).

d. Other FDA recommendations for patients with CKD and not receiving dialysis.

(1) Initiating ESA treatment should only be considered when the Hgb level ≤ 10g/dL.

(2) The rate of Hgb decline indicates the likelihood of requiring PRBC.

(3) The goal is to reduce the risk of allosensitization by decreasing the need for PRBC transfusion.

(4) If the Hgb level exceeds 12.0 g/dL, the dose of ESA should be reduced or interrupted.

e. Additional recommendations based on KDIGO guidelines (2012c).

(1) Reversible causes of anemia (e.g., iron deficiency and blood loss) should be evaluated before initiating ESA therapy.

(2) In adults with CKD and not receiving dialysis, consideration should be given to starting ESA when Hgb is < 10 g/dL, while also assessing the clinical presentation. The goal is to reduce the need for PRBC transfusion. ESA should not be initiated in a person with Hgb >10 g/dL.

(a) Initial dose is based on Hgb, body weight, and clinical circumstances.

(b) Usual doses.

i. Epoetin-alpha or epoetin-beta is 20 to 50 IU/kg of body weight given three times a week subcutaneously or intravenously.

ii. Darbepoetin-alpha is 0.45 μq/kg of

body weight administered once weekly subcutaneously or intravenously; or 0.75 µg/kg once every 2 weeks subcutaneously or intravenously. This is usually given once a week in patients with CKD before the individual starts dialysis.

(c) Determining frequency of administration should be based on CKD stage, treatment setting, efficacy consideration, patient tolerance, and preference and type of ESA.

(d) During the initiation phase, monitor Hgb at least once monthly and during the maintenance phase at least every 3 months.

(e) During the maintenance phase, it is recommended that an ESA not be used to maintain Hgb > 11.5 g/dL and to not intentionally increase Hgb > 13 g/dL.

f. Information and recommendations for hyporesponsiveness based on KDIGO guidelines (2012c).

(1) Definition: there is no increase in Hgb from baseline after the first month of ESA therapy and is on appropriate weight-based dose.

(a) Avoid increases in ESA dose beyond doubling the initial weight-based dose.

(b) Identify treatable causes of hyporesponsiveness including absolute iron deficiency, vitamin B12 deficiency, hypothyroidism, ACE-I or ARB therapy, infection/inflammation, bleeding, malignancy, malnutrition, and pure red cell aplasia (PRCA).

(c) PRCA is an antibody-mediated response against erythropoietin that can occur in persons receiving ESA for more than 8 weeks. Signs include a sudden rapid decrease in the Hgb at a rate of 0.5 to 1.0 g/dL per week; blood transfusions required at a rate of about 1 to 2 per week; normal platelet and white blood cell counts; absolute reticulocyte count less than 10,000 µl. Consideration should be given to discontinuing ESA therapy.

(d) Disorders that are impossible to correct are bone marrow disorders and hemoglobinopathies.

(e) For an individual who remains hyporesponsive despite treating correctable causes of anemia, individualizing approach to care is recommended. Consideration must be given to the risks and benefits of the

decline in Hgb level, continuing an ESA to maintain the target Hgb, and the need for PRBC transfusions.

(2) Iron supplementation based on KDIGO guidelines (2012c).

(a) The risks vs. benefits must be considered when starting iron therapy.

   i. Benefits include avoiding blood transfusions, minimizing ESA doses, and reducing symptoms of anemia.

   ii. Risks include potential anaphylactic reaction. There is a lack of data on long-term risks.

(b) Consider route of iron administration based on severity of iron deficiency, availability of venous access, response to prior oral iron therapy, side effects, adherence, and cost.

(c) With an adult who is not on iron or ESA therapy and not receiving dialysis.

   i. A trial of oral iron for 1 to 3 months with the goal being to increase the Hgb without starting ESA.

   ii. The patient's lab values should be: TSAT ≤ 30% and ferritin ≤ 500 ng/mL.

   iii. The decision is based on the individual's clinical presentation and overall clinical goals which include avoidance of PRBC and improvement in anemia-related symptoms.

   iv. The decision should be made after exclusion of active infection.

(d) With an adult receiving an ESA and not iron supplementation and not undergoing dialysis.

   i. A trial of oral iron for 1 to 3 months if an increase in Hgb or decrease in ESA dose is the goal.

   ii. The patient's lab values should be TSAT ≤ 30%, and ferritin level ≤ 500 ng/mL.

   iii. Consideration of iron supplementation is based on the individual's clinical presentation and overall clinical goals which include avoidance of PRBC and improvement in anemia-related symptoms.

   iv. The decision should be made after exclusion of active infection.

(e) If the person is not achieving the goal of increasing iron stores with oral iron, a trial of IV iron should be considered. The decision for iron supplementation in someone who has an active infection should consider the benefit vs. risk.

(f) Iron (oral or IV) should be started when TSAT ≤ 20% and ferritin ≤ 100 ng/mL.

(g) Subsequent doses of iron therapy require assessing the response to previous iron supplementation, ongoing blood losses, iron stores, ESA responsiveness, ESA dose, and the individual's clinical presentation.

(h) Caution.
  i. When administering an initial dose of iron dextran, it is recommended to monitor the patient for at least 60 minutes after the infusion and to have the ability to resuscitate the individual if needed.
  ii. Avoid administering IV iron during an active systemic infection. Whether or not to give IV iron is based on the patient's clinical presentation, the severity of the infection, and the potential benefit of giving the drug to this patient.

(3) Packed red blood cell transfusion (KDIGO, 2012b).
  (a) PRBC transfusions should be avoided when possible to minimize the general risks of transfusions.
  (b) Decisions made should not be based on an arbitrary Hgb threshold, but rather on the occurrence of symptoms caused by anemia.
  (c) In patients eligible for organ transplantation, PRBC transfusion should be avoided when possible to minimize the risk of allosensitization.
  (d) The benefit of transfusion outweighs the risks in the following circumstances.
    i. ESAs are ineffective, e.g., hemoglobinopathies, bone marrow failure, ESA resistance.
    ii. The risks of ESA therapy may outweigh ESA's benefits, e.g., previous or current malignancy, previous stroke.

B. Mineral and bone disorder (CKD-MBD). As kidney function declines, there is a progressive deterioration in mineral homeostasis.
  1. Definition of CKD-MBD and renal osteodystrophy (KDIGO, 2009, p. S4).
    a. CKD-MBD is a systematic disorder of mineral and bone metabolism due to CKD manifested by either one or a combination of:

(1) Abnormalities of calcium, phosphorus, PTH, or vitamin D metabolism.
(2) Abnormalities in bone turnover, mineralization, volume, linear growth, or strength.
(3) Vascular or other soft tissue calcification.
    b. Renal osteodystrophy is an alteration of bone morphology in patients with CKD and is one measure of skeletal component of the systematic disorder of CKD-MBD. It is quantifiable by histomorphometry of bone biopsy.
  2. Altered regulation of calcium, phosphate, and vitamin D homeostasis leading to secondary hyperparathyroidism, increased fibroblast growth hormone 23 (FGF23), metabolic bone disease, soft-tissue calcification, and other metabolic derangements increasing risk of mortality and morbidity (Quarles, 2014).
    a. Beginning in CKD stage 3, the kidneys have a diminished ability to excrete phosphate load leading to hyperphosphatemia, elevated PTH, and decreased 1,25(OH)D (calcitriol, an active form of vitamin D) with associated increase in FGF23 (KDIGO, 2009).
    b. Secondary hyperparathyroidism has a major role in the mineral bone disorder continuum (Martin & Gonzalez, 2007). Abnormalities in vitamin D metabolism and phosphate retention lead to hyperphosphatemia that directly or indirectly causes changes in calcium levels stimulating PTH.
      (1) High PTH in blood affects the bone, causing osteitis fibrosa (high-turnover bone disease), characterized by a greater number and size of osteoclasts (bone resorption cells) and abnormally high level of osteoblasts (bone-forming cells).
      (2) Elevated levels of PTH affect nonskeletal tissue, contributing to vascular and soft tissue calcification.
      (3) Decreased production of 1,25(OH)D.
        (a) Phosphate retention may directly suppress the activity of 1 alpha-hydroxylase, the substrate that converts 25-hydroxyvitamin D to 1,25 dihydroxyvitamin D.
        (b) FGF23 is a "key regulator of phosphate and vitamin D homeostasis, is perhaps the initial adaptive response to KD, and may also play a role in cardiovascular complications as well as progression of kidney disease" (Quarles, 2014, p. 477).
        (c) FGF23 levels are increased in early CKD and correlate with degree of hyperphoshatemia; however, more studies are noted to determine the

significance of FGF23 in CKD (Quarles, 2014, p. 477).

   (d) FGF23 inhibits 1-alpha-hydroxylase activity leading to a decrease in calcitriol (Martin & Gonzalez, 2007).

c. High-turnover metabolic bone disease (osteitis fibrosa) is the result of secondary hyperparathyroidism (KDIGO, 2009; Martin & Gonzalez, 2007; Quarles, 2014). Hyperplasia and resultant high levels of PTH cause:

   (1) Retention of phosphorus.
   (2) Decreased levels of calcitriol.
   (3) Changes within the parathyroid gland lead to further increases in the PTH levels.
   (4) Increased parathyroid growth.
   (5) Skeletal resistance to the actions of PTH.
   (6) Hypocalcemia.

d. Low-bone turnover (adynamic bone disease) is commonly observed in individuals with CKD but more common for those undergoing dialysis (Martin & Gonzalez, 2007).

   (1) Characterized by very low rates of bone formation (decreased numbers of osteoclasts and osteoblasts).
   (2) Osteomalacia, defective bone mineralization, may also be present.

      (a) Linked to aluminum toxicity from contamination of water used in mixing the dialysate and the use of aluminum-based binders.
      (b) 25-hydroxyvitamin D deficiency, due to poor dietary intake of vitamin D and calcium, lack of sunlight exposure, metabolic acidosis (inhibits osteoblasts and osteoclasts), extended hospitalization, and hypophosphatemia (e.g., as in Fanconi syndrome).

   (3) Factors contributing to low-bone turnover.

      (a) Administration of high calcium loads, e.g., calcium containing phosphate binders, use of dialysate fluid containing high levels of calcium.
      (b) Administration of vitamin D sterols.
      (c) Age.
      (d) Postmenopausal osteoporosis.
      (e) Osteopenia in association with systemic disease.
      (f) Increases in circulating peptides that may decrease bone formation (e.g., N-terminal truncated PTH fragments).
      (g) Undefined uremic toxins.
      (h) Metabolic acidosis.
      (i) Decreased expression of PTH receptors.
      (j) Alterations in growth factors and cytokines that affect bone turnover.

Table 2.6

Measurement of Vitamin D Deficiency

Normal	25(OH) D greater than 30 ng/mL
Insufficiency	25(OH) D 21 to 29 ng/mL
Deficiency	25(OH) less than 20 ng/mL

Adapted from Holick et al., 2011.

      (k) Previous corticosteroid therapy (e.g. induced osteoporosis).
      (l) General malnutrition.

3. Vitamin D.

a. Evolving evidence indicates that vitamin D plays a key role in immunity, vascular function, cardiomyocyte health, and insulin resistance (Al-Badr & Martin, 2008; Heaney, 2008; Jones, 2007).

b. Diagnosis of vitamin D deficiency or insufficiency (Table 2.6).

c. Vitamin D deficiency has been linked to hypertension, diabetes, heart failure, and higher frequency of cardiovascular disease and mortality (Al-Badr & Martin, 2008; Heaney, 2008; Jones, 2007; Mehrotra et al., 2009; Zhang et al., 2007).

d. As kidney function declines, the serum levels of 1,25(OH)2 also decrease.

e. There is a high prevalence of nutritional vitamin D deficiency. Serum levels of 25(OH)2 (calcidiol) begin to decrease in stage 2 (Reichel et al., 1991) and are prevalent in all stages of CKD (Pilz et al., 2011). In patients with diabetic nephropathy, vitamin D deficiency has been linked with accelerated progression of CKD (Fernández-Juárez, 2013).

f. It is important to measure 25(OH)2 levels and provide supplementation according to individual needs. This information regarding supplementation for nutritional vitamin D deficiency can be found in Module 2, Chapter 4.

4. Diagnosis of CKD-MBD.

a. Laboratory studies assessing for biochemical abnormalities are primary indicators of CKD-MBD.

b. When obtaining the laboratory studies, it is important to know assay type and precision, interassay variability, blood sample handling, and normal postprandial, diurnal, and seasonal variations in individual parameters. The mathematical construct of calcium X phosphorus product has limited clinical practice use because it is mainly derived from serum phosphorus levels and may not provide additional information beyond that level.

c. Recommendations for adults not on dialysis are based on KDIGO guidelines (2009).
  (1) Initial evaluation begins in stage 3; serum levels of calcium, phosphorus, PTH, and alkaline phosphate (ALP) should be obtained.
    (a) t-ALP is routinely done in clinical laboratories and is found throughout the body; b-ALP is bone specific; however, it is an expensive test so it is not recommended for routine testing but rather considered if the diagnosis is unclear.
      i. t-ALP can help in the diagnosis and assessment of CKD-MBD; if elevated, liver function tests should be checked.
      ii. Abnormal t-ALP can be due to abnormal liver function, increased bone activity, and bone metastases.
      iii. It is an inexpensive test that can be helpful in monitoring the response to therapy or determining bone turnover status when interpretations of PTH are not clear.
    (b) Frequency of testing is based on presence and degree of abnormalities. In patients receiving treatment, or when abnormalities are identified, the clinician may decide to monitor more frequently in an effort to evaluate trends, treatment efficacy, and side-effects.
      i. Stage 3: serum calcium and phosphorus every 5 to 12 months and PTH based on baseline level and CKD progression.
      ii. Stage 4: serum calcium and phosphorus every 3 to 6 months and PTH every 6 to 12 months.
      iii. Stage 5: serum calcium and phosphorus every 1 to 3 months and PTH every 3 to 6 months.
  (2) CKD stage 3 to 5 evaluate 25(OH)2 (calcidiol).
  (3) Bone biopsy (considered the "gold standard" for diagnosing renal osteodystrophy).
    (a) Can provide measurement of bone turnover, mineralization, and volume to assess bone quality and underlying physiology.
    (b) Histology varies and is influenced by stage of CKD, age, and treatments.
    (c) Consideration is given to obtaining a bone biopsy in patients who have clinical symptoms with no clear etiology and when laboratory studies are uncertain.
      i. Unexplained fractures.
      ii. Persistent bone pain.
      iii. Unexplained hypercalcemia.
      iv. Unexplained hyperphosphatemia.
      v. Possible aluminum toxicity.
      vi. Prior to administration of bisphosphonates in patients with CKD-MBD. Bone biopsy is the best way to identify adynamic bone disease. Once diagnosed, bisphosphonates are contraindicated (KDIGO, 2009).
5. Routine bone mineral density (BMD) does not predict fracture risk in this population and does not identify the type of renal osteodystrophy.
6. Clinical manifestations. Patients are often asymptomatic until later in the disease process and even then may have nonspecific symptoms (Martin & Gonzales, 2007).
  a. Musculoskeletal.
    (1) Predisposition to fractures.
    (2) Bone pain.
    (3) Proximal muscle weakness.
    (4) Spontaneous tendon rupture.
    (5) Periarticular pain and joint stiffness.
  b. Extraskeletal (affect soft tissues such as blood vessels, heart valves, and skin).
    (1) Coronary and peripheral vascular calcification.
    (2) Calciphylaxis or calcemia uremic arteriolopathy is extreme calcifications of the skin, muscles, and subcutaneous tissues. Symptoms can include:
      (a) Skin lesions, most often occurring on the breast, abdomen, and thighs.
      (b) Violaceous rash, skin nodules, skin firmness, eschars, livedo reticularis, and painful hyperesthesia of skin.
      (c) Nonhealing ulcerations and gangrene can lead to amputation, uncontrollable sepsis, and death (Quarles, 2014).
7. Pharmacotherapy treatment (more specific medication information can be found in Module 2, Chapter 5).
  a. Goals of treatment.
    (1) In stages 3 to 5: maintain serum phosphorus and calcium in normal range.
    (2) In stages 3 to 5: the optimal PTH is not known. KDIGO (2009) recommends maintaining level above the upper normal limit. Those with progressively rising PTH should be treated with calcitriol or vitamin D analogs.
    (3) The medication selection is based on serum calcium and phosphorus levels.

b. Treatment decisions should be made on trends and not just on one single laboratory study (KDIGO, 2009).

c. Vitamin D deficiency and insufficiency should be corrected.

d. The use of phosphate-binding agents in treatment of hyperphosphatemia.

   (1) Restrict the dose of calcium-based binders and/or the dose of calcitriol or vitamin D analog in the presence of persistent or recurrent hypercalcemia, arterial calcification, adynamic bone disease, and/or persistently low serum PTH levels.

   (2) Long-term use of aluminum-containing phosphate binders should be avoided.

   (3) Phosphate binders should be considered when dietary restriction is insufficient to control serum phosphorus levels (Cheng, 2011).

   (4) Phosphate binders should be given with meals and/or snacks.

      (a) Calcium-based binders, e.g., calcium carbonate/acetate.

         i. Commonly used as first-line agents in CKD stages 3 and 4.

         ii. Can lead to hypercalcemia and soft tissue calcification.

         iii. Should not be used if the serum calcium level is elevated.

         iv. In all patients, the dose should not supply more than 1.5 g/day of elemental calcium (Cheng, 2011).

      (b) Noncalcium-based binders have not been approved by the FDA for use in patients with CKD who are not on dialysis.

         i. The FDA requested more evidence of the efficacy and safety of these medications in the nondialysis CKD population (Winkelmayer & Chertow, 2010).

         ii. Some medical providers engage in "off-label" use of these binders in patients with CKD not undergoing dialysis (Winkelmayer & Chertow, 2010). The prescription is related to concern for increased exposure to calcium as previously discussed.

         iii. Block and colleagues (2012) reported that phosphate binders are effective in lowering serum phosphorus to normal or near normal levels; however, use of the binders promoted progression of vascular calcification.

         iv. Noncalcium-based binders have been shown to reduce the progression of vascular calcification in comparison to calcium-based binders (Cheng, 2011).

         v. There is a need for more evidence for treatment with noncalcium-based binders with this patient population.

   e. Active vitamin D and vitamin D analogs should be initiated to achieve the target PTH if the serum phosphorus, serum calcium, and vitamin D levels are at target.

      (1) Calcitriol is usually the first-line agent.

      (2) Monitor calcium and phosphorus monthly for 3 months and then every 3 months once stable.

8. Nonpharmacotherapy.

   a. Limit dietary intake of phosphorus. Dietary restriction of 800 to 1000 mg/day can be challenging, so it is important to take a person-centered approach to care by mutually establishing attainable goals (see Module 2, Chapter 4).

   b. Individualize approach to diet; consultation with dietitian for Medical Nutritional Therapy (MNT).

C. Elevated serum uric acid levels – hyperuricemia.

1. The kidney plays an important role in the elimination of about 70% of uric acid (Lipkowitz, 2012). A decreased GFR and albuminuria (Toto et al., 2010) are associated with hyperuricemia, a risk factor for gout (Kang & Chen, 2011).

2. Evidence supports that a decline in kidney function may occur before hyperuricemia is seen (Juraschek et al., 2013). It also supports an association between hyperuricemia with CKD and an adverse cardiovascular outcome. Hyperuricemia may also contribute to the progression of CKD (Obermayr et al., 2008).

3. In patients with CKD, who also have asymptomatic or symptomatic hyperuricemia, there is currently insufficient evidence to support or refute the use of medications to lower serum uric acid concentrations as an intervention to slow the progression of the disease (KDIGO, 2013a, p. 79).

D. Acid-base disturbances.

1. The kidneys play an essential role in acid-base homeostasis by controlling serum bicarbonate (HCO3-) concentration through excretion or reabsorption of filtered HCO3-, the excretion of metabolic acids, and synthesis of new HCO3- (Morrow & Malesker, 2013).

   a. Blood hydrogen concentrations are maintained at normal levels despite the daily acidic and/or alkaline loads from the intake and metabolism of foods.

b. The kidneys excrete less than 1% of the hydrogen ions generated on a daily basis. Patients with early stage CKD may not experience life-threatening imbalances until the individual reaches advanced CKD (Morrow & Malesker, 2013).

2. Metabolic acidosis is a major disorder in CKD that can lead to poor health outcomes.
   a. The best way to measure the acid-base status is through arterial blood gases, but this is usually not practical in the outpatient setting. In this case, measuring the serum HCO-3 by obtaining a venous carbon dioxide (CO_2) level (bicarbonate level) may be the best option.
   b. Metabolic acidosis is common in advanced CKD. As nephron mass decreases, the kidney's ability to excrete acid diminishes; typically occurs when the GFR falls < 20 to 25 mL/min.
   c. Some medications may impede renal acid excretion either directly or by interfering with sodium and potassium transport (Perumal & Argekar, 2011).
   d. Diets high in protein will increase acid load; discuss dietary intake with the patient and consider consultation with the renal dietitian.
   e. Complications of metabolic acidosis.
      (1) Increased protein catabolism.
      (2) Muscle wasting.
      (3) Chronic inflammation.
      (4) Impaired glucose homeostasis.
      (5) Impaired cardiac function.
      (6) Progression of kidney disease.
      (7) Increased mortality.
      (8) Insulin resistance.
   f. Metabolic acidosis should be identified early to prevent major complications. In extreme cases, it depresses cardiac function, impairs vascular response catecholamines, and causes arteriolar vasodilatation and venoconstriction leading to systemic hypotension and pulmonary edema (Perumal & Argekar, 2011).
   g. Treatment.
      (1) KDIGO guidelines (2012a) recommend that patients with CKD, whose serum bicarbonate concentrations are < 22 mmol/L, be given oral bicarbonate supplement. The goal, unless contraindicated, is to maintain serum bicarbonate within normal range; levels over 32 mmol/L are associated with increased risk of death.
      (2) Oral bicarbonate tablets ($NaHCO_3$), 0.5 meq/kg/day in divided doses, is recommended. Side effects include fluid retention, edema, exacerbation of heart failure, increased blood pressure.

3. Metabolic alkalosis: increase in HCO3-.
   a. Can be seen with gastric losses through vomiting and/or nasogastric suction, IV bicarbonate therapy, oral alkali therapy, hypokalemia, and mineralocorticoid excess (Morrow & Malesker, 2013). The most common cause in patients with CKD is diuretics (Permumal & Argekar, 2011).
   b. Symptoms.
      (1) Patients rarely have symptoms that can be attributed to alkalosis but rather have symptoms related to hypovolemia (muscle cramps, orthostatic dizziness, and weakness) or to hypokalemia (muscle weakness, polyuria, and polydipsia) (Morrow & Malesker, 2013).
      (2) In severe cases, can cause cardiac arrhythmias, neuromuscular irritability, and tissue hypoxemia (Permumal & Argekar, 2011).

4. Hyperkalemia is caused by positive potassium balance (increased potassium intake or decreased potassium excretion) or an increase in net potassium shift from intracellular to the extracellular compartment (Allon, 2014).
   a. Contributing factors.
      (1) Pseudohyperkalemia is not a true measure of serum potassium, but is due to release of potassium from the blood cells due to hemolysis, prolonged fist clenching, or severe leukocytosis (elevated WBCs).
      (2) Acute kidney injury or chronic kidney disease (most common in CKD stages 4 and 5).
      (3) Dietary indiscretions.
      (4) Constipation.
      (5) Hemorrhage.
      (6) Blood transfusions.
      (7) Medications.
         (a) ACE-I.
         (b) ARB.
         (c) Potassium-sparing diuretics.
         (d) NSAIDs.
         (e) Cyclosporine.
         (f) Beta blockers.
      (8) Physiologic changes.
         (a) Impaired tubular excretion of potassium.
         (b) Aldosterone deficiency can be seen with diabetic nephropathy, chronic interstitial nephritis, or obstructive nephropathy.
         (c) Volume depletion leading to poor perfusion.
         (d) Starvation.
      (9) Metabolic or respiratory acidosis.
      (10) Rhabdomyolysis or tumor lysis syndrome (see Module 4) (Allon, 2014).

b. Symptoms.
   (1) Can produce progressive electrocardio-graphic abnormalities; peaked T waves, flattening or absence of P waves, widening QRS complexes.
   (2) Severe hyperkalemia can cause muscle weakness to the point of paralysis and respiratory failure.
   (3) The most severe consequence of hyperkalemia is cardiac arrest.
c. Treatment (is based on etiology of hyperkalemia).
   (1) A consultation with the dietitian to discuss low potassium diet is recommended (see Module 2, Chapter 4).
   (2) Discontinue offending medications.
      (a) First actions should be to decrease dietary potassium, treat constipation, and stop other medications that may increase the potassium level.
      (b) It must be remembered that an ACE-I or ARB have a major role in slowing the progression of CKD. Therefore, before discontinuing the medication, a diuretic should be added or a decrease in the dose of the ACE-I or ARB should be tried (Allon, 2014).
   (3) Kayexalate (sodium polystyrene sulfonate) is a resin-exchanger that removes potassium from the blood via the gut.
      (a) It is a slow process that may take 1 to 2 hours before a decrease in serum potassium is seen. For those patients with a potential or actual life-threatening condition, other interventions will be needed.
      (b) Faster results are obtained when Kayexalate is given rectally; when given orally, results may take up to 4 hours.
      (c) In severe cases, when the patient has potential for developing life-threatening ventricular arrhythmias, hospitalization may be necessary for medical management and possible dialysis if the response to medical management is inadequate (see Module 4, Chapter 2).
   (4) Follow-up laboratory studies are highly recommended.
5. Malnutrition.
   a. Defined as hypoalbuminemia and/or body mass index of less than 18 kg/m².
      (1) Commonly occurs in patients with CKD (Goldstein-Fuchs & LaPierre, 2013).
      (2) Protein energy malnutrition (PEM) occurs when the supply of protein or calories are inadequate to maintain weight (Freshman, 2013).

b. Contributing factors.
   (1) Decreased dietary nutritional intake.
   (2) Financial or transportation difficulties.
   (3) Decreased appetite.
   (4) Uremic toxins.
   (5) Suboptimal protein intake because of concerns about progression of kidney disease (Personal communication, Hain, 2014).
   (6) Increased metabolic demands (fever, COPD, hyperthyroidism, malignant neoplasms).
   (7) Systemic inflammation.
   (8) Albuminuria.
   (9) Acute illness or infection.
   (10) Depression.
c. Clinical presentation.
   (1) Sacropenia (reduced muscle mass and strength).
   (2) Unintentional weight loss; loose-fitting clothes.
   (3) Low serum albumin.
   (4) Weakness/low energy level.
d. Treatment.
   (1) Contributing factors should be evaluated for and treated accordingly.
      (a) Ask about nutritional intake; requesting that the patient complete a dietary diary is another possibility.
         i. What is typical dietary intake?
         ii. What are the reasons for not eating? (e.g., weight loss, physical issues, psychosocial issues).
      (b) Determine if weight loss was intentional or unintentional.
      (c) Consider social issues (e.g., financial, living situation).
      (d) Evaluate access to food items.
   (2) The ideal protein intake for individuals with CKD is controversial.
      (a) Recommend consultation with the dietitian for a more comprehensive assessment.
      (b) Develop a shared nutritional plan that promotes health (see Chapter 4).

VI. Management of comorbidities associated with CKD.

A. Diabetes mellitus, a complex chronic disorder related to carbohydrate, fat, and protein metabolism and hyperglycemia, is due to deficits in insulin secretion, insulin action, or a combination of both.
1. Classification.
   a. Type 1 (T1DM), which is a metabolic disorder that is characterized by insulin deficiency related to beta-cell destruction, affects about

10% of the adults with diabetes (American Diabetes Association [ADA], 2010).

   b. Type 2 (T2DM), due to progressive insulin secretory defect related to insulin resistance (Golden et al., 2011), affects about 90% to 95% of persons with diabetes (ADA).

2. Epidemiological data from the 2014 National Diabetes Statistics Report (CDC, 2014).
   a. As of 2012, the prevalence of diabetes in the United States was about 29.1 million (9.3% of the population).
     (1) Of this population about 21.0 million have been diagnosed and 8.1 million remain undiagnosed.
     (2) Among adults 20 years and older, the prevalence is a bit higher in men (13.6%) as compared to women (11.2%).
     (3) 1.7 million new cases were identified between 2010 and 2012.
   b. The risk of T2DM increases with age and is higher among many ethnic groups.
     (1) Non-Hispanic whites – 7.6%.
     (2) Asian Americans – 9.0%.
     (3) Hispanics – 12.8%.
     (4) Non-Hispanic blacks – 13.2%.
     (5) American Indians/Alaska Natives – 15.9%.

3. Diabetic nephropathy.
   a. Most common cause of kidney failure in adults.
     (1) About 50% of the population starting dialysis has diabetes and of this population about 80% have T2DM.
     (2) There is an increased risk for mortality due to cardiovascular complications.
   b. Long-term hyperglycemia contributes to the development and maintenance of diabetic nephropathy (Dronavalli et al., 2008).
     (1) Hyperglycemic changes.
       (a) Alterations in glomerular feedback.
       (b) Forms advanced glycation end products (e.g., glycosylated proteins and polyols [alcohol sugars] that accumulate in the glomerulus).
     (2) Hormonal imbalances.
       (a) Increases in growth hormone and glucagon occur with poor glycemic control, hyperglycemia.
       (b) Glucose elevations cause glomerular hyperfiltration.
       (c) Changes in the levels of vasoactive hormones.
         i. Angiotensin II, catecholamines, and prostaglandins, or changes in the responsiveness to these hormones.
         ii. These changes lead to hyperfiltration.
     (3) Hemodynamic factors.
       (a) Glomerular hypertension leads to hyperfiltration.

       (b) Hyperfiltration leads to proteinuria and mesangial disposition of circulating proteins.
       (c) Mesangial expansion and glomerulosclerosis leads to progressive nephron loss.
   c. Progression of diabetic nephropathy.
     (1) Divided by clinical stages depending on the duration of the disease (see "d" below).
     (2) The prevalence of hypertension increases with higher levels of albuminuria (Mogensen et al., 2013; Suarez et al., 2013).
     (3) Uncontrolled diabetes, advanced age, cigarette smoking, and elevated lipid levels are risk factors for development of overt diabetic nephropathy (Bruno et al., 2003; Romero-Aroca et al., 2012).
     (4) The decline from one stage to another is about 2% to 3% per year (Adler et al., 2003).
   d. Stages of diabetic nephropathy (Suarez et al., 2013).
     (1) Stage 1.
       (a) Characterized by renal vasodilation and hyperfiltration.
       (b) Hyperfunction and hypertrophy.
       (c) ACR < 39 mg/g creatinine.
     (2) Stage 2.
       (a) Morphologic lesions develop without clinical signs of disease.
       (b) Glomerular basement membrane thickening.
       (c) ACR > 30 and < 300 mg/g creatinine.
     (3) Stage 3.
       (a) Microalbuminuria.
       (b) A slow and gradual increase of albuminuria for years is prominent feature of this stage.
       (c) ACR > 300 mg/g creatinine and/or persistent proteinuria with serum creatinine 2.0 mg/dL.
     (4) Stage 4.
       (a) Overt nephropathy.
       (b) Decrease in GFR.
       (c) Macroalbuminuria associated to the presence of proliferative retinopathy, coronary heart disease, and foot ulcers (Ismail et al., 1999).
       (d) Serum creatinine of 2.0 mg/dL with proteinuria.
     (5) Stage 5.
       (a) Kidney failure with uremia.
       (b) On dialysis.
   e. Screening and treatment (ADA, 2013).
     (1) The goals are to reduce the risk or slow the progression of nephropathy, optimize

glucose control, and achieve blood pressure control.

  (2) Screening.

    (a) Perform annual test to assess urine albumin excretion in T1DM with diabetes duration ≥ 5 years and in all individuals with T2DM starting at diagnosis.

    (b) Measure serum creatinine at least annually in all adults with diabetes regardless of the degree of urine albumin excretion. The serum creatinine should be used to estimate GFR and stage of CKD.

  (3) Treatment.

    (a) For adults with modestly elevated (30 to 299 mg/day) or higher (≥ 300 mg/day) of urinary albumin excretion, an ACE-I or ARB should be prescribed by the provider.

      i. Monitor serum creatinine and potassium.

      ii. Monitor urine albumin excretion to assess response to therapy and progression of disease.

    (b) Protein intake should be reduced to 0.8 to 1.0 g/kg of body weight per day in individuals with diabetes and earlier stages of CKD. Protein intake should be reduced to 0.8 g/kg of body weight in those with advanced stages of CKD. Consultation with a renal dietitian should be considered to individualize the approach to care.

    (c) A referral to a nephrologist should be initiated.

    (d) When eGFR < 60 mL/min/1.73 m², it is time to evaluate and manage potential complications of CKD.

B. Hypertension.

  1. Controlling blood pressure through lifestyle and pharmacologic strategies is an essential component of slowing the progression of kidney disease.

    a. Blood pressure targets and medications used to treat BP should be individualized with consideration given to the risks of CKD progression, age, coexistent CVD, other comorbid conditions, presence or absence of retinopathy, and tolerance to medications (Gansevoort et al., 2013).

    b. To achieve optimal health outcomes, it is essential to take a person-centered approach to care. This includes individualizing BP targets and treatment according to age, coexistent cardiovascular disease and other comorbidities, risk of progression of CKD, presence or absence of retinopathy (in patients with CKD and diabetes), and tolerance of treatment (KDIGO, 2012a, p. 347).

  2. Target blood pressure.

    a. Patients with diabetes and hypertension should be treated to a systolic blood pressure goal of < 140 mmHg and diastolic < 80 mmHg. And, if tolerated (e.g., younger patients), lower systolic targets, such as < 130 mmHg, may be appropriate (ADA, 2013).

    b. Patients with CKD nondialysis (ND) and urine albumin excretion of 30 to 300 mg/24 hours, should be treated to a goal of 130/80 mmHg. The treatment of choice is with ACE-I or ARB (KDIGO, 2012a).

    c. *The Clinical Practice Guidelines for the Management of Hypertension in the Community: A Statement by the American Society of Hypertension and the International Society of Hypertension* (Weber et al., 2014) reports that the goal of treatment is to manage hypertension by achieving a BP level of less than 140/90 mmHg and identifying and addressing risk factors for CVD (e.g., lipid disorders, glucose tolerance or diabetes, obesity, and smoking).

    d. In the past, guidelines have recommended BP values of less than 130/80 mmHg; however, there is a lack of evidence supporting these goals. Some experts still recommend BP less than 130/80 mmHg in patients with CKD and albuminuria. But there is concern over older adults and the possibility of orthostatic hypotension. Recent evidence supports cardiovascular and stroke protection with BP ≤ 150/90 mmHg in people 80 years or older. Currently, this is the recommended target BP for this population (Weber et al., 2014).

    e. African Americans are vulnerable to strokes and hypertensive kidney disease and are 3 to 5 times as likely as Caucasians to have renal complications and kidney failure (Weber et al., 2014).

  3. Older adults and individuals with diabetes who have autonomic neuropathy have a risk of orthostatic hypotension, putting them in danger of postural dizziness, syncope, falls, and reduced adherence. It is very important to check blood pressures sitting and standing and to monitor the effects of medications (KDIGO, 2012b).

  4. Pharmaceutical agents.

    a. Renin-angiotensin-aldosterone system blockers play a central role in treating blood pressure in patients with CKD. The blockade of angiotensin II with ACE-I or ARB leads to generalized vasodilation of the efferent and afferent glomerular arterioles with a subsequent decrease in the intraglomerular pressure. This leads to reduction in urine albumin excretion, which may provide some long-term renoprotection.

   (1) About 5% to 20% of individuals taking ACE-Is will experience a dry cough due to degradation of bradykinin. Angioedema, although rare, can occur with either ACE-Is or ARBs.

   (2) When initiating treatment, there can be about a 30% reduction in GFR as evidenced by an increase in the serum creatinine; this decline may be reversible. Greater reductions could indicate renal artery stenosis.

   (3) An ACE-I or ARB is recommended for patients with CKD who have urinary albumin excretion. The American Diabetes Association (2013) recommends that patients with diabetes and hypertension be treated with ACE-I or ARB. If one class is not tolerated, the other should be substituted. When administering these medications, it is important to monitor serum creatinine, eGFR, and serum potassium.

b. African Americans have differing blood pressure responses to antihypertensive agents.

   (1) These patients respond well to calcium channel blockers and diuretics but have smaller reductions with angiotensin-converting enzyme (ACE) inhibitors, angiotensin-receptor blockers (ARBs), and β-Blockers.

   (2) However, appropriate combination therapies provide powerful antihypertensive responses that are similar in Caucasians (Weber et al., 2014).

c. Most people will require more than one antihypertensive medication to achieve optimal control of blood pressure (Weber et al., 2014).

d. The Eighth Joint National Committee (JNC-8) *2014 Evidence-Based Guideline for the Management of High Blood Pressure in Adults* recommendations (James et al., 2014).

   (1) In the general population older than 60 years, initiate pharmacologic treatment when SBP is 150 mmHg or higher or DBP is 90 mmHg or higher and treat to a goal of SBP lower than 150 mmHg and goal of DBP lower than 90 mmHg. In some cases, if pharmacologic treatment for high BP leads to SBP < 140 mmHg, and treatment is not associated with adverse effects on health or quality of life, then treatment does not need to be adjusted. When prescribing medications for older adults, it is essential to consider the risk vs. benefit, what the desired outcome is, and monitoring for desired outcome or adverse drug events.

   (2) In the general nonblack population, including those with diabetes, initial antihypertensive therapy should include a thiazide-type diuretic, calcium channel blocker (CCB), ACEI, or ARB. In the general black-population, including those with diabetes, initial antihypertensive treatment should include a thiazide-type diuretic or calcium channel blocker.

   (3) In the general African-American population, including those with diabetes, initial antihypertensive treatment should include a thiazide-type diuretic or CCB.

   (4) In the population aged 18 years of older with CKD and hypertension, initial (or add-on) antihypertensive treatment should include an ACEI or ARB to improve kidney outcomes. This applies to all individuals with CKD regardless of race or diabetes status.

   (5) The goal of treatment is to attain and maintain target BP.

      (a) If the goal is not achieved in 1 month, the dose of initial drug should be increased or a second medication added from one of the classes stated above.

      (b) If the BP cannot be achieved with two medications, a third drug should be added and titrated from the same classes of medication as previously stated.

      (c) If there is the need for the use of more than three medications to reach BP goal, referral to a hypertensive specialist is indicated.

5. Lifestyle.

a. A fundamental component of controlling BP, reducing CVD risks, and slowing the progression of CKD is lifestyle management (Eskridge, 2010; KDIGO, 2012a).

   (1) Discovering strategies to help people successfully participate in self-management activities is a crucial aspect of lifestyle management (Eskridge, 2010).

   (2) The likelihood of getting people to engage in health promotion behaviors is greater when nephrology professionals establish a patient-provider partnership and engage in shared decision making by mutually establishing attainable goals (Hain & Sandy, 2013).

b. Exercise.
   (1) KDIGO guidelines (2012b) recommend participating in an exercise program that is compatible with cardiovascular health and individual tolerance.
      (a) At least 30 minutes a day, 5 times per week is suggested. However, some people may not be able to physically or psychologically achieve this goal, so it is important to engage in shared decision making to develop realistic goals.
      (b) There is a vast amount of evidence showing the benefits of exercise on general health, and this is similar for patients with CKD.
   (2) It is important to realize that taking an active role in an exercise plan takes personal commitment. Discovering "what matters most" (Hain & Sandy, 2013) to the patient may assist healthcare professionals in finding the best way to promote commitment.
   (3) Consultation with a physical therapist should be considered for those who have experienced a functional decline related to acute illness or other health problems.
c. Weight reduction.
   (1) A systematic review of clinical trials indicated that there are long-term (≥ 2 years) benefits for sustained weight loss.
      (a) Even a 3-kg weight loss can help lower BP (Aucott et al., 2009).
      (b) Neter and colleagues (2003) suggested that a kg of intentional weight loss can lead to 1 mmHg decrease in both systolic and diastolic BP.
   (2) Consultation with a renal dietitian should be considered to help with weight reduction and to maintain adequate nutritional status (see Chapter 4).
d. Diet.
   (1) Sodium restriction.
      (a) There is a link between sodium intake and blood pressure levels in individuals with CKD.
      (b) Individuals with a decreased eGFR, who have salt retention, tend to have higher blood pressures (KDIGO, 2012a).
      (c) The World Health Organization (WHO) recommends a reduction in salt intake to improve BP (http://www.who.int/cardiovascular_diseases/en/).
      (d) Lowering salt intake to < 90 mmol (< 2 grams) per day of sodium is recommended by KDIGO (2012b).
      (e) There are some forms of C[KD that may] be associated with salt wa[sting by] the kidney. These patients are at risk for higher than usual rate of volume depletion and electrolyte disturbances when placed on salt restriction diet.
         i. Careful monitoring of fluid and electrolyte status is important (KDIGO, 2012a).
         ii. Hypertension is common among African Americans, and they tend to be more sensitive to the blood pressure-raising effects of salt in the diet as compared to Caucasians (Weber et al., 2014).
   (2) Dietary Approaches to Stop Hypertension (DASH) (Sacks et al., 2001).
      (a) This diet is high in vegetables, fruits, low-fat dairy products, whole grains, poultry, fish, and nuts. It is low in sweets, sugar-sweetened beverages, and red meats (available at http://www.nhlbi.nih.gov/health/health-topics/topics/dash/). It has shown significant benefits of a low-sodium diet on lowering blood pressure.
      (b) Adults with prehypertension or stage 1 hypertension following the DASH diet who reduced sodium intake from 6 to 4 g/day had a greater decrease in BP, as compared to those who decreased sodium intake from 8 to 6 g/day (Sacks et al., 2001).
      (c) Caution should be taken for individuals with CKD, chronic heart failure, diabetes type 2, chronic liver disease, and those receiving renin-angiotensin-aldosterone system antagonists (Aaron & Sanders, 2013; Tyson et al., 2012).
         i. Clinicians should be aware that patients with severe CHF requiring high doses of diuretics may experience challenges with a low-sodium diet.
         ii. Monitoring fluids and electrolytes and tolerance to salt restriction is important (Aaron & Sanders, 2013).
      (d) The conflicts with the DASH diet (Tyson et al., 2012, p. 393).
         i CKD: high potassium, high protein usually contraindicated in patients with advanced CKD.
         ii T2DM: carbohydrate content may be higher than prescribed for the individual.

(e) Interventions (Tyson et al., 2012, p. 393).
  i. CKD: frequent monitoring of the potassium, phosphorus, calcium, and magnesium should be performed. If normal or elevated, DASH should not be started or should be discontinued if currently following.
  ii. T2DM: Adopt a low-carbohydrate version of DASH diet by substituting protein or monounsaturated fat for protein of the carbohydrate content. Select foods with a low glycemic index.
  e. Smoking cessation.
    (1) Cigarette smoke and exposure to environmental tobacco smoke are one of the most modifiable risk factors for CVD in the general population and those with CKD (KDIGO, 2012a).
    (2) Smoking cessation may not reduce blood pressure to a target BP, but because it is a major risk factor for CVD, strongly urging patients with CKD to discontinue this habit is a very important aspect of health promotion (Weber et al., 2014).
  f. Alcohol consumption.
    (1) Limiting alcohol intake to two drinks per day can be beneficial in protecting against cardiovascular events; women should limit intake to one drink per day (Weber et al., 2014).
    (2) Larger amounts of alcohol consumption can increase BP (Weber et al., 2014).
    (3) Emerging research is showing that moderate alcohol consumption is associated with less cardiovascular and renal risk (Schaeffner & Ritz, 2012). Until more evidence becomes available, it is recommended to follow the KDIGO guidelines (2012): limit alcohol intake to no more than two standard drinks per day for men and no more than one standard drink for women.

C. Dyslipidemia.
  1. It is well-known that dyslipidemia is common in patients with CKD and that it can occur early in the disease process (Harper & Jacobson, 2008).
  2. Research has demonstrated that a decreasing GFR was independently linked to the development of atherosclerotic CVD (Muntner et al., 2005). The association between dyslipidemia and the increased risk for CVD is challenging to identify. It is difficult to control for the many other cardiovascular risk factors that patients with CKD have, including:

  a. Oxidative stress.
  b. Inflammation.
  c. Physical inactivity.
  d. Anemia.
  e. Vascular calcification.
  f. Endothelial dysfunction.
  g. Reduced nitric oxide availability (Harper & Jacobson, 2008).
  h. Other determinants of dyslipidemia in CKD include diabetes mellitus, severity of proteinuria, and nutritional status (Kasiske, 1998).
3. Assessment of dyslipidemia (KDIGO, 2013a).
  a. Adults who have been recently diagnosed with CKD should have a lipid profile measured. Includes total cholesterol, low-density lipoprotein cholesterol (LDL-C), high-density lipoprotein (HDL-C), and triglycerides (LDL-C). *Note*: "does not reliably discriminate between those at low or high risk of cardiovascular events" (p. 269).
  b. Initial evaluation provides a baseline for further evaluation, but healthcare professionals should also consider secondary causes.
  c. Follow-up measurement is not recommended unless there would be a change in management.
  d. A lipid profile should be measured when the patient has been fasting. If abnormalities are identified, the patient should be referred to a specialist for further evaluation.
4. Causes of dyslipidemia (NKF, 2003).
  a. Medical conditions.
    (1) Nephrotic syndrome.
    (2) Hypothyroidism.
    (3) Diabetes.
    (4) Excessive alcohol intake.
    (5) Liver disease.
  b. Medications.
    (1) 13-cis-retinoic acid.
    (2) Anticonvulsants.
    (3) Highly active anti-retroviral therapy.
    (4) Diuretics.
    (5) Beta-blockers.
    (6) Androgens.
    (7) Oral contraceptives.
    (8) Corticosteroids.
    (9) Cyclosporine.
    (10) Siralimus.
5. Treatment with a statin.
  a. The primary goal of treatment is reducing mortality and morbidity. Lifestyle changes, although an important aspect of improving overall health, have not led to improved clinical outcomes in patients with CKD; thus, pharmacotherapy is an essential aspect of reducing mortality and morbidity. In particular, statins have shown the greatest effect

on reducing the risk of CV events (KDIGO, 2013b).
b. The initial therapeutic approach should be focused on nontraditional cardiovascular risk factors (Epstein & Vaziri, 2012). These include albuminuria, anemia, abnormal mineral metabolism, electrolyte imbalance, oxidative stress, inflammation, thrombogenic factors, and malnutrition (Sarnak et al., 2003).
c. Considering the high CVD risk for individuals with CKD, making the decision to prescribe lipid-lowering therapy for the nondialysis population should be based on absolute risk for coronary events and that the treatment would be beneficial (KDIGO, 2013b).
d. Adults ≥ 50 years with eGFR < 60 mL/min/1.73 m^2 who are not treated with kidney replacement therapy (KRT) (hemodialysis, peritoneal dialysis, or transplantation) should be treated with a statin or statin/ezetimibe combination.
e. For adults 18 to 49 years with CKD and not treated with KRT, a statin is recommended if one or more of the following are present.
   (1) Known coronary disease (MI or coronary revascularization).
   (2) Diabetes mellitus.
   (3) Prior ischemic stroke.
   (4) Estimated 10-year incidence of coronary death or nonfatal myocardial infarction >10% (KDIGO, 2013b).

D. Sleep disturbances.
   1. Current evidence suggests that there is a high prevalence of sleep disturbances in individuals with nondialysis-dependent CKD; in fact, sleep disturbances have a direct and indirect role in the development and progression of CKD (Turek et al., 2012).
   2. The prevalence of sleep disturbances is well-known in those undergoing dialysis, but less is known about the nondialysis CKD population.
      a. The wide range of sleep disturbances (14% to 85%) (Turek et al., 2012) supports how little available evidence there is about sleep problems in this population.
      b. The dearth of evidence warrants the need for further evidence regarding the direct and indirect impact of sleep disturbances on the development and progression of CKD as well as effective assessment and treatment measures.
      c. There are several reasons for sleep disturbances, including depression and obstructive sleep apnea (OSA).
   3. OSA can lead to intermittent hypoxia and re-oxygenation nocturnal blood pressure rise and sympathetic activation. This, in turn, promotes inflammation and systematic endothelial dysfunction (Lavie, 2003; Yamauchi & Kimura, 2008).
      a. Endothelial dysfunction, inflammation, and oxidative stress can have negative effects on the kidney, such as the development of arterial stiffness (van Bussel et al., 2011).
      b. Arterial stiffness contributes to decline in kidney function (Peralta et al., 2012).
      c. Research studies have shown a link between OSA and proteinuria.
         (1) Casserly and colleagues (2001) in a study of 148 participants found no association between the severity of OSA and proteinuria.
         (2) However, in a larger study (n = 496), researchers found that severe OSA was associated with increased urine albumin excretion independently of eGFR (Faulx et al., 2007).
      d. Over the past decade, plenty of evidence has shown the association between sleep disturbances and an increased risk for hypertension, type 2 diabetes, and obesity, and they all contribute to CKD (Turek et al., 2012).
      e. Current evidence supports the importance of recognizing OSA and other sleep disturbances in patients with CKD.
   4. Assessment for sleep problems involves asking questions that may indicate increased risk for OSA.
      a. The Epworth Sleepiness Scale (Johns, 1991, 1992, 1994) is a tool that can be used to screen for daytime sleepiness, which indicates a possible sleep disturbance. This tool can be found at http://epworthsleepinessssscale.com/about-epworth-sleepiness/
      b. Referral to a sleep specialist for consideration of additional diagnostic testing should be considered if the health professional suspects OSA or other health problems that may contribute to sleep disturbances, such as depression.

E. Depression.
   1. Individuals living with one or more chronic diseases are at risk for depression, making this an important condition to identify and treat.
      a. Determining the incidence and prevalence of depression in patients with CKD can be challenging, mainly because of variances in reporting mechanisms.
         (1) Self-report scales may actually overestimate the number of persons with depression (Palmer et al., 2012).
         (2) On the other hand, many people may not be diagnosed and thus not receive the necessary treatment.

Table 2.7

Diagnostic Criteria for Major Depressive Disorder

- Depressed or irritable mood most of the day (feeling sad or empty; appears tearful)
- Decreased interest or pleasure in activities
- Significant weight change (5%) or change in appetite
- Change in sleep (insomnia or hypersomnia)
- Change in activity (psychomotor agitation or retardation)
- Fatigue or loss of energy
- Guilt/worthlessness
- Concentration (diminished ability to think or concentrate, or more indecisiveness)
- Suicidality (thoughts of death or suicide)
- The symptoms cause clinically significant distress or impairment in social, occupational or other important areas of functioning
- The symptoms are not better accounted for by bereavement (i.e., after the death of a loved one)
- The symptoms are not due to the direct physiological effects of substance (e.g., drug abuse, prescribed medications, or a general medical condition (e.g., hypothyroidism)

Source: American Psychiatric Association (APA). (2000.) *Diagnosis and statistical manual of mental disorders* (4th ed.). Washington DC: Author.

    b. Palmer et al. (2013) concluded that about 25% of individuals with CKD may have some degree of depression, and the risk of depression increases with advancing disease.

2. Persistent depressive disorders (DSM-5).
    a. Chronic major depressive disorder (MDD).
      (1) MDD is a clinical syndrome in which five or more of the symptoms listed in Table 2.7 have been present every day during the same 2-week period and represent a change from previous functioning in at least one of the first two symptoms.
        (a) Depressed or irritable mood most of the day, *or*
        (b) Decreased interest or pleasure in most activities.
      (2) Do not include symptoms that are clearly due to a general medical condition.
    b. Dysthymic disorder is a depressed mood for a longer period of time – at least 2 years in adults.
3. Bereavement.
    a. Usually follows the death of a loved one.
    b. A severe psychosocial stressor can precipitate MDD.
    c. Symptoms.
      (1) Feelings of worthlessness.
      (2) Suicidal ideation.
      (3) Poor somatic health.
      (4) Difficulties with interpersonal relationships.
      (5) Functional deficits.

4. Grief is associated with a wide range of emotions.
    a. May be seen when an individual experiences the loss of a job or career, suffers a decline in physical function or ability to care for self, in health or the diminishing health of a loved one, or marital discord or divorce.
    b. Individuals with advancing kidney disease may experience grief related to deteriorating health and having to consider starting kidney replacement therapy.
5. Screening.
    a. Recommendation for screening for adults with depression.
      (1) Agency for Healthcare Research and Quality (AHRQ) http://www.ahrq.gov/professionals/clinicians-providers/resources/depsum1.html
      (2) U.S. Preventative Services Task Force Screening available at http://www.uspreventiveservicestaskforce.org/uspstf09/adultdepression/addeprrs.htm
    b. There are several instruments that can be used to assess for depression. The PHQ-2 and PHQ-9 are easy to administer and have been used in individuals with kidney disease. PHQ-9 can be found at http://www.integration.samhsa.gov/images/res/PHQ%20-%20Questions.pdf
6. Management.
    a. Depression is associated with increased risk of mortality in patients with CKD, making it very important for nephrology professionals to identify and treat (Palmer et al., 2013).
    b. Nonpharmacologic approaches.
      (1) Consultation with social worker, psychiatrist, psychologist, or psychiatric/mental health nurse practitioner for cognitive behavioral therapy and continued monitoring.
      (2) Engage in physical activities.
      (3) Music therapy.
      (4) Provide emotional support.
      (5) Relaxation therapy.
    c. Pharmacologic therapy.
      (1) More data is needed to determine the best antidepressant to prescribe for patients with CKD and depression.
      (2) At the time of this publication, a medication from the class of selective serotonin re-uptake inhibitors (SSRI) appears to be the most prudent choice for patients with CKD and CVD.
        (a) Once the medication is started, it is important to monitor the response before making a dose adjustment.
        (b) The dose should not be increased sooner than intervals of at least 1 to 2 weeks and only if tolerated.

(c) Monitoring for drug-drug interactions and suicidal ideation is essential when the medication is initiated (Hedayati et al., 2011).

(d) Additional considerations relating to SSRI therapy.

   i. Paroxetine should be avoided in individuals with CrCl < 30 mL/min and in older adults because of a prolonged half-life.

   ii. Fluoxetine has no dose adjustment, but has a long half-life, so should be prescribed cautiously and should be avoided in older adults.

   iii. Citalopram is not recommended in patients with eGFR < 20 mL/min.

   iv. Escitalopram should be used with caution in patients with advanced kidney disease.

   v. Sertraline requires no dose adjustment, but the active metabolite is excreted by the kidneys.

d. Collaboration with a psychiatrist or psychiatric/mental health APRN for medication management is recommended.

F. Sexual dysfunction.

1. Definition. *Sexual dysfunction* "is a set of disorders characterized by physical and psychological changes that result in inability to perform satisfactory sexual activities" (Theofulou, 2011, p. 76). Sexual dysfunction is highly prevalent in men and women with CKD, especially those undergoing dialysis (Navaneethan et al., 2010).

2. Factors contributing to sexual dysfunction.
   a. Hormonal disturbances.
   b. Anemia.
   c. The mineral and bone disorder of CKD.
   d. Psychological factors such as depression, anxiety, poor self-esteem, social withdrawal, body image, marital discord, and financial difficulties.
   e. Autonomic dysfunction.
   f. Medications such as antihypertensives, antidepressants, histamine receptor blockers.
   g. Comorbid conditions like diabetes mellitus, cardiovascular disease, and malnutrition.

3. Potential female sexual problems.
   a. DSM-IV-TR classifies female sexual dysfunction into four categories.
   (1) Sexual desire disorder includes hypoactive sexual desire disorder (HSDD) and sexual aversion.
      (a) HSDD is the most prevalent problem and is defined as diminished or absent feelings of sexual interest and a lack of responsive desire.
      (b) Sexual aversion disorder is a phobic aversion that in turn leads to avoidance of sexual contact. It is usually connected with an emotional issue that is often related to a history of physical or sexual abuse.
   (2) Sexual arousal disorder is an absent or an impaired genital sexual arousal.
   (3) Orgasmic disorder is an inability to achieve orgasm, markedly diminished intensity of orgasmic sensations, or marked delay of orgasm during any kind of sexual stimulation despite self-reported high sexual arousal.
   (4) Sexual pain disorder including dyspareunia (persistent or recurrent pain with vaginal entry or penile vaginal intercourse).

   b. Assessment of female sexual dysfunction.
   (1) Create an environment that promotes disclosure.
      (a) Take a nonjudgmental approach.
      (b) Ask open-ended questions such as: "Are you currently involved in a sexual relationship?" and "Are you having any problems?" (Bernice, 2013).
   (2) Ask about sexual partner(s).
   (3) Screening tools.
      (a) Decreased Sexual Desire Screener (DSDS): http://www.omniaeducation.com/whav/WHAV_Addenda2/Decreased_Sexual_Desire_Screener_DSDS_Female_Sexual_Dysfunction_Tool.pdf
      (b) Female Sexual Dysfunction Index (FSDI): http://www.fsfiquestionnaire.com/FSFI%20questionnaire2000.pdf

   c. Depending on the outcome of the health history, discuss with the nephrology provider possible referral to psychologist and/or gynecologist/women's health NP for further evaluation and treatment.

4. Potential male sexual problems.
   a. Disorders of desire: hypoactive means the individual has a lack of interest in sex or sexual activity, although the actual sexual experience is normal. Causes can be and often are a combination of biologic, psychological, and sociocultural factors.
   (1) Low levels of DHEA.
   (2) Chronic physical illness.
   (3) Pain medication, psychotropic drugs, cocaine, marijuana, and amphetamines.
   (4) Social pressures, such as job stress, marital discord, divorce, death in family, and infertility.

b. Disorders of excitement. Erectile dysfunction is the persistent inability to achieve and/or to maintain an erection sufficient to permit satisfactory performance. Causes can include:
   (1) Psychogenic: performance anxiety, depression, psychological stress, relationship problems.
   (2) Testosterone deficiency.
   (3) Cardiovascular disease: hypertension, congestive heart failure, peripheral vascular disease, hyperlipidemia, cigarette smoking.
   (4) Chronic disease: kidney disease and diabetes mellitus.
   (5) Neurologic: stroke, Parkinson's disease, peripheral neuropathy, spinal cord injury.
   (6) Medications such as antihypertensive drugs (e.g., beta blockers, ACE-inhibitors, calcium channel blockers, centrally acting agents, antiarrhythmic), antidepressants (selective serotonin reuptake inhibitors [SSRIs], serotonin and norepinephrine reuptake inhibitors [SNRIs]), anticholinergic medications.
c. Disorders of orgasm (i.e., problems with ejaculation) can be due to low testosterone level, neurologic disorders, and medications.
d. Assessment for male sexual dysfunction.
   (1) Obtain a history of any sexual or relationship concerns by asking open-ended questions.
   (2) Evaluate factors that may contribute to the problem.
   (3) A physical exam should consider endocrine, neurologic deficits, vascular assessment, and penile abnormality (DeNisco, 2013).
   (4) Laboratory studies may include CBC, metabolic panel, TSH, PSA, prolactin, serum testosterone, luteinizing hormone.
e. The treatment depends upon the underlying cause.
   (1) Referral of underlying or refractory medical problems to an appropriate specialist.
   (2) Counseling or psychotherapy.
   (3) Medications. *Note*: phosphodiesterase type 5 (PDE5) inhibitors (sildenafil, vardenafil, tadalafil) are contraindicated in individuals with cardiac failure, unstable angina, resting BP < 90/50 or > 170/110 mmHg. They should be used with caution with alpha blockers.

G. Pregnancy.
   1. Normal compensatory changes in the kidney.
      a. To provide sufficient fluid volume for effective placental exchange, total body water increases to about 7.5 L.
      b. To maintain osmolarity, sodium reabsorption increases in the tubules.
      c. Progesterone causes increased response for angiotensin-renin system, which increases aldosterone production that aids in sodium reabsorption (progesterone is potassium sparing so potassium levels remain adequate).
      d. During pregnancy, kidneys excrete fetal waste product along with the woman's waste products.
      e. Urine output gradually increases to 60% to 80%, specific gravity decreases.
      f. To meet the needs of the circulatory system, the GFR increases by 50% and renal plasma flow increases by 25% to 80%.
      g. The efficient GFR leads to lowered BUN and plasma creatinine level by about 25%.
      h. Renal threshold for glucose is decreased, allowing for minimal spillage (more than trace is considered abnormal unless proven otherwise) (Pillitteri, 2010).
   2. CKD and pregnancy.
      a. Pregnancy may be complicated by hypertension/preeclampsia, worsening proteinuria, and preterm delivery.
      b. Major concern is rapid progression of CKD and acute kidney injury (AKI).
      c. Failure to compensate for increased GFR when there is increased intraglomerular pressure.
      d. May lead to irreversible CKD/kidney failure.
      e. Those requiring KRT will most likely require dialysis postpartum (Vellanki & Hou, 2014).
   3. Cause of AKI in pregnancy.
      a. Volume depletion.
         (1) Hyperemesis gravidarum.
         (2) Postpartum bleeding.
         (3) Placental abruption.
      b. Sepsis.
         (1) Septic abortion.
         (2) Acute pyelonephritis.
      c. Severe preeclampsia.
      d. Thrombotic microangiopathies.
      e. Acute fatty liver of pregnancy.
      f. Urinary tract obstruction from gravid uterus (Vellanki & Hous, 2014).
   4. Assessment.
      a. Pregnant woman with CKD are considered high risk and will most likely be under the care of a perinatologist and nephrologist.
      b. Proteinuria may be first identified during pregnancy and may reflect preexisting or new-onset kidney disease.
      c. Observe for signs and symptoms of preeclampsia.
      d. At each medical visit and as needed, evaluate BP and weight. Assess for increasing edema or presence of proteinuria.
      e. Obtain laboratory studies.
         (1) CBC, CMP, uric acid, urinalysis.

(2) Liver function tests, coagulation studies.
f. Fetal assessment (Poole, 2014).
5. Preeclampsia is a multisystem complex health problem that is specific to pregnancy.
   a. New onset of hypertension (BP ≥ 140/90 mmHg) and proteinuria after 20 weeks of gestation often accompanied by edema and hyperuricemia.
   b. Common in first pregnancy and multigravidas with a new partner, family history, prior preeclampsia and underlying maternal medical conditions (e.g., hypertension, diabetes, CKD, obesity, and thrombophilias) (Vellanski & Hou, 2014).

VII. Medication management (See Chapter 5, Pharmacology, in this module).

A. Drug dosing.
  1. Understanding the pharmacokinetic and pharmacodynamic properties of medication is essential when determining the optimal dose of drugs and what medications to avoid.
  2. Drug absorption, bioavailability, protein binding, distribution volume, nonrenal clearance, and metabolism can be altered in individuals with CKD (Munar & Singh, 2007).
     a. Drug prescribing can become more complex in patients with advanced CKD.
     b. Inappropriate dosing in patients with CKD can cause toxicity or ineffective results.
     c. Many medications require dose adjustments to ensure efficacy and to reduce the risk of toxicity.
        (1) Calculate eGFR or creatinine clearance (Munar & Singh, 2007).
        (2) Fluid balance can affect pharmacokinetics of medications by altering volume distributions (Olyaei & Steffi, 2011).

B. There are some medications that should be avoided in individuals with CKD. Some pharmacologic agents have more active metabolites that accumulate, leading to complications.

C. Recommendations for successful medication self-administration.
  1. A systematic review of interventions to improve adherence to self-administration of medication revealed that this can be a complex issue that requires a multifaceted approach (Viswanathan et al., 2012). Some examples of interventions that have shown promise.
     a. Pharmacist-led.
     b. Reminders.
     c. Collaborative care.
     d. Telephone-based counseling.
     e. Decision aids.
  2. There are limitations to studies exploring interventions aimed at improving an individual's ability to successfully self-administer medication.

a. It is important to take ... approach to care.
b. Consideration must be g... physical functional status ... Module 5, Chapter 2 for m... about care of older adults).
c. Medications to avoid in older ...
   (1) BEERS Criteria for Potent... inappropriate Medication Use in Older Adults is available at: http://www.americangeriatrics.org/health_care_professionals/clinical_practice/clinical_guidelines_recommendations/2012
   (2) For more information: ConsultGeriRN.org

SECTION C
Kidney Disease Education Based on Stage of CKD

I. Medicare benefits.

A. Kidney disease education (KDE).
  1. The Medicare Improvements for Patients and Providers Act of 2008 Section 152(b) added KDE services under Medicare Part B coverage for Medicare beneficiaries diagnosed with stage 4 CKD who have received a referral from the physician who is managing the person's kidney disease.
     a. Educational content must be provided by a qualified professional defined as a physician, physician's assistant, nurse practitioner, or clinical nurse specialist.
     b. Dialysis facilities, hospitals, and skilled nursing facilities outside of rural areas are not considered qualified providers.
     c. Hospitals, home health agencies, outpatient rehabilitation facilities, hospices, or skilled nursing facilities located within a rural area are considered qualified providers.
  2. Under this benefit, a person with a documented ICD-9-CM code of 585.4 (stage 4 CKD) can receive up to six 1-hour sessions of KDE services in their lifetime. Each session must be at least 31 minutes to be billed and should include the following content.
     a. Management of comorbidities.
     b. Prevention of uremic complications.
     c. Therapeutic options, treatment modalities, and settings; advantages and disadvantages of each; how they replace the kidney.
     d. Opportunity to actively participate in the choice of therapy.

...ession should be tailored to meet the needs of the individual involved (CMS, 2010).

B. Diabetes education.
1. Medicare covers screening tests for diabetes for beneficiaries at risk for diabetes or who are diagnosed with prediabetes.
    a. These screening tests include a fasting blood glucose test and a postglucose challenge test.
    b. To be eligible, the beneficiary must have any of the following risk factors.
        (1) Hypertension.
        (2) Dyslipidemia.
        (3) Obesity.
        (4) Previous identification of an elevated glucose, or
    c. The beneficiary would have at least two of the following risk factors.
        (1) Overweight.
        (2) Family history of diabetes.
        (3) Age 65 or older.
        (4) History of gestational diabetes.
        (5) Delivery of an infant over 9 pounds.
2. For Medicare beneficiaries who have been diagnosed with diabetes, Medicare provides diabetes self-management training (DSMT) services to educate the individual on how to successfully manage diabetes. The DSMT program includes the following content.
    a. Instruction in blood glucose self-monitoring.
    b. Education about nutrition and exercise.
    c. Insulin treatment plan for insulin-dependent beneficiaries.
3. The physician or nonphysician practitioner (APRN or physician assistant) must certify that the DSMT services are necessary. The program must be accredited by a CMS-approved national accreditation organization such as the American Diabetes Association, the American Association of Diabetes Educators, or the Indian Health Service (CMS, 2013).

C. Medical nutritional therapies (MNT).
1. Medicare covers MNT for beneficiaries diagnosed with diabetes or chronic kidney disease. This service is not covered for patients on dialysis.
2. The MNT benefit is covered under Medicare Part B, and copayments and deductibles apply. The individual may receive 3 hours of 1:1 MNT services in the first year, and 2 hours each following year. The service is required for a change in condition, diagnosis, or treatment.
3. The MNT service must be provided by a registered dietitian or qualified nutritional professional.
    a. A referral for services is needed from the treating physician caring for the beneficiary.

The beneficiary must have also received the DSMT benefit.
    b. An individual may receive both DSMT and MNT services, but the sessions cannot be provided on the same day to the same beneficiary (CMS, 2013).

II. Education (see Chapter 3 in this module).

A. Pros and cons of kidney replacement therapies. Making a decision regarding best treatment options can be challenging.
1. Consider prognosis and comorbid condition as discussed throughout this chapter.
2. Engage in shared decision making by established patient-provider partnership (Hain & Sandy, 2013).
    a. Risk versus benefits of all modalities to help in the decision of which kidney replacement therapy is best for them.
    b. Hospice or palliative care.
    c. Discuss the person's typical day and how a modality fits into everyday living.

B. Reducing cardiovascular risk factors.
1. It is important to individualize CKD education and to develop strategies that fit into the person's everyday living. Educational interventions that are specific to the individual have been effective in helping persons with CKD understand management goals that support behaviors for optimal blood pressure control (Nunes-Wright et al., 2011).
2. Identify barriers to education; many barriers are modifiable (Williams-Joseph et al., 2014).
    a. Health literacy.
    b. Readiness to learn.
    c. Physical and cognitive limitations.
    d. Consider learning needs of older adults (Elliott, 2014).

References

Aaron, K.J. & Sanders, P.W. (2013). Role of dietary salt and potassium intake in cardiovascular health and disease: A review of the evidence. *Mayo Clinic Proceedings, 88*(9), 987-995).

Adler, A.I., Stevens, R.J., Manley, S.E., Bilous, R.W., Cull, C.A., & Holman, R.R. (2003). Development and progression of nephropathy in type 2 diabetes: The United Kingdom Prospective Diabetes Study (UKPDS 64). *Kidney International, 63*(1), 225-232.

Al-Badr, W., & Martin, K.J. (2008). Vitamin D and kidney disease. *Clinical Journal of the American Society of Nephrology, 3*(5), 1555-1560.

Allon, M. (2014). Disorders of potassium disorders. In S.J. Gilbert & D.E. Weiner (Eds.), *National Kidney Foundation primer on kidney disease* (6th ed.). Philadelphia: Elsevier Saunders.

American Academy of Pediatrics (AAP). (1993). Recommendations for preventive pediatric health care. In *Policy reference guide: A comprehensive guide to AAP policy statement.* Elk Grove Village, IL: American Academy of Pediatrics.

American College of Physicians (ACP). (2013). Screening, monitoring, and treatment of stage 1 to 3 chronic kidney disease: A clinical practice guideline from the clinical guidelines committee of the American College of Physicians. *Annals of Internal Medicine, 159*(12), 1-13.

American Diabetes Association (ADA). (2013). Standards of medical care in diabetes, *Diabetes Care, 36*, S4-S66.

American Nurses Association (ANA). (2012). The value of nursing care coordination: A white paper of the American Nurses Association. Available at http://www.nursingworld.org

American Psychiatric Association (APA). (2000.) *Diagnosis and statistical manual of mental disorders* (4th ed.). Washington, DC: Author.

Attkisson, C.C., & Greenfield, T.K. (2004). The UCSF Client Satisfaction Scales: I. The Client Satisfaction Questionnaire-8. In M.E. Maruish (Ed.), *The use of psychological testing for treatment planning and outcomes assessment* (3rd ed., Vol. 3). Mahwah, NJ: Lawrence Erlbaum Associates.

Aucott, L., Rothnie, H., McIntyre, L., Thapa, M., Waweru, C., & Gray, D. (2009). Long-term weight loss from lifestyle intervention benefits blood pressure? A systematic review. *Hypertension, 54*(4), 756-762.

Berwick, D.M., Nolan, T.W., & Whittington, J. (2008). The triple aim: Care, health, and cost. *Health Affairs, 27*(3), 759-769.

Beutler, E., & Waalen, J. (2006). The definition of anemia: What is the lower limit of normal of the blood hemoglobin concentration? *Blood, 107*(5), 1747-1750.

Beutler, E., & West, C. (2005). Hematologic differences between African-Americans and whites: the roles of iron deficiency and α-thalassemia on hemoglobin levels and mean corpuscular volume. *Blood, 106*(2), 740-745.

Block, G.A., Wheeler, D.C., Persky, M.S., Kestenbaum, B., Ketteler, M., Spiegel, D.M., … Chertow, G.M. (2012). Effects of phosphate binders in moderate CKD. *Journal of the American Society of Nephrology, 23*(8), 1407-1415.

Bruno, G., Merletti, F., Biggeri, A., Bargero, G., Ferrero, S., Pagano, G., & Perin, P. C. (2003). Progression to overt nephropathy in type 2 diabetes: The Casale Monferrato Study. *Diabetes Care, 26*(7), 2150-2155.

Caiulo, V., Caiulo, S., Gargasole, C., Chiriaco, G., Latini, G., Cataldi, L., & Mele, G. (2012). Ultrasound mass screening for congenital anomalies of the kidney and urinary tract. *Pediatric Nephrology, 27*, 949-953. doi:10.1007/s00467-011-2098-0

Camicia, M., Chamberlain, B., Finnie, R.R., Nalle, M., Lindeke, L.L., Lorenz, L., Hain, D., … McMenamin, P. (2013). The value of nursing care coordination: A white paper of the American Nurses Association. *Nursing Outlook, 61*(6), 490.

Casserly, L.F., Chow, N., Ali, S., Gottlieb, D.J., Epstein, L.J., & Kaufman, J.S. (2001). Proteinuria in obstructive sleep apnea. *Kidney International, 60*(4), 1484-1489.

Centers for Disease Control and Prevention (CDC). (2010). *National chronic kidney disease fact sheet: General information and national estimates on chronic kidney disease in the United States, 2010.* Atlanta: U.S. Department of Health and Human Services. Retrieved from http://www.cdc.gov/diabetes/pubs/factsheets/kidney.htm

Centers for Disease Control and Prevention (CDC). (2011). *Chronic kidney disease surveillance system.* Atlanta: U.S. Department of Health and Human Services. Retrieved from http://www.cdc.gov/ckd

Centers for Disease Control and Prevention (CDC). (2014). 2014 National diabetes statistics report. Atlanta: U.S. Department of Health and Human Services.Retrieved from http://www.cdc.gov/diabetes/data/statistics/2014statisticsreport.html

Centers for Medicare & Medicaid Services (CMS). (2010). *Coverage of kidney disease patient education services.* Retrieved from http://www.cms.gov/Outreach-and-Education/Medicare-Learning-Network-MLN/MLNMattersArticles/downloads/mm6557.pdf

Centers for Medicare & Medicaid Services (CMS). (2013). *Diabetes-related services.* Fact sheet. Retrieved from www.cms.gov/Outreach-and-Education/Medicare.../DiabetesSvcs.pdf

Cho, J., Lee, S., Reid, E., & Jee, S. (2013). Metabolic syndrome component combinations and chronic kidney disease: The severance cohort study. *Maturitas, 75*(1), 74-80. doi:10.1016/j.maturitas.2013.02.006

Chobanian, A.V., Bakris, G.L., Black, H.R., Cushman, W.C., Green, L.A., Izzo, J.L., … Roccella, E.J. (2003). Seventh report of the Joint National Committee On Prevention, Detection, Evaluation, and Treatment of High Blood Pressure. *Hypertension, 42*(6), 1206-1252.

Couser, W., Remuzzi, G., Mendis, S., & Tonelli, M. (2011). The contribution of chronic kidney disease to the global burden of major noncommunicable diseases. *Kidney International, 80*(12), 1258-1270.

Derose, S., Rutkowski, M., Levin, N., Liu, I., Shi, J., Jacobsen, S., & Crooks, P. (2009). Incidence of end-stage renal disease and death among insured African Americans with chronic kidney disease. *Kidney International, 76, 629-637.* doi:10.1038/ki2009.209

Dronavalli, S., Duka, I., & Bakris, G.L. (2008). The pathogenesis of diabetic nephropathy. *Nature Clinical Practice Endocrinology & Metabolism, 4*(8), 444-452.

Eckardt, K.U., Coresh, J., Devuyst, O., Johnson, R.J., Köttgen, A., Levey, A.S., & Levin, A. (2013). Evolving importance of kidney disease: From subspecialty to global health burden. *The Lancet, 382*(9887), 158-169.

Eckardt, K.U., Scherhag, A., Macdougall, I.C., Tsakiris, D., Clyne, N., Locatelli, F., … Drueke, T.B. (2009). Left ventricular geometry predicts cardiovascular outcomes associated with anemia correction in CKD. *Journal of the American Society of Nephrology, 20*(12), 2651-2660.

Edvardsson, V., Goldfarb, D., Lieske, J., Beara-Lasic, L., Anglani, F., Milliner, D., & Palsson, R. (2013). Hereditary causes of kidney stones and chronic kidney disease. *Pediatric Nephrology, 28*(10), 1923-1942. doi:10.1007/200467-012-2329-z

Epstein, M., & Vaziri, N.D. (2012). Statins in the management of dyslipidemia associated with chronic kidney disease. *Nature Reviews Nephrology, 8*(4), 214-223. doi:10.1038/nrneph.2012.33

Fernández-Juárez, G., Luño, J., Barrio, V., de Vinuesa, S. G., Praga, M., Goicoechea, M., … Oliva, J. (2013). 25 (OH) vitamin D levels and renal disease progression in patients with Type 2 diabetic nephropathy and blockade of the renin-angiotensin system. *Clinical Journal of the American Society of Nephrology, 8*(11), 1870-1876.

Furlong, W.J., Feeny, D.H., Torrance, G.W., & Barr, R.D. (2001). The Health Utilities Index (HUI®) system for assessing health-related quality of life in clinical studies. *Annals of Medicine, 33*(5), 375-384.

Gansevoort, R.T., Correa-Rotter, R., Hemmelgarn, B.R., Jafar, T.H., Heerspink, H.J.L., Mann, J.F., … Wen, C.P. (2013). Chronic kidney disease and cardiovascular risk: Epidemiology, mechanisms, and prevention. *The Lancet. 382*(9889), 339-352.

Hain, D. (2012). Fall prevent in adults undergoing incenter hemodialysis. *Nephrology Nursing Journal, 39*(3), 251-255.

Hain, D.J., & Sandy, D. (2013). Partners in care: Empowerment through shared decision making. *Nephrology Nursing Journal, 40*(2), 153-157.

Harambat, J., van Stralen, K., Kim, J., & Tizard, E. (2012). Epidemiology of chronic kidney disease in children. *Pediatric Nephrology, 27*(3), 363-373. doi:10.1007/200467-011-1939-1

Harper, A., & Power, M. (1998). Development of the World Health Organization WHOQOL-BREF quality of life assessment. *Psychological Medicine, 28*(3), 551-558.

Harper, C.R., & Jacobson, T.A. (2008). Managing dyslipidemia in chronic kidney disease. *Journal of American College of Cardiology, 51*(25), 2375-2384.

Hays, R.D., Amin, N., Apolone, G., Kamberg, C., Kallich, J., Coons, S., ... Mapes, D. (1997). *Kidney disease quality of life short form (KDQOL-SFTM), Version 1.2: A manual for use and scoring.* Retrieved from http://www.rand.org/pubs/papers/P7928z2.html

Heaney, R.P. (2008). Vitamin D in health and disease. *Clinical Journal of the American Society of Nephrology, 3*(5), 1535-1541.

Hemmelgarn, B.R., Zhang, J., Manns, B.J., James, M.T., Quinn, R.R., Ravani, P., ... Tonelli, M. (2010). Nephrology visits and health care resource use before and after reporting estimated glomerular filtration rate. *The Journal of the American Medical Association, 303*(12), 1151-1158.

Holick, M.F., Binkley, N.C., Bischoff-Ferrari, H.A., Gordon, C.M., Hanley, D.A., Heaney, R.P., ... Weaver, C.M. (2011). Evaluation, treatment, and prevention of vitamin D deficiency: An Endocrine Society clinical practice guideline. *The Journal of Clinical Endocrinology & Metabolism, 96*(7), 1911-1930.

Ismail, N., Becker, B., Strzelczyk, P., & Ritz, E. (1999). Renal disease and hypertension in non-insulin-dependent diabetes mellitus. *Kidney International, 55*(1), 1-28.

James, P.A., Oparil, S., Carter, B.L., Cushman, W.C., Dennison-Himmelfarb, C., Handler, J., ... Ortiz, E. (2014). 2014 evidence-based guideline for the management of high blood pressure in adults: Report from the panel members appointed to the Eighth Joint National Committee (JNC 8). *Journal of the American Medical Association, 311*(5), 507-520.

Jha, V., Garcia-Garcia, G., Iseki, K., Li, Z., Naicker, S., Plattner, B., ... Yang, C.W. (2013). Chronic kidney disease: Global dimension and perspectives. *The Lancet, 382*(9888), 260-272.

Johns, M.W. (1991). A new method for measuring daytime sleepiness: The Epworth sleepiness scale. *Sleep, 14*(6), 540-545.

Johns, M.W. (1992). Reliability and factor analysis of the Epworth Sleepiness Scale. *Sleep, 15*(4), 376-381.

Johns, M.W. (1994) Sleepiness in different situations measured by the Epworth Sleepiness Scale. *Sleep, 17*(8), 703-710.

Jones, G. (2007). Expanding role for vitamin D in chronic kidney disease: Importance of blood 25-OH-D levels and extra-renal 1alpha-hydroxylase in the classical and nonclassical actions of 1alpha, 25-dihydroxyvitamin D(3). *Seminars in Dialysis, 20*(4), 316-324.

Juraschek, S.P., Kovell, L.C., Miller III, E.R., & Gelber, A.C. (2013, June). Association of kidney disease with prevalent gout in the United States in 1988–1994 and 2007–2010. *Seminars in Arthritis and Rheumatism, 42*(6), 551-561. doi:10.1016/j.semarthrit.2012.09.009

Kang, D.H, & Chen, W. (2011). Uric acid and chronic kidney disease: New understanding of an old problem. *Seminars in Nephrology, 31*(5), 447-452.

Kasiske, B.L. (1998). Hyperlipidemia in patients with chronic renal disease. *American Journal of Kidney Disease, 32*(5 Suppl. 3), S142-156.

Katakam, R., Brukamp, K., & Townsend, R.R. (2008). What is the proper workup of a patient with hypertension? *Cleveland Clinic Journal of Medicine, 75*(8), 663-672.

Kennedy, S., Bailey, R., & Kainer, G. (2012). Causes and outcome of late referral of children who develop end-stage kidney disease. *Journal of Paediatrics and Child Health, 48*(3), 253-258. doi:10.1111/j.1440-1754.2011.02254.x

Kidney Disease Improving Global Outcomes (KDIGO) Blood Pressure Workgroup (2012a). KDIGO clinical practice guidelines for the management of blood pressure in chronic kidney disease. *Kidney International Supplements, 2*(5), 337-414.

Kidney Disease: Improving Global Outcomes (KDIGO). (2012b). Anemia Work Group. KDIGO clinical practice guideline for anemia in chronic kidney disease. *Kidney International Supplements, 2*(4), 279-335.

Kidney Disease Improving Global Outcomes (KDIGO). (2013a). CKD Work Group. KDIGO clinical practice guideline for the evaluation and management of chronic kidney disease. *Kidney International Supplements, 3*(1), 1-150.

Kidney Disease Improving Global Outcomes (KDIGO). (2013b). CKD Work Group. KDIGO 2012 clinical practice guideline for lipid management in chronic kidney disease. *Kidney International Supplements, 3*(3), 259-305.

Kroenke, K., Spitzer, R.L., & Williams, J.B. (2003). The patient health questionnaire-2: Validity of a two-item depression screener. *Medical Care, 41*, 1284-1292.

Lavie, L. (2003). Obstructive sleep apnoea syndrome – An oxidative stress disorder. *Sleep Medicine Reviews, 7*(1), 35-51.

Laville, M., & Juillard, L. (2010). Contrast-induced acute kidney injury: How should at-risk patients be identified and managed? *Journal of Nephrology, 23*(4), 387-398.

Mahmoodi, B.K., Matsushita, K., Woodward, M., Blankestijn, P.J., Cirillo, M., Ohkubo, T., ... Astor, B.C. (2012). Associations of kidney disease measures with mortality and end-stage renal disease in individuals with and without hypertension: A meta-analysis. *The Lancet, 380*(9854), 1649-1661.

Martin, K.J., & González, E.A. (2007). Metabolic bone disease in chronic kidney disease. *Journal of the American Society of Nephrology, 18*(3), 875-885.

McFarlane, S.I., Chen, S.C., Whaley-Connell, A.T., Sowers, J.R., Vassalotti, J.A., Salifu, M.O., ... Norris, K.C. (2008). Prevalence and associations of anemia of CKD: Kidney early evaluation program (KEEP) and National health and nutrition examination survey (NHANES) 1999-2004. *American Journal of Kidney Diseases, 51*(4), S46-S55.

Mehrotra, R., Kermah, D. A., Salusky, I.B., Wolf, M.S., Thadhani, R.I., Chiu, Y.W., ... Norris, K.C. (2009). Chronic kidney disease, hypovitaminosis D, and mortality in the United States. *Kidney International, 76*(9), 977-983.

Mindell, J., Moody, A., Ali, A., & Hirani, V. (2013). Using longitudinal data from the Health Survey for England to resolve discrepancies in thresholds for haemoglobin in older adults. *British Journal of Haematology, 160*(3), 368-376.

Mogensen, C.E., Christensen, C.K., & Vittinghus, E. (1983). The stages in diabetic renal disease: With emphasis on the stage of incipient diabetic nephropathy. *Diabetes, 32*(Suppl. 2), 64-78.

Morrow, L.E., & Malesker, M.A. (2013) Acid-base disturbances. In Chisholm, M.A., Wells, B.G., Schwinghammer, T.L., Malone, P. M., Kolesar, J.M. & Dipiro, J. T. *Pharmacotherapy: Principles and practice* (3rd ed.). New York: McGraw-Hill.

Munar, M.Y., & Singh, H. (2007). Drug dosing adjustments in patients with chronic kidney disease. *American Family Physician, 75*(10), 1487-1496.

Muntner, P., He, J., Astor, B.C., Folsom, A.R., & Coresh, J. (2005). Traditional and nontraditional risk factors predict coronary heart disease in chronic kidney disease: Results from the atherosclerosis risk in communities study. *Journal of the American Society of Nephrology, 16*(2), 529-538.

Murphree, D.D., & Thelen, S.M. (2010). Chronic kidney disease in primary care. *The Journal of the American Board of Family Medicine, 23*(4), 542-550.

National Kidney Foundation (NKF). (2002a). *KDOQI clinical practice guidelines for chronic kidney disease: Evaluation, classification, and stratification. Part 4. Definition and classification of stages of chronic kidney disease.* Retrieved from http://www.kidney.org/sites/default/files/docs/ckd_evaluation_classification_stratification.pdf

National Kidney Foundation (NKF). (2002b). *KDOQI clinical practice guidelines for chronic kidney disease: Evaluation, classification, and stratification. Part 5. Evaluation of laboratory measurements for clinical assessment of kidney disease. Guideline 6. Markers of chronic kidney disease other than proteinuria.* Retrieved from http://www.kidney.org/sites/default/files/docs/ckd_evaluation_classification_stratification.pdfv

National Kidney Foundation (NKF). (2003). KDOQI clinical practice guidelines for managing dyslipidemia in patients with kidney disease. *American Journal of Kidney Diseases, 41*(4, Suppl. 3), I-IV, S1-S91.

National Kidney Foundation (NKF). (2012). KDOQI clinical practice guideline for diabetes and CKD: 2012 update. *American Journal of Kidney Diseases, 60*(5), 850-886.

Neter, J.E., Stam, B.E., Kok, F.J., Grobbee, D.E., & Geleijnse, J.M. (2003). Influence of weight reduction on blood pressure: A meta-analysis of randomized controlled trials. *Hypertension, 42*(5), 878-884.

None, N., America, K.P., Funnell, M.M., Laffel, L., Center, J.D., Marks, J.B., ... None, V.N. (2014). Professional practice committee for the 2014 clinical practice recommendations. *Diabetes Care, 37*(Suppl. 1), S154-155. doi:10.2337/dc14-S154

Obermayr, R.P., Temml, C., Gutjahr, G., Knechtelsdorfer, M., Oberbauer, R., & Klauser-Braun, R. (2008). Elevated uric acid increases the risk for kidney disease. *Journal of the American Society of Nephrology, 19*(12), 2407-2413.

Palmer, S., Vecchio, M., Craig, J.C., Tonelli, M., Johnson, D.W., Nicolucci, A., ... Strippoli, G.F. (2013). Prevalence of depression in chronic kidney disease: Systematic review and meta-analysis of observational studies. *Kidney International, 84*(1), 179-191.

Peralta, C.A., Jacobs, Jr., D.R., Katz, R., Ix, J.H., Madero, M., Duprez, D.A., ... Shlipak, M.G. (2012). Association of pulse pressure, arterial elasticity, and endothelial function with kidney function decline among adults with estimated GFR > 60 mL/min/1.73 m²: The multi-ethnic study of atherosclerosis (MESA). *American Journal of Kidney Diseases, 59*(1), 41-49.

Perazella, M.A., & Shirali, A. (2014). Kidney disease caused by therapeutic agents. In S.J. Gilbert, & D.E. Weiner (Eds.), *National Kidney Foundation's primer on kidney disease* (6th ed.). Philadelphia: Elsevier Saunders.

Perumal, K. & Argekar, P. (2011). Acid-base status. In J.T. Daugirdas (Ed.), *Handbook of chronic kidney disease management.* Philadelphia: Wolters Kluwer; Lippincott Williams & Wilkins.

Pickering, T.G., Hall, J.E., Appel, L.J., Falkner, B.E., Graves, J., Hill, M.N., ... Subcommittee of Professional and Public Education of the American Heart Association Council on High Blood Pressure Research (2005). Recommendations for blood pressure measurement in humans and experimental animals: Part 1: Blood pressure measurement in humans: A statement for professionals from the Subcommittee of Professional and Public Education of the American Heart Association Council on High Blood Pressure Research. *Hypertension, 45*(1),142-61.

Pilz, S., Tomaschitz, A., Friedl, C., Amrein, K., Drechsler, C., Ritz, E., ... März, W. (2011). Vitamin D status and mortality in chronic kidney disease. *Nephrology Dialysis Transplantation, 26*(11), 3603-3609.

Pillitteri, A. (2010). Psychological and physiological changes in pregnancy. In A. Pillitteri (Ed.), *Maternal and child health nursing* (6th ed., pp. 237-240). Philadelphia: Wolters Kluwer Lippincott Williams & Wilkins.

Poole, J.H. (2014). Hypertensive disorders of pregnancy. In K.R. Simpson & P.A. Creehan (Eds.), *Perinatal nursing* (4th ed., pp. 122-142). Philadelphia: Wolters Kluwer Lippincott Williams & Wilkins.

Quarles, L.D. (2014). Bone disorders in chronic kidney diseases. In S.J. Gilbert, & D.E. Weiner (Eds.), *National Kidney Foundation premier on kidney disease* (6th ed., pp. 476-487). Philadelphia: Elsevier Saunders.

Recio-Mayoral, A., Banerjee, D., Streather, C., & Kaski, J.C. (2011). Endothelial dysfunction, inflammation and atherosclerosis in chronic kidney disease – A cross-sectional study of predialysis, dialysis and kidney–transplantation patients. *Atherosclerosis, 216*(2), 446-451.

Reichel, H., Deibert, B., Schmidt-Gayk, H., & Ritz, E. (1991). Calcium metabolism in early chronic renal failure: Implications for the pathogenesis of hyperparathyroidism. *Nephrology Dialysis Transplantation, 6*(3), 162-169.

Romero-Aroca, P., Baget-Bernaldiz, M., Reyes-Torres, J., Fernandez-Ballart, J., Plana-Gil, N., Mendez-Marin, I., & Pareja-Rios, A. (2012). Relationship between diabetic retinopathy, microalbuminuria and overt nephropathy, and twenty-year incidence follow-up of a sample of type 1 diabetic patients. *Journal of Diabetes and Its Complications, 26*(6), 506-12.

Sacks, F.M., Svetkey, L.P., Vollmer, W.M., Appel, L.J., Bray, G.A., Harsha, D., ... Cutler, J.A. (2001). Effects on blood pressure of reduced dietary sodium and the dietary approaches to stop hypertension (DASH) diet. *New England Journal of Medicine, 344*(1), 3-10.

Sanghavi, S., & Vassalotti, J.A. (2014). Practical use of home blood pressure monitoring in chronic kidney disease. *Cardiorenal Medicine, 4*(2), 113-122.

Schiffrin, E.L., Lipman, M.L., & Mann, J.F. (2007) Chronic kidney disease: Effects on the cardiovascular system. *Circulation, 116*(1), 85-97.

Shlipak, M.G., Fried, L.F., Cushman, M., Manolio, T.A., Peterson, D., Stehman-Breen, C., ... Psaty, B. (2005). Cardiovascular mortality risk in chronic kidney disease. *The Journal of the American Medical Association, 293*(14), 1737-1745.

Stenvinkel, P., Carrero, J.J., Axelsson, J., Lindholm, B., Heimbürger, O., & Massy, Z. (2008). Emerging biomarkers for evaluating cardiovascular risk in the chronic kidney disease patient: How do new pieces fit into the uremic puzzle? *Clinical Journal of the American Society of Nephrology, 3*(2), 505-521.

Stevens, L.A., Stoycheff, N., & Levey, A.S. (2009). Staging and management of chronic kidney disease. In S.J. Gilbert & D.E. Weiner (Eds.), *National Kidney Foundation primer on kidney disease* (6th ed., pp. 436-445). Philadelphia: Elsevier Saunders.

Stevens, L., Claybon, M., Schmid, C., Chen, J., Horio, M., Imai, E., ... Levey, A. (2011). Evaluation of the chronic kidney disease epidemiology collaboration equation for estimating the glomerular filtration rate in multiple ethnicities. *Kidney International, 79*(5), 555-562. doi:10/1038/ki.2010.462

Stokes, G.S. (2009). Management of hypertension in the elderly patient. *Clinical Interventions in Aging, 4*, 379-389.

Suarez, M.L.G., Thomas, D.B., Barisoni, L., & Fornoni, A. (2013). Diabetic nephropathy: Is it time yet for routine kidney biopsy? *World Journal of Diabetes, 4*(6), 245-255.

Tangri, N., Stevens, L.A., Griffith, J., Tighiouart, H., Djurdjev, O., Naimark, D., ... Levey, A.S. (2011). A predictive model for progression of chronic kidney disease to kidney failure. *Journal of the American Medical Associaiton, 305*(15), 1553-1559.

Toto, R.D., Greene, T., Hebert, L.A., Hiremath, L., Lea, J.P., Lewis, J.B., ... Wang, X. (2010). Relationship between body mass index and proteinuria in hypertensive nephrosclerosis: Results from the African American Study of Kidney Disease and Hypertension (AASK) cohort. *American Journal of Kidney Diseases, 56*(5), 896-906.

Turek, N.F., Ricardo, A.C., & Lash, J.P. (2012). Sleep disturbances as nontraditional risk factors for development and progression of CKD: Review of the evidence. *American Journal of Kidney Diseases, 60*(5), 823-833.

Tyson, C.C., Nwankwo, C., Lin, P.H., & Svetkey, L.P. (2012). The dietary approaches to stop hypertension (DASH) eating pattern in special populations. *Current Hypertension Reports, 14*(5), 388-396.

U.S. Preventive Services Task Force. (2012). Screening for chronic kidney disease: U.S. Preventive Services Task Force recommendation statement. *Annals of Internal Medicine, 157*(8), 567-570.

U.S. Renal Data Sytem (2013). *USRDS 2013 annual data report: Atlas of chronic kidney disease and end-stage renal disease in the United States.* Retrieved from http://www.usrds.org/atlas.aspx

van Bussel, B.C., Schouten, F., Henry, R.M., Schalkwijk, C.G., de Boer, M.R., Ferreira, I., ... Stehouwer, C.D. (2011). Endothelial dysfunction and low-grade inflammation are associated with greater arterial stiffness over a 6-year period. *Hypertension, 58*(4), 588-595.

Vellanski, K. & Hou, S. (2014). The kidney in pregnancy. In S.J. Gilbert & D.E. Weiner (Eds.), *National Kidney Foundation primer on kidney disease* (6th ed., pp. 427-436). Philadelphia: Elsevier Saunders.

Viswanathan, M., Golin, C. E., Jones, C. D., Ashok, M., Blalock, S. J., Wines, R. C., ... Lohr, K. N. (2012). Interventions to improve adherence to self-administered medications for chronic diseases in the United States: A systematic review. *Annals of Internal Medicine, 157*(11), 785-795.

Wauters, J.P., Lameire, N., Davison, A., & Ritz, E. (2005). Why patients with progressing kidney disease are referred late to the nephrologist: On causes and proposals for improvement. *Nephrology Dialysis Transplantation, 20*(3), 490-496.

Weber, M.A., Schiffrin, E.L., White, W.B., Mann, S., Lindholm, L.H., Kenerson, J.G., ... Harrap, S.B. (2014). Clinical practice guidelines for the management of hypertension in the community. *The Journal of Clinical Hypertension, 16*(1), 14-26.

Weisbord, S.D., Mor, M.K., Resnick, A.L., Hartwig, K.C., Sonel, A.F., Fine, M.J., & Palevsky, P.M. (2008). Prevention, incidence, and outcomes of contrast-induced acute kidney injury. *Archives of Internal Medicine, 168*(12), 1325-1332.

Williams-Joseph, N., Elwyn, G., & Edwards, A. (2014). Knowledge is not power for patients: A systematic review and thematic synthesis of patient-reported barriers and facilitators to shared decision making. *Patient Education and Counseling, 94*(3), 291-309.

Winkelmayer, W.C., & Chertwo, C. (2010). Off-label use of phosphate binders in non-dialysis dependent CKD. *American Journal of Kidney Disease, 56*(5), 813-816.

Wish, J.B. (2014). Anemia and other hematological complications of chronic kidney disease. In S.J. Gilbert & D.E. Weiner (Eds.), *National Kidney Foundation primer on kidney disease* (6th ed.). Philadelphia: Elsevier Saunders.

World Health Organization. (2012). *World Health Statistics 2012.* Retrieved from http://www.who.int/gho/publications/world_health_statistics/2012/en/index.html

Yamauchi, M., & Kimura, H. (2008). Oxidative stress in obstructive sleep apnea: Putative pathways to the cardiovascular complications. *Antioxidants & Redox Signaling, 10*(4), 755-768.

Zhang, Z., Yuan, W., Sun, L., Szeto, F.L., Wong, K.E., Li, X., ... Li, Y.C. (2007). 1, 25-Dihydroxyvitamin D3 targeting of NF-κB suppresses high glucose-induced MCP-1 expression in mesangial cells. *Kidney International, 72*(2), 193-201.

CHAPTER **3**

Individualizing the Care for Those with Kidney Disease

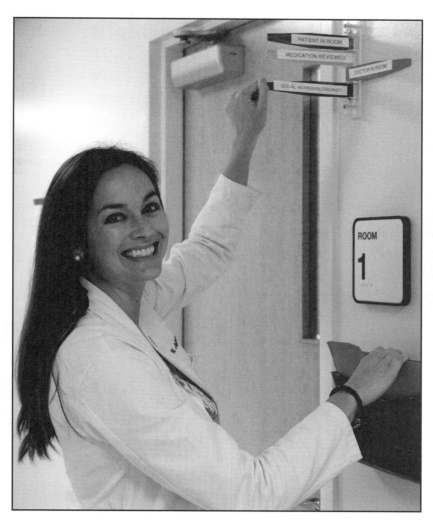

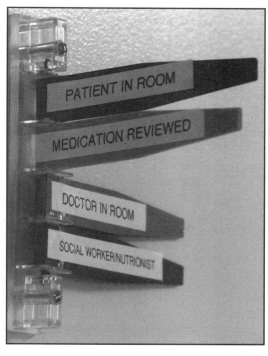

Chapter Editor
Donna Bednarksi, MSN, RN, ANP-BC, CNN, CNP
Authors
Donna Bednarski, MSN, RN, ANP-BC, CNN, CNP
Loretta Jackson Brown, PhD, RN, CNN
Molly Cahill, MSN, RN, APRN, BC, ANP-C, CNN
Deb Castner, MSN, APRN, ACNP, CNN
Daniel Diroll, MA, BSN, BS, RN
Cheryl L. Groenhoff, MSN, MBA, RN, CNN
Lisa Hall, MSSW, LICSW
Lois Kelley, MSW, LSW, ACSW, NSW-C
Sharon Longton, BSN, RN, CNN, CCTC

CHAPTER **3**
Individualizing the Care for Those with Kidney Disease

This offering for **2.1 contact hours** is provided by the American Nephrology Nurses' Association (ANNA).

American Nephrology Nurses' Association is accredited as a provider of continuing nursing education by the American Nurses Credentialing Center Commission on Accreditation.

ANNA is a provider approved by the California Board of Registered Nursing, provider number CEP 00910.

This CNE offering meets the continuing nursing education requirements for certification and recertification by the Nephrology Nursing Certification Commission (NNCC).

To be awarded contact hours for this activity, read this chapter in its entirety. Then complete the CNE evaluation found at **www.annanurse.org/corecne** and submit it; or print it, complete it, and mail it in. Contact hours are not awarded until the evaluation for the activity is complete.

Example of reference in APA format. Use author of the section being cited. This example is based on Section E – Caring for Veterans.

Brown, L.J. (2015). Individualizing the care for those with kidney disease: Caring for veterans. In C.S. Counts (Ed.), *Core curriculum for nephrology nursing: Module 2. Physiologic and psychosocial basis for nephrology nursing practice* (6th ed., pp. 189-254). Pitman, NJ: American Nephrology Nurses' Association.

Interpreted: Section author(s). (Date). Title of chapter: Title of section. In …

Cover photo by Counts/Morganello.

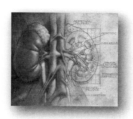

CHAPTER 3

Individualizing the Care for Those with Kidney Disease

Purpose

The overall purpose of this chapter is to provide nephrology nurses with information that enables them to deliver individualized care to patients with kidney disease. The chapter begins with the psychosocial impact of chronic kidney disease (CKD) on patients, identifying implications for practice, and exploring the influence of spirituality on adjustment to illness.

The chapter then diverts attention to the cultural and linguistic diversity of the United States and the challenges those differences bring to health care. Nurses caring for patients from unfamiliar sociocultural backgrounds have much to consider in understanding the needs of those patients and incorporating culturally competent care into their practice.

The chapter goes on to present the components of the teaching–learning process to assist nurses in the implementation of patient and family education. It is essential that nurses refine the process so it is effective and efficient in producing the desired patient outcomes and improving the patients' quality of life. The importance of patient and family engagement is identified as a priority within health care, and the chapter delivers information helpful in understanding the overall impact.

Attention is then given to the unique care needs of U.S. Veterans, and the distinct assessment and treatment approaches required in their care. The chapter offers basic information about financing the treatment of kidney disease and kidney failure, including financial burdens and resources available to help.

The next section addresses exercise guidelines as a component of care for all patients with kidney disease, the result being increased, safe participation in physical activity. Due to the high incidence of comorbidities in the CKD population, patients should receive a physical exam and permission from their primary provider/nephrologist/cardiologist (Smart et al., 2013) before engaging in an exercise program. An exercise program should be initiated in collaboration with the interdisciplinary team.

The final section reviews advance care planning and end-of-life issues and management. End-of-life care covers evidence-based predictors of morbidity and mortality and ethical considerations. Hospice is defined, including Medicare hospice benefits regulations, as well as a review of and management suggestions for symptoms seen at the end of life for the patient with CKD.

Objectives

Upon completion of this chapter, the learner will be able to:
1. Describe the psychosocial impact of kidney disease and kidney failure.
2. Define culture and culturally competent services for patients with kidney disease.
3. State how the stresses of war and deployment impact the health and well-being of military family members.
4. Summarize the definition of patient and family engagement.
5. Define the teaching–learning process, differentiating between teaching and learning.
6. Explain Medicare benefits including eligibility, when it starts and ends, and coverage for dialysis and transplantation.
7. Discuss the health benefits of increased physical activity.
8. Describe advance care planning as it relates to the patient with kidney disease.

SECTION A
Psychosocial Impact and Spirituality
Lisa Hall

I. Diagnosis of chronic illness: The patient's experience.

A. Lifestyle changes. Patients with chronic kidney disease (CKD) and kidney failure experience multiple losses, disruptions in usual valued activities and routines, and psychosocial risks associated with diagnosis and treatment. They require comprehensive services at various stages throughout the course of their illness and treatment. Some of the losses and other lifestyle changes related to CKD and its treatment are listed below.

1. Losses.
   a. Health.
   b. Libido, sexuality, and reproduction issues.
   c. Independence and autonomy (especially with in-center hemodialysis).
   d. Cognition.
   e. Physical strength.
   f. Body parts (amputation).
   g. Income and financial security.
   h. Sleep.
   i. Control over schedules, diet, fluid, and other lifestyle restrictions. A qualitative study by Ravenscroft (2005) found that the intrusion of hemodialysis on time was a major issue to participants. This included not only time spent on actual treatment but time spent on travel, waiting before and after treatments, preparing meals or snacks, and, in some instances, resting after treatments. The total time varied from approximately 6 hours to, for one participant, over 8 hours.

2. Vocational and economic.
   a. Ability to pay for treatment.
   b. Maintaining a job.
   c. Managing reduction in income related to change in employment status.
   d. Other financial stressors.

3. Social role.
   a. Social status.
   b. Loss of familial role functions.
   c. Feelings of isolation.
   d. Decrease in social contacts.
   e. Loss of familiar role identities.

4. Somatic symptoms.
   a. Nausea.
   b. Restless leg syndrome.
   c. Insomnia.
   d. Uremia.
   e. Anemia.

5. Pain.
   a. Diabetic neuropathy.
   b. Leg cramps.
   c. Pain with insertion of needles.
   d. Chronic pain such as back pain, exacerbated by being in the dialysis chair.

6. Lowered self-esteem. Any combination of the lifestyle changes mentioned in this section can result in lowered self-esteem.

7. Body image issues. Body image refers to the mental picture and attitudes one has toward his/her body and its structure and function.
   a. A unique kind of stressor in the population with kidney failure that is not shared by others with different chronic diseases is the presence of a fistula, graft, or catheter used to provide access to the circulatory system during hemodialysis (Al-Arabi, 2006).
   b. Gokal and Hutchison (2002) found that some patients with kidney failure worry about the integrity of the vascular access, fear that the access becomes damaged, and view it as an embarrassing disfigurement. Patients with CKD often delay vascular access placement due to these same concerns.
   c. Other aspects of kidney disease that may affect body image include ammonia breath, skin changes, hair changes, weight loss or gain, and surgical scars.

8. Tasked with decisions about treatment options.

B. Coping. True coping requires a person to give up previously held secure states of mind and adapt to the changes in circumstances (Mazella, 2004). Following are common themes related to coping with CKD and its treatment.

1. Denial regarding medical status is common among both CKD and patients whose kidneys have recently failed (CKD stage 5).
   a. Despite knowing about kidney failure, starting dialysis is frequently described as a surprise.
   b. Denial is one defense mechanism that can play an important role in the patients' ability to endure their illness (help them to cope).
   c. It may take time to let go of their past "ideal" state. However, it must be addressed when it interferes with their lives. Patients with CKD who are in denial may delay seeking treatment until they are symptomatic.

2. Grief. Bereavement over losses can be complicated by guilt or regret regarding health behaviors that may have led to progression of kidney disease.

3. Concerns about worsening health and facing issues of mortality.

4. Baseline coping prior to CKD diagnosis.
   a. Patients with CKD often have numerous comorbid conditions (such as diabetes,

hypertension, cardiovascular disease, and lupus) and related social concerns.

    b. Ravenscroft's (2005) review of the literature on diabetes and kidney failure indicated that the psychosocial issues of chronic illness (such as burden, fear, uncertainty, control, dependency, loss, depression, and guilt) are compounded in these individuals due to the preexistence of diabetes.

5. Dependency issues. These issues, including a feeling of being a burden on loved ones, can be debilitating for patients and can affect their self-esteem.

    a. When patients go on dialysis, or when they are soon to transition into therapy, they see their lives becoming controlled by a dependence on medical technology.

    b. This dependency can carry over into the relationship with healthcare providers, particularly if the patients are not provided with the information and opportunity to have an active role in their own care.

6. Stress.

7. Behavior changes. In response to the many lifestyle changes, many patients exhibit changes in behavior.

    a. Waiting to get on the dialysis machine, physical pain of cannulation, and other intrusions related to kidney failure can cause unhappiness, lack of cooperation, and complaining.

    b. Staff members tend to think of these patients as difficult, but their behaviors should be considered in the context of their adjustment phase.

C. Mood changes.

1. Depression. Depression has been shown to be a considerable problem for both patients with CKD and kidney failure.

    a. A recent study found that major depressive episode is common in patients with earlier stages of CKD (21% prevalence), before the onset of kidney failure and dialysis therapy (Hedayati et al., 2009).

    b. Depression in this population is a legitimate, expectable, and understandable reaction to a dramatic lifestyle change.

    c. It is the most commonly encountered psychological complication of chronic dialysis patients.

    d. Depression may pose increased risk for the development of poor kidney function and clinical progression to CKD stage 5 (Kop et al., 2011).

    e. The patient new to dialysis may require an initial period of adjusting. However, for some patients, the depression becomes chronic. If patients have the following symptoms, which

last for more than 2 weeks, or interfere with activities of daily life, they may be depressed.

    (1) Feeling sad or irritable most of the time.

    (2) Feeling worthless or guilty.

    (3) Feeling hopeless or like giving up.

    (4) Unable to enjoy things.

    (5) Difficulty remembering things, indecisiveness, or problems with concentrating.

    (6) Irritable or angry feelings.

    (7) Recurrent thoughts of suicide.

2. Adjustment disorder. Depression should be distinguished from adjustment disorder, which is sometimes called *situational depression*. An adjustment disorder is an intense reaction to an identifiable life stressor, or more distress than would be expected. An adjustment disorder can significantly impair social and work function.

3. Anxiety. Patients with CKD often express anxiety about their level of functioning once they initiate dialysis, particularly those who received little orientation before beginning treatment.

    a. Common concerns include ability to care for self, ability to perform usual daily tasks, concerns about feeling ill all the time, the amount of time that dialysis takes from normal daily routines, decreased feelings of control, and financial status (bills, cost of treatment and medications, ability to work).

    b. Anxiety can be quite normal, but problematic if protracted or excessive.

II. Impact on the caregiver.

A. Familial roles. When change occurs with one family member, the others have to step in and fill a role with which they may not be comfortable or for which they may not feel equipped. In relation to kidney disease, the caregiver is expected to perform some supportive functions. The caregiver is burdened with the following.

1. The daily demands of providing care and support.

2. Assisting with planning and preparation of the kidney diet.

3. Providing or arranging transportation.

4. Coping with mood and behavior changes.

B. Lifestyle. All of the lifestyle adjustments, losses, and stressors that affect patients are also observed by or experienced by the caregiver and can take their toll.

1. The impact of this burden may result in feelings of guilt, hopelessness, isolation, a loss of freedom to pursue personal and recreational interests, and fatigue, all of which can be the result of this added role demand (Campbell, 1998).

2. Caring for a person with a chronic illness impacts the caregiver's psychological and physical well-

being – their quality of life. This often manifests itself in experiences of depression and fatigue (LoGiudice et al., 1998).

3. Changes in family dynamics and disruptions in usual routines can impact relationships. Participants in Ravenscroft's (2005) qualitative study talked about intrusion of kidney failure into intimate relationships (sexual) and family relationships, including those with children.

III. Implications for practice.

A. Social and emotional problems that go unaddressed can manifest in numerous problems.
   1. Those manifestations can include:
      a. Substance abuse problems.
      b. Thought, mood, and personality disturbances.
      c. Impaired functioning because of anxiety, depression, or mania.
      d. Somatic complaints with no organic basis.
      e. Suicidal ideation or attempt.
      f. Eating disorders.
      g. Sexual dysfunction.
      h. Persistent psychological distress (anxiety, depression, hopelessness).
      i. Behavior problems and nonadherence to treatment (or treatment dropout).
   2. The impact of psychosocial factors on the outcome of patients with kidney disease has been receiving increased attention.
      a. The progressive increase in both the incidence and prevalence of patients with kidney failure has focused research interest on those aspects of care which affect patient outcomes and are potentially amenable to modification to improve these outcomes (Finkelstein & Finkelstein, 2000).
      b. In patients with kidney disease, treatment nonadherence and psychological distress are common and increasingly recognized as contributing to excess morbidity and mortality.

B. CKD education. Early intervention and education before kidney disease progresses are important.
   1. Patients who receive CKD education have higher mood scores, fewer mobility problems, fewer functional disabilities, a lower level of anxiety and are enabled to make decisions regarding modality type (Klang et al., 1999).
   2. Formal educational interventions in patients with CKD can delay the need for dialysis (Devins et al., 2003).
   3. It has also been noted to facilitate continued employment and aid in modality selection (Golper, 2001).
   4. Some dialysis facilities and nephrology practices use formal classroom formats to educate patients

while others use one-to-one meetings.
   5. Tours of the dialysis unit, including the home therapy program, provide the opportunities for the patient to see the treatment process and to ask questions of staff and patients. This allows the patient time to adjust to the eventual need for dialysis.
   6. Support. Support for patients and their families is available through the following.
      a. Patient organizations such as American Association of Kidney Patients (AAKP), National Kidney Foundation (NKF), American Kidney Fund (AKF), and Renal Support Network (RNS).
      b. Peer support is helpful in alleviating stress.
   7. If there is not a local support group, providers should consider incorporating a support group into their own CKD programs.

C. Transplantation.
   1. Education/referral.
      a. Provision of education about kidney replacement options, including transplantation, is recommended.
      b. Early referral for transplantation is optimal. When patients are listed early, they have fewer barriers to overcome as the disease progresses and symptoms worsen.
      c. The goal is to ensure access to transplantation for every individual who may be eligible.
   2. Coordination of process. Kidney transplantation requires teamwork and communication throughout the process, from the initial referral through the long-term care of the transplanted kidney.
      a. All disciplines should work together to provide optimal quality of life for the patients.
      b. Any barriers to the patients' transplant eligibility should be addressed with each patient by the team.
      c. Individual transplant centers have their own guidelines for selection of appropriate candidates.
      d. Dialysis facilities and the nephrologists, advanced practice registered nurses (APRNs), or physician assistants (PAs) working with patients with CKD can help those who could be kidney transplant candidates with factors that might affect their eligibility for transplant. These factors might include:
         (1) Addressing severe obesity.
         (2) Reinforcing adherence to prescribed medication or therapy.
         (3) Addressing social, emotional, and financial factors related to the ability to function posttransplant.

3. Organ donation. There is a national shortage of deceased donor organs.
   a. In spite of increased efforts at organ recovery and expanding guidelines, the number of patients waiting for a deceased donor kidney continues to grow.
   b. Living donor kidneys have a longer half-life than deceased donor kidneys, creating a significant benefit for the recipient without detriment to the donor. Therefore, transplant centers will make every effort to identify a suitable living donor for each recipient.
   c. There are now many paired exchange programs that help donor/recipient pairs with blood types who are otherwise compatible to find suitable donors.

D. Kidney failure (CKD stage 5).
   1. Participation in self-care and maintenance of an active lifestyle.
      a. Self-management has been defined as the positive efforts of individuals to oversee and participate in their health care to optimize health, prevent complications, control symptoms, marshal medical resources, and minimize the intrusion of the disease into their preferred lifestyles (Curtin & Mapes, 2001).
      b. Curtin et al. (2004) proposed that cooperative/participatory self-management behaviors can minimize the need for protective/proactive strategies. Further, increasing patients' knowledge of kidney disease may have long-term benefits.
      c. Curtin and Mapes (2001) found that the ability of patients on hemodialysis to self-manage aspects of their disease and its treatment may be positively associated with their overall functioning and well-being.
      d. Related research has shown that patients trained for self-care dialysis have higher role function, social function, and emotional well-being than similar patients who receive full care (Meers et al., 1996). Self-care modalities can include peritoneal dialysis, home hemodialysis, or self-cannulation.
   2. Focus on the strengths.
      a. Reinforcement of any positive changes in patient adjustment, lifestyle, or behavior is recommended.
      b. The strengths-based perspective makes several assumptions about the human condition.
         (1) One assumption is that all people have strengths that enable them to move forward.
         (2) Another assumption is that all people are more motivated to move toward things

they want and away from things that they don't want.
         (a) People are more motivated to work toward a goal they have set for themselves than one that an expert has set on their behalf.
         (b) This is self-determination, and when individuals are allowed to determine their own destiny, it is a powerful thing.
      c. The strengths model also assumes that all people have the capacity to change; it does not promise, however, that all will (McFarlane, 2006).
   3. Patient-centered care planning. To the extent possible, involve the patient in interdisciplinary team meetings.
      a. Allow the patient to share his/her perspective on care management and the agreed-upon goals for the patient and team to accomplish.
      b. Placing patients at the helm of the change process and letting them steer their own course has powerful ramifications and can lead to effectual treatment. Henry Ford said, "Whether you think you can or you think you can't, you're right."
      c. In addition, staff training in communication, professionalism, and patient sensitivity is beneficial. Training is available on the DPC (Dialysis Patient and Provider Conflict) tools by contacting your area's ESRD Network. The tools can be used when conflict occurs. To locate the ESRD Network in a particular area, go to http://www.esrdnetworks.org/

E. Considerations for working with caregivers.
   1. Treatment planning and education. Involvement of significant others in the care planning process and provision of education will serve to decrease the isolation the patient feels and bridge any gaps in knowledge about the patient's illness and treatment.
      a. Interactions with healthcare providers are perceived as more positive when there is mutual respect, trust, and collaborative decision making, and when healthcare providers share information with caregivers (Ravencroft, 2005).
      b. Communication and coordination of care are also important when the patient is in a nursing home or other long-term care setting.
   2. Provision of support. Promote early intervention with an identified caregiver. Involve the social worker in addressing family stressors and relationship concerns, including sexual intimacy.
      a. Participants in Ravencroft's 2005 study recalled there had been some discussion of sexual

concerns with healthcare providers, but this had not helped resolve problems. Referral to appropriate resources to address sexual relationships and performance should not be overlooked.

b. Additionally, caregivers should be encouraged to rest when able, use family or community resources, and reward themselves for their efforts.

c. With the number of patients on dialysis increasing each year, the staff is interacting with a growing number of caregivers.
   (1) It is essential that the staff remain sensitive to the burden and demands of family care for patients on dialysis.
   (2) Proactive intervention can help to prevent the conflict that can occur in the dialysis setting.

3. Tips for dealing with disruptive caregivers.
   a. Be certain that facility policies and possible consequences of violation are clearly communicated to caregivers; remember to equally enforce policies for all families.
   b. Be sure to consider the patient's needs and behaviors separate from the caregiver's.
   c. Refer to the social worker for assessment of the caregiver's emotional needs and intervene appropriately. Keep in mind that the controlling behavior on the part of the caregiver is often related to fears and anxiety.

F. Depression.
   1. Background information.
      a. Working with depressed patients can be draining.
      b. Some of these patients have a remarkable capacity for interpersonal insensitivity, manipulative behavior, and excessive demands.
         (1) These patients are often labeled as difficult, and staff often do everything possible to avoid them.
         (2) Unless one has the capacity to step back and reflect on the patient's state of mind, a vicious cycle can develop where a patient's demand or need can lead to an inconsistent or irrational response by the worker who feels taken advantage of or manipulated (Mazella, 2004).
   2. Prevalence. Literature on the topic has demonstrated that depression is highly prevalent in the CKD population and the ESRD setting.
      a. Hedayati et al. (2009) found that 1 in 5 patients with CKD had a major depressive episode.
      b. The 2012 Comprehensive Dialysis Study (USRDS 2012 Annual Data Report) reported that 27% of participants in the study met the criteria for depression.

c. In a 2007 study by Cukor et al., 29% of patients had a current depressive disorder (20% major depression and 9% dysthymia).

d. Depression has been linked to hospitalization and mortality rates (Panigua et al., 2005), an increased level of comorbid conditions, treatment nonadherence, rehabilitation outcomes, and overall patient adjustment.

e. Its prevalence varies widely across studies, which may reflect variation in the criteria and methodology used to diagnose depression.

f. Results from a study by Lopes et al. (2004) concluded:
   (1) Depression is highly prevalent among patients on hemodialysis, but is likely underdiagnosed and undertreated.
   (2) Higher scores on the quality of life (QOL) tool used in the study were significantly and independently associated with higher risk of all-cause death, hospitalization, and withdrawal from dialysis.

g. Kimmel et al. (2000) also linked depression with increased risk of mortality.

h. A national study of incident patients by Boulware et al. (2006) concluded that there is an increased risk for death and cardiovascular disease events in patients with depressive symptoms, particularly patients whose symptoms had persisted longer than 1 year.

3. Impact on outcomes.
   a. Depression can result in diminished motivation and apathy, and lead to a cascade effect of pervasive physical and mental deterioration. Often, when treating chronic illness, the mental components are lost within the context of multiple physiologic problems.
   b. Depression is related closely to nutritional status and could be an independent risk factor for malnutrition (Koo et al., 2005).
   c. It is also associated with poor compliance of fluid restriction and higher weight gain between treatments (Garcia Valderrama et al., 2002).
   d. Patients who are depressed and do not get treatment are also at a higher risk for hospitalization.
   e. Patients with kidney failure who feel they are less in control of their illness tend to cope less effectively and have a lower quality of life (Mapes et al., 2001).
   f. Depression may manifest itself in behaviors such as ignoring treatment recommendations, not taking medicines, skipping treatments, or other self-defeating behaviors.
   g. Many patients do not understand why they are experiencing the symptoms of depression and do not discuss them with their provider.

4. Diagnosis and quality-of-life assessment tools and resources.
   a. Because the patient on dialysis suffers from a variety of physical symptoms, it is easy to confuse them with the somatic symptoms that are commonly associated with depression.
   b. Sleep, sexual dysfunction, appetite changes, and fatigue are not enough to warrant a diagnosis of depression.
   c. Use of QOL assessment tools can be an important step in improving health, decreasing hospitalization, increasing adherence, improving relationship potential, and decreasing mortality rates.
   d. The dialysis social worker can screen the patient for depression and assist with a referral to available treatment.
   e. The following are some tools that clinical social workers can access to help assess the functional status of patients.
      (1) KDQOL-36. The Kidney Disease Quality of Life Survey Short Form (Rand Health, n.d.) is a disease-specific survey that includes generic functioning and well-being plus questions related to kidney disease burden of illness, satisfaction with care, sexual functioning, and more. Social workers can find the survey and associated scoring templates in English and Spanish, online at the KDQOL website: http://www.rand.org/health/surveys_tools/kdqol.html
      (2) The Geriatric Depression Scale (short form)(Aging Clinical Research Center, n.d.). This tool is easy to score, and scores can be prorated to remove the somatic components, such as energy, appetite, etc. A Spanish version is also available at http://web.stanford.edu/~yesavage/GDS.html
      (3) The Beck Depression Inventory Fast Screen for patients with medical conditions. The BDI Fast Screen was constructed to reduce the number of false positives for depression in patients with known biological, medical, or substance abuse problems. The BDI-FS is copyrighted and is available for a fee from various sponsored websites.
      (4) The Center for Epidemiologic Studies Depression Scale (CES-D). The CES-D is a tool that is frequently cited in research for screening of depression in people with kidney failure. Find this tool at http://counsellingresource.com/lib/quizzes/depression-testing/cesd/
      (5) There are numerous other QOL tools, including the nine questions Patient Health Questionnaire (PHQ-9), found at http://www.phqscreeners.com/, and the Cognitive Depression Index, Structured Clinical Interview for the DSM-IV (under revision for DSM-V at the time of publication).
   f. Depression may also be detected by the staff based on their observations and clinical suspicion. Overt symptoms or subjective complaints of depression, failure to respond to treatment, nonadherence, apathy, prior history of depression, anxiety, behavioral changes (especially irritability), and substance abuse are some indicators of depression.

5. Intervention. Depression is a treatable illness.
   a. There is a paucity of data relating to the effectiveness of therapeutic interventions in the treatment of depression occurring in patients with kidney failure.
   b. A recent publication by McCool et al. (2011) indicated that the practice of symptom-targeted intervention (STI) can help manage depression in patients on dialysis. STI can be used in brief intervals with patients while they are receiving dialysis treatments to help reduce depressive symptoms and improve quality of life. A pilot study of this intervention showed significant improvement in patients' mental health.
   c. Many patients feel initially friendlier toward the medical management of their moods while other patients prefer to stay away from any sort of medication management.
   d. The social worker, patient, nurse, APRN, PA, pharmacist, and nephrologist will find the combination that works best for each patient.
   e. Some barriers to treating depression can include:
      (1) The prescriber's comfort level with antidepressant medications.
      (2) The patient's resistance to assessment and/or treatment of depression. Patient resistance can be addressed with an educational handout detailing the benefits of working as a partner with the healthcare team to enhance adjustment to dialysis and quality of life.
   f. Some depressions do not require treatment and are limited to sporadic feelings or moods that change as time goes on. With this type of depression, the focus can be on educating the patient about their kidney disease, or connecting them to resources that can help them feel less isolated.
   g. Becoming involved with a support group or just talking to fellow patients may help to decrease their feelings of despair, loneliness, and isolation.

h. Social support for persons with kidney disease increases the quality of their lives. Two recent trials have focused attention on the impact of alterations in the dialysis treatment regimen on depressive symptoms in patients receiving hemodialysis (Chertow et al., 2010; Jaber et al., 2010). These studies indicate that more frequent hemodialysis can have a beneficial impact on various health related quality-of-life measures. Whatever the modality, treating depression can help patients with the following.
  (1) Relationships.
  (2) Work and other activities.
  (3) Transplant status.
  (4) Nutrition.
  (5) Ability to manage their illness.
  (6) Overall quality of life.

G. Adherence.
  1. Psychosocial barriers to adherence. Possible causes of nonadherence include lack of social support, lack of resources, feeling ineffective, low conscientiousness, high hostility or distrust, poor education about treatment, and untreated emotional or cognitive disorders.
  2. Nonadherence behaviors. These behaviors can include anything from not taking prescribed medications to missing appointments and treatments.
  3. Control issues. In Ravenscroft's 2005 study, participants indicated:
    a. They strove to find a balance between illness and their normal lives.
    b. Adherence to prescribed regimens was not always easy.
      (1) They described choosing, at times, to ignore treatment recommendations or make modifications to minimize the intrusive presence of these regimens.
      (2) This moves away from the more traditional perspective on compliance as patient conformity, to a prescribed regimen from a healthcare provider, and to concepts such as choice, self-management, and alliance.
  4. Tips.
    a. Assess the patient's capacity to understand the risks of nonadherence.
    b. Assess contributing factors to nonadherence.
    c. Provide education to the patient and family on the risks and optimal outcomes.
    d. Have the social worker address fears about treatment and social barriers.
    e. Detect depression early and refer for treatment.
    f. Ask team members to assist the patient in staying on track.
    g. Provide opportunities for the patient to make choices and maintain control.
    h. Develop a partnership with the patient.
    i. Minimize side effects of treatment.
    j. Identify creative ways to motivate the patient.
    k. If the patient's nonadherence disrupts daily operations, adjust schedules.
    l. Reinforce the patient's achievements or successes, no matter how small.

H. Anxiety. Anxiety has been studied extensively in patients with kidney failure on maintenance hemodialysis; however, there is limited research regarding the presence of anxiety in the CKD population. Based on staff observation and antidotal reports, it seems that anxiety is also common in patients who have not yet started dialysis treatments.
  1. Predialysis anxiety was investigated in a study by Iacono (2005), in which 44 people who attended a CKD educational class were evaluated for anxiety before and after attending the class. The class did appear to reduce the level of anxiety for most participants.
  2. Anxiety often occurs in patients with CKD and patients with kidney failure due to an overload of stress related to chronic illness.
  3. Many patients with CKD have an anxious reaction to the prospect of cannulation due to a fear of needle sticks. This anxiety can interfere with their vascular access decisions (i.e., an arteriovenous fistula versus a graft or catheter).
  4. Some interventions for anxiety are as follows.
    a. Reassurance and education.
      (1) Talking through, explaining, or educating patients during procedures in a calm, relaxed voice can help to alleviate anxiety and help patients become active partners in their treatments.
      (2) Allowing patients to discuss their fears and concerns can offer reassurance.
      (3) Assisting patients to assume control whenever possible.
    b. Relaxation. Relaxation techniques can include deep breathing exercises, sighing, humming, and systematic relaxation of muscle groups.
    c. Guided imagery. Guided imagery is a mind-body intervention aimed at easing stress, promoting a sense of peace and tranquility, and changing physiology.
      (1) It involves taking conscious control over imagination and guiding it in a desired direction.
      (2) Mental images are generated to evoke a psychophysiologic state of relaxation or a specific outcome.
      (3) Some indicators for using guided imagery include sleep, pain, grief, depression, anxiety, and side effects such as nausea or vomiting.

(4) Use of guided imagery can also enhance self-confidence and decrease acting out behaviors like substance abuse.

(5) A case study by Birnbaum & Birnbaum (2004) reported that spiritual concerns play a huge role among those who have attempted suicide. Yet spiritual concerns are poorly addressed, if at all, by the patients' psychotherapists.

    (a) The researchers designed a therapeutic group/workshop to incorporate relaxation and mindfulness meditation, along with guided imagery to access inner wisdom.

    (b) Many of the participants reported a significant positive experience, including connection to knowledge that was highly relevant to them in their current state of life.

    (c) The authors concluded that whether such insights were experienced as coming from within (a deeper part of the self) or from an external source (a guiding figure or divine presence), guided meditation appears to be a powerful resource.

(6) Richardson et al. (1997) studied the effects of guided imagery versus group support with breast cancer survivors. After 6 weeks, the imagery group had less stress, more vigor, and better quality of life than the support group.

(7) Guided imagery is used as a standard, complementary therapy to help reduce anxiety, pain, and length of stay among cardiac surgery patients at Inova Fairfax (Halpin et al., 2002).

(8) A study from the National Institute on Aging (Liu & Park, 2004) found that guided imagery helps elderly patients remember to take their medicine (picturing an action improves likelihood of performing the action).

d. Environment. Consider seating changes to reduce anxiety-provoking situations, and avoid seating anxious patients close together. Claustrophobia can be eased by seating the patient near a window or in a seat with a clear view of the exit. Avoid corners.

e. Referral to the MD, APRN, or PA for evaluation for potential medication therapy.

IV. Spirituality. The development of interventions that are relevant and sensitive to the patient's worldview is a foundational principle of cultural competence (Sue et al., 1992).

A. Cultural competence is exhibited by designing interventions that incorporate beliefs and practices from the client's worldview (including spiritual beliefs and practices) into the intervention.
1. The incorporation of the spiritual beliefs and practices of patients may foster increased patient investment in the healing process.
2. Addressing the spiritual needs of patients can assist them in their suffering.
3. The role of spirituality in health care, particularly in chronic illness and end-of-life care, should be recognized and addressed.

B. Spirituality defined. Spirituality is the dimension of a person that seeks to find meaning in his/her life; life as a spiritual journey.
1. Many patients view their spiritual and religious strengths as essential assets that can be tapped to foster healing and growth.
2. Healthcare providers can support patients in their suffering and in the midst of their existential pain.
3. The George Washington Institute for Spirituality and Health (2006, https://smhs.gwu.edu/gwish/) proposes that healthcare providers are entrusted with the care of the physical, the emotional, the social, and the spiritual aspects of their patients in all phases of patients' lives.
    a. Further, healthcare workers need to be aware of the importance of the spiritual needs of those who are ill and suffer; such awareness will lead to compassionate care.
    b. The Institute promotes inclusion of a spirituality component in medical education, research, policy decisions, and healthcare training for all disciplines.

C. Influence of spirituality on adjustment. Patients with kidney failure often suffer deeply in their lives – suffering that is difficult to both witness and experience.
1. A commitment to thinking positively has been noted to be an important activity in preparing oneself for dialysis. Mok, Lai, and Zhang (2004) observed this phenomenon as making an important contribution to ultimate acceptance of the treatment.
2. In 2006, Al-Arabi studied the quality of everyday life among patients on dialysis, and identified a conceptual category that emerged from participants' descriptions of ways they coped with having kidney failure.
    a. One theme that was revealed related to

spirituality. Participants described "trust in God," holding on to faith, and coming to terms with their illness through the knowledge and understanding they had gained with kidney failure and requiring dialysis.

b. Some in the study found a sense of purpose in their lives, inner peace, and the ability to accept being on dialysis by holding on to faith.

c. Prayer became more important to them at the onset of CKD stage 5 and gave them strength to keep going.

3. Patel et al. (2002) studied psychosocial variables, quality of life, and religious beliefs in patients with CKD stage 5 treated with hemodialysis.

a. Psychosocial and medical variables included perception of importance of faith (spirituality), attendance at religious services (religious involvement), the Beck Depression Inventory, Illness Effects Questionnaire, Multidimensional Scale of Perceived Social Support, McGill QOL Questionnaire scores, Karnofsky scores, dialysis dose, and predialysis hemoglobin and albumin levels.

b. The study concluded that religious beliefs are related to perception of depression, illness effects, social support, and QOL independently of the medical aspects of illness.

c. Additionally, the study suggested that religious beliefs may act as coping mechanisms for patients with kidney failure.

D. Assessment. Spiritual values and beliefs can be assessed as part of the routine medical or psychosocial history.

1. The George Washington Institute for Spirituality and Health uses the acronym FICA to help structure questions in taking a spiritual history by healthcare professionals.

a. F – Faith and belief. "Do you consider yourself spiritual or religious?" or "Do you have spiritual beliefs that help you cope with stress?" If the patient responds "No," the practitioner might ask, "What gives your life meaning?" Sometimes patients respond with answers such as family, career, or nature.

b. I – Importance. "What importance does your faith or belief have in your life? Have your beliefs influenced how you take care of yourself in this illness? What role do your beliefs play in regaining your health?"

c. C – Community. "Are you part of a spiritual or religious community? Is this of support to you and how? Is there a group of people you really love or who are important to you?" Communities such as churches, temples, mosques, or a group of like-minded friends can serve as strong support systems for some patients.

d. A – Address in Care. "How would you like me, your healthcare provider, to address these issues in your health care?"

2. Further recommendations by the Institute in taking a spiritual history include the following.

a. Consider spirituality as a potentially important component of every patient's physical well-being and mental health.

b. Address spirituality at each complete physical examination and continue addressing it at follow-up visits if appropriate. Spirituality is an ongoing issue.

c. Respect a patient's privacy regarding spiritual beliefs. Do not impose your beliefs on others.

d. As appropriate, make referrals to chaplains, spiritual directors, or community resources.

e. Be aware that your own spiritual beliefs can help you personally and will overflow in your encounters with those for whom you care to make the encounter a more humanistic one.

E. Healthcare provider self-assessment.

1. Recognize that healthcare providers have their own spirituality that plays a key role in their professional lives and affects interactions with patients and colleagues.

2. Self-examination is often helpful in respecting patient autonomy, and in some cases, referral to another healthcare provider whose value system is more congruent with that of the patient's is the most appropriate option.

F. Collaboration and referral. Form collaborative partnerships with chaplains, clergy, and other spiritual care providers.

SECTION B
Cultural Diversity
Molly Cahill, Cheryl L. Groenhoff

I. Terminology.

A. Ethnicity: someone's cultural background or where they came from (Webster 2010).

B. Culture: a group of shared set of beliefs, norms, and values (HRSA, 2013).

1. External: physical appearance of an individual or what can be observed, which makes up 10% of culture.

2. Internal: values, beliefs, world view, customs,

traditions, language, kinship patterns, food, art and music, which make up the other 90% of culture.

C. Race: describes populations or groups of people distinguished by different sets of characteristics and beliefs about common ancestry. The most widely used human racial categories are based on visible traits, such as skin color, facial features, and hair texture, as well as self-identification.

D. Cultural competency: recognition and developing awareness of the patient's culture and a set of skills, knowledge, and policies to deliver effective treatment.

E. Ethnocentrism: a person's belief in the inherent superiority of one's own culture over that of other cultures.

F. Cultural imposition: a situation where one culture forces its values and beliefs onto another culture or subculture.

G. Culture and nephrology nursing practice.
1. When nurses recognize, understand, and incorporate cultural values of their patients into practice, patients are less apt to become dissatisfied, withdraw, and/or have unfavorable health outcomes.
2. The nurse must first be aware of his/her own cultural values to understand another's culture in relationship to one's own. When there are identified shared meanings and common values, the patient-centered care plans are greatly facilitated. When there are not, conscious efforts to incorporate the patient's unique values into the care plan will enhance effectiveness of the plan and patient adherence with the prescribed treatment regimen.
3. Cultural diversity and variation occur among all humans. Professional, therapeutic care depends on the nurse's knowledge and recognition of subtle or major differences among cultural groups. Culturally specific care leads to patient satisfaction and achievement of therapeutic outcomes.
4. Culturally competent care includes the recognition that successful adaptation for a patient will be measured and judged by his/her cultural beliefs and values, which may or may not be shared by healthcare professionals.
5. Other reasons to increase knowledge in cultural competency.
    a. Improved communication with patients and families.
    b. Increased ability in negotiating differences.
    c. Greater likelihood of disclosure of patient information to the healthcare provider.
    d. More effective use of time with patients.
    e. Enhanced patient adherence to treatment.
    f. Decrease in healthcare worker and patient stress.
    g. Higher degree of trust in a relationship.
    h. Increase in patient and provider satisfaction.
    i. Adherence to increasingly stringent government regulations and standards.
    j. Improved clinical outcomes.

H. Cultural knowledge.
1. Obtaining information about patients' health beliefs and values to meet individual needs.
2. Understanding disease incidence and prevalence among specific ethnic groups.

I. Cultural assessment.
1. Gathering data about the culture of a patient.
2. Giger and Davidhizer (1991) suggest that the culture assessment should include six domains: communication, space, social organizations, time, environmental control, and biologic variation.

J. Health.
1. Absence of disease as defined by the patient's culture.
2. Includes a state of complete physical, mental, and social well-being with the ability to function in activities of daily living to achieve self-fulfillment or realize one's potential.

K. Disease.
1. In contrast to health, disease is defined in terms of pathology and as defined by the patient's culture.
2. Deviant behavior is determined by the culturally accepted value system to which one belongs, and therefore it is the culture, not the nature, that defines disease. Every society denotes what is normal and, therefore, healthy. What is considered normal is not universal.
3. Pathology relates to the biologic structure and functioning of the human body and is described in terms of systems related to the cells, tissues, organs, fluids, and various chemicals.

L. Illness: a subjective description by a person relaying symptoms of disease or discomfort.

M. Sickness.
1. Occurs when the person's state of illness becomes a social occurrence through either visibility or communication.
2. Each condition can occur in the absence of any others.
3. During the process of an illness, social roles change and behaviors are modified.
4. A given biologic condition may or may not be

considered a sickness depending on the cultural group in which it occurs.

5. When a deviation is fairly prevalent or widespread, it is considered an everyday occurrence and therefore a normal state rather than a sickness.

N. Acculturation.
   1. The process by which a given cultural group adapts to or learns how to take on the behaviors of another group.
   2. An unconscious fusion of attitudes in order to coexist within a community. However, complete acculturation to values and beliefs rarely happens, particularly when they are in conflict with one's own values and beliefs.

O. Assimilation: the process by which individuals or groups are absorbed into and adopt the dominant culture and society of another group.

P. Cultural diversity.
   1. Variety of ethnic groups in a specific region or in the world as a whole with independent sets of norms.
   2. Considerable variations in health and illness practices.

II. Prevalence and causation of CKD.

A. According to the USRDS (2014), as of December 31, 2012, prevalent population included 449,342 patients on dialysis and 186,303 patients with a functioning kidney transplant, and the 1-year growth of 3.6 percent to 636,905.

B. Prevalence: CKD in the U.S. adult population was 11% (19.2 million) (USRDS, 2013).
   1. Stage 1 – estimated 5.9 million individuals (3.3%) (persistent albuminuria with a normal GFR).
   2. Stage 2 – estimated 5.3 million (3.0%) (persistent albuminuria with a GFR of 60 to 89 mL/min/1.73 m^2).
   3. Stage 3 – estimated 7.6 million (4.3%) (GFR 30 to 59 mL/min/1.73 m^2).
   4. Stage 4 – estimated 400,000 individuals (0.2%) (GFR, 15 to 29 mL/min/1.73 m^2).
   5. Stage 5 – estimated 300,000 individuals (0.2%) described as kidney failure requiring kidney replacement therapy.

C. According to the 2014 USRDS, CKD is more prevalent in women than men.

D. Causation. There are typical medical and social risk factors associated with CKD according to the USRDS (2013).

1. Medical risk factors.
   a. Diabetes (30% of all patients diagnosed with CKD are diabetic). In the age category of 20 years and older, 35% of people with diabetes also have CKD.
   b. Hypertension. In the age category of 20 years and older, 20% of people with hypertension also have CKD.
   c. Autoimmune disease (e.g., lupus).
   d. Systemic infections.
   e. Frequent urinary tract infections.
   f. Recurring kidney stones.
   g. Malignancy.
   h. Family history.
   i. Trauma.
   j. Exposure to certain drugs during prolonged period of time (e.g., nonsteroidal antiinflammatory drugs).
   k. Hereditary or congenital defects.
2. Social risk factors.
   a. Age.
   b. Sex. According to the USRDS 2013, even though CKD is more prevalent in women, men with CKD are 50% more likely to progress to kidney failure.
   c. Ethnicity.
   d. Exposure to certain chemicals and environmental conditions.
   e. Low income.
   f. Education < 12 years.
   g. Drug abuse.
3. Risk factors for progression.
   a. Poor control of diabetes and hypertension increases risk for progressing to kidney failure.
   b. Multiple episodes of acute kidney injury (AKI) can increase risk for progressing to kidney failure.
   c. Variety of causes of AKI.
      (1) Infections.
      (2) Drugs or toxins.
      (3) Inflammation of the kidney.
      (4) Obstruction of the urinary tract.
      (5) Decreased renal blood flow.

E. Cultural risk factors.
   1. African American (AA)/Black American. *Note:* Terminology was used based on a study in the *Public Opinion Quarterly,* 2005. Of all respondents, 50% preferred the term African American, and 50% preferred the term Black American (*Public Opinion Poll Quarterly,* 2005).
      a. Diabetes and hypertension. According to the National Institutes for Health (Benjamin, 2010), diabetes and hypertension account for about 70% of kidney failure in African Americans.
      b. Diabetes and obesity. It is estimated more than 750,000 African Americans have undiagnosed

diabetes. Type 2 is most commonly caused by insulin resistance secondary to metabolic syndrome, obesity, hyperinsulinemia, gestational diabetes, and lack of physical exercise. Obesity is thought to play a role in 50% to 90% of type 2 diabetes. African American female obesity-related morbidity from diabetes has a relative risk of 2.5 deaths per 100,000 compared to whites (NIH, 2013).

   c. Cardiovascular disease, including coronary artery disease and hypertension. The age-adjusted prevalence for adults over 20 is 7.1 times higher for black men and 9 times higher for black women as compared to white men and women (NIH, 2013).

   d. Prostate cancer. Black males have the highest incidence and greatest mortality (NIH, 2013).

   e. HIV/AIDS. It is the leading cause of death in African Americans/Blacks between the ages of 25 and 44. The death rate is higher among men than women but the trend for this is changing (NIH, 2013).

2. Hispanic.
   a. Diabetes. According to the NIH (Benjamin, 2010), the prevalence of diabetes is 2 to 4 times greater in Latinos than non-Latino whites. Additionally, the incidence of type 2 diabetes in Mexican Americans is rising rapidly.

   b. Hypertension. The incidence of hypertension is equal in Hispanics and non-Latino whites.

   c. Breast cancer. Although there is no increase in the number of Hispanics with breast cancer, there is an increase in the number diagnosed at a later stage of the disease.

   d. HIV/AIDs. Latinos represented 19% of the HIV/AIDS cases reported in the 1990s. There is a notable increase in the heterosexual cases of HIV among foreign born Latino men and women and of American born Latino intravenous drug users. Latinos and African Americans have a higher death rate from HIV than whites.

3. Incidence by cultural and causation per Centers for Disease Control and Prevention (CDC, 2010).
   a. About 110,000 patients in the United States started treatment for kidney failure in 2007.
     (1) Leading causes of kidney failure are diabetes and hypertension.
     (2) In 2006, 7 out of 10 new cases of kidney failure in the United States had diabetes or hypertension listed as the primary cause.
     (3) Less common causes include glomerulonephritis, hereditary kidney disease, and malignancies such as myeloma.
     (4) Incidence of kidney failure is greater among adults older than 65 years.

   b. Racial disparities.
     (1) African Americans were four times more likely to develop kidney failure than whites in 2007. However, this disparity in kidney failure incidence has narrowed from 1998 to 2005.
     (2) Hispanics have 1.5 times the rate of kidney failure compared to non-Hispanic whites.
     (3) The incidence of kidney failure in African Americans has declined for the last 5 years. Rates also fell among Native Americans but are 13.5% higher than the Asian population – the smallest difference in more than 3 decades.
     (4) Areas with no improvement among those whose kidney failure is caused by diabetes; racial disparities persist, particularly among younger Blacks/African Americans.

III. Evidence-based treatment and minorities.

A. Treatment guidelines are often extrapolated from largely white populations, although applied to all, regardless of race or ethnicity.

B. The Minority Health Disparities Research and Education Act (2000) elevated the Office of Research on Minority Health to the National Center on Minority Health and Health Disparities.
1. Because of the above-noted disparities, the NIH increased programmatic and budget authority for research on minority health issues and health disparities (Benjamin, 2010).
2. The law also promotes additional training and education for healthcare professionals, the evaluation of data collection systems, and a national public awareness campaign.

IV. Coping styles.

A. Coping styles refer to those behaviors used in the management of an illness. There are cultural-specific behaviors viewed by various ethnic groups as acceptable in certain circumstances.

B. Chinese, Japanese, and other Asian cultures encourage harmony, and therefore they will agree with everything the physician/provider or nurse is saying. Therefore, it may be difficult to ascertain if the treatment plan is understood and acceptable to the patient.

C. Vietnamese may hesitate to ask a question in group settings. Questioning an authority figure is viewed as a sign of disrespect. As a result, education in a group setting may not be effective and one-on-one care planning more appropriate with this cultural group.

D. Gender may also influence how persons within certain cultures cope with illness.
   1. Female African Americans believe hypertension and stress are related and feel the need to discuss stress-related issues and not keep things inside.
   2. Male African Americans believe stress should be dealt with through action and are not likely to express their feelings or seek help, as it is viewed as a sign of weakness.

V. Spirituality and religion in health care (refer back to Section A for additional reading).

A. Spirituality is a person's individual journey in finding purpose and meaning. Religion is an organized system of beliefs encompassing cause, nature, and the purpose of the universe, especially pertaining to the worshiping of a higher power or god(s).

B. Patients' attitudes are the key to the healing process and are essential for self-fulfillment.

C. Beliefs and attitudes need to be understood by the nurse for optimal physical and emotional health, including the patient's spiritual well-being. Spirituality is often neglected when providing nursing care. This can be attributed to nurses:
   1. Viewing religion as a private subject and believing that spirituality should be kept between the person and his/her maker.
   2. Being uncomfortable about own beliefs.
   3. Having a knowledge deficit related to spirituality and religious concerns of others.
   4. Mistaking spiritual needs for psychosocial needs.
   5. Considering spiritual needs as the job of spiritual leaders and not that of the nurse.

VI. Cultural assessment.

A. Spiritual/religious beliefs and values.
   1. Meaning of kidney disease.
   2. Preferred treatment.
   3. Preferred outcomes.
   4. Preferences about palliative care and advanced directives.
   5. Role of medications.
   6. Sources of cultural stigma and esteem.
   7. Preferred personal role on treatment team.

B. Role of significant others.
   1. Caretaker's role and effects of affiliations with cultural organizations.
   2. Types of support as defined by cultural and family networks.
   3. Preferred role for those networks (e.g., do not resuscitate orders).
   4. Role of family vs. individual in decision making.

   5. Role of the authority figure within family or social group.
   6. Role of the community or spiritual leaders in decision making.

C. Lifestyle and practices. This information pertains to patients with CKD including kidney failure. The purpose is to encourage continued lifestyle practices such as working, continuing education, or even traveling.
   1. Family, and individual nutrition and dietary practices.
   2. Genetic risk patterns.
   3. Spiritual and religious practices.
   4. Substance use or nonuse.
   5. Activity levels.
   6. Stress generating or stress reduction practices.
   7. Practices affecting depression.
   8. Important cultural traditions.

D. Access to the healthcare system and other resources.
   1. Three high risk groups.
      a. Low socioeconomic status.
      b. Illegal immigrants for fear of deportation.
      c. Rural areas where logistics impede one's ability to seek or receive health care.
   2. Resources for transportation, medications, and nutritional requirements.
   3. Referrals to nephrologist, kidney education, kidney transplant evaluation, counseling for depression, loss and grief, crisis management, transition planning (e.g., beginning dialysis), and translation and literacy support.

E. Adherence.
   1. Adherence is the degree to which patients follow their medication and treatment regimen.
   2. Often, nonadherence is directly related to a knowledge deficit by the patient, and measures of a culturally competent teaching plan need to be implemented by the nurse (see Section C, Patient and Family Education, in this chapter for additional information). The term *noncompliance* should not be used.
   3. Adherence can also be impacted by lifestyle issues, values, medication side effects (cultural biology), and regimen complexity.
   4. Adjust the plan of care based on culturally unique needs, resources, and beliefs.
   5. Interventions to enhance adherence and service quality.
      a. Identify effects of own cultural background on providing patient care.
      b. Acknowledge cultural differences with patient and bridge similarities.
      c. Complete a cultural assessment regarding adherence potential.

d. Use cultural validation statements to support cultural strengths, needs, and goals.

e. Use challenges, identified through assessment questions, to focus on meeting individualized needs.

f. Use cultural exception questions to enhance coping and lifestyle practices.

g. Increase patient and social network involvement in treatment.

h. Develop patient-centered behavioral contracts.

VII. Mistrust.

A. Survey results from a study conducted by Halbert et al. (2006) suggest that African Americans and Caucasians who had fewer quality interactions with healthcare providers were likely to report low trust and that healthcare providers who communicate well may improve trust.

B. Research indicates that some minority groups are more likely than whites to delay seeking treatment until symptoms are more severe.

C. Immigrants and refugees from many regions of the world, including Central and South America and Southeast Asia, feel extreme mistrust of government. This mistrust is based on atrocities committed in their country of origin and fear of deportation.

D. Tips for managing mistrust.
1. Recognize prejudice and its effects.
2. Build trust and reassure the patient of your intentions.
3. Keep in perspective "what's at stake" for the patient, showing respect for patient's concerns.
4. Ask the patient what outcome he/she would like to achieve.

VIII. Communication.

A. Human interaction: culture is transmitted and is both verbal and nonverbal.

B. Poor communication is one of the biggest challenges when working with patients from diverse cultures.

C. Misunderstandings lead to lack of respect for persons whose cultural values are different from one's own and may cause harm to those persons, sometimes culturally, psychologically, physically, or spiritually.

D. In some cultures, words are sacred, pauses are common, and interruptions are considered rude. Speaking too loudly may be a sign of disrespect.

E. Communication tools must include sensitivity, awareness, knowledge, and alternatives to written communication.

IX. Healthcare disparities.

A. Patient factors.
1. Patient choice or preference.
2. Cultural beliefs about health and medical care.
3. Minority mistrust of the healthcare system (based in part on high reported rates of perceived instances of past discrimination).
4. Language barriers.
5. Difficulties in cross-racial/ethnic provider–patient communication.
6. Alleged biologic differences in clinical presentation or responses to treatments and medications.
7. Unmeasured aspects of socioeconomic status assumed to be associated with race or ethnicity.

B. Provider factors.
1. Lack of cultural competency.
2. Professional practice styles.
3. Clinical uncertainty about the findings in assessment, medical history, or symptom presentation of patients from diverse cultures.
4. Both conscious and unconscious racial/ethnic bias and negative stereotyping that influence clinical decisions.
5. Groups of professionals can be said to have a "culture" in the sense that they have a shared set of beliefs, norms, and values.
6. Culture is reflected by the language and terms used by members of a cultural group, emphasis in their textbooks, and their mindset or worldview.

X. Culture, society, and kidney disease.

A. With the range of effective treatments for kidney disease and the diversity of settings and sectors in which these treatments are offered, consumers can exercise choice in treatment.

B. Consumers can choose among treatment modalities such as hemodialysis, peritoneal dialysis, kidney transplantation, or no treatment based on cultural beliefs or societal pressure.

XI. Cultural variances.

A. Family influences are important resources for effective prevention and behavior changes. The family is broadly defined to include relationships rooted in lineage, descent or kinship.
1. Within the African-American culture.
a. There is the frequent use of given titles such as aunt, uncle, brother, or sister. These individuals

may be called upon during times of serious illness or to influence behavioral change.

   b. There is a greater proportion of females who are the head of the household. On the average, African-American women are the lowest wage earners of all race/gender groups; thus many live below poverty level, according to the Bureau of Labor statistics (2011).

2. Within Asian cultures.

   a. Often an individual puts the family's needs above his/her own.

   b. Extended families often live together as a single-family unit that includes grandparents, parents, children, and the families of paternal uncles.

   c. Family decision making usually includes extended family members.

   d. Children are expected to obey elders and to put the family's needs above their own.

3. Within American Indian and Pacific Islander cultures.

   a. Family is of paramount importance.

   b. The extended family structure of Indian communities reflects the importance of this socialization source.

   c. They may involve others who have experienced a disease or illness outside the family, as well as the use of communal ceremony that involves both healing and prevention.

B. Communication and language.

1. African Americans are a highly expressive people. The African-American language involves subtle patterns of verbal and body language that are often misunderstood by people unfamiliar with these patterns.

2. Middle Eastern cultures consider it disrespectful to look directly into the eyes of an authoritative figure when speaking. This is in stark contrast to Western cultures that consider it disrespectful not to look in a person's eyes during conversation.

3. Among Latinos, eye contact may not occur, especially among persons of low socioeconomic level, particularly if the patient does not agree with or understand the treatment plan.

4. Many cultures (e.g., Native American and Middle Eastern) still require the head of the household, most often a male, to communicate the wishes of the family. This can be challenging when attempting to maintain confidentiality and follow the Health Insurance Portability and Accountability Act (HIPAA) requirements.

5. Nonverbal communication in the form of hugs, handshakes, and smiles are considered personal expressions of warmth and caring by Hispanics/Latinos and are important priorities.

However, hand respect is valued, and handshakes may be seen as familiar or patronizing and experienced negatively.

C. Health beliefs.

1. Traditional medicine in most Hispanic countries includes an extensive list of folk remedies. For example:

   a. Using garlic to treat hypertension and cough.

   b. Consuming chamomile to treat nausea, gas, colic, and anxiety.

   c. Combining a purgative tea with stomach massage to cure lack of appetite, stomach pains, or diarrhea.

   d. Using peppermint to treat dyspepsia and gas.

2. Asian Americans believe the universe is composed of opposing elements held in balance.

   a. Thus, health is a state of balance between these opposing forces, known as *am* and *duong* in Vietnam and *yin* and *yang* in China.

   b. Chinese medicine is complex with well-established therapeutic traditions that use acupuncture, acupressure, and herbs, often in combination with dietary therapy, Western medicine, and supernatural healing.

   c. Some Chinese may believe that illness is a result of moral retribution by ancestors due to a person's misdeeds or negligence.

   d. Other health beliefs, held by patients from this group, include:

     (1) Cosmic disharmony due to a poor combination of year of birth, month of birth, day of birth, and time of birth.

     (2) Poor Feng Shui, such as improper placement of objects inside a room or orientation of the room or house itself.

3. In some Eastern religions, patients may feel that his/her illness is caused by karma (the law of cause and effect over countless lifetimes), even though the patient may understand that the actual illness has a biologic cause.

4. Some Hispanic people believe that disease is caused by an imbalance between hot and cold principles. Health is maintained by avoiding exposure to extreme temperatures and by consuming appropriate foods and beverages.

5. Some Cambodians may cup, pinch, coin, or rub an ill person's skin to treat a range of ailments. This may cause a skin alteration or scar, so it is important that these techniques not be labeled as abuse without further cultural assessment.

6. American Indians often rely on traditional healers.

   a. Some Native Americans/American Indians/Alaskan Natives believe that healing will result from sacred ceremonies that rely on having visions and using plants and/or objects symbolic of the individual, the illness, or the treatment.

  b. Native American herbal medicine is widely used by alternative medical practitioners. Examples include the use of echinacea, goldenseal, and burdock.

  c. Native Americans have a keen awareness of a sense of well-being, healing, and cultural context.

  d. To care for the Native American, the nephrology nurse must respect traditional healing practices that aim to restore balance and harmony to the mind, body, spirit, and community.

  e. Healthcare professionals must define and value health as they are defined and valued in traditional Native American communities.

7. Jehovah's Witnesses.

  a. The Jehovah's Witnesses faith does not allow the acceptance of transfusions from others.

  b. Conversations should start early in planning care of CKD to allow them an opportunity to donate their own blood to prevent negative consequences associated with severe anemia and/or blood loss (Panico et al., 2011).

D. Complementary alternative medicine (CAM).

1. Complementary medicine is used in conjunction with conventional medicine; for example, the use of aromatherapy to help lessen a patient's discomfort following surgery.

2. Alternative medicine is used in place of conventional medicine (for example, using a special diet to treat cancer instead of undergoing surgery, radiation, or chemotherapy that has been recommended by a conventional prescriber).

3. Five domains of CAM.

  a. Alternative medical systems are built upon complete systems of theory and practice.

   (1) Examples of alternative medical systems that have developed in Western cultures include homeopathic and naturopathic medicine.

   (2) Systems that have developed in non-Western cultures include traditional Chinese medicine and Ayurveda, which is holistic Indian medicine.

  b. Mind–body interventions use a variety of techniques designed to enhance the mind's capacity to affect bodily function and symptoms.

   (1) Some techniques that were considered CAM in the past have become mainstream (e.g., patient support groups and cognitive-behavioral therapy).

   (2) Other mind–body techniques, still considered CAM, include meditation,

prayer, mental healing, and therapies that use creative outlets such as art, music, or dance.

  c. Biologically based therapies use substances found in nature, such as herbs, foods, and vitamins; for example, dietary supplements, herbal products, and the use of other "so-called" natural, but not yet scientifically proven, therapies (e.g., using shark cartilage to treat cancer).

  d. Manipulative and body-based methods are based on manipulation and/or movement of one or more parts of the body, including chiropractic or osteopathic manipulation and massage.

  e. Energy therapies involve the use of energy fields and include two types: biofield and bioelectromagnetic-based therapies.

   (1) Biofield therapies are intended to affect energy fields that purportedly surround and penetrate the human body.

    (a) The existence of such fields has not yet been scientifically proven.

    (b) Some forms of energy therapy manipulate biofields by applying pressure and/or manipulating the body by placing the hands in, or through, these fields, including qi gong, Reiki, and therapeutic touch.

   (2) Bioelectromagnetic-based therapies involve the unconventional use of electromagnetic fields such as pulsed fields, magnetic fields, or alternating-current or direct-current fields.

  f. Patients should be warned that the use of dietary supplements, herbals, and natural products should be discussed with healthcare providers as there may be dangers associated with those with kidney disease. It is very important that nurses stay current on complementary and alternative practices and their risks (Fink et al., 2012).

E. Dietary considerations. Poor diet and exercise are modifiable risk factors to reduce cardiovascular morbidity and reduce obesity. Cultural impact on diet may alter the educational focus of care.

1. American-born African Americans enjoy pork products high in salt content and fried meats with heavy gravies, as compared to immigrant African Americans who have different dietary practices and preferences.

2. Kosher diets practiced by black Muslims exclude pork products.

3. Many island cultures (e.g., Haitian and Jamaican) have significant poverty. Therefore, obesity is a status symbol. It is considered a sign of health and

wealth. Behavior modification with regard to calorie reduction and weight loss may be a challenge within this ethnic group.

F. Religion and spirituality.
1. Although many Asian Americans are Christian, Islam, Hinduism, Confucianism, Taoism, and a host of other religions are practiced. Many follow Buddhist concepts.
   a. Buddhism is a philosophy of life that has profound impact on healthcare beliefs and practices.
   b. Buddhism encourages respect for elders and those in authority such as healthcare providers.
   c. Buddhism also teaches that life is a cycle of suffering and rebirth.
      (1) Pain and illness are sometimes endured, and health-seeking remedies may be delayed.
      (2) Healing is spiritual as well as scientific.
2. The Navajo Indians believe in the metaphysical premises of hozho/hochoo (hochxo), or beauty/harmony and ugliness/disharmony.
   a. While sometimes difficult for the nurse to understand, these are essential to conception of the "good life."
   b. Navajos, like many other American Indians, are not a homogenous group, and beliefs about religion and healing vary.
3. American Indians believe there is a Supreme Creator. Humans have a body, mind, and spirit, and illness affects all three realms. *Unwellness* is the disharmony of body, mind, and spirit. Unnatural illness exists.
   a. Intertribalism is the exchanging of traits between different American Indian nations.
   b. Pan-Indianism is a general sense of American Indian cultural identity that unites members of different American Indian nations.
   c. Religion and medicine are components of the Native North Americans that are inseparable.
4. Most Latinos are Roman Catholic, but an increasing number are Protestant. Additionally, a number of Jews settled in Latin America and have since immigrated to the United States.
   a. Many Catholics wear a crucifix as a symbol of faith and sometimes a protection against evil or illness.
   b. Arranging Last Rites or Sacrament of the Sick may be important to patients of Catholicism.
5. Some Latinos, particularly those from the Caribbean, practice Santeria, which synthesizes African religion and Christianity. This belief system also includes healing practices.
6. The topic of withdrawing treatment for kidney disease is covered later in this section, but it is important for the nurse to understand that several

religions or cultures associate this with suicide, and guidance is essential.

XII. Illegal immigrants.

A. Social patterns and family structure.
1. Settlement patterns of illegal immigrants have been a barrier to acculturation into American society.
   a. These settlement patterns provide aid and comfort, a network of support, and common linguistic forms of communication.
   b. However, their illegal status makes the immigrant at higher risk for inadequate wages and economic resources as well as limited, if any, access to health care.
2. Illegal immigrants are not captured in the collection of data by the United States Renal Data System (USRDS) where Medicare attributes its fiscal decisions based on these registries.
3. According to data collected by the United States Bureau of Labor Statistics and the Census Bureau, in 2005, 11.1 million unauthorized migrants lived in the United States.
   a. This was an increase from 8.4 million in 2000, a 32% increase in only 5 years.
   b. The Bureau additionally estimated 5,500 illegal immigrants have chronic kidney disease.

B. Health beliefs.
1. As with other cultures, cultural-specific health beliefs and practices affect the health and well-being of individuals in this group.
2. Therefore, it is important for the nurse to be aware of the individual practice patterns when providing care.

C. Communication and language.
1. Communication is imperative to gaining access to healthcare services. Languages such as Spanish are becoming more prevalent.
2. Ethnic groups such as Haitians who speak Creole have a linguistic disadvantage, as there are few health practitioners who are fluent in Creole.
3. Inability to understand creates embarrassment, frustration, and stress.
4. Many, therefore, choose not to seek health care or are unable to follow the prescribed treatment plan.

D. Barriers to care.
1. Economic.
2. Lack of healthcare insurance.
3. Geographic disadvantage. Rural areas lack healthcare workers and facilities, putting migrant workers at high risk.
4. Fear of deportation.

E. Major health issues. Poverty and poor living conditions are two major health risks facing illegal immigrants.

XIII. Patients as cultural consultants.

A. The patient is a teacher in disguise.

B. Allow patients to teach you about their culture and provide the necessary cultural resources for addressing their needs and enhancing adherence in their treatment.

XIV. Health literacy.

A. Background information.
1. Healthy People 2020 defined health literacy as the capacity to obtain, communicate, process, and understand basic health information and services.
   a. Health providers with health literacy skills are better able to share health information and improve outcomes.
   b. Only 12% of adults have proficient health literacy.
   c. Nine out of 10 adults may lack the skills needed to manage their health and prevent disease.
   d. 14% of adults (approximately 30 million people) have below-basic health literacy.
      (1) They are more likely to report their health as poor.
      (2) They are more likely to lack health insurance than adults with proficient health literacy.
2. The Centers for Disease Control and Prevention (CDC.gov) recommends and requests health professionals become educated about the following information presented in this section of the chapter.

B. Health literacy is dependent on both individual and systemic factors (HRSA, 2013).
1. Communication skills of lay people and professionals.
   a. Skills include reading, writing, and number.
   b. Oral and comprehension skills.
   c. Skills are content specific.
2. Knowledge of lay people and professionals of health topics.
   a. People with limited or inaccurate knowledge about the body and the causes of disease may not be able to:
      (1) Understand the relationship between lifestyle factors (such as diet and exercise) and health outcomes.
      (2) Recognize when they need to seek care.
   b. Health information can even overwhelm people with advanced literacy skills.

3. Culture and literacy.
   a. How people communicate and understand health information.
   b. How people think and feel about their health.
   c. When and from whom people seek care.
   d. How people respond to recommendations for lifestyle change and treatment.
4. Demands of the healthcare and public health systems.
   a. Individuals need to read, understand, and complete many kinds of forms to receive treatment and payment reimbursement.
   b. Individuals need to know about the various types of health professionals and services as well as how to access care.
5. Demands of the situation/context.
   a. Health contexts are unusual compared to other contexts because of an underlying stress or fear factor.
   b. Healthcare contexts may involve unique conditions such as physical or mental impairment due to illness.
   c. Health situations are often new, unfamiliar, and intimidating.
   d. Plain language is a technique for communicating clearly. It is one tool for improving health literacy.

C. Plain language is a strategy for making written and oral information easier to understand.
1. Key elements of plain language.
   a. Using simple language and defining technical terms.
   b. Using the active voice.
   c. Breaking down complex information into understandable pieces.
   d. Organizing information so the most important points come first.
2. A plain language document is one in which people can, with reasonable time and effort, find what they need, understand what they find, and act appropriately on that understanding (www.plainlanguage.gov).

D. Cultural competency is the ability of professionals to work cross-culturally. It can contribute to health literacy by improving communication and building trust.

E. Health literacy affects people's ability to complete the following tasks.
1. Navigate the healthcare system, including locating providers and services, and filling out forms.
2. Share personal and health information with providers.
3. Engage in self-care and chronic disease management.

4. Adopt health-promoting behaviors such as exercising and eating a healthy diet.
5. Act on health-related news and announcements.

F. Limited literacy leads to the following.
1. Higher use of treatment services.
   a. Hospitalizations.
   b. Emergency services.
2. Lower use of preventive services.
3. Higher use of treatment services results in higher healthcare costs.

G. People with limited health literacy often report feeling a sense of shame about their skill level.

H. Individuals with poor literacy skills are often uncomfortable about being unable to read well, and they develop strategies to compensate.

I. Measuring literacy.
1. Clinical: filling out a patient form.
2. Prevention: following guidelines for age-appropriate preventive health services.
3. Navigation of the healthcare system: understanding what a health insurance plan will pay for.

J. Evaluating literacy.
1. Proficient: can perform complex and challenging literacy activities.
2. Intermediate: can perform moderately challenging literacy activities.
3. Basic: can perform simple everyday literacy activities.
4. Below basic: can perform no more than the most simple and concrete literacy activities.

K. Measures of health literacy at the individual level were developed in the 1990s.
1. Rapid Estimate of Adult Literacy in Medicine (REALM). Medical word recognition and pronunciation test. Can be administered and scored in 3 minutes. Words are arranged in three columns by number of syllables, scores converted to reading levels.
2. Test of Functional Health Literacy in Adults (TOFHLA and S-TOFHLA). Includes 17 items for numerical ability and 50 for reading comprehension; total scores are divided into *inadequate, marginal*, and *adequate*. There is a 12-minute abbreviated version.
3. Health literacy measures based on functional literacy do not capture the full range of skills needed for health literacy. Current assessment tools (for populations and individuals) cannot differentiate among the following.
   a. Reading ability.

b. Lack of health-related background knowledge.
c. Lack of familiarity with language and materials.
d. Cultural differences in approaches to health.
e. Most tools do not account for the current demands of the healthcare system.

L. The problem of limited health literacy is greater among the following groups.
1. Older adults.
2. Persons with low or limited income.
3. People with limited education.
4. Minority populations.
5. Persons with limited English (ESL – English as second language).

M. Studies by the CDC revealed that persons with limited health literacy skills:
1. Are more likely to have chronic conditions and less likely to manage them effectively.
2. Have less knowledge of their illness (e.g., diabetes, asthma, HIV/AIDS, high blood pressure) and its management.
3. Experience more preventable hospital visits and admissions.
4. Are significantly more likely to report their health as "poor."

N. Strategies for improving health literacy.
1. Improve the usability of health information.
   a. Is the information appropriate for the users?
   b. Is the information easy to use?
   c. Are you speaking clearly and listening carefully?
2. Improve the usability of health services, particularly online.
   a. It is the nurse's responsibility to direct patients to reliable resources.
   b. People cannot find the information they seek on websites 60% of the time.
   c. Many elements that improve written and oral communication can be applied to information on the Web.
      (1) Plain language.
      (2) Large font.
      (3) White space.
      (4) Simple graphics.
   d. Many organizations have their own websites and encourage patients to engage them by making appointments, using resources, and clicking to other resources or reliable links.
   e. Health literacy has implications for web-based communication beyond written text.
      (1) Revise forms to ensure clarity and simplicity.
      (2) Test forms with intended users and revise as needed.
      (3) Provide forms in multiple languages.

(4) Offer assistance with completing forms and scheduling follow-up care.

f. Other options.
  (1) Apply user-centered design principles and conduct internal usability tests.
  (2) Include interactive features and personalized content.
  (3) Organize information to minimize scrolling.
  (4) Use uniform navigation (www.usability.gov).

3. Build knowledge to improve decision making.
4. Advocate for health literacy improvement.
5. Acknowledge cultural differences in health information.
  a. Accepted roles of men and women.
  b. Value of traditional vs. Western medicine.
  c. Favorite or forbidden foods.
  d. Manner of dress.
  e. Body language, especially touching or proximity.
  f. Involve diverse audiences, including those with limited health literacy, in development and rigorous user testing.

O. Cultural competency is the ability of health organizations and practitioners to recognize the following in diverse populations to produce a positive health outcome.
  1. Cultural beliefs.
  2. Values.
  3. Attitudes.
  4. Traditions.
  5. Language preferences.
  6. Health practices.
  (Based on the Office of Minority Health: The National Standards for Culturally and Linguistically Appropriate Services in Health and Health Care [the National CLAS Standards], 2014).

P. Improve access to accurate and appropriate healthcare information.
  1. Create new mechanisms for sharing and distributing understandable health education materials.
  2. Create audience or language-specific information. Partner with adult educators and schools.
  3. Finding new methods for disseminating information: smart phones, personalized and interactive tools, information kiosks, talking prescription bottles, etc.
  4. Form partnerships with civic and faith-based organizations trusted in the community.
  5. Ensure that the health information shared is accurate, current, and reliable. Offer resources to assist if identify poor quality information (cdc.gov).

XV. Other online resources.

A. www.culturediversity.org/cultcomp.htm

B. www.ethnomed.org

C. www.hrsa.gov/culturalcompetence

D. www.diversityresources.com

E. http://depts.washington.edu/pfes/CultureClues.htm

F. http://sis.nlm.nih.gov/outreach/multicultural.html

SECTION C
Patient and Family Education
Molly Cahill, Cheryl L. Groenhoff

I. The teaching–learning process.

A. Definition. The teaching–learning process involves the interaction of individuals and the environment for the purpose of achieving a specific goal.

B. Intervening variable. The nature of the teaching–learning process changes in complexity based on the number of relationships of the intervening variables present. Intervening variables are introduced into the process by both the participants and the environment. Examples of those variables include the following.
  1. Teacher variables.
    a. Abilities.
    b. Skills.
    c. Motivation.
    d. Intelligence.
    e. Creativity.
    f. Personality.
    g. Culture and values.
    h. Age.
    i. Gender.
  2. Learner variables.
    a. Abilities.
    b. Knowledge.
    c. Attitude.
    d. Motivation.
    e. Health state.
    f. Values and culture.
    g. Age.
    h. Gender.
  3. Environmental variables.
    a. Degree of quietness.
    b. Temperature of room.
    c. Number of human, inanimate, and other distracters.

d. Schedule conflicts.
e. Furniture arrangement.
f. Space. Respect personal boundaries and make sure there is plenty of room for family members and loved ones who the patient wishes to include in the decision-making process.

C. Components. Though related, two components of the teaching–learning process, teaching and learning, are independent of each other.
1. Teaching by definition is the intentional structuring of content to enhance human interactions to facilitate learning.
2. Learning is a change in behavior. In most instances, the degree of permanency of the behavior change is directly related to the amount of practiced reinforcement engaged in by the learner.

II. Theories of learning.

A. One approach to understanding human learning is to begin with a review of the major theories of learning and then to examine the progression or order of learning.

B. Table 3.1 presents an overview of several major classifications of learning theories, including the following.
1. A definition.
2. The major tenets.
3. Some major theorists.
4. An example of the learning represented.

Table 3.1

An Overview of the Major Classifications of Learning Theories

Classification	Definition	Major Tenets	Major Theorists	Example of the Learning
Behaviorist or Connectionist	Interprets human behavior as connections between stimuli and responses under the influence of reinforcement.	Respondent behavior results from a specific stimulus (S-R). Operant behavior is emitted as an instrumental act (R-R). Reinforcement increases the possibility of operant behavior recurring. Most human behaviors are operant in nature. Punishment decreases the possibility of a response recurring. Continuous reinforcement leads to faster learning. Intermittent reinforcement leads to longer retention of that which is learned.	Skinner Watson Thorndike Guthrie	Programmed instruction for skill development such as administering an insulin injection.
Cognitive, Organismic, or Gestalt	Interprets human behavior in terms of cognitive processes such as insight, intelligence, and organizational abilities.	Concerned with the process of decision making, cognitive structure, understanding, perception, and information processing. The emphasis is on the how of learning rather than what.	Bruner Piaget Ausubel	Exploring relationships such as those that exist between risk factors and the tendency to develop certain diseases.
Humanistic	Interprets human behavior as being self-centered and directly related to the process of self-actualization.	Learning is an individual internal process. People learn what they perceive to be helpful to maintaining their own structure. Self-actualization is the motivation for learning. Self-actualization and learning involve creative functioning. The organization of the self must not be threatened for new learning to occur.	Rogers Kohl	Exploring specific health promotion behaviors to stay healthy.

Table 3.2

Gagne's Hierarchy of Learning

Level of Learning	Definition	Example of the Learning
1. Signal learning	Learning to respond to a signal or developing a conditioned response.	Generating anxiety at the sight of a hypodermic needle.
2. Stimulus-response learning	Voluntary learning that involves making a specific response to a specified stimulus.	Responding "dialysis machine" when the stimulus of "artificial kidney" is given.
3. Chaining	Learning to connect sequentially two or more stimulus-response situations.	Performing each of the steps necessary for implementing home dialysis.
4. Verbal association	Learning to attach names or labels to objects or to translate words into other languages.	Translating medical terminology into lay terms for easy understanding.
5. Multiple discrimination	Learning an extensive series of simple chains and differentiating between similar stimuli.	Recalling the specific name of each medication when several different tablets or capsules are presented.
6. Concept learning	Learning to make a common response to a number of stimuli that may differ in appearance.	Recognizing that even though the substances presented are tablets, capsules, and elixirs, they are all medications.
7. Principle or rule learning	Learning a chain of two or more previously and separately learned concepts.	Recognizing that the concept of compliance represents a relationship between the concepts of adherence to a therapeutic regimen and feelings of being better.
8. Problem solving	Learning that requires considering previously learned principles to develop new, higher-level principles.	Deciding how frequently to institute home dialysis based on previously agreed-upon parameters.

C. Table 3.2 presents Gagne's hierarchy of learning.
   1. It includes the level of learning, a definition, and an example of the type of learning indicated for each level.
   2. The table can be used to assess and implement levels of learning required to meet specific objectives progressing toward mastery.
   3. Specific teaching strategies can be devised to produce the learning required to meet the objectives.

III. Principles of learning.

A. Understanding the theory related to how people learn is beneficial in the education process. When translating theoretical perspectives into learning principles, their applicability increases tremendously. Use of proven principles in patient and family education enhances learning.

B. Perception is a prerequisite to learning.

C. Perception is relative, selective, organized, and influenced by what is expected to be perceived.

D. Attention is a prerequisite to learning.

E. Attention is directed and captured by creative, innovative change in stimuli.

F. A person's perceptual capacity is about seven items at one time.

G. A person processes perceived information in chunks or clusters.

H. Organized information is more easily perceived and processed.

I. Familiar information is more easily perceived and processed.

J. Using more than one sensory organ enhances learning.

K. Accurate perception of information enhances subsequent cognitive processes using that information.

L. Learning that is personally relevant or meaningful is more easily acquired and retained longer.

M. Consolidating information enhances learning.

N. Repetition positively influences learning.

O. Concrete information is more easily learned and remembered than abstract information.

P. Correcting wrong information immediately facilitates learning.

Q. Learner maturity and motivation increases learning.

R. Information given at the beginning and end of instruction will be retained longer.

S. Active learner involvement in the learning process enhances learning.

T. Practicing use of information in different contexts fosters the utility and retention of that information.

U. Demonstration and return demonstration enhance the learning of psychomotor skills.

V. Using examples facilitates learning.

W. A learner's readiness to learn, or need to know, will increase the effectiveness of the learning.

IV. Adult learners.

A. The majority of our educational interaction occurs with adults, either the patient or family members. Those adults have specific characteristics that will influence learning. Nurses must be cognizant of those needs as educational interactions are planned.

B. Ability.
   1. In general, learning ability decreases with age, particularly in learning activities that are fast-paced or complex.
   2. However, adults in their 40s to 50s have a similar ability to learn as they did when they were in their 20s to 30s if they are able to control the pace.
   3. There appears to be significant decline in learning ability after age 60, consistent with the decreases in internal cognitive processes related to aging.
   4. Additionally, the ability to reason and make effective, efficient decisions appears to decrease.

C. Experiential base.
   1. Adults approach learning based on their previous experiences.
   2. They come with a wide experiential base that influences their cognitive structure and how they encode information for storage and retrieval.
   3. Thus, the learning needs to be relevant to their past experiences.

D. Perception.
   1. Adults use selective perception to deal with "new"

things. They try to make it meaningful to them within their perceptual context.
   2. When they are unable to incorporate the new information with existing cognitive structure, they are prone to misperceptions, and learning is hindered.

E. Memory.
   1. Memory includes the three phases of registration, retention, and recall.
   2. Registration includes exposure, acquisition, and encoding of information in the brain. Registration process, particularly visual information, decreases with age.
   3. Retention is the persistence of the encoded information, and it will decrease with age unless the information has direct meaning for the learner.
   4. Recall involves the search and retrieval processes used to remember information. Recall, particularly short-term recall, decreases with age.

F. Practice and repetition. Adults need repeated interactions with information coupled with appropriate, immediate feedback to learn.

G. Learning effectiveness.
   1. Learning effectiveness is decreased in adults because of their wide experiential base, and previous learning often interferes with their ability to cognitively organize new information.
   2. Time is required to sort through all of the old information to encode the new information. Therefore, learning usually takes longer for adults.

H. Self-pacing.
   1. Adults are self-directed and establish their own timelines for learning.
   2. They will learn more effectively if allowed to establish their own pace. Additionally, they need periodic breaks in the learning process.

I. Purposefulness.
   1. Adults engage in learning because they want to apply the information in their daily lives.
   2. The more practical and useful the information is to an adult, the easier it is for them to learn.
   3. They also learn to transfer the information to other situations more rapidly.

J. Resource interaction.
   1. The effectiveness of adult learning depends upon the availability, appropriateness, and utility of the resources for learning.
   2. Adults need easy access to and repeated opportunity to engage in interactions with educational resources.

K. Time perception.
   1. Adults tend to perceive time as being a valued, meaningful commodity.
   2. Their lives usually require them to manage their time appropriately to fulfill their responsibilities and meet their own needs.
   3. They recognize they take longer to learn, but they want their time spent learning to be meaningful and useful.

V. Activities of teaching.

A. Comparison to the nursing process. The process used in teaching patients is identical to the process used in delivering patient care.

B. The assessment/diagnosis phase.
   1. The teaching activities that occur during the assessment/diagnosis phase are determining the learning needs of the individual and assessing the individual's physical, psychological, and maturational readiness to learn.
   2. Assessment of learning needs.
      a. Assess a patient's behavior, asking specific questions regarding physiology, pathology, or the treatment regimen.
      b. Listen carefully to the patient's responses and questions.
   3. Assessment of readiness and ability to learn.
      a. The first step in the assessment of a patient's readiness to learn is to establish a record of the patient's baseline knowledge, related health experiences, written or verbal communication problems, current lifestyle, and significant others.
      b. The second step is to assess the patient's physical, psychological, and maturational readiness.
         (1) Physical readiness.
             (a) Physiologic state.
             (b) Pharmacologic therapy.
         (2) Psychological readiness.
             (a) Mental status.
             (b) Previous knowledge.
             (c) Past experiences.
             (d) Motivation for learning.
             (e) Attitude toward learning and health care.
             (f) Coping mechanisms.
         (3) Maturational readiness.
             (a) Life experiences.
             (b) Problem-solving ability.

C. The planning phase of the teaching process is critical to achieve a successful outcome. In most cases, this phase requires more time, energy, and deliberation than any other component of the entire process. The planning phase involves three parts: determining

purpose of the teaching, developing the teaching plan, and arranging the learning environment.
   1. Determine the purpose.
      a. In patient education, it is essential to be able to clearly articulate the precise nature of the learning to be accomplished.
      b. The purpose of the teaching serves as a broad guide for structuring the learning process, as well as for selecting the appropriate teaching strategy.
   2. Develop the teaching plan.
      a. Developing the teaching plan involves the following processes: identifying specific, measurable learning goals and behavioral objectives to meet specific learning activities.
      b. The teaching plan is crucial in identifying alternative teaching strategies to meet the needs of all learner variables such as auditory, tactile, and visual.
      c. Establish measurable and validated tools that can be used in evaluating the effectiveness of both the teaching and learning processes.
      d. Develop behavioral objectives.
         (1) Definition. Behavioral objectives are statements of specific learner behaviors that are expected to occur as a result of the teaching–learning process.
         (2) Characteristics. A behavioral objective always contains the performance behavior, the condition under which it is to occur, and the acceptable standard for the performance. In other words, it specifies what the learner should do, under what conditions, and how well.
         (3) Classifications. Behavioral objectives are classified according to three domains depending upon the type and level of learning that is to be achieved.
            (a) Cognitive domain deals with intellectual abilities and includes the hierarchical levels of knowledge, comprehension, application, analysis, synthesis, and evaluation.
            (b) Affective domain deals with the expression of feelings and includes the hierarchical levels of attentiveness, responsiveness, acceptance of values, organization of values, and characterization by a value.
            (c) Psychomotor domain deals with motor skills and includes the hierarchical levels of perception of a stimulus, preparation, guided response, mechanism (habit), complex overt response, adaptation, and organization of motor skills.
      e. Develop a content outline by consulting various

resources regarding the knowledge base essential for helping the learner achieve the desired behavioral objectives.

f. Identify specific learner activities.
   (1) Definition. *Learner activities* are those specific behaviors that are completed by the learner as part of the educational process. These activities may occur before, during, or after the specific teaching–learning session. It is important that the evaluation of the learning not occur until they have been completed.
   (2) Examples. Some examples of learning activities are reading specific items of information in preparation for the session, manipulating equipment, demonstrating a procedure, viewing various types of media, listening to audio tapes, and responding to practice situations.

g. Identify alternative teaching strategies.
   (1) Definition. *Teaching strategies* are those methods and media used by the teacher to facilitate learning.
   (2) Examples. Some examples of teaching methods are lecture, discussion, demonstration, and simulation.
      (a) Educational media include regular printed materials (such as textbooks), programmed instruction texts, still pictures, motion pictures, television, real objects or models, audio tapes and records, teaching machines, and computers.
      (b) The familiarity of most individuals with computers makes them a valuable asset in patient teaching, especially when the learner lives in remote locations.
         i. There are many online teaching modules that provide simulated scenarios and allow for learners to work at their own pace.
         ii. These modules should be monitored, however, for levels of literacy and to ensure they are appropriate resource tools.
   (3) Guidelines for use. As discussed, there are many methods of teaching methods and tools. The key to an effective learning process is assessing the needs of the learner and using those tools, which will foster the greatest cognitive retention. Examples include the following.
      (a) Using large colored pictures for older adult learners who may be visually impaired.
      (b) Using dolls to locate where the kidneys are located for pediatric learners.

(c) Teaching tools that are age appropriate.
(d) Information that is current and accurate.
(e) Information presented in an interesting manner to maintain the attention of the learner.
(f) Tools which are adaptable to be used in a variety of settings such as one-on-one and group venues.
(g) In addition, Table 3.3 suggests those methods, tools, and media that are most appropriate for producing the various hierarchical levels of the learning as described by Gagne.

h. Plan for evaluation.
   (1) Relationship to behavioral objectives.
      (a) If the behavioral objectives are specific enough, they can also be used as the evaluation criteria.
      (b) However, if they are not specific enough, then an additional criterion needs to be generated. For example, the objective, "Identify several foods that can be included on a low-sodium diet," is not specific enough to provide criteria for evaluation. A more specific

Table 3.3

Teaching Methods and Media Appropriate for Producing Specific Levels of Learning

Level of Learning	Appropriate Methods and Media
1. Signal learning	lecture, still pictures, motion pictures, television, audio recordings, texts
2. Stimulus-response learning	still pictures, motion pictures, models, television, demonstration
3. Chaining	motion pictures, programmed instruction, demonstration, still pictures, television
4. Verbal association	motion pictures, programmed instruction, demonstration, still pictures, television
5. Multiple discrimination	motion pictures, programmed instruction, still pictures, television, texts, lecture
6. Concept learning	motion pictures, television, still pictures, programmed instruction, texts, lecture
7. Principle learning	motion pictures, television, still pictures, programmed instruction, texts, lectures, simulation
8. Problem solving	lecture, motion pictures, television, texts, simulation

Table 3.4

Evaluation Tools Pros and Cons

Evaluation Tool	Pros	Cons
Evaluation matrix	Allows wide range of data to be collected.	Extra data not needed and may not be specific enough.
Anecdotal method	Narrative summation data.	Too subjective and difficult to validate.
Focus group	Information is easy to collect and open and honest.	Kind and quality of information may not be relevant and may also may be difficult to validate.
Questionnaire	Wealth of information can be obtained.	Questionnaires can be biased if not well-designed.
Likert Scale	Allows a respondent to rate a survey question at the level they agree or disagree. The categories represent an inherent order (more to less, stronger to weaker, bigger to smaller).	Numbers assigned to the categories do not indicate the magnitude of difference between the categories in the way that an interval or ratio scale would. Respondents may misread 1 to be 5 and vice versa, and the measurement may be altered.
Interval Scale	Numerical scales in which intervals have the same interpretation throughout.	Interval scales are not perfect, however. In particular, they do not have a true zero point even if one of the scaled values happens to carry the name "zero."
Ratio Scale	The ratio scale of measurement is the most informative scale. It is an interval scale with the additional property that its zero position indicates the absence of the quantity being measured.	None noted.

statement that would include the evaluation criteria would be: "After discussing sample menus, select in writing four foods that would be permitted on a 500 mg sodium diet and hand in at the end of the class." This objective states not only the behavior that is to be performed, but it also provides the conditions under which it must be performed and the degree of accuracy of the performance.

(c) These goals are SMART: specific, measurable, attainable, realistic, and timely.

(2) Measurement tools. According to Redman (2003), to evaluate the effectiveness of the educational processes, there needs to be valid and reliable tools that will measure what is intended to measure. There are many types of evaluation tools. The most effective tool needs to be determined when setting goals and objectives. Table 3.4 reviews the pros and cons of each of the following tools.

(a) Evaluation matrix.
(b) Anecdotal method.
(c) Focus groups.
(d) Questionnaire.
(e) Likert scale.
(f) Interval scale.
(g) Ratio scale.

3. Arrange the learning environment. The following factors are important when arranging the environment for learning.
   a. Structured time: a definite time period.
   b. Flexibility in both content and process.
   c. Climate: an acceptable atmosphere.
   d. Physical surroundings are comfortable and free of distraction.

D. The implementation phase.
   1. Teaching activities. The implementation phase is devoted to the following teaching activities.
      a. Teacher–learner mutual goals.
      b. Carrying out the teaching plan.
      c. Providing learning cues.
      d. Providing appropriate stimuli and maintaining attentiveness with learner.
      e. Fostering association of previously learned material.
      f. Providing opportunities for practice and return demonstration.
      g. Assisting the learner in associating new concepts with old ones.

2. Communication. Effective communication, both verbal and nonverbal, is essential in the process of patient education.
3. Evaluation phase. The evaluation phase is reserved for those activities needed to determine whether or not the objectives have been met and learning has occurred.

VI. Culturally sensitive approaches to patient education.

According to Price and Cordell, there are four-steps that help nurses promote cultural sensitivity when creating patient teaching programs, titled *Four Step Approach to Providing Culturally Sensitive Care.*

A. Examine personal culture. Be aware of potential barriers to learning.

B. Familiarity with client culture. It is essential that minority issues are explored and professionals of similar backgrounds are employed whenever possible to promote culturally sensitive care.

C. Identify adaptations made with client.
1. Incorporate continuing education programs to increase the knowledge of staff nurses about their own culturally based values, beliefs, and practices.
2. They can then integrate the cultural-specific, health-related beliefs and practices of others into the nursing process within their specialty areas of practice such as nephrology nursing.

D. Modify client teaching based from earlier steps.
1. Teaching must be based on culturological assessment, biocultural variations in health and illness, and cultural differences in communication, religious beliefs, nutrition, and aspects of the aging process.
2. Literacy and age-appropriate materials need to be incorporated to facilitate greater cognitive retention as well.

VII. Linguistic specific teaching strategies.

A. The most crucial element in the process of learning is the ability to understand language.

B. Linguistic-oriented theorists such as Cross and Brown specify there needs to be an association, reinforcement, and imitation.
1. One of the most effective methods of learning is first language learning.
2. Therefore, an interpreter is critical if the educator is not language specific for the targeted patient population.

C. Pictures and visual aids are extremely effective when language is a potential barrier to learning.

VIII. Retention of learning.

A. Initial learning is only part of the process of patient education. The second part is that of cognitive retention. The learning, which is retained, produces the long-term rewards in terms of behavior modification and patient care.

B. The retention of learning can be enhanced during the teaching–learning process through the use of the following specific types of learning activities or strategies.
1. Providing selective reinforcement immediately after the occurrence of an appropriate response.
2. Giving frequent, random reinforcement throughout the teaching–learning session.
3. Providing for repetitive practice of psychomotor skills and rote verbal learning.
4. Fostering the application of meaningful learning to commonly encountered situations.
5. Maintaining a high learner motivation level.
6. Offering organizing elements for categorizing information.
7. Encouraging the review or rehearsal of the information to be retained.

IX. Incorporating family-centered education.

A. The concept of "family" is more than people who are biologically related.
1. When viewed in the larger context, "family" might include two people of the same or different sex living together with or without sexual attachment, single-parent families, remarried families with children and stepchildren, and many other forms of family as defined by the patient.
2. When serious illness occurs, the entire family is affected. Other family members alter their lifestyles and take on role functions of the patient.
3. The extent of family disruption depends on the seriousness of the illness, the family's level of functioning before illness, socioeconomic considerations, and the extent to which family members can absorb the role of the patient.

B. No matter how the family is constructed, each is unique.
1. Assess family function and style by talking with patient and family and observing their interactions.
2. Gather information through their conversation about stressors, transition, family function, and expectations.
3. Involve the family in the teaching plan to avoid failure.
4. As noted in theories of adult learning, use case

studies of what other families have done in similar situations.

5. Include pertinent information about the disease process. Focus on planning, care giving, and problem solving.

6. If indicated, include education about planning for long-term care, respite care, support, and other available resources.

X. Application to patients with CKD.

A. When implementing the teaching–learning process with patients diagnosed with CKD, it is important to remember they have specific characteristics that occur as a result of their disease process that will influence their learning. In addition, it is important to recall some of the strategies that have been useful in assisting patients in their learning process. Characteristics of patients with CKD show information may be processed differently depending on the stage of their CKD. Variations in information processing are related to the following characteristics.

1. Depressed mentation: requiring repetition of information including objectives, content, and summary (OCS).
   a. Tell them what you are going to tell them (objectives).
   b. Tell them (content).
   c. Tell them what you told them (summary).
2. Short attention spans: usually tolerating only 10- to 15-minute teaching sessions.
3. Altered perceptual status: requires frequent clarification and reassurance.
4. Altered sensory systems: thus respond better to ideas that are repetitively presented in different audiovisual forms.
5. Decreased levels of concentration: may require additional stimulation, more repetition, and positive reinforcement as part of the educational process.

B. Strategies for enhancing learning: It has been noted that patients tend to learn more effectively if the following principles are adhered to whenever possible.

1. Brevity. Be brief in your educational interactions. About 50% of the statements made to a patient will be forgotten within 5 minutes of the interaction. This is particularly true if the other principles are not considered in the educational session.
2. Organization. Information that is structured and clearly organized enhances learning by facilitating the encoding of information for the adult.
3. Primacy. The items presented first are usually retained longer. This suggests that providing the

patient with the specific purpose of the educational session and some brief, but essential, components at the initiation of the session will enhance retention of the information.

4. Readability. Written or printed information that is given to a patient to supplement the educational process must be age specific and at an appropriate literacy level. Unfortunately, most educational tools are written at an 11th grade level, even though the research shows that the 8th grade level would be more appropriate for the majority of patients. Materials may need to be modified to accommodate the learner's characteristics.

5. Repetition. Adults need repetition to enhance learning. Information that is repeated is more readily retained and recalled. Repetition may take many forms, including printed or other visual materials and audio or videotapes. Repetition may also come from multiple healthcare professionals, which will augment learning from different perspectives.

6. Specificity. The more specific and useful the information is, the more powerful it is for the patient. In addition, specificity enhances retention and application of information.

SECTION D
Patient and Family Engagement
Sharon Longton

I. Definition of patient and family engagement.

A. Definition: actions or a set of behaviors that patients and family members take to obtain the greatest benefit from available healthcare services.

B. Healthcare professionals and organizational policies and procedures that foster the inclusion of patients and family members as active members of the healthcare team are important components in facilitating engagement.

C. Engagement is not synonymous with adherence. Engagement refers to an individual being involved in a process that matches information and professional advice with that person's own needs and abilities to prevent, manage, and cure disease.

D. Engagement promotes health and prevents illness and complications.

E. Physical and emotional status is monitored to enable the individual to make decisions based on self-monitoring.

F. The effects of illness are managed based on the individual's ability to function in important roles.

II. Tools used to evaluate patient engagement.

A. A limited number of tools are available to evaluate patient engagement. Most tools have demonstrated variable results.

B. Patient Activation Measure (PAM) is a measurement system developed by Hibbard and colleagues (2004, 2005) that assesses a patient's knowledge, skill, and confidence for self-management and reflects a developmental model of activation.
   1. Four stages of activation.
      a. Believing the patient's role is important.
      b. Having the confidence and knowledge necessary to take action.
      c. Taking action to maintain and improve one's health.
      d. Staying the course even under stress.
   2. Higher activation is associated with more needs being met and increased support from healthcare providers. Engaged patients are more likely to have improved health overall, better experiences with care, and better outcomes.

III. Strategies designed to engage patients.

A. The patient is the principal manager of his/her disease.
   1. Proficiency in specific skills and tasks is necessary to master this role.
   2. The role of the nurse and other members of the healthcare team cannot be underestimated.

B. Collaborative management means that the medical providers and the patient are able to have shared goals, a working relationship, and a mutual understanding of their roles.
   1. Clinicians can and should encourage patients to be active participants in their own care.
   2. Forming partnerships with the patient can be encouraged as follows.
      a. Ensuring the patient feels comfortable during visits.
      b. Avoiding rushed and insensitive interactions.
      c. Asking the patient to identify individual goals, current concerns, and progress to previously established goals.
      d. Encouraging the patient and family to ask questions.
      e. Spending time listening to the patient and less time offering advice.
      f. Showing concern for the patient first and the disease second.

g. Keeping the patient informed of the findings of an assessment and progress toward goals.

C. Characteristics that can impact engagement.
   1. The knowledge, attitudes, beliefs, skills, and self-efficacy of patients, families, and healthcare professionals can impact the level of success or number of barriers to engagement.
      a. Beliefs strongly influence self-management.
         (1) Encouraging individuals to change their lifestyles can be difficult.
         (2) Assessing the patient's perception is an important first step.
      b. Self-efficacy (confidence in one's ability to perform a task) must be developed. Thomas-Hawkins and Zazworsky (2005) identified four essential ingredients to building self-efficacy.
         (1) Performance mastery.
            (a) Helping patients to attain specific skills builds confidence.
            (b) Goals must be realistic.
            (c) One task must be mastered before new responsibilities are introduced.
         (2) Modeling.
            (a) Teaching materials should be appropriate to the patient's age, ethnicity, and, when appropriate, the person's gender.
            (b) Support groups provide opportunities for modeling.
         (3) Interpretation of symptoms.
            (a) If done in a negative way, the patient can be left feeling vulnerable and may have difficulty coping.
            (b) The patient may try new self-management behaviors if given alternative explanations for symptoms' causes.
         (4) Verbal persuasion.
            (a) A credible source should provide the patient with a "you can do it" attitude.
            (b) Classes and support groups are two venues in which this can occur.
   2. Demographics.
      a. Patients who are young, female, and highly educated are more likely to want involvement in healthcare decisions.
      b. Patients who have lower levels of education or have language or literacy difficulties may be less likely to engage.
      c. Providers may be more likely to facilitate and reinforce engagement based on certain patient qualities; e.g., age, education level, and location (urban vs. rural).
      d. Race may also influence a patient's willingness to be engaged.
   3. Experience. Patients and families may be more willing to be proactive if they:

a. Are familiar with the healthcare system.

b. Have experience with a particular condition.

c. Are familiar with a procedure or treatment.

D. An organization's culture, resources, facilitators, and constraints play a role in patient engagement.

E. Engagement can be facilitated as follows.
1. Communication.
   a. Self and staff introduction when approaching the patient and/or family and during rounds.
   b. Ask the patient what needs he/she has.
      (1) Encourage questions.
      (2) Coach patients on how to express concerns.
   c. Bedside report during change of shift.
      (1) Increased ability to prioritize work.
      (2) Decreases staff time.
      (3) An increase in nurse and physician satisfaction has been reported.
   d. Use whiteboards to convey and share information.
      (1) Staff names.
      (2) Telephone numbers.
      (3) Visiting times.
      (4) Meal times, etc.
   e. Shared care plans for collaboration of problem identification, priorities, treatment plans, and goals.
   f. Determine preferred contact method.
      (1) Email.
      (2) Text message.
      (3) Telephone.
      (4) Mail.
      (5) Patient portals/online access.
2. Invite participation.
   a. Invite patients and families to participate in rounds.
      (1) Allows patients and families to be involved in decision making.
      (2) Orders and discharge paperwork can be clarified.
   b. Sit down when talking with the patient or family member.
3. Provide educational material in a variety of languages and venues.
   a. Written materials, videos, pictures, hands-on displays, etc.
   b. Determine preferred learning method.
   c. Use "teach back" to ascertain understanding.
4. Open visitation policy.
5. Allow access to medical records or online portals for information.
6. Be accessible at the different stages of readiness and confidence to support patient and family engagement.
7. Patient and Family Advisory Councils (PFAC) allow facility partnering.
   a. Participation in quality and safety policies.
   b. Organizational assessments.
   c. Education and training.
   d. Develop and improve patient information materials.
8. Facilitate transition planning.
   a. Engage patients and family members in discharge planning beginning when the patient is admitted.
   b. Provide medication lists.
   c. Encourage participation in medication reconciliation.
   d. Establish a resource center for educational materials.

F. Anticipated outcomes.
1. Improved communication.
2. Improved provider–patient partnerships.
3. Improved patient experiences of care.
4. More efficient use of resources.
5. Improved provider satisfaction.
6. Better patient experiences, outcomes, and health.

IV. Barriers to patient and family engagement.

A. Fear and feelings of intimidation.

B. Uncertainty on how to be involved.

C. Health literacy.

D. Lack of provider support.

E. Unwillingness to change.
1. Transtheoretical model (TTM) of intentional change focuses on the decision making of the individual.
   a. Developed by Prochaska, DiClemente, and colleagues in 1977. Research based on a variety of problem behaviors.
   b. Behavioral change is a process rather than a discrete event. Relapse may occur. Individuals go through a series of changes on the road to adopting healthy behaviors and/or cessation of unhealthy behaviors.
2. Five stages of change.
   a. Precontemplation: lack of awareness that a situation/problem can be improved by change in behavior.
      (1) The individual has no intention of changing in the near future, i.e., the next 6 months.
      (2) The patient is often characterized as resistant or unmotivated.
      (3) The person tends to avoid information, discussion, or thought about the situation or problem.
      (4) Traditional programs are often not designed for such individuals, and their needs can go unmet.

b. Contemplation: recognition of the problem.
   (1) Initial consideration is given to change in behavior.
   (2) Gathering information about potential solutions and actions begins.
   (3) Often seen as ambivalent to change or as a procrastinator.
   (4) Like those in the precontemplation stage, these individuals are not ready for traditional action-oriented programs.
c. Preparation: introspection about the decision.
   (1) Reaffirms the need and desire to change a behavior(s), usually within the next 30 days.
   (2) Completes the final pre-action steps.
   (3) A transition stage rather than a stable stage.
d. Action: implementation of the practices needed for successful behavior change (e.g., taking antihypertensive medication as prescribed).
   (1) Lifestyle modifications for fewer than 6 months.
   (2) Vigilance against relapse is critical.
e. Maintenance: consolidation of the behaviors initiated in the action stage.
   (1) Report the highest level of self-efficacy.
   (2) Less frequently tempted to relapse.
f. Termination: problem behaviors are no longer desirable.

3. Processes of change are covert, and individuals use overt actions to progress through the stages of change. The processes of change are important guides for intervention programs to help the individual move through these stages.
a. Consciousness-raising: increasing the awareness about the causes, consequences, and cures for a particular problem, e.g., CKD. Potential interventions: feedback, education, confrontation, media campaigns.
b. Dramatic relief: emotional arousal; produces increased emotional experiences followed by reduced affect if appropriate action can be taken. Potential interventions: role-playing, grieving, personal testimonies, media campaigns.
c. Environmental reevaluation: social reappraisal; assesses how the problem affects one's social environment. It can also include the awareness that one can serve as a role model in a positive or negative way. Potential interventions: empathy training, documentaries, and family interventions.
d. Social liberation: environmental opportunities; requires an increase in social opportunities or alternatives especially for people who are relatively deprived or oppressed. Potential interventions: advocacy, empowerment procedures, appropriate policies.

e. Self-reevaluation: self-reappraisal; assessment of an individual's self-image with and without a particular unhealthy habit. Potential interventions: value clarification, appropriate role models, imagery techniques.
f. Stimulus control: reengineering; remove cues for unhealthy habits and add prompts for healthier alternatives. Potential interventions: avoidance, environmental reengineering, self-help groups.
g. Helping relationships: supporting; combine caring, trust, openness, acceptance, and support for healthy habits. Potential interventions: rapport building, therapeutic alliance, counselor calls, buddy system.
h. Counter conditioning: substituting; learning healthier behaviors that can substitute problem behaviors. Potential interventions: e.g., substitute hard candy for fluid to accommodate limitations in intake.
i. Reinforcement management: rewarding; self-changers rely more on rewards than on punishments. Potential interventions: contingency contracts, positive self-statements, group recognition.
j. Self-liberation: committing; the belief that one can change as well as the commitment and recommitment to act on that belief.

4. Enhancing change with motivational interviewing.
a. Background. Motivational interviewing was developed by William Miller and Stephen Rollnick in the early 1990s. Its aim is to help someone make changes in behavior. Motivational interviewing can be integrated with other methods for facilitating change.
b. Definition. Motivational interviewing is a client-centered, directive method for enhancing intrinsic motivation to change by exploring and resolving ambivalence (Miller & Rollnick, 2002).
   (1) It is person-centered and focuses on the concerns and perspectives of the individual. It relies heavily on the work of Carl Rogers.
   (2) It intentionally seeks to resolve ambivalence, often in a particular direction of change. The interviewer selectively responds to speech in a way that resolves ambivalence and moves the person toward change.
   (3) It is a method of communication rather than a set of techniques; it is a facilitative approach to communication that evokes natural change.
   (4) The focus is on eliciting the person's intrinsic motivation for change.
   (5) It cannot be used to impose change that is inconsistent with the individual's own values and beliefs.

5. Goals of motivational interviewing.
  a. Create a safe and supportive rapport with a person and facilitate thinking about one's own behavior(s).
  b. Help the individual explore the behavior(s).
  c. Make a cost-benefit analysis of the status quo.
  d. Decrease potential resistance to change.
  e. Clarify goals.
  f. Help develop realistic strategies for facilitating behavioral changes.
6. Addresses whether and/or how the individual might make changes.
7. Recognizes that if the idea of change was entirely positive, then it would be easy.
8. Motivational interviewing techniques recognize both positive and negative aspects of change.
9. Situations to avoid during a motivational interview.
  a. The question/answer routine: prevents elaboration and exploration.
  b. Confrontation/denial: almost always demands the individual insist on the opposite perspective. Avoid arguments, struggles, or debates about what the person should do.
  c. The expert trap: can lead the individual into a passive role. The person will not work on his/her own to explore and resolve ambivalence.
  d. Labeling: e.g., troublemaker, can provoke resistance. If a person should ask about a label, the response should indicate that a label is not of interest. The person's behavior and what it means to him/her is the important component.
  e. Blaming: is not relevant or important to the goals of the interview.
  f. Preaching: does not encourage change or engagement. Avoid scolding, lecturing, or talking down to. Give suggestions and feedback.

SECTION E
Caring for Veterans
Loretta Jackson Brown

I. Overview.

A. Career military.
1. A career in the military often involves deployment to war zones.
2. Upon return, many military members are able to quickly bounce back from the stresses of war.
3. Some are not as resilient, and many experience signs of combat stress, to include traumatic brain injury (TBI) and posttraumatic stress disorder (PTSD).

B. In years past, U.S. service members would receive care in military treatment centers; however, with the realignment and closure of military installations, most service members and their family members receive medical care in primary care setting within their local community.
1. There are an estimated 22.2 million veterans in the United States, and this means that a large number of them are being treated by civilian healthcare providers.
2. To provide service members with the best opportunity to recover from combat stress and to live a full and healthy life, it is important for civilian healthcare providers to be familiar with the unique care needs of veterans and their family members.

II. Traumatic brain injury (TBI).

A. Has been called the "signature injury" for Operation Enduring Freedom and Operation Iraqi Freedom (Afghanistan and Iraq wars).

B. An alteration in brain function, or other evidence of brain pathology caused by an external force (Menon et al., 2010).

C. Results from blunt or penetrating trauma to the head or indirect acceleration and deceleration forces or blast – does not require direct impact.

D. Extent and severity of TBI after an initial mechanical event depends on several factors.
1. Magnitude of direct or indirect forces applied to the head.
2. Direction of the force.
3. Subsequent direction, duration, and amplitude of angular accelerations to which the brain is subjected.

III. Causes of traumatic brain injury in the U.S. military.

A. Blast injury results from pressure waves interacting with the body following exposure to a high-order explosive event where the blast creates a surge of high pressure followed by a vacuum.
1. Primary. Blast wave shoots through body and brain, compressing blood vessels and transmitting damaging energy pulses into the brain.
2. Secondary. Shrapnel and debris propelled by the blast hits a soldier's head resulting in a closed-head injury from blunt force or penetrating head injury that damages brain tissue.
3. Tertiary. Abrupt deceleration of the head occurring when a soldier is impelled through the

air following a blast, and the brain keeps moving after the skull is stopped.

B. Falls.

C. Motor vehicle crashes.

D. Assaults.

IV. Functional consequences of TBI.

A. Range from transient, reversible alterations in brain function to extensive disability or death.

B. Recovery of neurologic functioning after TBI might or might not occur and varies in its recovery progress from a few minutes to many years.

C. In cases of mild TBI, 38% to 80% of individuals may develop postconcussion syndrome, a syndrome characterized by headaches, depression, irritability, sleep disorder, poor concentration, and fatigue (Hall et al., 2005).

V. Signs and symptoms of traumatic brain injury.

A. Physical: headache, nausea, vomiting, dizziness, blurred vision, sleep disturbance, weakness, paralysis, sensory loss, spasticity, disorders of speech or language, swallowing disorders, balance disorders, disorders of coordination, seizure disorder.

B. Cognitive: difficulty with attention, concentration, memory, speed of processing, new learning, planning, reasoning, judgment, language, and abstract thinking.

C. Behavioral/emotional: depression, anxiety, agitation, irritability, impulsivity, aggression and violence, social inappropriateness, emotional outbursts, childishness, impaired self-control, impaired self-awareness, inability to take responsibility or accept criticism, alcohol or drug abuse/addiction, apathy, paranoia, confusion, frustration, agitation, sleep problems, or mood swings (American Psychiatric Association, 2000).

VI. TBI assessment, diagnosis, and treatment.

A. TBI may not always have obvious signs and may not be recognized in the field; therefore, screening should also occur upon return from deployment.

B. Diagnosis should be compared and contrasted with other conditions that may alter consciousness such as hypoglycemia, cardiac arrhythmia, stroke, and alcohol and drug intoxication.

C. The Glasgow Coma Scale can help to determine if there is an acute alteration in alertness or consciousness. The Glasgow Coma Scale has three components: eye opening, verbal response, and motor response (National Center for Injury Prevention and Control, 2003).
 1. Scores of 8 or less – classified as severe TBI.
 2. Scores of 9 to 12 – moderate TBI.
 3. Scores of 13 to 15 – mild TBI.

D. Positive TBI screening should be followed up with a comprehensive evaluation. The diagnosis of TBI is usually made clinically, and neuroimaging is commonly used to identify bleeding inside the skull.

E. Bleeding is not associated with all TBI; however, posttraumatic bleeding is associated with poorer prognosis and can be life threatening.

F. Intensive care medicine is used to manage hemodynamically unstable cases of TBI. This includes the use of ventilators, intracranial pressure monitoring, and management of coexisting injuries.

G. Combat veterans with suspected TBI should be referred to a specialist who has been trained in managing TBI in combat veterans.

VII. Posttraumatic stress disorder (PTSD).

A. PTSD is an anxiety disorder that some people develop after seeing or living through an event that caused or threatened serious harm or death.
 1. PTSD has been with those serving in the military since the beginning of military service.
 2. PTSD can also occur outside of the military in people who have experienced other kinds of traumas.
 3. Each case is unique to the affected individual.

B. About one third of soldiers with mild TBI also have PTSD (Brenner et al., 2009; Hoge et al., 2008).

C. Lifetime prevalence of PTSD among male combat veterans is about 39% compared to 3.6% lifetime prevalence for PTSD in the general population of men.

D. PTSD prerisk factors include being a younger adult, being a minority, being a female, and having a prior psychiatric history.

E. Postrisk factors for PTSD include lack of social support and subsequent life stresses.

F. Individuals with PTSD are likely to have other

psychological disorders to include depression, other anxiety disorders, and substance abuse.

VIII. Symptom clusters of PTSD.

A. Re-experiencing: reliving the trauma.
1. Memories of the trauma may return at any time.
2. An individual may experience intrusive thoughts and flashbacks; the person may become physically and emotionally upset when reminded of the trauma.

B. Numbing and avoidance.
1. Tactics that allow an individual to avoid thinking about the trauma.
2. Individuals may turn down their emotions to block out fear responses and may not be able to recall parts of the trauma.

C. Arousal.
1. Difficulty sleeping and concentrating along with anxiety are the results of an individual trying to manage intrusive thoughts from the trauma.
2. Other symptoms include an exaggerated startle response and hypervigilance.

IX. PTSD diagnosis and treatment.

A. To be diagnosed with PTSD, an individual should have one re-experiencing symptom, one numbing/avoidance, and two arousal symptoms.

B. Diagnosis of PTSD cannot be made until a month after a traumatic event.

C. Once diagnosed, new trauma or life events may reactivate PTSD symptoms.

D. The two main types of treatment for PTSD are pharmacologic and psychotherapy counseling.
1. Selective serotonin reuptake inhibitors (SSRIs) are a type of antidepressant medicine.
   a. They raise the level of serotonin in the brain by inhibiting uptake of serotonin by the central nervousness system neuronal.
   b. The two SSRIs that are currently approved by the FDA for the treatment of PTSD are sertraline (Zoloft®) and paroxetine (Paxil®).
2. Psychotherapy treatment for PTSD.
   a. Cognitive behavioral therapy: cognitive processing and prolonged exposure therapy.
   b. Integrative therapy: eye movement desensitization and reprocessing (EMDR).

X. Impact of deployment on families.

A. Characteristics of families at high risk for deployment crisis.
1. Dysfunctional family dynamics.
2. Young families with no history of deployment.
3. Foreign-born spouse.
4. Pregnancy.
5. Single parent or jointly deployed parents.

B. Children of deployed service members may experience emotional and behavioral difficulties and health complaints.
1. Emotional: sadness, anxiety, depression, loneliness, numbness, overwhelmed, poor coping.
2. Behavioral: school performance problems, peer-related difficulties, disrespecting authority figures, sleep disturbances, regression in stages of development, sexual acting out.
3. Health: rapid heart rates and systolic pressure, decreased appetite, weight loss.

C. Helping families cope with deployment.
1. Screen individuals on admission to learn if they are military veterans or members of a military family.
2. Assess for psychosocial stressors and functional impairment.
3. Assess family readiness plan to prepare for deployment and resilience plan to support recovery from deployment.
4. Refer to trained counselors familiar with military families.

SECTION F
The Financial Impact
Lois Kelley, Donna Bednarski

I. Costs of treating kidney disease.

A. Costs and chronic kidney disease (CKD).
1. In 2011, patients with CKD represented 9.2% of the Medicare prevalent population and accounted for 18.2% of total Medicare expenditures (USRDS, 2013), which increased to 19.6% in 2012 (USRDS, 2014).
2. Costs per person with CKD reached $20,162 for Medicare patients 65 years of age and older. Costs were higher if the patient had hypertension or diabetes or both (USRDS, 2014).
3. In 2012, costs for patients with CKD reached $44.6 billion (USRDS, 2014).

B. Costs of dialysis and transplant. In 2011, as a primary payer, Medicare paid $87,945 per hemodialysis patient, $71,630 per peritoneal dialysis patient, and $32,922 per transplant recipient (USRDS, 2013).

II. Paying for treatment.

A. Medicare is health insurance for select groups of people.
  1. Qualifications include the following groups.
     a. People 65 and older.
     b. Those who have received Social Security Disability Insurance (SSDI) checks for 24 months.
     c. Those patients who have kidney failure requiring dialysis or transplant for survival.
  2. To be eligible for ESRD Medicare, patients must be certified by a physician to have kidney failure requiring dialysis or transplant for survival. In addition, each patient must also have worked long enough to qualify on his/her own work record, his/her spouse's (or in some cases, an ex-spouse's) work record, or parent's work record if the patient is a child.
     a. Social Security can advise a patient if he/she is eligible for Medicare.
     b. Dialysis and transplant providers must complete the ESRD Medical Evidence Report Medicare Entitlement & Patient Registration form (CMS 2728). This registers the patient in the ESRD program and alerts Social Security that the patient may be eligible for Medicare. Applications are available at the local Social Security office and can be completed in person, by phone, or by mail.
  3. Medicare Part A.
     a. Covers hospital room, board, and care; transplant evaluation and surgery for recipients and donors; hospice care; and limited care in a skilled nursing facility.
     b. Hospital stays.
        (1) As a primary payer, Part A pays 100% for the first 60 days after the hospital deductible is paid. Medicare Part A hospital days are limited.
        (2) After 60 days, there is a copay for each hospital day.
        (3) After a 90-day hospital stay, Medicare will pay for only 60 more days (called lifetime reserve days), and there is a higher copay.
        (4) Although the first 90 Medicare Part A days can be renewed if someone stays out of the hospital at least 60 days, once used, lifetime reserve days are gone. If someone remains out of the hospital over 60 days, it starts a new benefit period with a new Part A deductible.
        (5) Part A also pays up to 100 days in a skilled nursing facility. There is no daily charge for the first 20 days, but after that, there is a daily charge.
        (6) Part A is premium free for anyone with enough work credits. Those 65 and older, without enough work credits, can purchase Part A. The cost is dependent upon how many credits have been earned.
  4. Medicare Part B.
     a. Covers outpatient charges including doctors' and surgeons' fees, outpatient surgery, in-center and home dialysis, durable medical equipment, rehabilitation therapy, home health care, ambulance (if "medically necessary"), and some prescription drugs.
     b. As a primary payer, Part B pays 80% of the allowed charge after the annual deductible is met.
     c. The Part B annual deductible increases every year. The guidelines may change over time. (www.medicare.gov).
  5. Patients with Employer Group Health Plan (EGHP) coverage may not want to pay the premium for Medicare Part B.
     a. If patients do not sign up for Part A or B, they can sign up at any time without penalty.
     b. However, if they sign up for Part A (free) and waive Part B (premium), they can only sign up for Part B from January to March of each year, and Medicare would start the following July. Signing up late for Part B may also result in higher Part B premiums.
     c. Patients should talk with Social Security before deciding not to sign up for Medicare.
  6. There are several Medicare plans available for patients to choose from.
     a. Original Medicare is provided by the government. In this plan, patients can choose their healthcare providers and know what percent or fees that will be owed.
     b. Patients who join Medicare Advantage (MA) plans purchase them through private insurance companies that contract with Medicare.
        (1) In comparison to Original Medicare, MA plans may offer extra benefits or have different copays or coinsurance without any cap.
        (2) Some plans offer a higher cost option to cover copays and coinsurance while others do not.
     c. Patients can stay in an MA plan when they start dialysis, but dialysis patients cannot sign up for an MA plan unless it is a "special needs plan" that has agreed to accept people on dialysis.

d. Transplant patients who do not need dialysis can stay in or join an MA plan.

7. The type of treatment the patient chooses governs when Medicare can start.
   a. If the patient starts a home training program before the third full month of dialysis, Medicare coverage can be backdated to the first day of the month chronic dialysis started, regardless of location (hospital or clinic) of initiation of dialysis.
   b. If in-center dialysis is the patient's choice of treatment, Medicare starts the first day of third full month of dialysis.
   c. If a patient receives a preemptive transplant, Medicare starts the month of the transplant or can be backdated up to 2 months if the patient was admitted for evaluation that month.

8. When Medicare ends is also dependent on the patient's type of treatment and whether or not he/she has Medicare for more than one reason.
   a. As long as someone is on dialysis, he/she can receive Medicare indefinitely.
   b. If kidney function recovers and dialysis is no longer needed, Medicare coverage can continue for 12 months.
   c. If a patient is transplanted and has Medicare solely based on kidney failure, Medicare coverage will end after 36 months.
   d. If someone is eligible for Medicare due to age or disability, as well as kidney failure, even if he/she gets a transplant, Medicare continues indefinitely.

B. Medicare savings programs can help Medicare beneficiaries with limited income and assets to get state help to pay Medicare premiums and, in some cases, to pay secondary benefits for Medicare covered services. State medical assistance offices can screen patients for these programs.
   1. Qualified Medicare Beneficiary program (QMB) pays Medicare premiums and Medicare coinsurance or copays, but it does not cover other Medicaid-only services.
   2. Specified Low-Income Medicare Beneficiary (SLMB) pays Medicare Part B premiums only, but it does not cover Medicare copays or coinsurance or provide other Medicaid-only services.
   3. Qualified Individual program (QI), like SLMB, pays Medicare Part B premiums only.
   4. Qualified Working Disabled Individual (QWDI) program helps those with disabilities who would lose Medicare due to work pay Part A premiums.
      a. Those with Part A are eligible for Part B.
      b. Transplant patients who have a disability other than kidney failure and continue to work may qualify for QWDI.

c. QDWI is one of the Medicare Savings Programs. For financial qualifications for 2013, refer to http://www.medicare.gov/your-medicare-costs/help-paying-costs/medicare-savings-program/medicare-savings-programs.html
d. Someone who works with a disability can keep free Medicare Part A (and can still buy Part B and D) under Continuation of Medicare for 93 months after the 9-month trial work period ends.
e. The SSA Red Book includes information about various work incentive programs and can be found at www.socialsecurity.gov/redbook/index.html

C. Every state has state medical assistance or Medicaid (Medi-Cal in California).
   1. To qualify for full Medicaid benefits, patients must meet eligibility criteria including state income and asset guidelines.
      a. Determining who is eligible for help and income requirements varies from state to state.
      b. Some states allow patients with incomes above state Medicaid guidelines to pay some of the costs of their medical care (called *spend down* or *share of costs*) with state Medicaid paying the remainder.
   2. The federal government mandates that states provide certain benefits and offers states the flexibility to cover additional services.
      a. Patients with limited income and assets may have Medicaid alone if they do not qualify for Medicare, usually because they have not earned enough work credits.
      b. Some states cover undocumented aliens on dialysis with 100% state funds. Most do not pay for transplants for these individuals.
   3. Some patients are "dual eligible." This means they have both Medicare and Medicaid.
      a. Medicare is considered the primary insurance and always pays first.
      b. Medicaid is considered secondary and therefore pays the deductible and coinsurance for Medicare-covered services and services that are covered by Medicaid.
      c. Like Medicare, states have payment limits for covered services.

D. Medigap or Medicare supplement plans help to cover costs for Medicare covered services.
   1. Medigap plans are sold by private insurance companies and can pay all or part of Medicare deductibles and coinsurance for Part A and Part B covered services, including Part B covered drugs.
   2. Medigap plans in all but Massachusetts, Minnesota, and Wisconsin use the National

Association of Insurance Commissioners (NAIC) model plan to structure benefits.
  a. In the NAIC model, plans are designated by letters A through L.
  b. All A plans offer the same benefits.
  c. All L plans offer the same benefits.
  d. This makes it easy to compare plans because the premium is the only difference.
3. Under federal law, a Medigap plan must accept anyone 65 or older, even those with preexisting conditions, during the first 6 months he/she has Medicare.
  a. Those with Medicare who are under 65 may be denied Medigap coverage or may have to wait for coverage for kidney disease.
  b. State insurance department health experts can advise patients about Medigap coverage in their state.

E. Some patients have an Employer Group Health Plan (EGHPs) when their kidneys fail.
  1. An EGHP usually has more benefits and pays more than Medicare allows on Medicare covered services.
  2. An EGHP may also cover prescription drugs as well as or better than Medicare Prescription Drug Coverage (Part D).
  3. An EGHP is the primary payer for the first 30 months that a dialysis patient is eligible for Medicare whether or not they enroll in Medicare. Providers can bill Medicare as a secondary payer for EGHP deductibles, copays and coinsurance, and services that Medicare covers but the EGHP denies.
  4. Having Medicare with an EGHP limits the amount a patient can be charged by providers that accept assignment to 100% of the Medicare allowable charge. Paying the Part B premium may save money as the EGHP pays at least 100% of Medicare's allowed charge because the patient is not liable for the difference between the charge and Medicare's allowable rate.

F. Some people have an individual (nongroup) health plan when their kidneys fail.
  1. Coverage varies and may not be as comprehensive as group plans. Premiums and cost shares may be higher.
  2. Medicare is always the primary insurance before a nongroup health plan.

G. High risk health insurance plans are available in some states.
  1. High risk health plans help people who have been denied coverage because of preexisting medical conditions. Although expensive, with possible

waiting periods for preexisting conditions coverage, they do, however, immediately cover any new health conditions.
  2. Some states do not have high risk plans and others do not allow those with Medicare to buy them.
  3. State insurance department health experts can advise patients about this coverage.

H. Federal Employees Health Benefit (FEHB) Plans are available to federal employees.
  1. There are several choices of plans from managed care plans to fee-for-service.
  2. Federal employees have an opportunity to change plans every year.
  3. People can have both an FEHB plan and Medicare if they meet the qualifications for both.
  4. FEHB plans may cover services that Medicare does not and Medicare can help to pay FEHB deductibles, copays, or coinsurance. For more information about FEHB, see http://www.opm.gov/healthcare-insurance/healthcare/

I. Health benefits are available for veterans.
  1. Those eligible for Veterans Administration (VA) health benefits include anyone who served on active duty without dishonorable discharge as well as those who were in the National Guard and called to active duty by executive order.
  2. VA provides care in VA health facilities or pays for the care of veterans at local healthcare facilities, including dialysis and transplant facilities.
  3. Veterans do not have to have service-connected disabilities to receive certain health benefits. For more information about VA benefits, see www.va.gov/health

J. TRICARE is the military health benefit for service members and dependents.
  1. Those eligible for TRICARE include active military duty, their dependents, and retirees and dependents.
  2. What is covered and where coverage must be received depends on the TRICARE plan selected: TRICARE Prime, TRICARE Extra, TRICARE Standard, and TRICARE for Life. The latter is for those 65 or older with Medicare.
  3. TRICARE applications are accepted at veterans health centers, by calling 877-222-VETS or accessing online at http://www.mytricare.com/internet/tric/tri/mtc_nprov.nsf/PGS/Frms_IndvdlApplctns_1

K. The Indian Health Service (IHS) funds health care for those who are members of American Indian tribes or Alaska natives corporations.
  1. Health care is provided to American Indians or

Alaska natives living on or near reservations as well as some care of those living in urban areas. For eligibility, see www.ihs.gov

2. IHS provides care for prevention and treatment of diseases, including kidney failure.
3. Care is provided through IHS facilities or private providers through purchase of services. For general information on health benefits see www.ihs.gov

L. State Child Health Insurance Program (SCHIP) is a program of services to children.
   1. SCHIP provides basic health care, physicians, hospitals, immunizations, and emergencies.
   2. To qualify, children must be under 19, and their families must meet eligibility requirements. In most states, families of four with no health insurance can earn up to $36,200 and still qualify for SCHIP. For more information, see www.insurekidsnow.gov

M. Program of All-Inclusive Care for the Elderly (PACE) provides services to the elderly. The goal of this program is to allow the elderly to stay in their communities rather than in nursing facilities.
   1. PACE programs are not available in all states.
   2. Where available, people must be 55 years old or older to obtain PACE help.
   3. PACE programs provide comprehensive primary care services, social services, restorative therapies, personal care and supportive services, nutritional counseling, recreational therapy, and meals 24 hours a day, 7 days a week, 365 days a year in an adult day program or in-home. For more information about where PACE services are offered, see www.cms.hhs.gov/PACE/LPPO/list.asp

N. State kidney programs are state-funded programs for people with kidney disease and kidney failure.
   1. All states do not have state kidney programs, and in those states that do, eligibility guidelines vary.
   2. State kidney programs may help with such things as the cost of access surgery, treating kidney failure, medications, and treatment-related transportation. Covered services, in states with kidney programs, are determined by state funds and program guidelines.
   3. Most nephrology social workers know if their state has a state kidney program. To get a directory and/or to find out if your state has one, call Missouri Kidney Program at 800-733-7345 or download the 2005 Directory of State Kidney Programs from http://som.missouri.edu/mokp/docs/noskp/index.html

O. Health Savings Accounts (HSA) allow people to set aside money, tax-free, to pay for qualifying medical costs.
   1. HSAs are designed to help patients afford health care, particularly if they only qualify for high deductible health plans (HDHPs).
   2. Those with Medicare and those who can be claimed as a dependent on someone else's health plan are not eligible for an HSA.
   3. Those with cafeteria plans set up by their employers can save money on taxes by setting aside pretax dollars from their paycheck to pay their share of health insurance premiums, out-of-pocket medical or dental costs, and child care. In a traditional cafeteria plan, employees must spend the money they set aside for the year or lose what remains in the account at the end of the year. However, some HSAs do allow funds to carry over from year to year.
   4. Funds in an HSA are portable if the person changes jobs.

P. Exchange plans.
   1. The Affordable Care Act (ACA), passed in 2010, was designed to make it possible for all Americans to obtain affordable health insurance; it began in 2014. States are implementing this act in different ways. Some states use the Federal Marketplace and other states set up their own.
   2. Policies are available on four levels: Bronze, Silver, Gold, and Platinum, which vary on coverage and level of cost sharing. Lower income Americans may qualify for subsidies and tax credits that make the insurance more affordable. Some states have expanded Medicaid to allow more low income Americans to have health care at low cost. For more information, go to https://finder.healthcare.gov
   3. The law has little impact on the dialysis-dependent kidney failure population who are Medicare eligible, but has significant impact on CKD (pre-ESRD) and transplant population.
      a. CKD.
         (1) No longer excluded from coverage due to CKD diagnosis, which will allow access to screening and hopefully delay or avoid kidney failure.
         (2) No longer need to be employed to have access to coverage.
         (3) Depending on income, can be eligible for subsidies and tax credits.
         (4) Once they have kidney failure, may have the option of transitioning to Medicare or maintaining their current coverage.
      b. Transplant.
         (1) Transplant recipients who were eligible for Medicare solely on the basis of kidney

failure would no longer lose their coverage 3 years posttransplant.

(2) Cannot be denied due to preexisting condition.

(3) Transplant recipients could buy coverage through the marketplace and could be eligible for subsidies and tax credits.

(4) Marketplace plans drug benefits to cover immunosuppressants that are critical to maintaining graft function.

4. Patients can access information and apply for health insurance by going to https://finder.healthcare.gov

III. Legal protections for health benefits.

A. Medigap. There are legal protections that allow patients with Medicare and Medigap plans who return to work and obtain coverage through their job to put their Medigap plan "on hold" and return if their employer plan coverage ends.

B. Consolidated Omnibus Budget Reconciliation Act (COBRA). Certain "events" grant continuation coverage if someone works for a company with 20 or more employees.

1. If someone loses his/her job or experiences a reduction in hours/benefits, he/she is eligible for 18 months of COBRA coverage.

2. In cases of separation or divorce, death, or the obtainment of Medicare from the employee, the spouse and dependent children are eligible for 36 months of COBRA coverage.

3. If a child is no longer considered a dependent due to age, he/she is eligible for 36 months of COBRA coverage.

4. The premium for COBRA is 102% of the full premium. The employee is responsible for paying the total premium and the employer pays nothing.

5. Employees who are disabled before or within 60 days after the COBRA event can have an extra 11 months of coverage for a premium of 150% of the full premium. The employee is responsible for paying the total premium, while the employer pays nothing.

6. Someone who has Medicare before he/she has COBRA must be offered COBRA coverage. An employer can terminate COBRA coverage if an employee signs up for Medicare after he/she has COBRA.

7. A COBRA plan is the primary payer for the first 30 months when patients have kidney failure and are eligible for Medicare.

C. Americans with Disabilities Act (ADA). The ADA applies to employers with 15 or more employees.

1. The ADA does not require that any employer offer health insurance coverage to employees.

2. If an employer has 15 or more employees and provides health benefits to others in the same job, the employer must provide health insurance to the person with a disability.

3. It is not legal for plans to have caps on coverage for certain diagnoses unless they do this for everyone within that group (Employment retirement Income security Act of 1974).

D. Health Insurance Portability and Accountability Act (HIPAA). This federal law allows those with preexisting conditions to get group or individual health insurance on the commercial market.

1. HIPAA applies to anyone losing Medicare, Medicaid, TRICARE, or VA benefits.

2. Proof of coverage is needed, and people must sign up for their new plan before 63 days elapse.

3. When faced with the loss of health insurance, the plan must send a letter stating the loss coverage. This letter proves "creditable coverage" and when the clock is started for the open enrollment period.

4. The new health plan must count time that the patient was covered in the previous plan toward any preexisting condition waiting period.

5. HIPAA is the law that also protects the confidentiality of patients' personal health information.

IV. Paying for medications.

A. Insurance companies may offer coverage for prescription drugs.

1. Out-of-pocket expenses vary by health plan.

2. Some plans have formularies and coinsurance or copays.

3. Plan enrollment packets and websites provide information on patient rights and responsibilities, including how to file an exception request to get a nonformulary drug covered.

B. Medicare Part D provides prescription drug coverage sold by private insurance companies.

1. Anyone with Medicare Part A and/or Part B is eligible. Those who have current prescription coverage that is as good as or better than Part D coverage can wait to join Part D when needed.

2. Anyone can enroll in Part D during the 3 months following eligibility for Medicare.

a. If they join after the 3-month period, they could have a higher premium when they join.

b. In some cases, Medicare beneficiaries can join or switch outside the annual coordinated election period from November 15 to December 31. However, most can only join or switch during this period.

3. Most drug coverage for patients with Medicare and Medicaid (dual eligible) is under Medicare Part D. Coverage depends on whether the patient's drugs are on the Part D formulary. Patients eligible for both can switch plans any month to get the best coverage. Medicaid may still pay for drugs that are excluded under Part D.

4. Drugs covered under Part A or Part B are still covered by Part A or Part B regardless of the patient's chosen Medicare plan: Original Medicare or Medicare Advantage.

5. Those with limited income and assets are eligible for additional assistance called "extra help" to pay premiums and cost shares for covered drugs. Others pay premiums, deductibles, and coinsurance or copays. Social Security accepts applications for the low-income subsidy.

6. Unless someone qualifies for extra help, low-income subsidy, standard Part D plan have a coverage gap.
   a. Once those with Medicare Part D have paid the annual "true out-of-pocket" (TrOOP) costs for Part D, they receive catastrophic coverage.
   b. Help from family, friends, qualified state pharmacy assistance programs, and charities to pay these TrOOP costs can assist people in reaching the catastrophic benefit, at which time the plan pays 95% of the cost of covered drugs.
   c. Some Part D plans do not have a coverage gap while others cover generic drugs or even brand-name drugs during the gap. However, these plans have a higher premium.
   d. The ACA provides the coverage gap to grow smaller each year, disappearing entirely by year 2020. The coverage gap closes by maintaining the 50% discount the manufacturers offer and increasing what Medicare drug plans cover.

7. Part D plans limit their costs by negotiating prices with drug companies, limiting drug coverage, requiring prior authorization, step therapy, or limiting the number of pills a patient can obtain per month.
   a. If the patient's health or functioning may be harmed, patients or providers can request an expedited coverage determination and receive a response from the plan within 24 hours.
   b. There is a standard template that prescribers can use to request expedited coverage determination from the plan. However, Part D plans are not required to accept it.
   c. Medicare requires that Part D plans post their exception request forms online.

8. Nurses can encourage patients to take the time to compare plans every year and choose the one with the best coverage for their current medication regimen, taking into consideration future needs.
   a. Patients can call the Medicare Helpline at 1-800-MEDICARE or use the Prescription Drug Plan Finder at www.medicare.gov to compare plans offered in their state and even sign up for a plan during their initial enrollment or the annual enrollment period.
   b. The Formulary Finder on the Medicare Web site and Epocrates at www.epocrates.com can help nurses and other healthcare providers see what drugs are on a plan's formulary.

C. State Pharmacy Assistance Programs (SPAPs) are not available in every state. To determine which states offer these programs, refer to http://www.medicare.gov/(X(1)S(jkrhxx5503e052j2jky2vsmd))/pharmaceutical-assistance-program/state-programs.aspx?AspxAutoDetectCookieSupport=1
   1. Where available, these state-funded programs are intended to help pay for certain drugs for patients meeting identified guidelines.
   2. Help from qualified SPAPs for people with Medicare Part D counts toward the TrOOP costs patients must have before the Part D catastrophic benefit. Some state kidney programs are qualified SPAPs.

D. Pharmaceutical patient assistance programs (PAPs) are established by drug companies to help people without health or drug coverage get their drugs.
   1. Each program has its own application form, eligibility guidelines, and frequency to reapply. More information can be found on http://rxassist.org
   2. Some PAPs will not help those who have Part D.

E. Charities and foundations may help those who qualify to pay for drugs. For resources that help pay for drugs, see www.rxassist.org or www.needymeds.com
   1. Guidelines for eligibility vary. Some require that the patient has a certain diagnosis and is taking medications for that diagnosis.
   2. Some obtain funds from pharmaceutical companies to run their PAP.
   3. Because funding is limited, everyone who needs help to get their drugs may not get the help they need.
   4. Help from charities can count toward the true out-of-pocket TrOOP costs patients must have before the Part D catastrophic benefit.

V. Income and income support.

A. Socioeconomic status and patient outcomes.
   1. Low socioeconomic status is linked to premature births, diet, diabetes, hypertension, smoking, alcohol, and/or drug usage. All of these are risk factors for kidney disease.

2. Kidney function decline in African Americans with diabetes is three times faster than in Caucasians. Eighty percent of the difference is explained by socioeconomic status, behaviors, and poor control of blood pressure and blood sugar.

3. For every $1,000 of higher income in African Americans on dialysis, there was a 3.3% lower relative risk of dying.

4. Income less than 200% of the federal poverty level was associated with microalbuminuria, a factor in the progression of kidney disease.

5. Financial status affects access to transplantation.

B. Employment improves socioeconomic status and provides benefits for patients, providers, and the system.

1. Employment is one factor that predicts how well African-American patients with hypertension and CKD function physically and emotionally.

2. For patients, employment provides a better standard of living, improved income, a sense of self-worth, socialization opportunities, and a better chance of having health insurance that covers preventive health care as well as treatment for known illnesses.

   a. Working helps patients have the financial resources to overcome healthcare access barriers and assure early identification and treatment of kidney disease.

   b. Working patients have the money to afford lifestyle changes and treatments to prolong kidney function or keep someone with kidney failure healthy.

   c. Once kidneys fail, working improves the chances for transplant and for better dialysis.

   d. Even though Medicare will not routinely pay for more than three treatments a week, their EGHP may pay for more frequent dialysis treatments performed at home or in the dialysis clinic and ongoing prescription coverage.

3. For facilities, having working patients who can more easily afford their treatment plan reduces frustration that nurses and other healthcare providers often feel when they recommend treatments that patients do not follow. Staff working in dialysis clinics where patients function at a higher level, including working, have higher job satisfaction and lower turnover.

4. When patients work, they are taxpayers as well as recipients of government benefits. When a working patient has EGHP coverage, it saves Medicare money for 30 months when Medicare is the secondary payer.

5. It takes a team to keep patients working and to return patients who are not working to the workforce.

   a. The physician/provider and nurse play an important role in keeping patients with CKD and kidney failure working by assessing work-limiting symptoms and making sure that patients know they can work with kidney disease and kidney failure.

   b. The nurse and other dialysis team members can help assure that working patients are offered home dialysis and transplant and/or are assigned shift times that fit their work schedule.

   c. Nurses need to educate patients about what symptoms to report and to whom. Advise the physician about work-limiting symptoms as soon as the patient reports them.

   d. Nurses can assist with early referral for nutritional counseling. Dietitians can help patients learn how to eat healthy meals to stay strong and be physically able to work.

   e. Nurses can also refer patients expressing financial concerns to the social worker to help address financial issues and evaluate work ability. The social worker can help working patients and those seeking employment to understand their legal rights and advocate with an employer for workplace accommodations.

   f. Social workers can also offer emotional counseling and refer patients to physical and vocational rehabilitation services to help them keep their jobs or become job ready.

C. Government disability benefits are available for those with a disability that is expected to last a year or result in death.

1. Social Security has a booklet that describes which conditions are considered potentially disabled. Some conditions that accompany kidney damage and kidney failure are listed.

2. Although government disability programs do not provide temporary disability benefits, there are work incentive programs to help people with disabilities return to work. For more information on work incentive programs, see www.socialsecurity.gov/work

3. Social Security can advise patients about disability benefits and work incentive programs.

4. Social Security Disability Insurance (SSDI) is a government-funded disability program for people who meet work requirements.

   a. Other income does not affect eligibility for SSDI.

   b. There is a 5-month waiting period during which no checks are paid.

   c. On average SSDI pays an average of 35% of the patient's past earnings.

   d. SSDI replaces more of a low-income worker's wages than the wages of a high-income worker.

e. A spouse and children may be eligible for SSDI family benefits.

f. Because someone receiving SSDI is eligible for Medicare after receiving SSDI checks for 24 months, some people with CKD may already have Medicare due to disability.

5. Supplemental Security Income (SSI) is a disability program for people who have limited income and assets, meet the disability qualifications, and have no or a limited work record.

a. People who qualify can get SSI during the SSDI waiting period.

b. SSI pays a very limited amount of income that is less than the federal poverty level.

c. There are no family benefits with SSI.

d. In most states, having SSI qualifies the patient for Medicaid.

D. Some people may receive private disability benefits through a job or private policy.

1. These plans may provide short- or long-term benefits.

2. To promote return to work, these plans usually pay only 60% of one's current income.

3. When the patient also qualifies for Social Security benefits, these benefits reduce private disability benefits.

E. Other financial assistance programs may help those patients who qualify for programs to pay for housing, utilities, food, transportation, living expenses, etc. Programs may be funded by the federal or state government, by local agencies, or national kidney charities like the American Kidney Fund or local affiliates of the National Kidney Foundation.

1. Patients must apply for assistance and meet the identified guidelines.

2. Some programs assist patients as long as they qualify while others provide temporary assistance to meet emergency needs.

3. Nephrology social workers often are aware of these programs and help patients access them.

VI. Resources.

A. Nurses can collaborate with social workers to help patients reach their maximum level of functioning.

1. Nurses and technicians see patients every day. Nurses are one of the best referral sources for social workers to identify patients' concerns and target interventions to assist them.

2. The social worker should assess patients' coping and offer counseling to patients and families, evaluate patients' psychosocial needs including financial concerns, assist patients to access helpful resources, provide directly or refer patients to agencies that can help them keep their jobs or find

new ones, recommend care based on patients' individual psychosocial needs, and assess and address barriers that keep patients from following their treatment plan.

B. Other resources.

1. Centers for Medicare and Medicaid Services. End Stage Kidney Disease (ESRD) Center, www.cms.hhs.gov/center/esrd.asp

2. Home Dialysis Central, www.homedialysis.org

3. Kidney School, www.kidneyschool.org

4. Life Options Rehabilitation Program, www.lifeoptions.org

5. Life Options, Employment: A Kidney Patient's Guide to Working and Paying for Treatment, www.lifeoptions.org/catalog/pdfs/booklets/employment.pdf

6. Health Well Foundation for help with premiums or prescription drug costs, www.healthwellfoundation.org

7. Social Security Administration. 2006 Red Book: A Summary Guide to Employment Support for Individuals with Disabilities under the Social Security Disability Insurance and Supplemental Security Income Programs, SSA Pub. No. 64-030, www.socialsecurity.gov/redbook

Section G
Physical Rehabilitation
Daniel Diroll

I. Definitions.

A. Physical activity – bodily movement that is produced by the contraction of skeletal muscle and that substantially increases energy expenditure.

B. Physical fitness – a set of attributes that people possess or achieve that relates to the ability to perform physical activity.

C. Physical functioning – an individual's ability to perform activities required in his/her daily life.

D. Exercise prescription – specifies the frequency, intensity, duration and mode of exercise training. When applied over time, it is designed to elicit adaptation to cumulative overload.

E. Exercise frequency – refers to the number of exercise session conducted per week.

F. Exercise duration – refers to the length of the exercise session.

G. Exercise mode – refers to the type of exercise being employed, such as walking, cycling, swimming, etc.

H. Exercise intensity – refers to the effort involved in an exercise session; can be measured using heart rate or rating of perceived exertion (Borg Scale).

I. Borg scale – a 15-point scale for rating of perceived exertion (RPE) during exercise (see Table 3.5).

J. Cardiorespiratory fitness – the ability to perform large muscle, dynamic, moderate-to-high intensity exercise for prolonged periods.

K. Exercise training – the planned, structured, and repetitive bodily movement done to improve or maintain one or more components of physical fitness or other health benefits.

L. Resistance training – physical exercise using resistance to induce muscular contraction that improves muscular strength, size, and endurance.

M. Heart rate reserve – a method used to determine exercise intensity using heart rate. It is also known as the Karvonen method and is calculated: (HRmax–HRrest) x (40% to 80%)+HRrest.

N. Body mass index (BMI) – calculated by dividing body weight in kilograms by height in meters squared and used to assess weight relative to height.

O. VO_2 max – reflects the volume of oxygen in milliliters of oxygen per minute that can be used in a maximal aerobic effort. It is closely related to the functional capacity of the heart.

P. VO_2 peak – the highest value of oxygen consumption attained during a graded exercise test; it does not necessarily define the highest value attainable by the individual (this would be the VO_2 max).

Q. Maximal exercise test – a graded test in which the patient exercises to a point of volitional fatigue. It is designed to elicit a maximal effort and allows for the accurate assessment of VO_2 max.

R. Submaximal exercise test – a test designed to determine the heart rate response to one or more submaximal work rates which can be used to predict VO_2 max.

S. Left ventricular ejection fraction (LVEF) – the percent of blood a full left ventricle pumps into the aorta with each cardiac cycle. It provides an assessment of cardiac efficiency and health.

Table 3.5

Borg's 15-point Scale for Rating of Perceived Exertion (RPE)

6 – 20% effort	
7 – 30% effort	Very, very light (Rest)
8 – 40% effort	
9 – 50% effort	Very light, gentle walking
10 – 55% effort	
11 – 60% effort	Fairly light
12 – 65% effort	
13 – 70% effort	Somewhat hard, steady pace
14 – 75% effort	
15 – 80% effort	Hard
16 – 85% effort	
17 – 90% effort	Very hard
18 – 95% effort	
19 – 100% effort	Very, very hard
20 – Exhaustion	

Borg RPE scale © Gunnar Borg, 1970, 1985, 1994, 1998

Source: Jung, T., & Park, S. (2011). Intradialytic exercise programs for hemodialysis patients. *Chonnam Medical Journal, 47*(2), 61-65. doi:10.4068/cmj.2011.47.2.61 Copyright © Chonnam Medical Journal, 2011. (Open Access article [http://creativecommons.org/licenses/by-nc/3.0]).

T. Protein energy wasting – a specific form of muscle wasting in patients with kidney failure, characterized by increased muscle protein catabolism relative to protein synthesis.

U. Uremic myopathy – a muscle disease in CKD that causes proximal muscle weakness and wasting. It is predominant in the muscles of the lower limbs and associated with fatigability and reduced exercise capacity.

II. Benefits of exercise.

A. Many studies have shown positive health benefits from increased physical activity without structured exercise training. There may be other benefits of regular physical activity that could positively impact other factors, specifically muscle wasting, cardiovascular risk, oxidative stress, and chronic inflammation.

B. Improved aerobic capacity.
  1. The results of a study by Heiwe and Jacobson (2011) showed that regular exercise significantly

improved aerobic capacity. It is hypothesized that this could be due to an improvement in anemia since hemoglobin (Hgb) levels affect oxygen-carrying capacity.
2. Exercise training in patients on hemodialysis has been shown to increase the hematocrit and hemoglobin concentrations (Goldberg, 1980).

C. Improved cardiovascular risk.
1. Regular cardiovascular exercise has a positive influence on cardiovascular risk profile. In patients on dialysis, early studies showed improvements in fasting glucose, insulin levels, and BP with exercise training.
2. Improvement in lipid and carbohydrate metabolism.
   a. Goldberg (1980) showed that exercise training lowers triglyceride levels and increases high-density lipoprotein (HDL) levels.
   b. He also demonstrated a 23% improvement in glucose tolerance and a 40% reduction in hyperinsulinism.
3. Decreased use of antihypertensives. The average relative benefit of exercise was a 36% reduction in antihypertensive medications with an annual cost savings of $885/patient/year in the exercise group (Miller et al., 2002).
4. Improved blood pressure (BP).
   a. Reductions in BP have been reported with cardiovascular exercise training by Hagberg et al. (1983) and Painter et al. (1986), with reductions in antihypertensive medication requirements.
   b. Both interdialytic ambulatory BP and treatment-related BP were significantly improved by exercise training during HD in a study by Anderson et al. (2004).

D. Improved inflammation.
1. Inflammation has been associated with atherosclerotic cardiovascular disease (CVD) and anemia which may lead to left ventricular impairment via myocardial hypertrophy and/or ischemia (El-Agroudy & El-Baz, 2010).
2. Better VO_2 max was associated with lower frequency of elevated C-reactive protein (CRP) levels in subjects with CKD. The current study strengthens previous findings and reinforces the hypothesis of cardiovascular benefits with a better aerobic capacity in patients with CKD (Shiraishi et al., 2012).
3. Patients with coronary artery disease submitted to adequate chronic training with increase in VO_2 max have lower levels of CRP compared with basal levels (Fernandes et al., 2011).
4. Cheema et al. (2007) showed that resistance

training in patients on hemodialysis resulted in decreased levels of CRP.
5. Although cardiorespiratory fitness has not been directly associated with improvement in cardiovascular risk in the patient with CKD, it has been shown to reduce the inflammatory marker, C-reactive protein (CRP). Furthermore, elevated CRP levels have been associated with higher risk for vascular disease (Martins, 2010).
6. Secondary pulmonary hypertension in patients with CKD is strictly related to pulmonary circulation impairment together with chronic volume overload and increased levels of cytokines and growth factors (DiLullo et al., 2013).

E. Decreased risk of sudden cardiac death (SCD). Exercise was shown to improve some indicators or risk of SCD (Kouidi et al., 2009). Indicators were calculated, and included LVEF and VO_2 peak.

F. Improved sense of well-being.
1. Quality of life scores, as measured by The Functional Assessment of Chronic Illness Therapy-Spirituality Scale Quality of Life Tool (FACIT-Sp), showed an improved score in domains concerned with physical quality of life and health after 1 month in an exercise group. This study focused on patients with CKD stages 4 and 5 and included a walking program where the patients were to walk 30 minutes, 5 days a week (Kosmadakis et al., 2012). These improvements in quality of life and health and exercise tolerance achieved by 1 month were maintained through 6 months.
2. A short and practical exercise training program was shown to improve health-related quality of life (HRQL) in individuals with pulmonary artery hypertension (Shoemaker et al., 2009). A 40% prevalence of pulmonary hypertension was found in patients on hemodialysis due to vascular access (both central venous catheter and arteriovenous fistula) and a 10% prevalence in patients on peritoneal dialysis or prior to starting dialysis (Yigla et al., 2003).
3. Progressive resistance training showed a statistically significant improvement in quality of life in two of eight domains using the Medical Outcomes Trust Short Form-36 (SF-36) survey (Cheema et al., 2007).
4. Physical rehabilitation improves physical proficiency, the performance of daily activities, and quality of life (Golebiowski et al., 2009).

G. Improved body composition. Exercise training and lifestyle intervention in patients with CKD produces improvements in cardiorespiratory fitness, body composition, and diastolic function (Howden et al., 2013).

H. Improved strength.
1. Cycle exercise during dialysis is safe even in older patients on hemodialysis with multiple comorbidities. It results in a significant increase in general patient walking ability and in a gain in lower extremity muscle strength (Golebiowski et al., 2012).
2. Muscle strength is likely to increase with both aerobic and resistance type exercises, but more with resistance training (Heiwe & Jacobson, 2011).
3. Exercise is one of the possible preventive means to reduce muscle protein loss from protein–energy wasting and maintain muscular function (Jung & Park, 2011). Muscle wasting is a strong risk factor for mortality in ESRD patients (Carrero, 2008).

I. Improved physical functioning and outcomes.
1. Physical inactivity is one of the strongest predictors of physical disability in older persons (Buchner et al., 1992; Carlson et al., 1999).
2. Regular physical exercise has been shown in longitudinal observational studies to extend longevity and to reduce risk of physical disability in later life (Ferrucci et al., 1999; LaCroix et al., 1993; Leveille et al., 1999; Strawbridge et al., 1996; Wu et al., 1999).
3. Low exercise capacity as measured by treadmill testing is also predictive of outcomes. Seitsema et al. (2004) reported the prognostic value of exercise capacity as measured by VO_2 peak in 175 ambulatory patients on hemodialysis over a 3½-year follow-up period. They also reported that exercise capacity was the strongest predictor of survival over the 3½-year follow-up, even when corrected for other contributing variables.
4. In the Established Populations for Epidemiologic Studies of the Elderly (EPESE) of 6,200 older persons free of baseline disability, those with a low level of regular physical activity were 1.8 times more likely to develop disability in activities of daily living or mobility over 6 years than those with a high level of physical activity.
5. Cardiovascular exercise training has also been shown to result in significant improvement on physical performance tests in patients on dialysis (Mercer et al., 2002; Painter et al., 2000a, 2000b).
6. In the Kidney Exercise Demonstration Project (Painter et al., 2000a, 2000b), there were significant differences in the change over time in normal and fast gait speed and sit-to-stand tests between the exercise intervention group and no intervention group. The changes were most pronounced in patients who had low self-reported physical function scores.
   a. Results indicated that the natural course is for deterioration of physical functioning over time. Thus, maintenance of functioning is a positive

outcome that can be obtained with increasing physical activity.
   b. The project also resulted in significant improvements in self-reported physical functioning in the exercise intervention group.

J. Improved dialysis efficacy.
1. A low-intensity intradialytic exercise program has been shown to be a viable therapy, improving hemodialysis (HD) efficacy and physical function in patients on HD (Parsons et al., 2006). The primary findings of the study found an overall 11% increase in serum urea clearance and a 14% improvement in functional performance, as measured by the distance walked by the participants.
2. A simple aerobic exercise program increases dialysis effectiveness and may be considered as a safe, complementary, effective modality for patients on hemodialysis. A 38% improvement in single-pool model of urea kinetics (spKt/V) and an 11% increase in urea reduction ratio (URR) was found after 8 weeks of a regular, structured, 15-minute exercise program during dialysis. It is thought that the exercise increases the movement of urea from the tissue compartment into the vascular compartment (Mohseni et al., 2013).

III. Limitations to exercise.

A. CKD is associated with high morbidity, mortality, and community costs. It affects multiple organs and systems, and physical inactivity is known to be a major risk factor. The physical inactivity and CKD relationship is outlined in Figure 3.1.

B. Endocrine: diabetes and the risk of hypoglycemia.
1. According to Henderson et al. (2003), severe hypoglycemia is highly associated with frequent occurrences of low blood sugar glucose readings.
2. Those most at risk for hypoglycemia.
   a. Those with low and variable glucose readings.
   b. Patients who have a longer duration with type 2 diabetes.
   c. Patients with a lower body mass index.
   d. Those with impaired awareness of hypoglycemia, such as pediatric patients.

C. Neurologic: peripheral neuropathy.
1. In the presence of peripheral neuropathy, it may be best to encourage nonweight-bearing activities such as swimming, bicycling, or upper arm ergometry.
2. If a patient is ambulating, it may be beneficial to avoid high-impact activity. Load may also be reduced by slowing the walking speed or by using prostheses for load transfer.

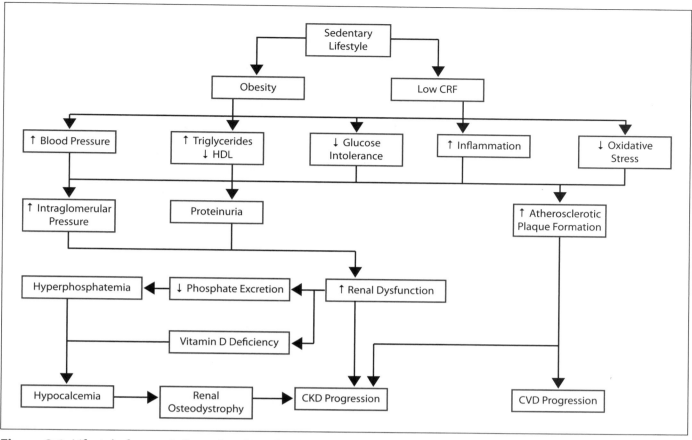

Figure 3.1. Lifestyle factors influencing CKD development and progression (Smart et al., 2013).

Source: Smart, N.A., Williams, A.D., Livinger, I., Selig, S., Howden, E., Coombes, J.S., & Fassett, R.G. (2013). Exercise & Sports Science Australia (ESSA) position statement on exercise and chronic kidney disease. *Journal of Science and Medicine in Sport, 16,* 406-411. Used with permission from Elsevier.

3. Regular foot inspection may also be beneficial (Armstrong et al., 2004).

D. Anemia.
1. Anemia leads to reduced oxygen-carrying capacity, compromising oxygen delivery to the muscle mitochondria, consequently reducing VO_2 and increasing lactic acid production (Sala et al., 2001).
2. Anemia is not considered to be a limiting factor as long as patients are adequately treated with an erythropoiesis-stimulating agent (Painter & Johansen, 2006; Painter et al., 2002).
3. The correlation between VO_2 and hemoglobin (Hgb) is statistically significant (Pattaragarn et al., 2004).

E. Uremia. Uremia has been found to suppress myocardial contractility (El-Agroudy & El-Baz, 2010) and therefore decreases the heart's ability to pump blood into the aorta.

F. Microvascular disease. Due to the risk of causing vitreous hemorrhage or retinal detachment, individuals with proliferative retinopathy should avoid any activity that may result in a Valsalva maneuver such as anaerobic activities (American Diabetes Association, 2008).

G. Peripheral artery disease.
1. Walking exposes the feet to impact and can be an important contributor to the development of foot ulceration, especially in subjects with neurovascular disease.
2. Active individuals seem to be less likely to develop foot ulceration; this may be due to better glycemic control and better vascular function in active individuals (Armstrong et al., 2004).
3. When foot ulceration does occur, it appears to be associated with greater variability in activity.

H. Musculoskeletal.
1. Uremic myopathy.
   a. *Uremic myopathy* is a term commonly used to describe a host of skeletal muscle structural and physiologic abnormalities seen in patients

with chronic kidney failure. The most common characteristics of this problem are fatigue, muscle weakness, and limited exercise tolerance (Sala et al., 2001).
  b. A treatment that may improve exercise tolerance and muscle function in patients with CKD is optimization of dialysis efficacy (Fahal et al., 1997).
  2. Orthopedic.
  a. There may be an increased risk for bone fracture in patients with CKD as a result of hyper-parathyroidism and bone disease (Alem, 2000).
  b. Furthermore, spontaneous quadriceps tendon ruptures have been reported (Shah, 2002). This is quite possibly also due to secondary hyper-parathyroidism.

I. Psychosocial: lack of time.
  1. Children receiving hemodialysis spend 43% of their waking time in treatment and travel. It is not surprising they have little time for exercise.
  2. It may be beneficial under these circumstances to implement a routine exercise program during hemodialysis (Goldstein & Montgomery, 2009).

IV. Components of physical fitness.

A. Muscular endurance.
  1. It is the muscle's ability to perform for successive exertions or many repetitions.
  2. It is beneficial for walking or other prolonged aerobic activity.

B. Muscular strength.
  1. The ability of the muscle to exert force.
  2. This component is necessary for activities of daily living such as rising from a chair, opening heavy doors, or entering or exiting a vehicle.

C. Cardiorespiratory fitness. As stated in the American College of Sports Medicine's (ACSM) Guidelines for Exercise Testing and Prescription (2006), "Cardiorespiratory fitness is related to the ability to perform large muscle, dynamic, moderate-to-high intensity exercise for prolonged periods. Performance of such exercise depends on the functional state of the respiratory, cardiovascular, and skeletal muscle systems."
  1. Objectively measured using laboratory measures of oxygen uptake including VO_2 peak during maximal exercise tests.
  2. Stress testing performed on a cycle ergometer or treadmill.

D. Flexibility.
  1. The ability to move a joint through its complete range of motion.

2. Important in athletics as well to perform activities of daily living.

E. Body composition.
  1. Body composition is the percentage of body mass that is fat relative to total body mass.
  2. Body Mass Index (BMI) has been generally accepted as a surrogate for body composition even though it does not distinguish between body fat, muscle mass, or bone. Increased BMI, above 30, has been associated with increased risk of hypertension, total cholesterol/high-density lipoprotein cholesterol ratio, coronary disease, and mortality rate (Rimm et al., 1995).

V. Exercise recommendations.

A. General guidelines.
  1. Studies reporting exercise benefits have not reported any safety issues arising from exercise interventions (Heiwe & Jacobson, 2011).
  2. Exercise appears to be safe in the patient population with CKD if begun at moderate intensity and increased gradually (Johansen & Painter, 2012).
  3. According to the American College of Sports Medicine and American Heart Association, to reduce risk of cardiovascular events, individuals with chronic illnesses should perform moderate-intensity physical activity, 30 minutes, five times weekly (Nelson et al., 2007).
  4. Current scientific evidence supports exercising regularly for greater than 30 minutes per session, three times per week to improve physical fitness, cardiovascular dimensions, and health-related quality of life (Heiwe & Jacobson, 2011).
  5. Patients on hemodialysis.
  a. Larger adaptations may occur when exercise is completed on nondialysis days.
  b. Intradialytic exercise training.
    (1) Intradialytic exercise training may produce better adherence rates.
    (2) Intradialytic exercise is an ideal setting to provide the opportunity for increased physical activity, since patients are there 3 times/week using their time quite unproductively.
    (3) That exercise should be conducted within the first 3 hours of dialysis initiation when blood pressure control is best (Smart & Steele, 2011).
    (4) Cheema et al. (2005) have made the argument for incorporation of regular intradialytic exercise into the routine dialysis care. They support the practice of using stationary cycles during the hemo-dialysis treatment and purport it to be safe.

The experience of the author using cycling during dialysis is extensive, with exercise training in over 400 hemodialysis patients.
(a) There have been no untoward events.
(b) There were no negative hemodynamic events.
(c) Systolic blood pressure stabilized during the exercise time.
(d) Patients typically experienced less cramping and hypotensive episodes.
c. Patients on HD should avoid upper limb activity with temporary or healing AV fistulas.
d. Fistulas should not be used for functional assessment, thus avoiding false blood pressure testing; using the fistula arm for blood pressure measurement is contraindicated (Smart et al., 2013).
6. Patients on peritoneal dialysis (PD).
a. Patients perform exercise more comfortably with abdominal cavities emptied of dialysis fluid, reducing diaphragmatic pressure, breathlessness, and, in some types of PD, chest discomfort (Smart et al., 2013).
b. It is recommended that their abdominal cavities be emptied of dialysis fluid which may alleviate these problems (Smart & Steele, 2011).

B. Contraindications.
1. Unstable angina.
a. Workload and exercise angina are associated with cardiac events.
b. A majority of those with unstable angina have an underlying ruptured plaque and significant coronary artery disease (Gibbons et al., 2002).
2. Poorly controlled blood pressure.
a. Exercise tolerance is decreased in patients with poor BP control.
b. Severe systemic hypertension may cause exercise-induced ST-depression in the absence of atherosclerosis (Gibbons et al., 2002).
3. Electrolyte abnormalities: especially hypo/hyperkalemia.
4. Recent changes to electrocardiogram, especially symptomatic tachyarrhythmias or bradyarrhythmias.
5. Excess interdialytic weight gain greater than 4 kilograms since last dialysis or exercise session.
6. Unstable on dialysis treatment and changing/titrating medication regimen.
7. Pulmonary congestion.

C. Reducing barriers to exercise.
1. Individuals with a chronic illness have more to deal with, including the illness and symptoms, clinical status, and physical limitations. Barriers to exercise are well documented in the general population also, and include:

a. Time commitment.
b. Lack of interest.
c. Lack of support from family members, etc.
2. Physical functioning in patients with CKD is not routinely assessed, and physical activity recommendations and follow-up are not part of the routine care.
a. This results in a situation in which interventions such as physical therapy are incorporated only when the patient becomes nonambulatory or when it is too late.
b. Results in a misunderstanding about what the patient can and cannot do.
3. When physical activity is not mentioned by the healthcare provider and reinforced regularly, the patient and family will most likely become (or remain) sedentary.
a. There is a justifiable fear of exertion on the part of the patient and family members.
b. There is a very real fear that exertion will make the condition worse, will make the individual tired/fatigued, and/or is just not OK for someone with CKD.
c. It takes very specific instructions and encouragement to increase physical activity.
4. In addition to the message sent by providing information on physical activity, there are many other messages that are inadvertently transmitted to patients by healthcare providers.
a. "Take it easy" is easily interpreted to mean "Don't do anything strenuous." "Taking it easy" means different things to different people. Thus, the healthcare provider should be very specific in what is meant by "take it easy." Say instead: "Why don't you cut back your walking to 20 minutes instead of 60 minutes?" or "When you go out for your walk, don't push yourself until <a given clinical situation> is taken care of."
b. "Don't overdo it." We must remember that an individual with a chronic disease probably does not know how much he/she can do and has probably experienced severe fatigue and malaise. Thus, it is justifiable for them to think that anything may be "overdoing" it. Specify recommendations on how to start out with physical activity and how to progress gradually so they will experience benefits and enjoy it.
5. Contradictory messages from various healthcare providers also present a barrier to adoption of physical activity.
a. All individuals involved in the care of a patient must consistently understand what is recommended for a patient and encourage and support the patient in adopting those recommendations.
b. Likewise, including assessment of activity and

recommendations for adoption and participation in physical activity into the routine care and follow-up will assure consistent messages from all healthcare providers.

c. Consistent recommendations and encouragement may alleviate misunderstanding on the part of the patient and families regarding physical activity, and possibly reduce future disability.

d. The ongoing opportunity of encouraging physical activity for patients seen regularly for dialysis should be capitalized on.

6. Low expectations for physical functioning, as if the inability to be physically active is an inevitable consequence of the disease.

a. It is not surprising that patients adapt to this low level of functioning by modifying what they do and how they do it and by enlisting assistance from others for their activities.

b. Once this low level of functioning is accepted by patients, their family, and the healthcare professionals working with them, the expectation is fulfilled.

c. The healthcare team has an enormous influence on whether patients become physically active and try to maintain, and possibly improve, their level of functioning or they accept the low functioning that is expected to accompany their chronic illness.

D. Implementation of an exercise program.

1. A common sense, gradually progressing approach for starting activity, which is individualized and considers the symptoms, clinical status, medications, and treatments of each patient is recommended.

2. When planning aerobic exercise, heart rate reserve or rate of perceived exertion, Borg's 15-point scale should be considered to match exercise intensity to individual patients (see Table 3.5).

3. The challenge for the kidney community is finding the resources to provide counseling and encouragement as a routine part of the patient care, whether it is in the provider's office or at the dialysis clinic.

4. Medical order for exercise. If there is an order for exercise participation, then the patient should receive information/education about how to start a program and how to progress.

a. Providing this information could be in the form of educational materials or referral to a physical therapist or exercise specialist.

b. Patients who qualify for cardiac rehabilitation (e.g., postmyocardial infarction, bypass surgery, angioplasty) should be referred to cardiac rehabilitation.

5. Regular follow-up and documentation of participation.

a. Ask about exercise participation at the time of every patient encounter, e.g., as a part of the assessment done before putting the patient on dialysis, at every clinic visit, or phone contact.

b. Incorporate physical functioning assessment and participation into the routine short- and long-term care plans to facilitate regular review of participation at the time of the patient review.

c. If, at the time of patient review, there is a change in participation, it should be addressed to identify problems and concerns with participation or the program.

6. Dialysis staff education on the benefits of regular physical activity for patients and how to encourage patient participation in regular physical activity should be a part of the staff training for new employees and could become a part of the unit quality assurance program.

7. A starting, sample program for exercise for patients on dialysis can be found in the free materials "Exercise for the Dialysis Patient" on the following website: www.lifeoptions.org

8. Proposed guidelines for an exercise training program can be found in Table 3.6 (Jung & Park, 2011) and Table 3.7 (Smart et al., 2013).

VI. Summary.

A. Patients with CKD have low levels of physical functioning that negatively affect overall health, quality of life, and outcomes.

B. Incorporation of regular assessment and encouragement of physical activity and exercise as a part of the routine care of patients with kidney disease and kidney failure is needed to facilitate increased physical activity.

C. This will be a challenge within the existing system of CKD, including dialysis care, and will necessitate a change in the mindset on the part of the nephrology healthcare providers. It will require a change in administrative procedures and staff training, as well as patient and family training and education.

D There is ample evidence that increasing physical functioning through increased physical activity will improve quality of life, may improve outcomes, and could improve survival through improvement in overall health and cardiovascular risk profile. This is true, not only for all stages of CKD, but also for all ages and populations.

Table 3.6

Proposed Exercise Programs for Patients on Hemodialysis

Component	Mode	Intensity Measure	Intensity	Frequency	Duration	Time to Goal
Aerobic	Cycling	HR or RPE	40% HRR at start 60% HRR in first 1 month 80% HRR in next 1 month RPE 13-14, if not using HR	3 days/week	60 min/day	At least 2 months

Source: Jung, T., & Park, S. (2011). Intradialytic exercise programs for hemodialysis patients. *Chonnam Medical Journal, 47*(2), 61-65. Copyright © Chonnam Medical Journal, 2011. (Open Access article [http://creativecommons.org/licenses/by-nc/3.0]).

Table 3.7

Guidelines for Aerobic and Resistance Exercise Prescriptions in Patients Undertaking (Non-Nocturnal Haemodialysis)

	ESRD interdialysis	ESRD intradialysis	Nondialysis
Aerobic			
Session duration	Build up to 30–45 min	Build up to 30–45 min.	Build up to 30–45 min.
Session timing	Nondialysis days	During first 2 hr of dialysis	According to patient needs
Intensity (% max HR or RPE)	55–70% max HR or RPE 11–13 moderate	55–70% max HR or RPE 11–13 moderate	55–90% max HR or RPE 11–16 mod. to vigor.
Frequency	Up to 180 min	Up to 180 min	Up to 180 min
Resistance			
Initial frequency/week	2 nonconsecutive days	2 nonconsecutive days	2 nonconsecutive days
Different muscle groups/ Exercises	8–12 exercises prioritizing major muscle groups	Up to 12, as many as practical in dialysis session	8–12 exercises prioritizing major muscle groups
Initial volume	1 set to fatigue, 12–15 reps or 60–70% Repetition Maximum	1 set to fatigue, 12–15 reps or 60–70% Repetition Maximum	1 set to fatigue, 12–15 reps or 60–70% Repetition Maximum
Timing	Nondialysis days	Before or during dialysis	As comfortable
Modality	Weight-bearing activity, thera-bands, weight cuffs, light dumbbells, weight machines	Weight-bearing activity, thera-bands, weight cuffs, light dumbbells – as practical in dialysis	Weight-bearing activity, thera-bands, machine and free weights
Indications	Cachexia, poor bone density, low BMI or lean body mass	Cachexia, poor bone density, low BMI or lean body mass	Cachexia, poor bone density, low BMI or lean body mass
Flexibility	5–7 days per week for a duration of about 10 minutes per session. Where possible combine with aerobic or resistance exercise session and include exercises for those at risk of falls.		

Both resistance and aerobic activity should be completed (although not necessarily in the same session); recommendations assume no contraindications to exercise. Abbreviations: Reps – repetitions; BMI – body mass index; RPE – rate of perceived exertion; HR – heart rate.

Source: Smart, N.A., Williams, A.D., Livinger, I., Selig, S., Howden, E., Coombes, J.S., & Fassett, R.G. (2013). Exercise & Sports Science Australia (ESSA) position statement on exercise and chronic kidney disease. *Journal of Science and Medicine in Sport, 16*, 406-411. Used with permission from Elsevier.

SECTION H
Advance Care Planning and Palliative/End-of-Life Care
Deb Castner

I. Patient Self-Determination Act (PSDA) 1991.
How the act was passed can be found at
http://www.ncbi.nlm.nih.gov/pubmed/1588296

A. A federal mandate for facilities that receive Medicare or Medicaid funding requires each state to address the issue of identifying care wishes of all patients on admission to acute care facilities, nursing homes, home health agencies, and hospice programs, including the following.
   1. Providing each incoming patient with a statement of rights regarding making healthcare decisions.
   2. Asking patients if they have an advance directive and, if one is available, this fact must be documented in the medical record.
   3. Providing the patient an explanation of the facility's policy regarding advance directives.
   4. Ensuring compliance with the requirements of state law.

B. Dialysis centers often have the nephrology social worker or registered nurse ask about medical directives during admission process to the outpatient center and during the comprehensive care planning session.

II. Advanced Care Planning (ACP) process.

A. Not a form, but a process of proactive communication to identify patient wishes related to medical decisions and care.

B. ACP evolves over many conversations with the patient and provider or healthcare team.

C. It helps identify and formulate the patients' plans related to medical decision making when they may no longer be able to do so for themselves.

D. Predicting what patients may want at the end of life is complicated by the following factors.
   1. The patient's age.
   2. The status of the chronic illness.
   3. The ability to sustain life with the medications and treatment regimens available.
   4. The emotions of the family and/or significant others when the patient disease progresses and end of life approaches.

E. Families may find it difficult to make decisions on whether to continue medical treatment, and if so,

how much and for how long. ACP can help guide the family in following the patient's wishes.

F. The nurse is often the facilitator of the conversation. Patients rely on trusted healthcare professionals for guidance.
   1. Therefore, it is important to discuss, not only for those who are terminally ill or whose death is imminent, but for those with chronic illness, including CKD.
   2. With chronic illness, the disease trajectory is more uncertain, and the patient has an increased likelihood of a shortened life span with a slow progressive decline in health with sudden episodes of disease exacerbation, possibly requiring hospitalization. This pattern usually repeats itself with the patient's overall health steadily declining until the patient dies.
   3. It is also important in situations where patients have experienced comorbid complications or a new terminal or complicated diagnosis in addition to kidney disease.

G. To see research results on ACP go to "ACP Preferences for Care at End of Life" at http://www.ahrq.gov/research/findings/factsheets/aging/endliferia/index.html

H. A formal process and policy for ACP is helpful.
   1. Should be a team effort including not only the nurse but the nephrology social worker, physician/advanced provider, technician, and dietitian, in addition to those persons identified by the patient as important to the process.
   2. Initiate guided discussions when initiating care, whether in the clinic, dialysis center, or hospital setting.
   3. Introduce the subject of ACP. Inform the patient that these conversations occur with all patients, and provide education and information to clarify any misconceptions.
   4. Have Advanced Care Planning (ACP) documents ready and available (see Tables 3.8 and 3.9).
      a. Advanced Medical Directive.
      b. Living Will.
      c. Physician Orders for Life Sustaining Treatment (POLST).
   5. Review the patient's preferences on a regular basis and update documentation. Discussions should be held at regular intervals as well as when there is a change in patient condition.

I. Components of ACP.
   1. Discussion topics.
      a. Treatment options.
         (1) Length of time the treatment may be required.

(2) Invasiveness of the treatment.

(3) Consideration for the benefits and burdens of treatment options, including what the patient would regard as worthwhile and what treatments as overly burdensome.

(4) Chance of success.

b. Overall prognosis.

c. Reflection on the patient's values, beliefs, and goals in life.

d. Quality of life during and after the treatment.

2. Prepare the environment. Attempts should be made to create a supportive environment that would facilitate discussions, including the following.

a. Adequate privacy.

b. Ensuring patient comfort.

(1) Timing of discussion. Ensure adequate time so the patient and family do not feel hurried or rushed.

(2) Adequate space for all participants.

(3) Proper position of all participants. Healthcare providers should be relaxed and comfortable. Avoid standing and looking down on the patient.

c. Maintaining therapeutic communication. Convey warmth, caring, respect, sensitivity, active listening, and empathy.

d. Ensuring discussions are at the patient's level of understanding.

e. Consider conference calling for family member(s) or provider(s) who cannot be present, if agreeable with the patient.

f. For more information on how to use effective communication techniques, refer to PowerPoint "Techniques to Facilitate Discussion for Advance Care Planning" at http://www.annanurse.org/resources/cne-opportunities/education-modules

J. Pediatric ACP.

1. The pediatric population needs to be included in ACP. Children/adolescents can participate in planning and decision making.

2. They should have the same rights as adults to information and involvement in discussions, which are age appropriate and suited to the child's stage of development.

3. In pediatric palliative care, there is usually time for these discussions as death is rarely sudden.

4. Parents often try to protect their child from knowledge regarding the severity of their illness. However, children usually know and want to talk about it.

5. Children are often more ready to talk about death than their parents. They are more able to face the truth about illness and death. The child may, in fact, guide the parents in the process by talking about their condition and asking questions.

6. There are a variety of therapies that can be used to help children express their feelings and desires including play, music, and art therapy.

Table 3.8

Physician Orders for Life Sustaining Treatment (POLST) (http://www.caringinfo.org)

For persons with serious illness — at any age.
Provides medical orders for **current** treatment.
Guides actions by Emergency Medical Personnel when made available.
Guides inpatient treatment decisions when made available.

Table 3.9

Advance Directive (www.caringinfo.org)

For anyone 18 and older.
Provides instructions for **future** treatment.
Appoints a Health Care Representative.
Does not guide Emergency Medical Personnel.
Guides inpatient treatment decisions when made available.

III. Advance Medical Directive (AMD).

A. The AMD is a form that asks under what circumstances the patient would or would not want care initiated related to medical/emergent health needs. There are two types of AMD: health care proxy and living will. A lawyer is not necessarily needed to complete either one. They are usually written but could be given verbally if patient is still able to do so.

1. Health care proxy is also known as a medical power of attorney or durable power of attorney for health care; assigns a surrogate to make health decisions if the patient cannot. This legal document overrides the "next of kin" decision-making power. It does not allow for proxy to make legal or financial decisions.

2. Living will is a legal document also called an instructive directive; expresses the treatment of the patient related to end-of-life care. The patient specifies what is to be done or not done and in what situations.

3. State-by-state considerations.

a. All 50 states have passed laws related to AMD.

b. Each state has specific requirements of what makes up an AMD.

c. It is your professional responsibility, as a nurse, that you become familiar with your state's specific requirements that cover terminology used, appropriate forms to use, and any special circumstances.

4. For a free brochure from the National Kidney Foundation, *Advance Directives: A Guide for Patients and Their Families,* go to http://www.kidney.org/atoz/pdf/AdvanceDirect.pdf

5. Specific AMD forms can be found at http://www.americanbar.org/content/dam/aba/migrated/2011_build/law_aging/st_spec_adv_dirs_update_2-11.authcheckdam.pdf

B. Do not resuscitate (DNR).
   1. Laws regarding DNR include the process for obtaining, recording, and recognizing that status varies across states.
   2. The DNR process allows patients to not receive cardiopulmonary resuscitation (CPR) in the event of cardiac arrest and relieves emergency services staff, other health professionals, or good Samaritans from the responsibility of "not treating."
   3. Allow a Natural Death (AND) is a term being used to describe DNR. Some believe this term better reflects what is trying to be accomplished and does not imply that you are not "treating" or caring for a patient at the time of their death.

C. Physician Orders for Life Sustaining Treatment (POLST).
   1. "The National POLST Paradigm Program is an approach to end-of-life planning that emphasizes patients' wishes about the care they receive. The POLST Paradigm is both a holistic method of planning for end-of-life care and a specific set of medical orders that ensure patients' wishes are honored.
      a. The POLST paradigm is built upon conversations between patients, loved ones, and healthcare professionals, during which patients can determine the extent of care they wish to receive.
      b. As a result of these conversations, patients may elect to create a POLST form, which translates their wishes into actionable medical orders.
      c. The POLST form assures patients that healthcare professionals will provide only the care that patients themselves wish to receive, and decreases the frequency of medical errors.
      d. POLST is not for everyone. Only patients with serious, progressive, chronic illnesses should have a POLST form. For these patients, their current health status indicates the need for standing medical orders.

e. For healthy patients, an Advance Directive is an appropriate tool for making future end-of-life care wishes known to loved ones. Find info at http://www.polst.org/about-the-national-polst-paradigm/

2. A POLST is not intended to replace an AMD; it is meant to complement it (refer to Tables 3.8 and 3.9 on previous page).
   a. A POLST form should accompany an Advance Directive when appropriate.
   b. For more information, see www.caringinfo.org

IV. Palliative care/end-of-life care.

A. Palliative care definition. The World Health Organization defines it as "an approach which improves quality of life of patients and their families facing life-threatening illness through prevention, assessment, and treatment of pain and other physical, psychosocial, and spiritual problems."

B. It begins when the patient is diagnosed with a serious illness and the start of a life-prolonging therapy.

C. The goal for the patient may still include remission or cure with a focus on relief of symptoms.

D. Predictors of morbidity and mortality.
   1. There are several tools available to use in assessment of patients to predict which patients would benefit from palliative or hospice referral and care.
   2. Refer to http://www.annanurse.org/resources/cne-opportunities/education-modules module 4
   3. Another tool called the "HD Mortality Calculator" uses the "Surprise Question"(Moss, 2008) that asks you to assess if you feel the patient would still be alive in the next 6 months, and other patient parameters to develop an evidence-based mortality risk score, available at http://touchcalc.com/calculators/sq

E. Other factors associated with increased mortality risk.
   1. Elevated C-reactive protein levels.
   2. Low BMI < 18.5, undernourished, cachexic appearance.
   3. Increased protein catabolic rate (PCR).
   4. Elevated Malnutrition Inflammation Score (MIS).
   5. Subjective Global Assessment of Nutritional Status (Detsky et al., 1987).
   6. Low cholesterol.
   7. Low serum phosphorus.
   8. Low vitamin D levels.
   9. Decreased skinfold measurement.
   10. Elevated troponin, BNP.

11. Low blood pressure.
12. Use of a central venous catheter for dialysis access.
13. Poor functional status – walking, transferring, activities of daily living, etc.

F. Statistics related to survival rates and end of life in the population with kidney failure.
   1. Each year, 1 out of 5 patients withdraws from dialysis.
   2. For a free brochure from the National Kidney Foundation, *When Stopping Dialysis Treatment Is Your Choice*, go to: https://www.kidney.org/atoz/content/dialysisstop
   3. Annual rate (23%) or > 70,000 deaths.
   4. 16 to 37% life expectancy (age and sex matches).
   5. 8% CPR survival to hospital discharge.
   6. High in-hospital deaths.
   7. High percentage of comorbidities (Cohen & Davis, 2006).

G. Evidence-based predictors in kidney failure.
   1. 50% survival first year of dialysis if albumin level < 3.5mg/dL.
   2. 40% to 72% increased risk of death if amputation in last year.
   3. 50% survival rate if acute myocardial infarction in last year.
   4. Late referral to start of dialysis.
   5. Race, sex, and age.
      a. African Americans have longer survival than Caucasians on dialysis but higher incidence.
      b. Older age at start of dialysis associated with higher morbidity.
      c. Women in age bracket 20 to 54 years old have higher death rates than males (USRDS, 2010).

V. Hospice.

A. Definition: A subset of palliative care, where patient comfort takes precedence over other goals and treatments are simplified.
   1. The goals are the same as in palliative care, but the patient is in the terminal phase of disease.
   2. The focus is on providing for a "good" death.

B. Hospice benefit.
   1. Medicare enacted the hospice benefit in 1982 (CMS, 2010). Hospice services may also be covered by private insurance.
   2. Physician certification is required to document patient life expectancy of 6 months or less, and it is not limited to cancer diagnoses.
   3. If hospice benefit is based on a diagnosis unrelated to kidney disease, such as cancer or late-stage emphysema, the patient may stay on dialysis while in hospice, if that is his/her wish and it meets the individual hospice program requirements.
   4. Patients with kidney disease are also entitled to hospice benefit. Hospice programs may ask that they stop all life-sustaining treatments, including dialysis, to enroll. In certain circumstances patients can stay on dialysis while they adjust to the hospice option.
   5. Kidney failure may be used as a terminal diagnosis.
      a. If the patient is not seeking dialysis or transplant.
         (1) Cr clearance < 10 mL/min (15 for DM).
         (2) Serum creatinine > 8 (6 for DM).
         (3) Signs and symptoms of kidney failure.
      b. If the hospice provider agrees to be responsible for the cost of the dialysis treatments, should the patient wish to continue with dialysis.

C. The hospice referral process requires a physician order for hospice evaluation.

D. The nursing role is to expedite patient requests for information about hospice and to keep the lines of interdisciplinary communication open.

E. Hospice is given in periods of care. Patients can get hospice care for two 90-day periods followed by an unlimited number of 60-day periods. At the start of each period of care, the hospice medical director or other hospice doctor must recertify that the patient is terminally ill to continue hospice care. Hospices are paid a per diem rate based on the number of days and level of care provided during the election period. Levels of care are defined as follows.
   1. Routine Home Care.
   2. Continuous Home Care.
   3. Inpatient Respite Care.
   4. General Inpatient Care (CMS, 2010).

VI. Ethical considerations.

A. Guiding principles.
   1. Beneficence: to do good or receive benefit from something rendered.
   2. Nonmalifience: to prevent harm.
   3. Autonomy: patient right to self-govern his/her care; respect of patient wishes.

B. Guidelines and standards for care guiding nursing practice related to end-of-life care include the following.
   1. *American Nurses Association Code of Ethics for Nurses with Interpretive Statements* (2001).
   2. ANNA *Nephrology Nursing Standards of Practice and Guidelines for Care* (Gomez, 2011).
   3. Clinical Practice Guideline – "*Shared Decision-Making in the Appropriate Initiation and Withdrawal from Dialysis.*"

4. *Clinical Practice Guidelines for Quality Palliative Care* (National Consensus Project, 2010).

C. Ethical issues at end of life.
1. Futile care. Medical futility can be considered care that serves no useful purpose and provides no immediate or long-term benefit; or treatment that, even though having physiologic effects, is nonbeneficial to the patient as a person. Aspects of futile care include the following.
   a. There is no hope for improvement and no treatment to improve an incapacitating condition. It is dissimilar to the idea of euthanasia or assisted suicide because assisted suicide involves active intervention to end life, while withholding futile medical care does not encourage the natural onset of death.
   b. Serves only to prolong death.
   c. There are no physical or spiritual benefits.
   d. Prolongs the grieving process and frequently raises false hope.
2. The issue of cost in medical futility involves the expenditure of resources that could be used for those with a greater likelihood of achieving a positive outcome. Traditionally, discussions about medical futility do not include the ability of the patient to pay for treatment.
3. Assisted suicide is the practice of providing a means to terminate the life of a person. Usually the person has an incurable disease, intolerable suffering, or a possibly undignified death with the purpose to limit suffering. Laws regarding assisted suicide vary greatly.
   a. Physician-assisted suicide generally refers to the practice in which the physician provides a patient with a lethal dose of medication, upon the patient's request to end his/her own life. The significant difference is whether a lethal dose of medication is administered by the patient or by the physician.
   b. Passive-assisted suicide is the withdrawal or withholding of life-sustaining medical treatment in accordance with a competent patient who has made an informed decision to refuse treatment.
   c. Often terminally ill patients require dosages of pain medication that impair respiration or have other effects that may hasten death. Administering pain medications to achieve the desired patient comfort, even if the medication may compromise vital functions, is generally held by most professional societies, and supported in court decisions, justifiable as long as the intent is to relieve suffering.
   d. Providers are faced with balancing these concerns with their legal duty and moral obligation to treat pain in the suffering patient.

4. Informed consent is the process where fully informed patients can make choices in their health care. There are four general standards to informed consent including the ability of the patient to do the following.
   a. Express a choice.
   b. Understand information relevant to the decision about treatment.
   c. Understand the significance of the information provided.
   d. Analyze the relevant information and weigh the treatment options.

VII. Personal considerations.

A. Your personal past experience and values associated with death affect how you will care for patients. You need to have a clear understanding of situations in which you, ethically, are unable to assist in patient care and refer the care to a colleague who is able to work with the patient if you cannot based on your personal ethics.

B. Cultural diversity. As discussed in a previous section, reviewing cultural impact related to death customs, traditions, and beliefs specific to individual populations is critical in developing the patient-focused plan of care. Clarify and ask the patient or family member about any preferences.
1. Research has identified three basic dimensions in end-of-life treatment that vary culturally.
   a. Communication of "bad news."
   b. Views regarding decision making.
   c. Attitudes toward advance directives and end-of-life care.
2. Cultural considerations.
   a. By assessing the patient's values, spirituality, and relationship dynamics, healthcare providers can incorporate and follow cultural preferences.
   b. It is not uncommon for healthcare professionals from outside the United States to conceal serious diagnoses from patients, as disclosure may be viewed as disrespectful, impolite, or even harmful to the patient.
   c. Among some cultures, emphasizing patient autonomy in decision making may contrast with preferences for more family or physician-based decision making.
   d. Completion of advance directives is lower among patients of various ethnic backgrounds. This may be due to the distrust of the healthcare system, healthcare disparities, cultural perspectives on death and suffering, and family dynamics.

VIII. Symptoms seen at end of life in kidney patient (Castner & Bednarski, 2011).

A. Fatigue, pruritis, anorexia, dyspnea, difficulty concentrating.

B. Nausea, vomiting.

C. Myoclonic movements, convulsions, coma.

D. Pain is usually related to other causes of death, such as a cancer diagnosis or neuropathic pain.

E. Most have few symptoms: usually more fatigue, lengthening sleep cycle, then coma.

IX. Treatment of symptoms.

A. Pain.
   1. Be mindful of the method of excretion for medications used and the effects of metabolites from the breakdown of medications, especially narcotics and hypnotics.
   2. Methadone, hydromorphone (Dilaudid®), or fentanyl are excreted by the liver, making them a better choice for pain control in late kidney failure.
   3. Morphine products can cause symptoms due to metabolites produced in long-term use and may cause confusion.
   4. Refer to available drug tables to adjust dosing or schedule appropriate for kidney failure.
   5. Always develop a plan for bowel hygiene when using pain medication by adding a daily stool softener or other agent. The goal is to treat prophylactically versus waiting until constipation occurs.
   6. As with many other medications used in patients with kidney failure, they may have side effects not commonly seen in the typical population.
      a. Frequent patient assessment of response to medications is important.
      b. The direction of the treatment of symptoms based on the patient's individual response.

B. Other.
   1. Simple measures can give relief such as using fans for patients with feeling of dyspnea or using a clear liquid diet for nausea and vomiting.
   2. Food and fluids. It is best to avoid force-feeding or fluids; let the patient guide you. A decrease in appetite is common in later stages of impending death. It is also an area where families and friends feel the need to "feed" the patient so they can "maintain their strength." Food is symbolic of health, family, and pleasurable memories. Yet, feeding or offering fluids may be detrimental as gag reflex becomes suppressed or as the level of consciousness changes.
   3. Relaxation. Guided meditation techniques or massage can be helpful in coping with symptoms such as anxiety, pain, or nausea.
   4. Treating symptoms should be on an individual basis as they occur, using simplest measures first and progress based on patient feedback.
   5. Depression. Be aware that many terminal patients may have depression and can benefit from treatment.

X. Grief counseling and bereavement period.

A. Nephrology nursing allows for a unique connection to the patients.

B. Following patient from diagnosis to death can be emotionally straining.

C. Nephrology nurses need to develop support systems within their work, personal, or professional environments to assist with coping with these feelings.

D. Hospice programs offer bereavement counseling to family survivors for the first year following the death of a patient.

E. There are grief/bereavement groups available in most counties.

F. Though patients have a serious illness, death may come as a surprise to families and even nephrology staff.

G. Do not forget to anticipate the grief response of other patients who have known the deceased, and support their needs for sharing their feelings or referral for counseling.

H. Some dialysis centers offer memorial services to recognize patients who have died, allowing for staff and families to participate.

References

Adsit, K.I. (1996). Multimedia in nursing and patient education. *Orthopaedic Nursing, 15*(4), 59-63.

Agency for Healthcare Research and Quality (AHRQ). (2003). Advance care planning: preferences for care at end of life *Research in Action*, Issue 12. Retrieved from http://www.ahrq.gov/research/findings/factsheets/aging/endliferia/endria.pdf

Agency for Healthcare Research and Quality (AHRQ). (2010). Literacy and health outcomes. *AHRQ Archives*. Retrieved from http://www.ahrq.gov/clinic/epcsums/litsum.htm

Aging Clinical Research Center (ACRC). *Geriatric depression scale.* Retrieved from http://www.stanford.edu/~yesavage/GDS.html

Al-Arabi, S. (2006). Quality of life: Subjective descriptions of challenges to patients with end stage kidney disease. *Nephrology Nursing Journal, 33*(3), 285-293.

Aldrige, M. (2004). Writing and designing readable patient education materials. *Nephrology Nursing Journal, 31*(4), 373-377.

Alem, A.M., Sherrard, D.J., Gillen, D.L, Weiss, N.S. Beresford, S.A., Heckbert, S.R., & Stehman-Breen, C. (2000). Increased risk of hip fracture among patients with end-stage renal disease. *Kidney International, 58,* 396-399.

American College of Sports Medicine (2006). *Guidelines for exercise testing and prescription* (7th ed.). Philadelphia: Williams & Wilkins.

American Diabetes Association (ADA). (2002). *Diabetes mellitus and exercise.* Retrieved from http://care.diabetesjournals.org/content/25/suppl_1/s64.full

American Medical Association (AMA). (2012-2013). *AMA code of medical ethics.* Retrieved from http://www.ama-assn.org/ama/pub/physician-resources/medical-ethics/code-medical-ethics.page

American Nurses Association (ANA). (2001). *Code of ethics for nurses with interpretive state*ments. Washington, DC: Author. http://www.nursingworld.org/MainMenuCategories/EthicsStandards/CodeofEthicsforNurses/Code-of-Ethics.pdf

American Nurses Association (ANA). (2012). *Nursing care and do not resuscitate (DNR) and allow natural death (AND) decisions.* Retrieved from http://nursingworld.org/dnrposition.

American Nurses Association (ANA). (2013). *Ethics and human rights position statements: Assisted suicide.* Retrieved from http://nursingworld.org/euthanasiaanddying.

American Psychiatric Association (APA). (2013). *Posttraumatic stress disorder.* Retrieved from http://www.psychiatry.org/File%20Library/Practice/DSM/DSM-5/DSM-5-PTSD.pdf

Anderson, J.E., Boivin, M.R., & Hatchett, L. (2004). Effect of exercise training on interdialytic ambulatory and treatment-related blood pressure in hemodialysis patients. *Renal Failure, 26,* 539-544.

Andrews, M.M., & Boyle, J.S. (2002). Transcultural concepts of nursing care. *Journal of Transcultural Nursing, 13*(3), 178-180.

Andrews, M.M., & Boyle, J.S. (2007). *Transcultural concepts of nursing care* (5th ed.). Philadelphia: Lippincott Williams & Wilkins.

Antai-Otong, D. (2006). *Nurse-client communication: A life span approach.* Sudbury, MA: Jones and Bartlett Publishers.

Armstrong, D.G., Lavery, L.A., Holtz-Neiderer, K., Mohler, M.J., Wendel, C.S., Nixon, B.P., & Boulton, A. (2004). Variability in activity may precede diabetic foot ulceration. *Diabetes Care, 27*(8), 1980-1984. doi:10.2337/diacare.27.8.1980

Atherton, H., Sawmynaden, P., Meyer, B., & Car, J. (2012). Email for the coordination of healthcare appointments and attendance reminders. *Cochrane Database of Systematic Reviews.* Retrieved from http://www.ncbi.nlm.nih.gov/pubmed/22895971

Baer, C. (2001). Principles of patient education. In L. Lancaster (Ed.), *Core curriculum for nephrology nursing (4th ed.).* Pitman, NJ: American Nephrology Nurses' Association.

Bastable, S.B. (2003). *Nurse as educator: Principles of teaching and learning for nursing practice* (2nd ed.). Sudbury, MA: Jones and Bartlett Publishers.

Bastable, S.B. (2006). *Essentials of patient education.* Sudbury, MA: Jones and Bartlett Publishers.

Bednarski, D. (2009). Integrating a culture of caring into a technological world. *Nephrology Nursing Journal, 36*(6), 261.

Benjamin, R. (2010). Improving health by improving health literacy. *Public Health Reports, 125*(6), 784-785. Retrieved from http://www.ncbi.nlm.nih.gov/pmc/articles/PMC2966655/

Birnbaum, L., & Birnbaum, A. (2004). In search of inner wisdom: Guided mindfulness meditation in the context of suicide. *Scientific World Journal, 4,* 216-217.

Blanchard, W.A. (1998). Teaching an illiterate transplant patient. *ANNA Journal, 25*(1), 69, 70, 76.

Boulware, L.E., Liu, Y., Fink, N.E., Coresh, J., Ford, D.E., Klag, M.J., & Powe, N.R. (2006). Temporal relation among depression symptoms, cardiovascular disease events, and mortality in end-stage kidney disease: contribution of reverse causality. *Clinical Journal of the American Society of Nephrology, 1*(3), 1-9.

Boyd, M.D., Gleit, C.J., Graham, B.A., & Whitman, N.J. (1998). *Teaching in nursing practice: A professional model* (3rd ed.). Norwolk, CT: Appleton-Century-Crofts.

Boyle, J.S., & Andrews, M.M. (2011). *Transcultural concepts in nursing care* (6th ed.). Philadelphia: Lippincott Williams & Wilkins.

Brenner, L.A., Ivins, B., Schwab, K., Warden, D., Nelson L.A., Jaffee, M., & Terrio, H. (2010). Traumatic brain injury, post traumatic stress disorder, and post concussive symptom reporting among troops returning from Iraq. *Journal of Head Trauma Rehabilitation, 25*(5), 307-312.

Brown, H.D. (1980). *Principles of language learning and teaching.* Retrieved from http://tip.psychology.org/language.html

Brundage, D.J., & Swearengen, P.A. (1994). Chronic kidney failure: Evaluation and teaching tool. *ANNA Journal, 21*(5), 165-270.

Buchner, D.M., Beresford, S.A., Larson, E.B., LaCroix, A.Z., & Wagner, E.H. (1992). Effects of physical activity on health status in older adults II: Intervention studies. *Annual Review of Public Health, 13,* 469-488.

Bureau of Labor Statistics. (2011). *United States Department of Labor.* Retrieved from http://www. bls.gov

Burrows-Hudson, S., & Prowant, B.F. (2005). *Nephrology nursing standards or practice and guidelines for care.* Pitman, NJ: American Nephrology Nurses' Association.

Campbell, A. (1998). Family caregivers: Caring for aging ESRD partners. *Advances in Kidney Replacement Therapy, 5*(2), 98-108.

Campbell, G.A., Sanoff, S., & Rosner, M.H. (2010). World Kidney Forum: Care of the undocumented immigrant in the United States with ESRD. *American Journal of Kidney Diseases, 55*(1), 181-191. Retrieved from http://www.medscape.com/viewarticle/715289_2.

Carlson, M.C., Fried, L.P., Xue, Q.L., Bandeen-Roche, K., Zeger, S.L., & Brandt, J. (1999). Association between executive attention and physical functional performance in community dwelling older women. *Journals of Gerontology Series B: Psychological Sciences and Social Sciences, 54,* S262-S270.

Carrero, J.J., Chmielewski, M., Axelsson, J., Snaedal, S., Heimbürger, O., Bárány, P., ... Qureshi, A.R. (2008). Muscle atrophy, inflammation and clinical outcome in incident and prevalent dialysis patients. *Clinical Nutrition, 27*(4), 557-564. doi:10.1016/j.clnu.2008.04.007

Castner, D., & Bednarski, D. (2011). The intersection of the medicare ESRD hospice benefit: An overview for home care/hospice clinicians. *Home Healthcare Nurse, 29*(8), 464-476. doi:10.1097/NHH.0b013e31821fea6f

Center for Advancing Health. (2010). A new definition of patient engagement: What is engagement and why is it important? A white paper with excerpts from Gruman, J., Holmes-Rovner, M., French, M.E., Jeffress, D., Sofaer, S., Shaller, D., & Prager, D.C. (2010, March). From patient education to patient engagement: Implications for the field of patient education. *Patient Education and Counseling, 78*(3), 350-356. Retrieved from http://www.cfah.org/pdfs/CFAH_Engagement_Behavior_Framework_current.pdf

Centers for Disease Control and Prevention (CDC). (2010). *National chronic kidney disease fact sheet: General information and national estimates on chronic kidney disease in the United States, 2010.* Atlanta GA: Author.

Centers for Disease Control and Prevention, National Institutes of Health, the Department of Defense and the Department of

Veterans Affairs. (2013). *The report to Congress on traumatic brain injury in the United States: Understanding the public health problem among current and former military personnel.* Retrieved from http://www.cdc.gov/traumaticbraininjury/pdf/Report_to_Congress_on_Traumatic_Brain_Injury_2013

Center for Epidemiologic Studies Depression Scale-Short Form (CESD-SF). Retrieved from http://counsellingresource.com/lib/quizzes/depression-testing/cesd

Centers for Medicare & Medicaid Services (2013). *Toolkit for making written materials clear and effective.* Retrieved from http://www.cms.gov/Outreach-and-Education/Outreach/WrittenMaterialsToolkit/index.html?redirect=/writtenmaterialstoolkit

Chambers, J., Germain, M., & Brown, E. (2005). *Supportive care for the renal patient.* New York: Oxford.

Cheema, B., Abas, H., Smith, B., O'Sullivan, A., Chan, M., Patwardhan, A., & Singh, M.F. (2007). Progressive exercise for anabolism in kidney disease (PEAK): A randomized, controlled trial of resistance training during hemodialysis. *Journal of the American Society of Nephrology, 18*(5), 1594-601.

Cheema, B.S.B., Smith, B.C.F., & Singh, M.A. (2005). A rationale for intradialytic exercise training as standard clinical practice in ESRD. *American Journal of Kidney Diseases, 45,* 912-916.

Chertow, G.M., Levin, N.W., Beck, G.J., Depner, T.A., Eggers, P.W., Gassman, J.J., … Kliger A.S. (2010). In-center hemodialysis six times per week versus three times per week. *New England Journal of Medicine, 363*(24), 2287-300.

Cohen, L., & Davis, M. (2006). Did this patient die with hospice? New questions in caring for patients with ESRD (PowerPoint). Retrieved from http://www.kidneysupportivecare.org/files/presentations/davisppt.aspx

Cross, K.P. (1990). *Adult learning.* Retrieved February 6, 2008, from http://tip.psychology.org/cross.html

Cukor, D., Coplan, J., Brown, Cl, Friedman, S., Cromwell-Smith, A., Peterson, R., & Kimmel, P (2007). Depression and Anxiety in Urban Hemodialysis Patients. *Clinical Journal American Society of Nephrology, 2,* 484-490.

Cukor, D., Coplan, J., Brown, C., Peterson, R., & Kimmel, P. (2008). Course of depression and anxiety diagnosis in patients treated with hemodialysis: A 16-month follow-up. *Clinical Journal American Society of Nephrology, 3,* 1752-1758.

Curtin, R.B., & Mapes, D.L. (2001). Health care management strategies of long-term dialysis survivors. *Nephrology Nursing Journal, 28*(4), 385-394.

Curtin, R.B., Bultman Sitter, D.C., Schatell, D., & Chewning, B.A. (2004). Self-management, knowledge, and functioning and well-being of patients on hemodialysis. *Nephrology Nursing Journal, 31*(4), 378-387.

Deccache, A. (1995). Teaching, training, or educating patients? Influence of contexts and models of education and care on practice in patient education. *Patient Education and Counseling, 26*(1-3), 119-129.

De Jongh, T., Gurol-Urganci, I., Vodopivec-Jamsek, V., Car, J., & Atun, R. (2012). Mobile phone messaging for facilitating self-management of long-term illnesses. *Cochrane Database of Systematic Reviews.* Retrieved from http://www.ncbi.nlm.nih.gov/pubmed/23235644

Detsky, A.S., McLaughlin, J.R., Baker, J.P., Johnston, N., Whittaker, S., Mendelson, R.A., & Jeejeebhoy, K.N. (1987). What is subjective global assessment of nutritional status? *Journal of Parenteral and Enteral Nutrition, 11*(1), 8-13.

Devins, G.M., Mendelssohn, D.C., Barre, P.E., & Binik, Y.M. (2003). Predialysis psychoeducational intervention and coping style influence time to dialysis in chronic kidney disease. *American Journal of Kidney Diseases, 42*(4), 693-703.

DiLullo, L., Floccari, F., Rivera, R., Barbera, V., Granata, A., Otranto,

G., & Ronco, C. (2013). Pulmonary hypertension and right heart failure in chronic kidney disease: New challenge for 21st-century cardionephrologists. *Cardiorenal Medicine, 3*(2), 96-103. doi:10.1159/000350952

Dinwiddie, L., & Colvin, E., (2006). End of life care in the chronic kidney disease population. In A. Molzahn & E. Butera (Eds.), *Contemporary nephrology nursing: Principles and practice* (2nd ed., pp. 361-367). Pitman, NJ: American Nephrology Nurses' Association.

Doss, S., DePascal, P., & Hadley, K., (2011). Patient-nurse partnerships. *Nephrology Nursing Journal, 38*(2), 115-125.

Eble, K.E. (1988). *The craft of teaching* (2nd ed.). San Francisco: Jossey-Bass Publishers.

El-Agroudy, A.E., & El-Baz, A. (2010). Soluble Fas: A useful marker of inflammation and cardiovascular diseases in uremic patients. *Clinical and Experimental Nephrology, 14,* 152-157. doi:10.1007/s10157-009-0261-8

Ethnicity. (n.d.). In *Webster's new world college dictionary.* Retrieved from http://www.yourdictionary.com/ethnicity

Fahal, I.H., Bell, G.M., Bone, J.M., & Edwards, R.H. (1997). Physiological abnormalities of skeletal muscle in dialysis patients. *Nephrology Dialysis Transplantation, 12,* 119-127.

Ferell, B., & Coyle, N. (2005). *Textbook of palliative care nursing* (2nd ed.). New York: Oxford Press.

Fernandes, J.L., Serrano, C.V., Toledo, F. Hunziker, M.F., Zamperini, A., Teo, F.H., & Negrao, C.E. (2011). Acute and chronic effects of exercise on inflammatory markers and B-type natriuretic peptide in patients with coronary artery disease. *Clinical Research in Cardiology, 100*(1), 77-84. doi:10.1007/s00392-010-0215-x

Ferrucci, L., Izmirlian, G., Leveille, S., Phillips, C.L., Corti, M.C., Brock, D.B., & Guralnik, J.M. (1999). Smoking, physical activity, and active life expectancy. *American Journal of Epidemiology, 149*(7), 645-653.

Fink, J.C., Joy, M.S., St. Peter, W.L., Wahba, I.M., & ASN Chronic Kidney Disease Advisory Group. (2012). Finding a common language for patient safety in CKD. *Clinical Journal of the American Society of Nephrology, 7*(4), 689-695. doi:10.2215/CJN.12781211

Finkelstein, F.O., & Finkelstein, S.H. (2000). Depression in chronic dialysis patients: Assessment and treatment. *Nephrology Dialysis & Transplantation, 15,* 1911-1913.

Gagne, R. (1985). *The conditions of learning* (4th ed.). Retrieved from http://tip.psychology.org/gagne.html

Garcia Valderrama, F.W., Fajardo, C., Guevara, R., Gonzales Perez, V., & Hurtado, A. (2002). Poor adherence to diet in hemodialysis: Role of anxiety and depression symptoms. *Nefrologia, 22,* 244-252.

Gerstle, D.S. (1999). Grab their attention! Make your point! *MCN – The American Journal of Maternal/Child Nursing, 24*(5), 257-261.

Giacome, T., Ingersoll, G.L., & Williams, M. (1999). Teaching video effect on kidney transplant patient outcomes. *ANNA Journal, 26*(1), 29-33, 81.

Gibbons, R.J., Balady, G.J., Bricker, J.T., Chaitman, B.R., Fletcher, G.F., Froelicher, V.F., … Smith, S.C. (2002). ACC/AHA 2002 guideline update for exercise testing: Summary article. A report of the American College of Cardiology/American Heart Association Task Force on Practice Guidelines (Committee to Update the 1997 Exercise Testing Guidelines). *Journal of the American College of Cardiology, 40*(8), 1531-1540. doi:10.1161/01.CIR.0000034670.06526.15

Giger, J.N., & Davidhizar, R.E. (1991). *Transcultural nursing: Assessment and intervention.* St. Louis: Mosby.

Gokal, R., & Hutchison, A. (2002). Dialysis therapies for end stage kidney disease. *Seminars in Dialysis, 15*(4), 220-226.

Golberg, A.P., Hagberg, J.M., Delmez, J.A., Haynes, M.E., & Harter, H.R. (1980). Metabolic effects of exercise training in hemodialysis patients. *Kidney International. 18*, 754-761. doi:10.1038/ki.1980.194

Goldfield, N.I., McCullough, E.C., Hughes, J.S., Tang, A.M., Eastman, B., Rawlins, L.K., & Averill, R.F. (2008). Identifying potentially preventable readmissions. *Health Care Financing Review, 30*(1), 75-91.

Goldstein, S.L., & Montgomery, L.R. (2009). A pilot study of twice-weekly exercise during hemodialysis in children. *Pediatric Nephrology, 24*(4), 833-9. doi:10.1007/00467-008-1079-4

Golebiowski, T., Kusztal, M., Weyde, W., Dziubek, W., Wozniewski, M., Madziarska, K., … Klinger, M. (2012). A program of physical rehabilitation during hemodialysis sessions improves the fitness of dialysis patients. *Kidney and Blood Pressure Research, 35*(4), 290-296. doi:10.1159/000335411

Golebiowski, T., Weyde, W., Kusztal, M., Szymczak, M., Madziarska, K., Penar, J., … Klinger, M. (2009). Physical exercise in the rehabilitation of dialysis patients. *Postępy Higieny i Medycyny Doświadczalnej* (Online), 6(63), 13-22.

Golper, T. (2001). Patient education: Can it maximize the success of therapy? *Nephrology Dialysis & Transplantation, 16*(7), 20-24.

Gomez, N. (2011). *Nephrology nursing standards of practice and guidelines for care* (7th ed.). Pitman, NJ: American Nephrology Nurses' Association.

Hagberg, J.M., Goldberg, A.P., Ehsani, A.A., Heath, G.W., Delmez, J.A., & Harter, H.R. (1983). Exercise training improves hypertension in hemodialysis patients. *American Journal of Nephrology, 3*, 209-212.

Hain, D.J., & Sandy, D. (2013). Partners in care. Patient empowerment through shared decision making. *Nephrology Nursing Journal, 40*(2), 153-157.

Halbert, C.H., Armstrong, K., Gandy, O.H., & Shaker, L. (2006). Racial differences in trust in health care providers. *Journal of the American Medical Association, 166*(8), 896-901.

Halpin, L.S., Speir, A.M., CapoBianco, P., & Barnett, S.D. (2002). Guided imagery in cardiac surgery. *Outcomes in Management & Nursing Practice, 6*(3), 132-137.

Hansen, M., & Fisher, J.C. (1998). Patient-centered teaching from theory to practice. *American Journal of Nursing, 98*(1), 56, 58, 60.

Harwood, L., Locking-Cusolito, H., Spittal, J., Wilson, B., & White, S. (2005). Preparing for hemodialysis: Patient stressors and responses. *Nephrology Nursing Journal, 32*(3), 295-302.

Health Resources and Services Administration (HRSA). (2013). *Culture, language and health literacy.* Retrieved from http://www.hrsa.gov/culturalcompetence/index.html

Healthy People 2020. (2014). U.S. Department of Health and Human Services, Office of Disease Prevention and Health Promotion, Washington, DC. Retrieved from http://www.healthypeople.gov

Hedayati, S., Minhajuddin, A., Toto, R., Morris, D., & Rush, A. (2009). Prevalence of major depressive episode in CKD. *American Journal of Kidney Disease, 54*(3), 424-432.

Heiwe, S., & Jacobson, S.H. (2011). Exercise training for adults with chronic kidney disease. *Cochrane Database of Systematic Reviews, 10,* CD003236. doi:10.1002/14651858.CD003236.pub2

Henderson, J.N., Allen, K.V., Deary, I.J., & Frier, B.M. (2003). Hypoglycaemia in insulin-treated Type 2 diabetes: Frequency, symptoms and impaired awareness. *Diabetic Medicine, 20*(12), 1016-1021.

Hibbard, J.H., & Cunningham, P.J. (2008). How engaged are consumers in their health and health care, and why does it matter? *HSC Research Brief No. 8.* Retrieved from http://www.hschange.com/CONTENT/1019/#ib2

Hibbard, J.H., Mahoney, E.R., Stockard, J., & Tusler, M. (2005). Is patient activation associated with outcomes of care for adults with chronic conditions? *Health Services Research, 40*(6), 1918-1930.

Hibbard, J.H., Stockard, J., Mahoney, E.R., & Tusler, M. (2004). Development of the patient activation measure (PAM): Conceptualizing and measuring activation in patients and consumers. *Health Services Research.* Retrieved from http://www.ncbi.nlm.nih.gov/pmc/articles/PMC1361049

Hilgard, R.R., & Bower, G. H. (1966). *Theories of learning.* New York: Appleton-Century-Crofts.

Hodge, D.R. (2006). Spiritually modified cognitive therapy: A review of the literature. *Social Work: A Journal of the National Association of Social Workers, 51*(2), 157-165.

Hoge, C.W., McGurk, D., Thomas, J.L., Cox, A.L., Engel, C.C., & Castro, C.A. (2008). Mild traumatic brain injury in U.S. soldiers returning from Iraq. *New England Journal of Medicine, 358*(5), 453-63.

Howden, E.J., Leano, R., Petchey, W., Coombes, J.S., Isbel, N.M., & Marwick, T.H. (2013). Effects of exercise and lifestyle intervention on cardiovascular function in CKD. *Clinical Journal of the American Society of Nephrology, 8*(9), 1494-1501. doi:10.2215/CJN.10141012

Iacono, S.A. (2005). Predialysis anxiety: What are the concerns of patients? *The Journal of Nephrology Social Work, 24,* 21-24.

Institute of Medicine (IOM). (2004). *Report – Health literacy: A prescription to end confusion.* Retrieved from http://www.iom.edu/Reports/2004/Health-Literacy-A-Prescription-to-End-Confusion.aspx

Jaber, BL., Lee, Y., Collins, A.J., Hull, A.R., Kraus, M.A., McCarthy, J., Miller, B.W., Spry, L., Finkelstein, F.O., & FREEDOM Study Group. (2010). Effect of daily hemodialysis on depressive symptoms and postdialysis recovery time: Interim report from the FREEDOM (Following Rehabilitation, Economics, and Everyday-Dialysis Outcome Measurements) Study. *American Journal of Kidney Disease, 56*(3), 531-539. doi:10.1053/j.ajkd.2010.04.019

Johansen, K.L., & Painter, P. (2012). Exercise in individuals with CKD. *American Journal of Kidney Diseases, 59*(1), 126-34. doi:10.1053/j.ajkd.2011.10.008

Jung, T., & Park, S. (2011). Intradialytic exercise programs for hemodialysis patients. *Chonnam Medical Journal, 47*(2), 61-65. doi:10.4068/cmj.2011.47.2.61

Kimmel, P., Peterson, R., Weihs, K., Simmens, S., Alleyne, S., Cruz, I., & Veis, J. (2000). Multiple measures of depression predict mortality in a longitudinal study of chronic hemodialysis patients. *Kidney International, 57,* 2093-2098.

Kinzbrunner, B., Weinreb, N.J., & Policzer, J.S. (2011). *End of life care a practical guide* (2nd ed.). New York: McGraw-Hill.

Klang, B., Bjorvell, H., & Clyne, N. (1999). Predialysis education helps patients choose dialysis modality and increases disease-specific knowledge. *Journal of Advanced Nursing, 29*(4), 869-876.

Knox, A.B. (1986). *Helping adults learn.* San Francisco: Jossey-Bass Publishers.

Koo, J.R., Yoon, J.Y., Joo, M.H., Lee, H.S., Oh, J.E., Kim, S.G., …Son, B.K. (2005). Treatment of depression and effect of antidepression treatment on nutritional status in chronic hemodialysis patients. *The American Journal of the Medical Sciences, 329*(1), 1-5.

Kop, W., Seliger, S., Fink, J., Katz, R., Odden, M., Fried, L., … Gottdiener, J. (2011). Longitudinal association of depressive symptoms with rapid kidney function decline and adverse clinical renal disease outcomes. *The Clinical Journal of the American Society of Nephrology, 6*(4), 834-844. doi:10.2215/CJN.03840510

Kouidi, E.J., Grekas, D.M., & Deligiannis, A.P. (2009). Effects of exercise training on noninvasive cardiac measures in patients undergoing long-term hemodialysis: A randomized controlled trial. *American Journal of Kidney Diseases, 54*(3), 511-521.

Kosmadakis, G.C., John, S.G., Clapp, E.L., Viana, J.L., Smith, A.C., Bishop, N.C., & Feehally, J. (2012). Benefits of regular walking exercise in advanced pre-dialysis chronic kidney disease. *Nephrology Dialysis Transplantation, 27,* 997-1004.

Krop, J.S., Coresh, J., Chambless, L.E., Shahar, E., Watson, R.L., Szklo, M., & Brancati, F.L. (1999). A community-based study of explanatory factors for the excess risk for early kidney function decline in blacks vs. whites with diabetes: The Atherosclerosis Risk in Communities study. *Archives of Internal Medicine, 159*(15), 1777-1783.

Kuebler, K., Berry, P., & Heidrich, D. (2007). *Palliative care and end of life care clinical practice guidelines* (2nd ed.). Philadelphia: Saunders.

Kusek, J.W., Greene, P., Wang, S.R., Beck, G., West, D., Jamerson, K., ... Level, B. (2002). Cross-sectional study of health-related quality of life in African Americans with chronic kidney insufficiency: The African-American study of kidney disease and hypertension trial. *American Journal of Kidney Diseases, 39*(3), 513-524.

LaCroix, A.Z., Guralnik, J.M., Berkman, L.F., Wallace, R.B., & Satterfield, S. (1993). Maintaining mobility in late life II: Smoking, alcohol consumption, physical activity and body mass index. *American Journal of Epidemiology, 137,* 858-869.

Lane, D. (2003). *Levels of measurement: Connexions module.* Retrieved from http://cnx.org/content/m10809/latest/

Leveille, S.G., Guralnik, J.M., Ferrucci, L., & Langlois, J.A. (1999). Aging successfully until death in old age: Opportunities for increasing active life expectancy. *American Journal of Epidemiology, 149,* 654-653.

Liu, L.L., & Park, D.C. (2004). Aging and medical adherence: The use of automatic processes to achieve effortful things. *Psychology and Aging, 19*(2), 318-325. Retrieved from http://agingmind.utdallas.edu/publications?f=year&v=all

LoGiudice, D., Kerse, N., Brown, K., & Gibson, S.J. (1998). The psychosocial health status of caregivers of persons with dementia: A comparison with the chronically ill. *Quality of Life Research, 7,* 345-351.

Lopes, A.A., Albert, J.M., Young, E.W., Satayathum, S., Pisoni, R.L., Andreucci, V.E., ... Port, F.K. (2004). Screening for depression in hemodialysis patients: Associations with diagnosis, treatment, and outcomes in the DOPPS. *Kidney International, 66,* 2047-2053. doi:10.1111/j.1523-1755.2004.00977.x

Mapes, D.L., Callahan, M.B., & Richie, M.F. (2001). Psychosocial and rehabilitative aspects of kidney failure and its treatment. In L. Lancaster (Ed.), *Core Curriculum for nephrology nursing* (4th ed., pp. 159-189). Pitman, N.J.: American Nephrology Nurses' Association.

Martin, J.A., Smith, B.L., Mathews, T.J., Ventura, S.J., & Division of Vital Statistics. (1999). Births and deaths: Preliminary data for 1998. *National Vital Statistics Reports* (from the Centers for Disease Control and Prevention), *47*(25), 1-48. Retrieved from http://www.cdc.gov/nchs/data/nvsr/nvsr47/nvs47_25.pdf

Martins, D., Tareen, N., Zadshir, A., Pan, D., Vargas, R., Nissenson, A., & Norris, K. (2006). The association of poverty with the prevalence of albuminuria: Data from the Third National Health and Nutrition Examination Survey (NHANES III). *American Journal of Kidney Diseases, 47*(6), 965-971.

Maurer, M., Dardess, P., Carman, K.L., Frazier, K., & Smeeding, L. (2012). Guide to patient and family engagement: Environmental scan report. (Prepared by American Institutes for Research under contract HHSA 290-200-600019). AHRQ Publication No. 12-0042-EF. Rockville, MD: Agency for Healthcare Research

and Quality: May 2012.

Maynard, A.M. (1999). Preparing readable patient education handouts. *Journal for Nurses in Staff Development, 15*(1), 11-18.

Mazella, A. (2004). Psychosocial factors in treating the depressed kidney patient. *The Journal of Nephrology Social Work, 23,* 40-47.

McCool, M., Johnstone, S., Sledge, R., Witten, B,. Contillo, M., Aebel-Groesch, K., & Hafner, J. (2011). The promise of symptom-targeted intervention to manage depression in dialysis patients. *Nephrology News & Issues, 25*(6), 32-33.

McFarlane, C.D. (2006). My strength: A look outside the box at the strengths perspective. *Social Work: A Journal of the National Association of Social Workers, 51*(2), 175-176.

Meers, C., Singer, M.A., Toffelmire, E.B., Hopman, W., McMurray, M., Morton, A.R., & MacKenzie, T.A. (1996). Self-delivery of hemodialysis care: A therapy in itself. *American Journal of Kidney Diseases, 27*(6), 844-847.

Menon, D.K., Schwab, K., Wright, D.W., & Maas A.I. (2010). Demographics and Clinical Assessment Working Group of the International and Interagency Initiative toward Common Data Elements for Research on Traumatic Brain Injury and Psychological Health. Position statement: Definition of traumatic brain injury. *Archives Physical Medicine and Rehabilitation, 91*(11), 1637-1640.

Mercer, T.H., Crawford, C., Gleeson, N.P., & Naish, P.F. (2002). Low-volume exercise rehabilitation improves functional capacity and self-reported functional status of dialysis patients. *American Journal of Physical Medicine and Rehabilitation, 81,* 162-167.

Miller, B.W., Cress, C.L., Johnson, M.E., Nichols, D.H., & Schnitzler, M.A. (2002). Exercise during hemodialysis decreases the use of antihypertensive medications. *American Journal of Kidney Diseases, 39,* 828-833.

Mohseni, R., Zeydi, A.E., Ilali, E., Adib-Hajbaghery, M., & Makhlough, A. (2013). The effect of intradialytic aerobic exercise on dialysis efficacy in hemodialysis patients: A randomized controlled trial. *Oman Medical Journal, 28*(5), 345-349. doi:10.5001/omj.2013.99

Mok, E., Lai, C., & Zhang, Z. (2004). Coping with chronic kidney failure in Hong Kong. *International Journal of Nursing Studies, 41*(2), 205-213.

Molzahn, A.E. (1996). Changing to a teaching paradigm for teaching and learning. *ANNA Journal, 23*(2), 217-221.

Mosen, D.M., Schmittdiel, J., Hibbard, J., Sobel, D., Remmers, C., & Bellows, J. (2007). Is patient activation associated with outcomes of care for adults with chronic conditions? *Journal of Ambulatory Care Management, 30*(1), 21-29.

Moss, A., Ganjoo, J., Sharma, S., Gansor, J., Senft, S., Weaner, B. ... Schmidt, R. (2008). Utility of the "surprise" question to identify dialysis patients with high mortality. *Clinical Journal of the American Society of Nephrology, 3,* 1379-1384.

Nápoles-Springer, A.M., Santoyo, J., Houston, J., Pérez-Stable, E J., & Stewart, A.L. (2005). Patients' perceptions of cultural factors affecting the quality of their medical encounters. *Health Expectations, 8*(1), 4.

National Center for Education Statistics. (2003). *Health literacy: Statistics-at-a-glance.* Boston, MA. Retrieved from http://nces.ed.gov/naal/health.asp

National Center for PTSD. (2013). *Understanding PTSD treatment.* Retrieved from http://www.ptsd.va.gov/public/understanding_TX/booklet.pdf

National Conference of State Legislatures. (2011). The affordable care act: A brief summary. Retrieved from http://www.ncsl.org/portals/1/documents/health/hraca.pdf

National Consensus Project. (2010). *Clinical practice guidelines for quality palliative care.* Retrieved from http://www.nationalconsensusproject.org

National Standards for Culturally and Linguistically Appropriate Services in Health and Health Care (the National CLAS Standards). (2014). Retrieved from https://www.thinkculturalhealth.hhs.gov/content/clas.asp

Nelson, M.E., Rejeski, W.J., Blair, S.N., Duncan, P.W., Judge, J.O., King, A.C., & Castaneda-Sceppa, C. (2007). Physical activity and public health in older adults: Recommendations from the American College of Sports Medicine and the American Heart Association. *Medicine & Science in Sports and Exercise, 39*(8), 1435-1445. Retrieved from http://circ.ahajournals.org/content/116/9/1094.full.pdf

Painter, P.L., Carlson, L., Carey, S., Paul, S.M., & Myll, J. (2000a). Low functioning patients improve with exercise training. *American Journal of Kidney Diseases, 36*(3), 600-608.

Painter, P.L., Carlson, L., Carey, S., Paul, S.M., & Myll, J. (2000b). Physical functioning and health related quality of life changes with exercise training in hemodialysis patients. *American Journal of Kidney Diseases, 35*(3), 482-492.

Painter, P., & Johansen, K.L. (2006). Improving physical functioning: Time to become a part of the routine care. *American Journal of Kidney Diseases, 48*(1), 167-170.

Painter, P.L., Messer-Rehak, D., Hanson, P., Zimmerman, S.W., & Glass, N.R. (1986). Exercise capacity in hemodialysis, CAPD and kidney transplant patients. *Nephron, 42*, 47-51.

Painter, P., Moore, G.E., Carlson, L., Paul, S., Myll, J., Phillips, W., & Haskell, W.(2002). The effects of exercise training plus normalization of hematocrit on exercise capacity and health related quality of life. *American Journal of Kidney Diseases, 39*(2), 257-265.

Paniagua, R., Amato, D., Vonesh, E., Guo, A., & Mujais, S. (2005). Health-related quality of life predicts outcomes but is not affected by peritoneal clearance: The ADEMEX trial. *Kidney International, 67*(3), 1093-1094.

Panico, M., Jeng, G., & Brewster, U. (2011). When a patient refuses life-saving care. *American Journal of Kidney Diseases, 58*(4), 647-653.

Parsons, T.L., Toffelmire, E.B., & King-VanVlack, C.E. (2006). Exercise training during hemodialysis improves dialysis efficacy and physical performance. *Archives of Physical Medicine and Rehabilitation, 87*, 680-687. doi:10.1016/j.apmr.2005.12.044

Patel, S.S., Shah, V.S., Peterson, R.A., & Kimmel, P.L. (2002). Psychosocial variables, quality of life, and religious beliefs in ESRD patients treated with hemodialysis. *American Journal of Kidney Disease, 40*(5), 1013-1022.

Pattaragarn, A., Warady, B.A., & Sabath, R.J. (2004). Exercise capacity in pediatric patients with end-stage renal disease. *Peritoneal Dialysis International, 24*, 274-280.

Payne, G.M. (2013). We can do better: By changing culture to improve care. *Nephrology Nursing Journal, 40*(1), 11, 27.

Physicians Health Questionnaire (PHQ-9). Retrieved from http://www.phqscreeners.com/

Port, F.K., Wolfe, R.A., Levin, N.W., Guire, K.E., & Ferguson, C.W. (1990). Income and survival in chronic dialysis patients. *ASAIO Transplantation, 36*(3), M154-157.

Puchalski, C. (2006). *The George Washington Institute for Spirituality and Health.* Retrieved from https://smhs.gwu.edu/gwish

Ramsdell, R., & Annis, C. (1996). Patient education: A continuing repetitive process. *ANNA Journal, 23*(2), 217-221.

Rand Health. (n.d.) Kidney Disease Quality of Life survey (KDQOL). Retrieved from http://www.rand.org/health/surveys_tools.kdqol.html

Ravenscroft, E.F. (2005). Diabetes and kidney failure: How individuals with diabetes experience kidney failure. *Nephrology Nursing Journal, 32*(4), 502-509.

Redman, B. (1997). *The process of patient education* (8th ed.). St Louis: Mosby.

Redman, B.K. (2003). *Measurement tools in patient education* (2nd ed.). New York: Springer Publishing Company.

Renal Physicians Association (RPA) and American Society of Nephrology (ASN). (2010). *Clinical practice guideline: Shared decision-making in the appropriate initiation of and withdrawal from dialysis.* Washington, DC: Author.

Richardson, M.A., Post-White, J., Grimm, E.A., Moye, L.A., Singletary, S.E., & Justice, B. (1997). Coping, life attitudes, and the immune responses to imagery and group support after breast cancer treatment. *Alternative Therapy Health Medicine, 3*(5), 62-70.

Rimm, R.B., Stampfer, M.J., Giovannucci, E., Ascherio, A., Spiegelman, D., Colditz, G.A., & Willett, W.C. (1995). Body size and fat distribution as predictors of coronary heart disease among middle-aged and older US men. *American Journal of Epidemiology, 141*(12), 1117-27.

Robert Wood Johnson Foundation End-Stage Renal Disease Workgroup. (2009). *Completing the continuum of nephrology care recommendations to the field.* Retrieved from http://www.promotingexcellence.org

Robinson, K., & Ricca, L. (2002). AAKP reviews 30 years of the Medicare ESRD Program. *Kidney Life, 17*(6).

Ross, P.E., Groenhoff, C., & Zin, P. (2004). Chronic kidney disease, now what! *American Association of Occupational Health Nurses Journal, 52*(7), 287-297.

Sala, E., Noyszewski, E.A., Campistol, J.M., Marrades, R.M., Dreha, S. Torregrossa, J.V., & Roca, J. (2001). Impaired muscle oxygen transfer in patients with chronic renal failure. *American Journal of Physiology – Regulatory, Integrative and Comparative Physiology, 280*, R1240-8.

Sandrick, K. (1998). Teach your patients well. *Health Management Technology, 19*(3), 16-18.

Satayathum, S., Pisoni, R.L., McCullough, K.P., Merion, R.M., Wikstrom, B., Levin, N., … Port, F.K. (2005). Kidney transplantation and wait-listing rates from the international Dialysis Outcomes and Practice Patterns Study (DOPPS). *Kidney International, 68*(1), 330-337.

Sietsema, K.E., Amato, A., Adler, S.G., & Brass, E.P. (2004). Exercise capacity as a prognostic indicator among ambulatory patients with end stage kidney disease. *Kidney International, 65*(2), 719-724.

Shah, M.K. (2002). Simultaneous bilateral quadriceps tendon rupture in renal patients. *Clinical Nephrology, 58*(2), 118-21.

Shiraishi, F.G., Belik, F.S., Silva, V.R., Martin, L.C., Hueb, J.C., Goncalves, R.S., & Franco, R.J. (2012). Inflammation, diabetes, and chronic kidney disease: Role of aerobic capacity. *Experimental Diabetes Research, Vol. 2012*, Article ID 750286, 6 pages. doi:10.1155/2012/750286

Shoemaker, M.J., Wilt, J.L., Dasgupta, R., & Oudiz, R.J. (2009). Exercise training in patients with pulmonary arterial hypertension: A case report. *Cardiopulmonary Physical Therapy Journal, 20*(4), 12-18.

Shoham, D.A., Vupputuri, S., & Kshirsagar, A.V. (2005). Chronic kidney disease and life course socioeconomic status: A review. *Advances in Chronic Kidney Disease, 12*(1), 56-63.

Smart, N., & Steel, M. (2011). Exercise training in hemodialysis patients: A systematic review and meta-analysis. *Nephrology, 16*(7), 626-632.

Smart, N.A., Williams, A.D., Livinger, I., Selig, S., Howden, E., Coombes, J.S., & Fassett, R.G. (2013). Exercise & Sports Science Australia (ESSA) position statement on exercise and chronic kidney disease. *Journal of Science and Medicine in Sport, 16,* 406-411. doi.org/10.1016/j.jsams.2013.01.005

St. Peter, W. (2005). United States Kidney Data System. Presentation by the American Society of Nephrology.

Strawbridge, W.J., Cohen, R.D., Shema, S.J., & Kaplan, G.A. (1996). Successful aging: Predictors and associated activities. *American Journal of Epidemiology, 144*(2), 135-141.

Sue, D.W., Arrendondo, P., & McDavis, R.J. (1992). Multicultural counseling competencies and standards: A call to the profession. *Journal of Counseling and Development, 70,* 477-486.

Swartzendruber, D. (1994). Gaming: A creative strategy for staff education. *ANNA Journal, 21*(1), 21-25.

Tang, P.C., & Newcomb, C. (1998). Informing patients: A guide for providing patient health information. *Journal of the American Medical Informatics Association, 5*(6), 563-570.

Tattersall, R. (1995). Patient education 2000: Take-home messages from this congress. *Patient Education and Counseling, 26*(1-3), 373-377.

Ulrich, B., (2009). Providing culturally competent nursing care. *Nephrology Nursing Journal, 36*(4), 367.

United States Renal Data System (USRDS). (2012). *USRDS 2012 annual data report, comprehensive dialysis study, chapter 9: Rehabilitation/quality of life & nutrition special studies,* 309-318.

United States Renal Data System (USRDS). (2013). *USRDS 2013 annual data report: Atlas of chronic kidney disease and end-stage renal disease in the United States.* National Institutes of Health; National Institute of Diabetes and Digestive and Kidney Diseases. Bethesda, MD. Retrieved from http://www.usrds.org

United States Renal Data System (USRDS). (2014). *USRDS 2014 annual data report: An overview of the epidemiology of kidney disease in the United States.* National Institutes of Health; National Institute of Diabetes and Digestive and Kidney Diseases. Bethesda, MD. Retrieved from http://www.usrds.org/adr.aspx

Van den Borne, H.W. (1998). The patient from receiver of information to informed decision-maker. *Patient Education and Counseling, 34*(2), 89-102.

Wingard, R. (2005). Patient education and the nursing process: Meeting the patient's needs. *Nephrology Nursing Journal, 32*(2), 211-215.

Wu, S.C., Leu, S.Y., & Li, C.Y. (1999). Incidence of and predictors for chronic disability in activities of daily living among older people in Taiwan. *Journal of American Geriatric Society, 47*(9), 1082-1086.

Yigla, M., Nakhoul, F., Sabag, A., Tov, N., Gorevich, B., Abassi, Z., & Reisner, S.A. (2003). Pulmonary hypertension in patients with end-stage renal disease, *Chest, 123,* 1577-1582.

Internet Resources

http://www.annanurse.org/resources/cne-opportunities/education-modules

End of Life Decision Making and the Role of the Nephrology Nurse
Module 1: Techniques to Facilitate Discussion for Advance Care Planning (ACP)
Module 2: Ethical and Legal Aspects of Advanced Care Planning (ACP)
Module 3: Cultural Diversity: Different Cultures, Different Solutions
Module 4: Coordination of Hospice and Palliative Care in ESRD

http://www.eperc.mcw.edu/EPERC/FastFactsandConcepts End of life/palliative care education resource center

http://www.adec.org (Association of Death Education and Counseling)

http://www.aacn.nche.edu/ELNEC (End of Life Nursing Education Consortium)

http://www.hpna.org (Hospice and Palliative Nurses Association)

http://www.americanbar.org/content/dam/aba/migrated/2011_build/law_aging/st_spec_adv_dirs_update_2-11.authcheckdam.pdf (State Specific AMD Forms)

Toolkit for Nurturing Excellence at End-of-Life Transition (TNEEL) CD-rom. Funded by the Robert Wood Johnson Foundation. Download at http://www.tneel.uic.edu/tneel.asp

Foundations in Nutrition and Clinical Applications in Nephrology Nursing

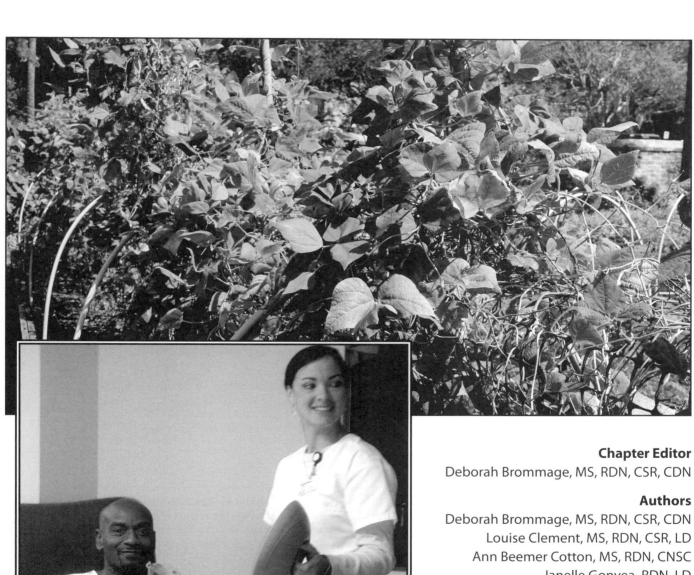

Chapter Editor
Deborah Brommage, MS, RDN, CSR, CDN

Authors
Deborah Brommage, MS, RDN, CSR, CDN
Louise Clement, MS, RDN, CSR, LD
Ann Beemer Cotton, MS, RDN, CNSC
Janelle Gonyea, RDN, LD
Mary Kay Hensley, MS, RDN, CSR
Pamela S. Kent, MS, RDN, CSR, LD
Maureen P. McCarthy, MPH, RDN, CSR, LD
Jessie M. Pavlinac, MS, RDN, CSR, LD
Jean Stover, RDN, CSR, LDN

CHAPTER **4**

Foundations in Nutrition and Clinical Applications in Nephrology Nursing

This offering for **1.4 contact hours** is provided by the American Nephrology Nurses' Association (ANNA).

American Nephrology Nurses' Association is accredited as a provider of continuing nursing education by the American Nurses Credentialing Center Commission on Accreditation.

ANNA is a provider approved by the California Board of Registered Nursing, provider number CEP 00910.

This CNE offering meets the continuing nursing education requirements for certification and recertification by the Nephrology Nursing Certification Commission (NNCC).

To be awarded contact hours for this activity, read this chapter in its entirety. Then complete the CNE evaluation found at **www.annanurse.org/corecne** and submit it; or print it, complete it, and mail it in. Contact hours are not awarded until the evaluation for the activity is complete.

Example of reference for Chapter 4 in APA format. Use author of the section being cited. This example is based on Section C – Special Considerations in Kidney Disease.

Brommage, D., Cotton, A.B., Gonyea, J., Kent, P.S., & Stover, J. (2015). Foundations in nutrition and clinical applications in nephrology nursing: Special considerations in kidney disease. In C.S. Counts (Ed.), *Core curriculum for nephrology nursing: Module 2. Physiologic and psychosocial basis for nephrology nursing practice* (6th ed., pp. 255-290). Pitman, NJ: American Nephrology Nurses' Association.

Interpreted: Section authors. (Date). Title of chapter: Title of section. In …

The Academy of Nutrition and Dietetics' Board of Directors and the Commission on Dietetic Registration have approved the optional use of the credential "registered dietitian nutritionist" (RDN) by registered dietitians (RD). The option was established to further enhance the RD brand and more accurately reflect to consumers who registered dietitians are and what they do. This will differentiate the rigorous credential requirements and highlight that all registered dietitians are nutritionists but not all nutritionists are registered dietitians. Inclusion of the word "nutritionist" in the credential communicates a broader concept of wellness (including prevention of health conditions beyond medical nutrition therapy) as well as treatment of conditions. The RDN credential is offered as an option to RDs who want to emphasize the nutrition aspect of their credential to the public and to other health practitioners. The RD and RDN credential have identical meanings and legal trademark definitions. *Source*: Academy of Nutrition and Dietetics (AND). (2014), *RDN credential: Frequently asked questions*. Retrieved November 10, 2014, from http://www.eatright.org/RDN/

Cover photos by Counts/Morganello and Sandra Cook.

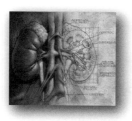

CHAPTER 4

Foundations in Nutrition and Clinical Applications in Nephrology Nursing

Purpose

The focus of this section is to examine nutrition issues related to chronic kidney disease, dialysis, and transplantation. This review looks at the nutrition care process in managing kidney disease, including nutrition assessment, nutrition diagnosis, nutrition intervention, and nutrition monitoring and evaluation (Writing Group of the Nutrition Care Process/Standardized Language Committee, 2008).

Nutrition assessment encompasses interpretation and evaluation of food/nutrition-related history, medications, biochemical data, medical tests/procedures, anthropometric measurements, nutrition-focused physical exam findings, and medical history.

Nutrition diagnosis involves recognizing nutrient deficits or excesses that result in complications such as protein-energy wasting, bone disease, and anemia. The identification of nutrition problems is necessary for determining the nutritional needs for chronic kidney disease, different types of dialysis, kidney transplantation, and for special life stages such as pregnancy and older adults.

Nutrition intervention includes strategies to meet the special nutrition needs associated with kidney disease for adults, the elderly, patients with diabetes, and culturally diverse populations. Patient adherence to nutrition intervention and improved patient outcomes relies on overcoming low health literacy and applying sound education strategies.

Nutrition monitoring and evaluation uses selected outcome indicators such as biochemical markers and clinical data to ensure that nutrition goals are being met for patients with kidney disease.

Objectives

Upon completion of this chapter, the learner will be able to:
1. Interpret the results of biochemical tests and procedures used for assessing nutritional status in patients with kidney disease.
2. Identify signs, symptoms, and indices of protein-energy wasting in patients with kidney disease.
3. Explain nutrition recommendations for patients of varying ages and comorbidities with chronic kidney disease and those who are receiving kidney replacement therapies.
4. Identify cultural factors that impact food practices and the implications for nutrition care of patients with kidney disease.
5. Explain the adverse effects of excessive sodium intake on target organs and the benefits of a sodium-controlled diet, when appropriate.
6. Outline stages of behavioral changes that influence patients with kidney disease to adjust to the renal nutrition regimen.

SECTION A
Nutrition Screening and Assessment
Jessie M. Pavlinac

I. Nutrition screening is a process used to identify nutrition-related problems.

A. Patients identified as either at high risk of developing or are currently malnourished should be referred to the nephrology dietitian for a comprehensive nutrition assessment. Screening criteria include (Charney & Marian, 2008):
1. Height and weight.
2. Unintentional change in weight.
3. Food allergies.
4. Diet.
5. Biochemical data.
6. Change in appetite.
7. Nausea/vomiting.
8. Bowel habits.
9. Chewing and swallowing ability.
10. Medical diagnosis.

B. No single measure can diagnose malnutrition or identify the different aspects of protein-energy wasting (PEW) (See Section C.I. Malnutrition and protein-energy wasting in kidney disease).

II. Nurses may assist in identification of risk for malnutrition and/or PEW in patients with chronic kidney disease (CKD).

A. Simple clinical signs include loose-fitting clothes, rings, or ill-fitting dentures as a result of weight loss secondary to inadequate caloric intake.

B. Loss of muscle mass can be evident when taking blood pressure.

C. Decreased strength and endurance may be noted in assisting the patient with mobilization.

III. Identifying patients at risk for poor nutritional status – elements of a nutrition assessment (DiBenedetto & Brommage, 2013).

A. Medical history.
1. Chronic disease that affects ingestion, digestion, or absorption of nutrients (e.g., scleroderma, Crohn's disease, amyloidosis, diabetic gastroparesis, GI bleeding, bowel obstruction).
2. Significant change in usual body weight or weight when patient started kidney replacement therapy. (Was weight change intentional and over what period of time?)
3. Increased metabolic needs related to dialysis, sepsis, fever, infection, inflammation, or medications.
4. Increased nutrient losses from open wounds, draining fistulas, chronic blood loss, or peritonitis.
5. Recent major surgery or hospitalization with clear liquid diet or NPO status for greater than 5 days.
6. Neurologic impairment or presence of dysphagia.

B. Social history.
1. Lives alone without family or peer support.
2. Depression.
3. Limited financial resources.
4. Physical or psychological disabilities that limit ability to prepare meals or shop for food.
5. Alcoholism or drug and/or tobacco abuse.
6. Behavioral barriers.
7. Limited literacy skills that affect the ability to follow oral/written instructions.

C. Food and nutrition history.
1. Dietary interviews and/or diaries that indicate inadequate intake compared to estimated nutrient needs.
2. Multiple dietary restrictions or modifications that make the kidney diet more difficult to follow.

3. Anorexia, nausea, vomiting, or change in bowel habits.
4. Impaired sense of taste or smell.
5. Poor dentition.
6. Religious, ethnic, or cultural beliefs that influence intake.
7. Food allergies, preferences, or intolerances.
8. Medications (prescribed and over the counter) with food–drug interactions, drug–nutrient interactions, and nutrient–nutrient interactions.
9. Dietary supplements or alternative therapies.

IV. Identifying nutritional risk from biochemical data.

A. Serum albumin less than 4.0 g/dL, using the bromcresol green method laboratory assay (BCG) (National Kidney Foundation [NKF], 2000).
1. Readily available and widely accepted nutritional parameter in most patient groups; strongest prognostic indicator in dialysis patients.
2. Slow response to depletion or repletion; altered by factors other than malnutrition since it is a negative acute phase reactant (may be a reflection of illness or inflammation rather than visceral protein stores). Half-life is 21 days.
3. Low levels may be secondary to infection, inflammation, trauma, decreased synthesis related to liver disease, peritoneal/urinary albumin losses, hydration status, and/or acidemia.
4. High levels may be secondary to severe dehydration and albumin infusion.
5. Clinical status must be considered when evaluating changes in serum albumin concentration.

B. Serum total cholesterol less than 100 mg/dL (Fouque et al., 2008).
1. Low levels may be secondary to acute infection, starvation, and PEW.
2. Maintenance hemodialysis patients with a low normal serum total cholesterol level have a higher mortality rate than hemodialysis patients with higher cholesterol.
3. Serum total cholesterol should be used only for nutrition screening purposes. Patients with low levels should be evaluated for other comorbidities in addition to nutritional deficits.

C. Prealbumin less than 30 mg/dL predialysis (NKF, 2000).
1. Marker of protein energy malnutrition.
2. Low levels have been associated with increased mortality risk and correlates with other markers of malnutrition in dialysis patients.
3. High levels may be secondary to administration of corticoids.

4. May be falsely elevated in patients with significantly decreased kidney function secondary to impaired degradation by the kidney.
5. Negative acute-phase reactant; levels can decline as a response to inflammation or infection.

D. Serum bicarbonate less than 22 mEq/dL (NKF, 2000).
   1. Metabolic acidosis is associated with increased oxidation of branch chain amino acids.
   2. Metabolic acidosis decreases albumin synthesis and increases muscle protein catabolism.
   3. Acidosis affects bone mineral content, increases osteoclast activity, and decreases osteoblast activity.
   4. Acidosis disrupts potassium homeostasis, leading to a shift of potassium from intracellular to extracellular.

E. For patients undergoing dialysis, predialysis serum creatinine less than 10 mg/dL (anuric) (NKF, 2000).
   1. Creatinine is a reflection of somatic (skeletal muscle mass) and dietary protein (muscle) intake.
   2. Residual kidney function and dose of dialysis must be considered when using serum creatinine as a marker of dietary intake.

V. Nutrition-focused physical examination
(Hammond, 1997; Hammond, 1999; Seidel et al., 2011).

A. Using a systems approach, a nutrition-focused physical exam can be integrated into the complete physical assessment of kidney patients.

B. General survey.
   1. Nutrition focus.
      a. Body weight and height compared with normal height–weight chart.
      b. General wasting of muscle and/or loss of adipose tissue.
      c. Alertness, orientation.
      d. Any deviation from normal growth or development.
      e. Note skin condition throughout exam. Check for signs of dryness/scaling and overall skin pigmentation.
   2. Nutritional implications.
      a. Insufficient calories and protein.
      b. Inability to feed self.
      c. Food preparation.
      d. Other activities of daily living.
      e. Poor wound healing and pressure ulcers associated with protein, vitamin C, and zinc deficiencies; purpura associated with vitamins C and K deficiencies.

C. Vital signs.
   1. Temperature. Fever increases energy and fluid needs.
   2. Respirations. Increased rate or work of breathing can impact calorie and protein requirements, quantity of food eaten, and acid-base status.
   3. Pulse. Heart rate may increase with anemia.
   4. Blood pressure. May indicate need for diet modification, such as weight reduction and sodium or fluid management.

D. Head and face.
   1. Nutrition focus.
      a. Inspect and palpate shape and symmetry.
      b. Note texture, distribution, and quantity of hair (check for signs of thin, sparse hair with easy pluckability).
      c. Palpate temporomandibular joint (TMJ) while patient opens and closes mouth.
      d. Assess CN V (trigeminal) and CN VII (facial).
   2. Nutritional implications.
      a. Bilateral temporal wasting may reflect protein–calorie deficiency.
      b. Problems with TMJ may influence the ability to eat.
      c. Weakness, asymmetry, or pain related to CN V and CN VII problems can affect chewing or may result in holding food in mouth.
      d. Sparse hair with easy pluckability may suggest protein, biotin, or zinc deficiencies.

E. Eyes.
   1. Nutrition focus.
      a. Inspect appearance of sclerae, conjunctivae, and corneae. Is the eye drying or tearing?
      b. Inquire about problems with adjustments to darkness or visual impairment.
   2. Nutritional implications.
      a. May suggest vitamin A deficiency or B-carotene deficit, though very rare in dialysis-dependent patients. *Note*: Hypervitaminosis A occurs in kidney failure so caution should be taken with any form of supplementation.
         (1) Dull, rough appearance to inner lids (conjunctival xerosis).
         (2) Softening of cornea (keratomalacia).
         (3) Foamy or cheesy raised lesions noted on the temporal side of the sclera (bitot's spots).
         (4) Dull, milky, hazy/opaque appearance of cornea (corneal xerosis) or night blindness.
      b. Vision impairment can affect ability to cook, shop, eat, or follow written dietary guidelines.

F. Nose.
   1. Nutrition focus.
      a. Determine patency of each nostril; inspect mucosa, septum, and turbinates.

b. Test CN I (olfactory).
2. Nutritional implications.
   a. Patency of nostrils may influence decision on feeding tube placement.
   b. Sense of smell influences foods eaten and may alter appetite.

G. Mouth and oropharynx.
   1. Nutrition focus.
      a. Inspect lips, buccal mucosa, gums, hard and soft palates, and floor of mouth for color and surface characteristics.
      b. Inspect teeth for color, number, and surface characteristics.
      c. Inspect and palpate tongue, noting color, characteristics, symmetry, and movement.
      d. Test CN IX (glossopharyngeal), CN X (vagus), and CN XII (hypoglossal).
   2. Nutritional implications.
      a. Bilateral cracks and redness of lips (angular stomatitis) or vertical cracks of lips (cheilosis) may suggest riboflavin, niacin, and pyridoxine deficiency.
      b. Dryness of mucosa can reflect hydration status.
      c. Condition of teeth influences ability to chew.
      d. Spongy, swollen, bleeding gums may be secondary to vitamin C deficiency.
      e. Slick or beefy-red tongue (glossitis) suggests riboflavin, niacin, folate, iron, or vitamin B12 deficiency.
      f. Note any evidence of dysphagia or risk for aspiration.

H. Neck.
   1. Nutrition focus.
      a. Inspect symmetry and smoothness of neck.
      b. Palpate thyroid and parotid glands.
   2. Nutritional implications.
      a. Enlarged thyroid may reflect iodine deficiency.
      b. Bilateral enlargement of parotids may reflect protein deficiency. Consider bulimia.

I. Upper extremities.
   1. Nutrition focus.
      a. Inspect skin and nail characteristics.
      b. Palpate hands, arms, and shoulders.
      c. Assess amount of subcutaneous fat in triceps and biceps and any evidence of interosseous wasting.
      d. Check range of motion in wrists, elbows, and shoulders.
      e. Assess muscle and grip strength bilaterally.
   2. Nutritional implications.
      a. Fat and muscle wasting reflect protein and calorie deficiency.
      b. Swollen painful joints may suggest vitamin C deficiency.

c. Range of motion in upper extremities affects ability to feed independently.
d. Muscle and grip strength may indicate malnutrition or need for assistive devices or assistance with food preparation.

J. Chest and lungs.
   1. Nutrition focus. Inspect, palpate, percuss, and auscultate.
   2. Nutritional implications.
      a. Prominent bony skeleton with muscle and fat wasting reflect inadequate calorie and protein intake.
      b. Crackles and wheezes suggest fluid overload and may influence fluid requirements and nutrition regimen.
      c. Increased work of breathing increases energy needs.

K. Cardiovascular.
   1. Nutrition focus. Inspect, palpate, and auscultate.
   2. Nutritional implications.
      a. Jugular venous distention (JVD) and edema will influence fluid requirements.
      b. Edema may be related to protein deficiency, malnutrition, or fluid status.
      c. Dysrhythmias may be related to potassium, calcium, magnesium, or phosphorus imbalances.
      d. Tachycardia and heart failure have been associated with thiamin deficiency. Sodium and fluid intake related to heart failure.
      e. Cardiac cachexia is associated with inability to eat and digest adequate quantities of food; loss of lean body mass may not be detected if hidden by fluid overload.

L. Abdomen.
   1. Nutrition focus.
      a. Inspect skin, contour, and muscle development.
      b. Auscultate for bowel sounds.
      c. Percuss for tone.
      d. Palpate all quadrants.
   2. Nutritional implications.
      a. Poor wound healing may reflect inadequate calories, protein, zinc, or vitamin C.
      b. Presence of ascites may impact fluid, sodium, and protein requirements.
      c. Absent or hypoactive bowel sounds will influence feeding route.
      d. Hepatomegaly may reflect protein deficiency or excessive vitamin A intake.

M. Lower extremities.
   1. Nutrition focus.
      a. Inspect skin and nails.
      b. Palpate thigh, calf, and feet bilaterally.

c. Evaluate range of motion (ROM) and muscle strength of lower extremities.
d. Test deep tendon reflexes (DTRs) bilaterally.
e. Sensory exam in three dermatomes.
2. Nutritional implications.
   a. Muscle wasting and prominent skeleton suggest inadequate calorie and protein intake.
   b. Poor wound healing associated with inadequate calorie, protein, zinc, vitamin C intake, or poor glucose control.
   c. Motor weakness in lower extremities associated with thiamin deficiency.
   d. Hypoactive reflexes may reflect thiamin or vitamin B12 deficiency.
   e. Peripheral neuropathy associated with thiamin, vitamin B12, and pyridoxine deficiency.

VI. Anthropometric data (NKF, 2000).

A. Determine percentage of usual body weight (UBW). Unintentional weight loss greater than 10% is clinically significant.

B. Determine percentage of standard body weight (SBW) determined from NHANES II data (average 50th percentile weights for men and women by age, height, and frame size in the United States).

C. Determine body mass index (BMI).
1. BMI = weight in kg/height in m^2.
2. BMI of 14 to 15 kg/m^2 is associated with significant mortality in general populations.
3. BMI of 23.6 for women and 24 for men is associated with increased survival in hemodialysis patients.
4. BMI greater than 27 is associated with increased risk for all-cause mortality.

D. Determine adjusted edema-free body weight (aBWef) for assessing or prescribing calorie and protein intake for patients less than 95% or greater than 115% of the median standard weight as determined from NHANES II data.
Equation to calculate aBWef:

aBWef = BWef + [(SBW – BWef) x 0.25]

BWef is the actual edema-free body weight and SBW is the standard body weight as determined from the NHANES II data.

E. Patients whose edema-free body weight is between 95% and 115% of the median standard weight should have calorie and protein needs assessed or prescribed based on actual edema-free body weight.

F. Determine triceps skinfold thickness (TSF), mid-arm circumference (MAC), mid-arm muscle circumference (MAMC), and mid-upper arm muscle area (MAMA).

G. Measure waist circumference (WC) and waist-to-hip ratio (WHR).
1. WC associated with higher risk for disease (NIH, 2014).
   a. Greater than 102 cm (40 inches) for men.
   b. Greater than 88 cm (35 inches) for women.
2. WHR = WC ÷ hip circumference. WHR associated with metabolic complications (World Health Organization [WHO], 2008).
   a. Greater than 9.0 for men.
   b. Greater than 8.5 for women.

H. Other measures of body composition not typically done in the clinical setting include:
1. Dual energy x-ray absorptiometry (DEXA).
   a. DEXA is a validated method to assess body composition in patients with CKD.
   b. DEXA is affected by hydration and tissue density.
2. Hydrodensitometry or underwater weighing.
3. Bioelectric impedance (BIA).
4. Near infrared interactance.

SECTION B
Chronic Kidney Disease
Mary Kay Hensley, Maureen P. McCarthy

I. Nutrition care for the patient with CKD stages 1–4 (Academy of Nutrition and Dietetics [AND], 2010).

A. Goal of therapy: achieve or maintain optimal nutritional status and preserve remaining kidney function through alterations in protein and electrolyte intake, blood glucose, and blood pressure control.

B. Nutrition interventions.
1. Protein restriction.
   a. Protein-restricted diets reduce the accumulation of metabolic waste products that may suppress the appetite and stimulate muscle protein wasting (Kidney Disease Improving Global Outcomes [KDIGO], 2013a).
   b. The Modification of Diet in Renal Disease (MDRD) study did not show conclusively that protein restriction slows the progression of kidney disease (Klahr et al., 1994).

c. Suggested protein restriction is 0.8 g/kg/day in adults with diabetes or without diabetes and GFR less than 30 mL/min/1.73m^2 (KDIGO, 2013a).

d. A plant-based diet, low in concentrated sweets and saturated fats, may decrease CKD progression as well as metabolic complications but more interventional studies are needed (Filipowicz & Beddhu, 2013).

e. There is a spontaneous decline in protein intake as GFR falls, so the indices of malnutrition should be followed closely.

f. With the increased incidence of malnutrition at initiation of kidney replacement therapy, low protein diets should not be generalized for all patients.

g. Low-protein diets should only be planned and implemented by registered dietitians with experience and expertise in nephrology care.

2. Energy intake.
   a. A prescribed low-protein diet for patients not yet on dialysis must provide adequate calories to maintain neutral nitrogen balance and prevent a decline in nutritional status.
   b. Recommended caloric intake: 23 to 35 kcal/kg/day based on the following factors:
      (1) Weight status and goals.
      (2) Age and gender.
      (3) Level of physical activity.
      (4) Metabolic stressors.

3. Prevention of CKD mineral bone disorder (KDIGO, 2009a).
   a. Control of calcium and phosphate metabolism should be considered in patients with CKD stages 3–4.
   b. Limited dietary phosphate intake and the use of phosphate binders may help prevent secondary hyperparathyroidism.
   c. The addition of calcitriol or other vitamin D analogs should be considered in patients with CKD stages 3–4 if serum PTH is progressively rising and remains above the upper limit of normal.
   d. Supplement with calcitriol to correct vitamin D deficiency as determined by serum 25 (OH) levels less than 30 ng/ml.
   e. Goals of therapy (CKD stages 3–4).
      (1) Serum phosphorus level within the normal range for the laboratory used.
      (2) Corrected serum calcium level within the normal range for the laboratory used. *Equation to calculate corrected calcium:*

Corrected serum calcium =
Total calcium mg/dL + 0.8 x (4.0 – serum albumin (g/dL)

      (3) The optimal PTH level is not known.

4. Control of metabolic acidosis (KDIGO, 2013a).
   a. Dietary protein restriction reduces hydrogen ion generation.
   b. Correction of metabolic acidosis is necessary because acidosis increases muscle protein catabolism, reduces albumin synthesis, and can lead to negative nitrogen balance.
   c. Goal of therapy: serum CO_2 22 mEq/L or greater, prescribing oral bicarbonate supplementation as needed.

C. Other interventions to slow progression of CKD (NKF, 2012; KDIGO, 2013a).
   1. In patients with diabetes a target HbA1C of ~ 7% is recommended.
   2. Use of angiotensin-converting enzyme inhibitors (ACE-I) or an angiotensin receptor blocker (ARB) in normotensive patients with diabetes is suggested for patients with albuminuria 30 mg/g or greater, who are at high risk of diabetic kidney disease and its progression. Monitor serum potassium with the use of ACE-I or ARB; may need dietary potassium restriction.
   3. Individualize blood pressure targets based on age, comorbidities, risk of CKD progression, retinopathy in diabetics, and tolerance to treatment:
      a. Urine albumin less than 30 mg/24 hours: 140/90 mmHg or less.
      b. Urine albumin greater than 30 mg/24 hours: 130/80 mmHg or less.
      c. Limit sodium intake to less than 2,000 mg/day to improve blood pressure control, unless contraindicated.

II. Nutrition care for the patient receiving dialysis (CKD stage 5).

A. Goals of therapy through consumption of prescribed diet and prescribed medications.
   1. Meet nutritional requirements.
   2. Prevent malnutrition.
   3. Maintain acceptable blood chemistries, blood pressure, and fluid status.

B. Hemodialysis (NKF, 2000).
   1. Amino acid and peptide losses average 10 to 13 g/dialysis session.
   2. Recommended protein intake for stable patients is 1.2 g/kg/day; protein from plant-based sources may be considered, depending on patient's preferences.
   3. Protein requirements for acutely ill patients are at least 1.2 to 1.3 g/kg/day.
   4. Recommended caloric intake is 35 kcal/kg/day for patients less than 60 years of age, and 30 to 35 kcal/kg/day for patients 60 years of age or older.

5. The adjusted edema-free body weight (aBWef) should be used to calculate calorie and protein needs, and the weight should be obtained postdialysis.

C. Peritoneal dialysis (McCann, 2013).
1. Average protein loss is 9 g/day for CAPD; 4 to 6 g of amino acids and peptides are lost each day. Protein losses can double with peritonitis.
2. Recommended protein intake for stable patients is 1.2 to 1.3 g/kg/day; protein from plant-based sources may be considered, depending on patient preferences.
3. Protein requirement for acutely ill patients is at least 1.3 g/kg/day.
4. Protein intake can be monitored in the stable patient by assessing the protein equivalent of nitrogen appearance (PNA).
5. Recommended caloric intake is 35 kcal/kg/day for patients less than 60 years of age and 30 to 35 kcal/kg/day for patients 60 years of age or older.
6. The adjusted edema-free body weight (aBWef) should be used to calculate calorie and protein needs and should be obtained after draining dialysate fluid.
7. Patients with normal peritoneal transport capacity absorb approximately 60% of the dextrose calories on CAPD and 40% of dextrose calories on ADP from their PD exchanges.
8. Dialysate.
   a. 1.5% dextrose solution contains 15 grams of monohydrous dextrose per liter.
   b. 2.5% dextrose solution contains 25 grams of monohydrous dextrose per liter.
   c. 4.25% dextrose solution contains 42.5 grams of monohydrous dextrose per liter.
9. To estimate calories absorbed from PD dialysate.
   a. Total the grams of dextrose from all exchanges for 24 hours.
   b. Multiply by 3.4 calories/gram (conversion factor for monohydrous dextrose).
   c. Multiply total calories by 60% for CAPD and 40% for APD (average absorption) to estimate calories patient receives from dialysate fluid.

D. Daily and nocturnal hemodialysis (McPhatter, 2013).
1. Fewer dietary restrictions and increased energy and protein intake, which may result in an increase in dry weight and improved serum albumin levels.
   a. Energy and protein requirements have yet to be established.
   b. Use guidelines for hemodialysis patients (see C.2. Hemodialysis).
2. No need for phosphorus restriction for most patients.
   a. May require increased dietary phosphorus

when serum levels are below the normal range.
   b. Normalizing bone parameters has the potential to reverse vascular calcification and reduce cardiovascular disease risk.
3. Dietary sodium restriction is based on the patient's volume and hypotensive state.
   a. Hypotensive: may benefit from additional dietary sodium.
   b. Normotensive: may need only a healthy dietary limitation of 1,500 to 2,300 mg sodium/day.
4. Dietary potassium needs may be increased, resulting in more liberal dietary potassium intake.
5. Benefits include improved blood pressure, fluid control, anemia management, and quality of life.

E. Survival skills for new patients on dialysis.
1. Potassium and fluid are two important elements of the kidney diet to implement immediately until the patient can be seen by the dietitian.
   a. Potassium: Limit servings of fruits, vegetables, and juices to a total of 4 to 6 half-cup servings per day. Avoid salt substitutes and any other form of potassium chloride.
   b. Fluid: Allow 4 cups of fluid plus the amount equal to urine output. Fluids are any foods or beverages that are liquid at room temperature (e.g., ice, soup, tea, coffee, gelatin dessert).
2. Protein: If the patient was on a low-protein diet prior to dialysis, more protein foods can now be consumed (unsalted meats, fish, poultry, eggs). Limit dairy products to ½ cup per day until needs are determined.
3. Sodium. Avoid the salt shaker, convenience foods, "fast foods," and cured or processed meats.

F. Frequent problems for patients on dialysis (Hutson & Stewart, 2013).
1. Thirst.
   a. Suck on cold, sliced fruit, lemon wedges, mints, or sour candy.
   b. Use spray mouthwash, sports gum, or rinse mouth with chilled mouthwash.
   c. Add lemon juice to drinking water.
   d. Use small cups and glasses for beverages.
   e. Limit high-sodium foods.
   f. Keep blood glucose under good control if diabetic.
2. Constipation.
   a. Increase dietary fiber with allowed fruits, vegetables, grains, and cellulose fiber.
   b. Stool softeners or bulk laxatives as needed.
   c. Increase exercise and activity as tolerated.
3. Poor appetite. (Also see Section C.I. Protein–energy wasting in kidney disease.)
   a. Assess adequacy of dialysis.
   b. Small, frequent meals (adjust binders accordingly).

c. Maintain good oral care to improve taste.

d. Appetite stimulant such as megesterol acetate may be used.

4. Hyperkalemia related to causes other than diet (Beto, 1992).

   a. Inadequate dialysis.

   b. Dialysis potassium concentration is too high.

   c. Hemolysis of lab specimen.

   d. Metabolic acidosis.

   e. Hyperglycemia.

   f. Tissue destruction.

   g. Drug interactions.

   h. Severe constipation.

   i. GI bleeding.

5. Wound healing (Hutson & Stewart, 2013).

   a. Vitamin A. Should only be supplemented if usual intake is inadequate or deficiency is present; then supplement 900 mcg per day for 7–10 days.

   b. Vitamin C. Supplementation should not exceed 250 mg per day to prevent the risk of oxalosis and soft tissue calcification.

   c. Zinc. Supplement 50 mg of elemental zinc provided by 220 mg of zinc sulfate.

   d. Calories. Energy intake of 30 to 35 kcal/kg to achieve protein-sparing effect and positive nitrogen balance.

   e. Protein. Intake of 1.2 to 2.0 grams per day to meet the nitrogen needs of wound healing. Higher protein intake appropriate for stage 3 and stage 4 wounds.

6. Pica (Ward & Kutner, 1999).

   a. Pica is an appetite or craving for non-nutritive substances such as ice, clay, dirt, ashes, starch, paper, or many other items.

   b. Can be related to cultural tradition, acquired taste, neurologic condition, or chemical imbalance.

   c. Assess to determine if behavior is impacting or has the potential to impact the following:

      (1) Laboratory values.

      (2) Interdialytic fluid gains.

      (3) Dry weight gain/loss.

      (4) GI injury, i.e., perforation or obstruction.

      (5) Dental injury.

      (6) Bowel habits.

      (7) Drug interactions.

      (8) Toxicity.

III Nutrition care for the kidney transplant recipient.

A. Pretransplant nutrition.

1. Conditions of Participation from Centers for Medicaid and Medicare Services (CMS) specify that nutrition services must be available to all potential transplant recipients (CMS, 2014).

   a. Some transplant centers provide nutrition services to all pretransplant candidates.

   b. Other transplant centers screen all candidates and provide direct nutrition services for those at nutritional risk.

2. Patients should attempt to maintain optimal nutritional status.

   a. Serum albumin is not reliable as a nutrition marker (Fuhrman & Charney, 2004). It may be reduced due to proteinuria as part of the disease process, by recent access procedures or infection, and other causes.

   b. Serum albumin is a good indicator of morbidity and mortality (Beindorff & Ulerich, 2013).

   c. Stable baseline functional status and muscle stores, with stable dry weight, are markers of nutritional status (Hasse & Matarese, 2012).

   d. Unintended weight loss prekidney transplant has been linked with higher posttransplant mortality (Molnar et al., 2011).

3. Pretransplant nutrition evaluations assess food and nutrition-related history (including complementary and alternative medications), anthropometric measurements, biochemical data, nutrition-focused physical findings, and client history (Academy of Nutrition and Dietetics, 2013).

4. Nutritional status including underweight or obesity can affect kidney transplant outcomes. Weight criteria, though controversial, are used by some transplant centers (Potluri et al., 2010).

   a. Body mass index (BMI) less than 18.5 kg/m^2 or greater than 35 kg/m^2 has been linked with negative outcomes.

   b. Central obesity, as measured by waist circumference or by waist-to-hip ratio, has been linked with poor outcomes in patients with kidney failure, including kidney transplant recipients (Postorino et al., 2009).

   c. BMI of the donor has been shown to affect graft function.

   d. Problems secondary to immunosuppression and malnutrition may arise when underweight patients are transplanted. The results can lead to decreased graft survival.

   e. Obese kidney transplant recipients appear to be at risk for decreased graft survival marked by (Meier-Kriesche et al., 2002):

      (1) Increased risk of delayed graft function.

      (2) Increased length of hospital stay.

      (3) More wound infections.

      (4) Increased chance for acute rejection and graft loss; surmised to be an immunologic problem.

f. Morbidly obese patients who desire kidney transplantation may opt for surgery.
   (1) Pretransplant obesity has been shown to retard wound healing (Meier-Kriesche et al., 2002).
   (2) The safety and effectiveness of weight loss medications in the pretransplant patient are not well studied (DiCecco, 2007).
   (3) There are reports of successful kidney transplants after bariatric surgery. Roux-en-Y gastric bypass surgery is the most common bariatric surgery procedure in kidney transplant recipients (Modanlou et al., 2009).

B. Posttransplant nutrition.
   1. Initial recovery period, 4 to 6 weeks after the transplant (Beindorff & Ulerich, 2013).
      a. Transplant recipients are adjusting to their new medication regimen, healing the transplant wound, and beginning the new phase of their life without dialysis.
      b. See Table 4.1 for nutrition recommendations for kidney transplant recipients.
      c. Initially the protein allowance is greater for wound healing (Beindorff & Ulerich, 2013).
         (1) The transplant wound must granulate from bottom up.
         (2) Certain immunosuppresive medications,

Table 4.1

Daily Nutrient Recommendations for Adult Kidney Transplant

Nutrient	Acute Period	Chronic Period
Protein	1.3–2 g/ kg[a]	0.8–1 g/kg Limit with chronic graft dysfunction.
Energy	30–35 kcal/kg[a] or BEE x 1.3 May increase with postoperative complications.	Adjust calories to maintain desirable body weight.
Carbohydrate	Limit simple carbohydrate intake with elevated blood glucose levels and/or unwanted weight gain.	Emphasize complex carbohydrate intake and distribution.
Fat	Remainder of calories.	Emphasize PUFA and MUFA.
Sodium	Restrict if blood pressure/fluid status dictates.	2–4 g with hypertension and/or edema.
Potassium	2–4 g if hyperkalemic.	Unrestricted unless hyperkalemic.
Calcium	1,200–1,500 mg	1,200–1,500 mg
Phosphorus	DRI May need supplementation to normalize serum levels.	DRI[b]
Other vitamins	DRI[b]	DRI[b]
Other minerals	DRI[b]	DRI[b]
Trace elements	DRI[b]	DRI[b]
Fluid	Limit only by graft function; generally unrestricted	Limit only by graft function; generally unrestricted

Abbreviations: BEE = basal energy expenditure; DRI = Dietary Reference Intake (recommended dietary allowance or adequate intake); MUFA = monounsaturated fatty acids; PUFA = polyunsaturated acids.

[a] Based on standard or adjusted body weight.

[b] Due to lack of research, no specific recommendations are available for this population. Currently the DRI is used as a guideline.

Source: Data are reference 19 and Academy of Nutrition and Dietetics Evidence Analysis Library CKD Guidelines. Available at: http://andevidencelibrary.com/topic.cfm?cat=3929. Accessed December 15, 2012.

This table was reprinted from *A Clinical Guide to Nutrition Care in Kidney Disease* © Academy of Nutrition and Dietetics 2013. Reprinted with permission.

such as prednisone, can complicate healing (McPartland & Pomposelli, 2007).
d. Potassium.
   (1) Serum potassium can be elevated as a side effect of calcineurin inhibitors such as cyclosporine and tacrolimus (McPartland & Pomposelli, 2007).
   (2) A low potassium diet of 2–4 g per day may be indicated if serum levels are increased (Beindorff & Ulerich, 2013).
   (3) Kayexalate may be used depending on the potassium level.
e. Phosphorus.
   (1) Serum phosphorus levels may be low due to wasting in the renal tubule.
   (2) Posttransplant patients are generally encouraged to increase intake of high phosphorus foods (Beindorff & Ulerich, 2013).
   (3) A phosphorus supplement may be used but can cause diarrhea.
f. Magnesium.
   (1) Cyclosporine and tacrolimus promote magnesium-wasting by the kidney (Beindorff & Ulerich, 2013).
   (2) While high magnesium foods may improve serum levels, magnesium supplements are often needed (McPartland & Pomposelli, 2007).
   (3) Magnesium may decrease absorption of mycophenolate mofetil; they must be taken separately (Beindorff & Ulerich, 2013).
g. Blood glucose.
   (1) Blood glucose may be acutely elevated from the transplant surgery or infection (Beindorff & Ulerich, 2013).
   (2) Some immunosuppressive agents, especially prednisone, tacrolimus, and cyclosporine, may cause insulin resistance or reduced insulin secretion, leading to increased glucose levels (Hasse & Matarese, 2009).
   (3) New-onset diabetes after transplant (NODAT) is diagnosed when fasting plasma glucose is 126 mg/dL or greater, or when patient is symptomatic and has random glucose greater than 200 mg/dL on two or more occasions (Davidson et al., 2003).
   (4) Risk factors for NODAT include age older than 40 years, obesity, family history of diabetes, certain ethnicities, history of hepatitis C, and prior type 2 diabetes mellitus (Rodrigo et al., 2006).
   (5) Blood glucose levels and other factors will determine whether the recipient is placed on an oral agent or insulin.

   (6) A consistent carbohydrate diet may be part of managing NODAT (Karosanidze, 2014).
   (7) Blood glucose checks three to four times per day are usual practice.
h. Hypertension.
   (1) Both cyclosporine and tacrolimus can exacerbate high blood pressure (Beindorff & Ulerich, 2013).
   (2) Blood pressure medications may be discontinued as the transplanted kidney begins to regulate blood pressure through the renin-angiotensin system.
   (3) Sodium should be limited to 2 to 4 grams per day if the kidney transplant recipient is retaining fluid and taking several blood pressure medications (Beindorff & Ulerich, 2013).
i. Excessive weight gain.
   (1) Weight gains of 3 to 10 kg are reported after kidney transplant (Karosanidze, 2014).
   (2) A well-balanced diet and physical activity are important for weight control. Referral to a registered dietitian nutritionist (RDN) is recommended (Karosanidze, 2014).
   (3) Weight-loss medications have not been well studied in the posttransplant patient. Some act by causing fat malabsorption, which may interfere with immunosuppressive medications (DiCecco, 2007).
j. Dyslipidemia.
   (1) Immunosuppresive medications that contribute to dyslipidemia include cyclosporine, tacrolimus, sirolimus, and corticosteroids (Phillips & Heuberger, 2012).
   (2) Dyslipidemia may be seen in 60% or more of kidney transplant recipients (Karosanidze, 2014). It includes at least one of the following:
       (a) Cholesterol greater than 200 mg/dL.
       (b) Low-density lipoprotein greater than 130 mg/dL.
       (c) Triglycerides greater than 150 mg/dL.
       (d) High-density lipoprotein less than 40 mg/dL.
   (3) In general, patients are counseled to lose excess weight, consume lower fat and low-cholesterol diet, and stop smoking (Beindorff & Ulerich, 2013).
   (4) The Mediterranean diet has been linked with improved cardiovascular outcomes after kidney transplant (Barbagallo, 1999).
   (5) Lipid-lowering medications may be prescribed (Ward, 2009).

k. Medication interactions and herbal remedies.
   (1) Postkidney transplant patients should avoid grapefruit, mandarin oranges, pomegranate, and other foods that may interfere with therapeutic levels of tacrolimus or cyclosporine (Nowack, 2008).
   (2) Generally herbal remedies are contraindicated after organ transplant due to the undesirable nature of the improved immune response they create (e.g., ginseng) and due to drug–drug interactions that affect use of tacrolimus or cyclosporine (Cooke, 2004).
l. Food safety.
   (1) Kidney transplant recipients are 15–20% more vulnerable to foodborne illness than the general population due to immunosuppression (Obayashi, 2012).
   (2) Sources of foodborne illness include (Obayashi, 2012):
      (a) Contaminated water.
      (b) Unpasteurized dairy products.
      (c) Undercooked meat/fish/poultry/eggs.
      (d) Food prepared in unsanitary conditions.
      (e) Improperly stored food.
   (3) Steps to assure food safety include (USDA-FDA, 2011):
      (a) Wash hands and food preparation tools and surfaces often.
      (b) Separate raw foods from cooked foods to avoid cross-contamination.
      (c) Cook food to safe temperatures (check USDA-FDA references).
      (d) Refrigerate foods promptly after shopping and/or after cooking.
2. Long-term nutrition concerns, from 6 weeks posttransplant to the end of the transplanted kidney's function (Beindorff & Ulerich, 2013).
   a. The major goals for this period are to maintain graft function and overall health.
   b. Table 4.1 summarizes the nutrient needs for the long-term posttransplant recipient. Needs are closer to those of normal adults (Beindorff & Ulerich, 2013).
   c. Hypertension is seen in 50–85% of kidney transplant recipients (Chatzikyrkou, 2011).
      (1) A 2- to 4-gram sodium diet is recommended if the patient is hypertensive.
      (2) Most patients are used to having less sodium in their diets so do not necessarily mind this modification.
   d. Obesity continues to be a problem.
      (1) Weight gains in the first year after kidney transplant range from 8 to 14 kilograms (Potluri & Hou, 2010).

   (2) Some patients gain weight with every visit.
      (a) Nutrition counseling and physical activity promote weight loss and maintenance (Karosanidze, 2014).
      (b) Keeping a food diary can be a helpful tool.
   e. NODAT can occur at any time after kidney transplant.
      (1) Age, obesity, ethnicity, family history, and transplant medications contribute to the development of NODAT (Davidson et al., 2003).
      (2) Glucose monitoring and medication adherence are imperative to manage glucose levels and to retain graft function (Phillips & Heuberger, 2012).
   f. Cardiovascular disease is the number one cause of death for kidney transplant recipients.
      (1) A major study in which kidney transplant recipients received folic acid and vitamins B12 and B6 showed that homocysteine levels improved. However, there was no effect on risk of cardiovascular disease (Bostom et al., 2011).
      (2) Keep hyperlipidemia in check with medication and nutrition (see Table 4.1).
   g. Long-term bone problems.
      (1) Hyperparathyroidism may still be a problem.
      (2) Serum 25-OH vitamin D levels should be monitored and repleted if necessary (Beindorff & Ulerich, 2013).
      (3) Since prednisone reduces intestinal absorption and increases urinary output of calcium, osteoporosis is a common posttransplant problem (Beindorff & Ulerich, 2013).
      (4) Calcium supplement should be taken if the patient does not consume dairy products (see Table 4.1 for amount).

Section C

Special Considerations
in Kidney Disease

*Deborah Brommage, Ann Beemer Cotton,
Janelle Gonyea, Pamela S. Kent,
Jean Stover*

I. Malnutrition and protein–energy wasting in kidney disease.

A. Malnutrition is defined as any nutrition imbalance. Lack of adequate calories, protein, or other nutrients needed for tissue maintenance and repair results in undernutrition (White et al, 2012).
   1. Causes of nutrition disorders.
      a. Inadequate or unbalanced diet.
      b. Digestive difficulties.
      c. Absorption problems.
      d. Hypercatabolism or other medical conditions.
   2. Older adults, nursing home residents, hospitalized persons, and homeless persons are most at risk for undernutrition.
   3. For the diagnosis of malnutrition, there must be evidence of two or more of the following six characteristics.
      a. Insufficient energy intake.
      b. Weight loss.
      c. Loss of muscle mass.
      d. Loss of subcutaneous fat.
      e. Localized or generalized fluid accumulation that may sometimes mask weight loss.
      f. Diminished functional status as measured by handgrip strength.

B. Protein-energy wasting (PEW) is the loss of body protein mass and fuel reserves not related to nutrient intake alone. These abnormalities cannot be corrected solely by increasing the diet (Fouque et al., 2008).
   1. Given the name PEW by the International Society of Renal Nutrition and Metabolism (ISRNM) in 2008.
   2. PEW refers to the interrelationship of mechanisms causing a syndrome of wasting, malnutrition, and inflammation in individuals with CKD.
   3. For the diagnosis of PEW, there must be evidence of one or more indicators in at least three of the four categories as follows:
      a. Serum chemistry.
         (1) Serum albumin less than 3.8 g/dL (bromocresol green method).
         (2) Serum prealbumin (transthyretin) less than 30 mg/dL for maintenance dialysis patients.
         (3) Serum cholesterol less than 100 mg/dL.
         (4) Do not use inflammatory markers such as C-reactive protein or interleukin-6 as evidence of PEW.
      b. Body mass.
         (1) Body mass index (BMI) less than 23: (BMI=weight [kg]/height[m^2]).
         (2) Unintentional weight loss of 5% over 3 months, or 10% over 6 months.
         (3) Total body fat percentage less than 10%.
      c. Muscle mass.
         (1) Reduced muscle mass of 5% over 3 months, or 10% over 6 months.
         (2) Reduced mid-arm muscle circumference area as a reduction of greater than 10% in relation to the 50th percentile of the reference population.
         (3) Creatinine appearance.
      d. Dietary intake.
         (1) Unintentional low dietary protein intake (DPI) of less than 0.8g kg/day for at least 2 months for patients on dialysis.
         (2) Unintentional low DPI of 0.6g/kg/day for patients with CKD stages 2 to 5.
         (3) Unintentional low dietary energy intake of less than 25 kcal/kg/day for at least 2 months.
   4. Causes of PEW in patients with CKD (Carrero et al., 2013).
      a. Decreased protein and energy intake.
         (1) Anorexia.
            (a) Dysregulation in circulating appetite mediators.
            (b) Hypothalamic amino acid sensing.
            (c) Nitrogen-based uremic toxins.
         (2) Dietary restrictions.
         (3) Alterations in organs involved in nutrient intake.
         (4) Depression.
         (5) Inability to obtain or prepare food.
      b. Hypermetabolism.
         (1) Increased energy expenditure.
            (a) Inflammation.
            (b) Increased circulating proinflammatory cytokines.
            (c) Insulin resistance secondary to obesity.
            (d) Altered adiponectin and resistin metabolism.
         (2) Hormonal disorders.
            (a) Insulin resistance of CKD.
            (b) Increased glucocorticoid activity.
      c. Metabolic acidosis.
      d. Decreased physical activity.
      e. Decreased anabolism.
         (1) Decreased nutrient intake.

(2) Resistance to growth hormone/insulin-like growth factor-1 (GH/IGF-1).
(3) Testosterone deficiency.
(4) Low thyroid hormone levels.
f. Comorbidities and lifestyle.
g. Dialysis.
(1) Nutrient losses into dialysate.
(2) Dialysis-related inflammation.
(3) Dialysis-related hypermetabolism.
(4) Loss of residual kidney function.

II. Diabetes and kidney disease.

A. Prevalence and incidence (United States Renal Data Systems [USRDS], 2013).
1. Diabetes is a primary cause of CKD, and is the major cause of kidney failure in the United States.
2. The prevalence of diabetes in the dialysis population is 44.2%, and the incidence of diabetes in patients new to dialysis is 44.7%.

B. Importance of glucose control.
1. Controlling blood glucose helps prevent the onset of diabetes.
2. The Diabetes Prevention Program produced a 58% risk reduction in persons with prediabetes from progressing to diabetes. This study used lifestyle modification consisting of weight loss facilitated by diet and exercise (Knowler et al., 2002).
3. Tight glucose control may benefit persons with type 1 diabetes. The Diabetes Control and Complications Trial (DCCT) Research Group (1993) demonstrated a 34% risk reduction of microalbuminuria and a 56% risk reduction in persons with microalbuminuria from progressing to proteinuria.
4. A similar decrease in the rate of complications in persons with type 2 diabetes was noted in the United Kingdom Prospective Diabetes Study (UKPDS, 1998).
5. In persons with diabetes on dialysis, intensive diabetes education and care management produced significant decreases in hemoglobin A1C (HbA1C), amputations, and diabetes-related or vascular-related hospital admissions (McMurray et al., 2002).

C. Making diabetic meal plans kidney friendly.
1. Modifying a traditional meal plan that had a focus on carbohydrate, protein, and fat to one with restrictions on sodium, potassium, phosphorus, and fluid can be challenging and should be planned by an experienced nephrology dietitian (NKF, 2012).
2. Many foods considered "free" on the diabetic food lists, due to their low caloric content, are high in

sodium, potassium, phosphorus, and/or fluid.
a. High-sodium "free" foods: bouillon, broth, many condiments such as soy sauce, dill pickles, commercial taco sauce, seasoned salt, and other salt and spice blends.
b. High-potassium "free" foods: low-sodium bouillon cubes or granules, mushrooms, spinach, and tomatoes.
c. High-phosphorus "free" foods: diet colas.
d. High-fluid "free" foods: broth, coffee, tea, sugar-free beverages, water, diet gelatin dessert, ice and sugar-free popsicles.
3. The carbohydrate content of breads, cereals, fruit, and milk is similar per serving at 12–15 grams, but the potassium content of fruit and milk is much higher. A higher percentage of carbohydrate needs to come from breads and cereals for persons on a potassium restriction.
4. Another issue in potassium control is seen in the starch/bread list. Potatoes, sweet potatoes, winter squash, dried beans, lentils, and lima beans are in the diabetic starch/bread list, but are all high in potassium.
a. Peeling, cutting into small cubes or shredding, and then boiling potatoes can remove 50 to 75 percent of potassium respectively in white potatoes. When the cooking process is complete, the potassium-rich water must be discarded before the potatoes can be used (Bethke & Jansky, 2008).
b. This process does not work for Yukon Gold potatoes (Burrowes & Ramer, 2008).
5. Traditionally, "diabetic snacks" have included a protein source, often from cheese, peanut butter, nuts, or milk. These foods are all high in potassium and/or phosphorus. Furthermore, protein does not prevent blood glucose from dropping and does not prevent subsequent hypoglycemia when used to treat low blood sugar.

D. Alcohol.
1. The effect of alcohol on blood glucose levels is related to the quantity of alcohol and its timing with other food consumed. Alcohol is a source of energy but is not converted to glucose. Alcohol can suppress gluconeogenesis, especially in a fasting state. Therefore, hypoglycemia may result if alcohol is taken while fasting by persons on insulin or oral insulin secretagogues (sulphonylureas).
2. For persons with diabetes choosing to drink, alcohol should be limited to one drink per day or less for adult women and two drinks per day or less for adult men (Evert et al., 2013).
3. One drink contains 15 g of alcohol, equivalent to 12 oz of beer, 5 oz of wine, and 2 oz of distilled spirits. Persons should be cautioned regarding any

drink mixers used, as they may contain excessive amounts of sodium, potassium, or phosphorus.

4. When diabetes is well-controlled, moderate use of alcohol should not affect blood glucose levels. Alcohol does not need insulin for its metabolism.

E. Monitoring glucose and HbA1C.
1. The risk of hypoglycemia is increased in patients with advanced CKD (stages 4 and 5) due to decreased clearance of insulin and of some oral hypoglycemic agents, and impaired gluconeogenesis with reduced kidney mass (Gerich et al., 2001).
   a. Oral hypoglycemic medications and insulin should be adjusted accordingly.
   b. Patients and their caregivers should be more alert to the signs, symptoms, and possibility of hypoglycemia.
2. The KDOQI diabetes guidelines (NKF, 2012):
   a. Recommend a target HbA1C of ~7.0% to prevent or delay progression of the microvascular complications of diabetes, including diabetic kidney disease.
   b. Recommend not treating to an HbA1C target of less than 7.0% in patients at risk of hypoglycemia.
   c. Suggest that target HbA1C be extended above 7.0% in patients with comorbidities or limited life expectancy and risk of hypoglycemia.
3. Only certain assays can be accurately used to test HbA1C when uremia is present, including affinity chromatography, colorimetric, or enzyme-linked immunoassays. In-house units commonly used in physician offices are acceptable.
4. The HbA1C reflects average blood glucose of 3 months in non-CKD patients. This time frame is reduced in uremia to 4 to 6 weeks, due to the reduced red blood cell survival rate.
5. Monitoring HbA1C levels on a quarterly basis is reasonable, considering the fragile medical condition and frequent history of uncontrolled blood sugars in many persons in this population.

F. Treating hyperglycemia and hypoglycemia.
1. Because of the increased sensitivity to insulin in CKD, the treatment of hyperglycemia is usually modified, compared to a patient's previous care. An altered sliding scale schedule may become necessary also (Schatz & Pagenkemper, 2013).
2. Due to the reduction or absence of urine output in persons on dialysis, the "safety valve" effect of glucosuria is also reduced or absent. Severe hyperglycemia with glucose levels greater than 1000 mg/dL may develop as a result. However, severe hyperosmolality is unusual since the kidney cannot compensate with osmotic diuresis. Therefore, the treatment does not include large amounts of fluid, but does involve insulin administration and potassium monitoring.
3. Treating low blood glucose with orange, prune, or vegetable juice is contraindicated in patients on a potassium restriction.
4. Appropriate foods to treat low blood glucose are high in sugar and dissolve quickly in the stomach. They may need to be low in salt, potassium, phosphorus, and fluid, depending on the patient's dietary restrictions. "Safe" choices, according to the Renal Dietitians Practice Group (RPG) (2013), to provide 15 g of carbohydrate include:
   a. Plain table sugar: 1 tablespoon (or 3 teaspoons), 3 packets, or 3 sugar cubes.
   b. ½ cup regular lemon-lime soda or gingerale.
   c. ½ cup regular lemonade.
   d. ½ cup apple, grape, or cranberry juice.
   e. 6 pieces of regular hard candy.
   f. 3 glucose tablets or 1 tube of glucose gel.
5. Foods usually NOT appropriate include:
   a. Milk or milk products.
   b. Chocolate.
   c. Salty crackers and salty snack foods.
   d. Peanuts, peanut butter, and other nuts.
   e. Many fruits and fruit juices.
6. The 15/15 rule is appropriate to treat hypoglycemia. Take 15 g of a safe carbohydrate, wait 15 minutes and retest. Repeat until blood glucose normalizes.
7. Persons on peritoneal dialysis are exposed to a high glucose load, both on CAPD and APD, due to the peritoneal absorption of dextrose. This can create confusion on behalf of the patient as they no longer have truly fasting blood glucose levels in the morning due to the exposure to glucose throughout the night.

G. Retinopathy (American Diabetes Association [ADA], 2012).
1. Diabetes is the most common cause of blindness among adults.
2. Adequate blood glucose and blood pressure management will decrease the risk or rate of progression of retinopathy.
3. Comprehensive eye exams should be completed annually.
4. Loss of vision can have a negative impact on a person's ability to prepare food properly, on appetite as they cannot appreciate the presentation of the food, and on ability to adhere to diet as they cannot read education materials provided or food labels while shopping.
   a. Verbal repetition of diet parameters and educational materials are needed to improve adherence.
   b. Adaptive equipment such as magnifiers and talking glucose meters might be needed.

H. Gastrointestinal autonomic neuropathy (Schatz & Pagenkemper, 2013).
   1. Gastroparesis, or delayed stomach emptying, is a common complication of diabetes during any stage of CKD.
      a. Usual symptoms include early satiety, bloating, nausea, vomiting of undigested food, and heartburn.
      b. Dietary treatment includes frequent small meals and snacks, four to six times daily, which are low in fat and fiber.
      c. Hyperglycemia slows gastric emptying, thus optimizing glycemic control, which is key in treating gastroparesis.
      d. Commonly used medications to treat gastroparesis include prokinetic agents, antiemetics, and proton pump inhibitors or hydrogen blockers.
   2. Diabetic diarrhea.
      a. Can be watery and often nocturnal. At times can alternate with constipation.
      b. Treatment includes antidiarrheal medications such as loperamide (Imodium®), diphenoxylate and atropine (Lomotil®), and cholestyramine resin (Questran®).
   3. Constipation due to dysfunction of intestinal neurons.
      a. Treatment includes stool softeners and laxatives.
      b. Fleet® Enema containing phosphorus and magnesium containing laxatives should not be used.
      c. These affect nutrient intake and absorption and result in unpredictable blood glucose levels.
   4. More frequent blood glucose monitoring with related adjustments in insulin or oral medications may be necessary to optimize glucose control.

I. Medications for diabetes (NKF, 2012).
   1. Safe oral hypoglycemic agents for persons with CKD are primarily metabolized in the liver rather than the kidney, and are short-acting.
   2. First-generation sulfonylureas, such as acetohexamide (Dymelor®), chlorpropamide (Diabinese®), tolazamide (Tolinase®), and tolbutamide (Orinase®), are largely excreted in the urine, and should not be used in persons on dialysis.
   3. The second-generation sulfonylurea glipizide (Glucotrol®) is preferred for persons on dialysis as it does not have active metabolites and thus does not increase the risk of hypoglycemia.
   4. The biguanide metformin (Glucophage®) or the metformin combination (Glucovance® and Avandamet®) are contraindicated in the dialysis population due to the potential for lactic acidosis.
   5. The thiazolidinediones pioglitazone (Actos®) and rosiglitazone (Avandia®) do not increase the risk

for hypoglycemia; thus, no dose adjustment is necessary for persons on dialysis, but they have the potential to worsen fluid retention.
   6. Rapid, short, intermediate, and long-acting insulin may all be used in CKD, while considering the longer half-life of insulin.

J. Enteral and oral supplements.
   1. Some kidney-specific enteral or oral supplements were designed for persons on hemodialysis and are therefore limited in potassium and phosphorus content, but are higher in calories.
   2. Predialysis formulations are lower in protein and higher in carbohydrate in comparison.
   3. Most diabetes-specific enteral and oral supplements contain significant amounts of potassium and phosphorus, while controlling for carbohydrate type and amount.
   4. Choosing an appropriate formula for a person with both diabetes and CKD requires the skills and assessment ability of an experienced nephrology dietitian. Formula content, cost, and availability should be matched with the prioritized medical and nutrition needs of the patient.
   5. See Table 4.2. Comparison of Renal and Diabetic Enteral and Oral Formulations.
   6. For dialysis patients who are on both insulin and a tube-feeding formula, care must be taken to match the insulin timing with the formula administration.
      a. Continuous tube-feeding formulas are usually stopped for dialysis treatments. This period might be approximately 6 hours (4 for dialysis and 2 for transit time).
      b. To provide 100% of the formula volume in 18 hours rather than 24, the tube-feeding pump speed must be increased accordingly.
      c. To prevent hypoglycemia: if a patient is on the morning shift, and the tube feeding is stopped at 6 a.m. in preparation for dialysis, the morning insulin needs to be moved to a later time to when the patient has resumed the formula.
      d. To maintain consistency and make it easier for caregivers, use the same formula and insulin schedule 7 days a week, instead of different ones on dialysis days.

K. Diabetes self-management training (DSMT).
   1. Some people on dialysis were diagnosed with diabetes before the DSMT classes became popular.
   2. Patients may or may not have been referred to these or to alternate comprehensive training programs, either at diagnosis, or at a subsequent time.
   3. Because many persons with diabetes have lived with their disease for many years, they are unaware of their lack of updated or even basic knowledge.

Table 4.2

Comparison of Renal and Diabetic Enteral and Oral Formulations

Product	Company	Nutrients per 1000 calories						
		Pro g	Carb g	Fat g	Na mg	K mg	Ca mg	P mg
Diabetic								
Glucerna 1.0	Abbott	41.8	95.6	54.4	930	1570	705	705
Glucerna 1.2	Abbott	50	95.6	50	931.8	1688	668	668
Glucerna 1.5	Abbott	55	88.7	50	920	1980	667	667
Glytrol	Nestle	45	100	47.5	740	1400	720	720
Diabetisource AC	Nestle	50	83	49	883	1333	667	667
Resource DiabetaShield	Nestle	46.7	200	0	533	400	666	3330
Boost Glucose Control	Nestle	84.2	84.1	36.8	1157	894	1841	1578
Predialysis								
Renalcal	Nestle	17.2	145.2	41.2	30	40	30	50
Suplena with Carb Steady	Abbott	25	109.6	53.4	447	635	580	400
Dialysis								
NovaSource Renal	Nestle	45.4	91.5	50	473	473	420	410
Nepro with Carb Steady	Abbott	45	89.2	53.4	588	588	588	400
Renament	Medtrition	41.5	100	47.8	213	149	426	107

a. Many persons with diabetes initially arrive at dialysis facilities lacking adequate diabetes education, skill development, and glucose control, and may or may not have a close working relationship with an endocrinologist.
b. They are often frustrated with the additional dietary restrictions imposed by their failing kidneys.
4. The Centers for Medicare and Medicaid Services (CMS), on a one-time basis, will cover 80% of the cost of approved DSMT programs for all Medicare recipients who have diabetes, regardless of the diagnosis date.
a. This includes 9 hours of group training and 1 hour of individual training or assessment. In addition, 2 hours of individual or group training are allowed annually.
b. These resources, especially the annual retraining hours, are underused in the diabetic dialysis population.

L. Supplies and reimbursement.
1. CMS covers blood glucose testing supplies for Medicare recipients who have Part B.
a. This includes strips, lancets, and control solution.
b. Glucose monitors are allowed every 5 years, although many suppliers will provide these free of charge to their clients.
c. Batteries and lancet injectors may be provided every 6 months.

2. Therapeutic shoes and thermal foot gauntlets are allowed once every calendar year for certain diagnoses, including peripheral neuropathy and poor circulation, under Part B.
3. Part B will not cover insulin (unless required for use in an insulin pump), syringes, skin care products, or therapeutic socks. Medicare Part D will cover insulin, and some Part D plans will cover syringes.
4. CMS will cover 80% of the cost of allowed supplies. Suppliers may or may not bill a patient separately for the 20% copay who has no secondary insurance.

III. Older adults with kidney disease.

A. General considerations.
1. Inadequate energy and protein intakes in older patients on hemodialysis have been associated with lower markers of nutrition and functional status, as well as higher comorbidities than with younger patients (Barboza, 2008; Chauveau et al., 2001; Johansson et al., 2013).
2. Malnutrition in elderly patients on hemodialysis has been shown to influence overall survival despite adequate dialysis treatment (Chauveau et al., 2001).

B. Nutrition needs.
1. Energy: 30 kcal/kg/day for individuals over 60 years (NFK, 2000). Range of 23–35 kcal/kg body weight; use actual weight with clinical judgment for the increase or decrease of kcals needed (AND, 2006, 2009, 2010).
2. Protein.
   a. CKD (without dialysis) (AND, 2010; NKF, 2000).
      (1) Stages 1 and 2: 0.8 to 1.4 g/kg/day.
      (2) Stages 3 and 4: 0.6 to 0.8 g/kg/day.
      (3) Stage 5: 0.6 g/kg/day.
      (4) Protein restriction for older adult patients should be individualized based on nutritional status, other comorbidities, prognosis, and appetite.
   b. Dialysis: at least 1.2 g/kg/day (hemodialysis); 1.2 to 1.3 g/kg IBW/day (PD) (NKF, 2000).
3. Vitamins/minerals.
   a. General multivitamin until later stages of CKD/dialysis, then change to water soluble vitamins for Dietary Reference Intake (DRI) or renal multivitamin (AND, 2010). May need to use liquid renal vitamin if difficulty swallowing.
   b. Vitamin D (25 OH vitamin D) status is generally monitored closely in patients with CKD prior to initiating dialysis and supplemented if needed (NKF, 2000); active vitamin D analogs (and possibly cinacalcet)

may also be used in latter stages of CKD and for dialysis patients if PTH exceeds accepted goals (KDIGO, 2009a).
   c. Calcium supplements and/or calcium-containing phosphorus binders if needed based on lab values and tolerance. Determine best binder if difficulty swallowing or tube feeding required (Greene & Gutekunst, 2013).
   d. Sodium restriction generally advised to be less than 2.4 g/day for most CKD patients, prior to and while undergoing HD or PD (AND, 2010); work with patient and/or caregivers to keep diet as palatable as possible while controlling hypertension/volume status.
   e. Potassium restriction may or may not be necessary, even in stage 5 CKD. Older adult patients who eat poorly or have diarrhea may not require strict dietary potassium limitation; monitor serum potassium levels (McCann, 2009).
   f. Fluid intake. Probably no need to restrict until stage 5 CKD, and then individualize based on hypertension/volume status; work with patient and/or caretakers if difficulty eating due to limited fluid allowed (McCann, 2009).

C. Factors affecting nutritional status in older adults.
1. Living situation.
   a. Home. If living alone or with an older adult spouse, obtaining food and meal preparation may be difficult or impossible.
      (1) Work with a social worker to obtain delivered meals or assistance with grocery shopping and meal preparation.
      (2) Nutritional supplements (if possible to obtain) may be an easy meal replacement.
   b. Long-term care (LTC) facility. These issues need to be explored and addressed if nutritional status declines.
      (1) Many older adult patients live in LTC facilities where they may dislike the food and, therefore, eat very little; nutritional supplements may be needed.
      (2) Diet may be too restrictive.
      (3) Patients needing to be fed may not always be helped or receive enough feeding assistance due to insufficient staffing.
2. Comorbid conditions.
   a. Dentition. Consistency of food may need to be modified if dentition is poor or dentures do not fit.
   b. Wounds.
      (1) Pressure sores occur frequently with immobility. Protein, vitamin, and mineral needs are then increased to facilitate healing.
      (2) Nutritional supplements often needed (see

Nutrition care for the patient receiving dialysis: Section B. II. F. 5. Wound healing).
c. Cerebrovascular accident (CVA).
(1) Residual loss of swallowing ability causing risk for aspiration and inability to consume adequate amounts of food and/or dislike of food consistency required.
(2) Work with caretaker or LTC facility staff to have patient evaluated periodically to upgrade food consistency if possible.
d. Depression (Johansson et al., 2013).
(1) Can cause anorexia.
(2) Antidepressant therapy may be needed.
(3) Patient may need to be referred to primary care physician and/or geriatric psychiatry for treatment.
e. Dementia.
(1) May interfere with adequate nutrition if memory loss causes decreased food intake.
(2) Reminders to eat or help with eating (in later stages) may be needed.
3. Other issues.
a. Decreased sense of smell, taste, and saliva production in older adult patients.
(1) If sodium does not have to be strictly limited, intake of food may be better with a more liberal sodium intake.
(2) Use a variety of herbs, spices, and seasonings to enhance taste of food.
(3) Encourage allowed liquids with foods.
b. Constipation.
(1) Ensure that stool softeners are used regularly.
(2) Consider fiber supplements that do not require large amounts of fluid.
(3) Consider fruit versus juice, if tolerated.
(4) Incorporate prunes into meal plan, keeping in mind potassium content.
c. Diarrhea.
(1) Need to determine reason and treat if possible.
(2) During or after antibiotic therapy consider probiotics such as acidophilus or lactobacillus and/or check for *C. difficile*.
(3) If no treatable cause, consider soluble fiber added to oral diet or tube feeding (if receiving) and products containing glutamine.
d. Drug interactions or inappropriate medication use.
(1) Can lead to confusion, memory loss, and anorexia in older adults.
(2) Frequent medication review.
(3) Aid with organizing medications may be needed.

D. Nutrition management.
1. Communication with caretakers.
a. Family.
(1) Need to ensure that family is aware of patient's nutrition needs and dietary modifications.
(2) Need to call or meet with family frequently if nutritional status is suboptimal or labs are abnormal.
b. LTC staff.
(1) Monthly review of labs necessary.
(2) Frequently the dialysis dietitian will send labs to the nursing home dietitian with a nutrition note on a monthly basis.
(3) Inservices to LTC facility staff, if possible, may be helpful regarding needs of the dialysis patient (including nutrition).
2. Obtaining nutritional supplements.
a. Patients at home.
(1) If feasible, have patients and/or family purchase supplements.
(2) If unable to afford, work with social worker to obtain financial assistance through medical insurance plans, monetary grants, kidney funds, or other agencies.
b. Patients in LTC facilities.
(1) Work with LTC dietitian to obtain available supplements suitable for the patient.
(2) Renal-specific supplements may not be necessary based on laboratory values.
3. Liberalization of diet restrictions.
a. Diet restrictions should not be imposed if not necessary, especially in LTC facilities.
b. Individualized needs must be encouraged based on labs, fluid retention, and nutritional status.
4. Use of appetite stimulants (Greene & Gutekunst, 2013).
a. Megesterol acetate has been used to stimulate appetite for some older adult patients on dialysis, but caution must be taken with side effects, especially if the patient is immobile.
b. Other medications used for this purpose such as dronabinol and mirtazapine may be investigated as well.

IV. Pregnancy in dialysis and transplantation.

A. Dialysis.
1. Energy/protein needs.
a. Kilocalories.
(1) ~35/kg pregravida IBW + 300 kcal/day (2nd and 3rd trimesters) (AND, 2008; NKF, 2000).
(2) Kcals from absorption of glucose in PD dialysis solutions should be estimated and included (NKF, 2000).

(3) Intakes should be evaluated frequently by the dietitian.
(4) May need nutritional supplements to meet needs.
  b. Protein needs.
    (1) HD: 1.2 g/kg pregravida IBW + 10 to 25 g/day (AND, 2008; NKF, 2000).
    (2) PD: 1.3 g/kg pregravida IBW + 10 to 25 g/day (AND, 2008; NKF, 2000).
    (3) 1.5 g/kg/d also recommended for patients on HD and 1.8 g/kg/d for patients on PD; pregravida weight or IBW not specified (Reddy & Holley, 2007).
    (4) Evaluated frequently by the dietitian.
    (5) May need protein supplements to meet needs.
    (6) Keep in mind that the expected serum albumin decrease during pregnancy for women without CKD is at least 1 g/dL (Fredericksen, 2001).
2. Minerals.
  a. Sodium, potassium, and phosphorus.
    (1) Restrict sodium according to fluid retention, fluid weight gains, and BP.
    (2) Potassium content of diet often liberalized with more frequent dialysis; dialysate content often increased to 3 K+.
    (3) Phosphorus may not need restriction with more intensive dialysis; monitor lab values.
  b. Calcium.
    (1) Calcium needs of the fetus are increased, thus, calcium-containing phosphate binders are usually given.
    (2) If the phosphorus is below goal range, these medications are given apart from meals, primarily for calcium supplementation.
  c. Iron.
    (1) IV iron has been used without complications; usually given as iron gluconate or iron sucrose.
    (2) Dose given depends on iron studies used for nonpregnant dialysis patients.
    (3) Although not as well absorbed, oral iron preparations have also been used instead of intravenous iron, either alone or in combination with a vitamin.
  d. Zinc.
    (1) At least 15 mg/day given to prevent increased risks of fetal malformation, preterm delivery, low birth weight, and pregnancy-induced hypertension.
    (2) May be given alone or included in the renal vitamin prescribed.
3. Vitamins.
  a. Water-soluble vitamins are usually preferred over prenatal vitamins due to the need to avoid

excess vitamin A. With increased requirements for water-soluble vitamins during pregnancy, as well as increased losses anticipated with more intensive dialysis, a standard renal vitamin containing 1 mg folic acid is often doubled and now even additional folic acid prescribed to ensure at least 2–4 mg of folic acid per day (Hou, 2008).
  b. Vitamin D analogs have been given IV during dialysis to treat high PTH and to maintain normal serum levels of calcium.
    (1) There does not seem to be definitive information available about whether these forms of vitamin D cross the placental barrier and, if so, whether they are safe relative to fetal development.
    (2) Doxercalciferol is considered a Category B drug during pregnancy.
4. Other medications.
  a. Antihypertensives (Hou, 2008; Hou & Grossman, 2014).
    (1) Agents considered safe during pregnancy include α-methyldopa, beta blockers, labetelol, and calcium channel blockers. There is less experience with clonidine and beta-blockers; with the exception of atenolol, these drugs are probably safe.
    (2) Angiotensin-converting enzyme inhibitors (ACEIs) and angiotensin-receptive blockers (ARBs) are contraindicated during pregnancy.
    (3) Hydralazine can be added to any of the first line drugs but is not effective as a single agent when given orally.
  b. Epoetin alfa has been used safely to treat anemia, and frequently needs to be increased as the pregnancy progresses.
5. Weight gain is difficult to determine due to fluid retention (Hou, 2008; Nadeau-Fredette et al., 2013).
  a. Approximately 1.6 kg usually occurs in the first trimester.
  b. It has been suggested that estimated dry weight (EDW) be increased by .5 kg/week in the 2nd and 3rd trimesters, but weight gain throughout the pregnancy needs regular, careful evaluation by the nephrology interdisciplinary team.
6. Dialysis modifications.
  a. Hemodialysis (Hou, 2010; Nadeau-Fredette et al., 2013).
    (1) Usually 5 to 6 times per week with 20 to 24 hr/week or greater to assimilate more normal kidney function during fetal development.
    (2) Dialysate may need to have a higher K^+ content with more frequent dialysis, but calcium content is usually ~2.5 mEq/L.
    (3) Transfer to inpatient dialysis setting for

fetal monitoring during treatment at approximately 24 weeks gestation.
    b. Peritoneal dialysis (Chang et al., 2002).
        (1) Smaller volumes with more exchanges needed.
        (2) Tidal PD may be more efficient and comfortable

B. Transplantation.
    1. Energy/protein needs (AND, 2008; Institute of Medicine [IOM], 2010).
        a. Kilocalories: 25 to 35/kg pregravida IBW + 300 per day (2nd and 3rd trimesters).
        b. Protein: 1.1 g/kg pregravida IBW/day.
    2. Minerals (guidelines for normal pregnancy) (AND, 2008).
        a. Sodium: usually 2,300 mg/day.
        b. Potassium: liberal intake unless serum levels increased.
        c. Calcium: at least 1,000 mg/day.
        d. Phosphorus: at least 700 mg (1,250 mg/day less than 19 years of age).
        e. Zinc: at least 11 mg/day (12 mg/day less than 19 years of age).
        f. Iron: at least 27 mg/day.
    3. Vitamins (guidelines for normal pregnancy) (AND, 2008).
        a. Vitamin A: ~ 800 μg/day.
        b. Folic Acid: at least 600 mcg/day.
        c. Thiamin: 1.4 mg/day.
        d. Riboflavin: 1.4 mg/day.
        e. B6: 1.9 mg/day.
        f. B12: 2.6 mg/day.
        g. Biotin: 30 μg/day.
        h. Vitamin C: 85 mg/day.
        i. Vitamin D: 5 μg/day.
        j. Vitamin E: 15 mg/day.
    4. Weight gain (normal pregnancy) (AND, 2008).
        a. Underweight (BMI less than 19.8): 28 to 40 lb.
        b. Normal weight (BMI 19.8 to 26): 25 to 35 lb.
        c. Overweight (BMI 26 to 29): 15 to 25 lb.
        d. Obese (BMI greater than 29): at least 15 lb.
        e. Other: Young adolescents and black women should strive for gains at the upper end of the recommended range. Short women (157 cm) should aim for gains at the lower end of the range.

V. The impact of culture on food-related behavior.

A. Culture.
    1. Culture is an accumulation of behaviors shared by a social, ethnic, racial, or religious group (Goody & Drago, 2010).
    2. Culture determines how a person defines health, recognizes an illness, and seeks treatment (Sucher & Kittler, 2007).
    3. Each culture has different attitudes, beliefs, and practices about health and prevention, health care and treatment, and healthcare provider interactions.
    4. Culture not only influences health, healing, and wellness belief systems, but food-related behaviors. In all cultures, staple or core foods form the foundation of the diet.
    5. There are many cultural determinants of food choices including biological, environmental, social, physiologic, personal, and psychological influences (Schlenker, 2011). All of these influences need to be assessed to assist the healthcare professional in incorporating cultural competencies to improve cross-cultural interaction and improve health outcomes.

B. Acculturation may involve altering traditional eating behaviors to fit in to the dominant culture (Graves & Suitor, 1998).
    1. Addition of new foods in the diet occurs due to economic status and food availability.
    2. Substitution may occur because new foods are convenient to prepare, more affordable, or better liked than traditional foods.
    3. Rejection of traditional foods occurs more frequently in children and adolescents since it makes them feel different.

C. Nutrition assessment: determinants of food choices.
    1. Biology.
        a. Hunger and satiety.
        b. Sensory aspects.
        c. Palatability.
    2. Environmental factors.
        a. Agriculture.
            (1) Food availability.
            (2) Food technology.
            (3) Season and climate.
            (4) Geography.
        b. Housing and sanitation.
        c. Storage and cooking facilities.
    3. Social factors.
        a. Religion and social customs. Religion is a key aspect of culture that often prescribes or proscribes food patterns.
        b. Food traditions.
            (1) Identification of foods.
            (2) Methods of food preparation.
            (3) Condiment selection.
            (4) Timing and frequency of meals.
            (5) Fasting and meditation practice.
            (6) Feasting and special occasions.
            (7) Avoidance of certain foods at certain times.
            (8) Ritual, social, and symbolic use of foods.
        c. Education, food, and nutrition knowledge.
        d. Media.

e. Political and economic policies.
f. Socioeconomic status.
g. Social class role.
h. Social problems, poverty, substance abuse, mental health.
i. Use of complementary and alternate medicine (CAM).
4. Physiologic factors.
   a. Allergies, food intolerance.
   b. Physical disabilities.
   c. Health–disease status.
   d. Macronutrient and micronutrient needs.
5. Personal factors.
   a. Health literacy.
   b. Perceptions and expectations about food.
   c. Food preferences.
   d. Food preparation.
   e. Feeding practices.
   f. Attitudes and feelings.
   g. Motivations and values.
   h. Social relationships.
   i. Family and social networks.
   j. Alternative healing practices.
   k. Physical activity.
6. Psychological factors.
   a. Stress.
   b. Mood.
   c. Body image.
   d. Eating disorders.

D. Keys to cross-cultural communication (Graves & Suitor, 1998).
   1. Consider the patient's learning style, health literacy level, and preferred language.
   2. Use trained interpreters instead of family members because of several factors.
      a. Uncertain proficiency across both languages.
      b. Issues of confidentiality.
      c. Cultural norms may prohibit discussion of certain topics between particular family, age, or gender roles.
   3. Respect personal space.
   4. Learn and follow cultural rules about touching, including rules based on gender.
   5. Pay attention to body language.
   6. Express interest in people.
   7. Listen carefully. Health professionals must listen carefully and not interrupt or try to put words in the individual's mouth.
   8. Respect silence. People need a moment to gather their thoughts, especially when they are trying to speak in a nonprimary language.
   9. Notice how people make eye contact. Many cultures consider it impolite to look directly at the person who is speaking.
   10. Assess family and community dynamics on healthcare decision making (value of decision of

elders, differing gender roles, traditional healers, tribal leaders, spiritual leaders, and role of extended family members).
   11. Reach the appropriate family. For example, in some cultures the oldest male is considered the head of the family, while in others, an elderly female has this role.
   12. Address cultural beliefs, healthcare traditions, and misconceptions.
   13. Identify complementary alternative medicine (CAM) practices. Discuss potential side effects of CAM and kidney disease. May need to limit or restrict use, if not appropriate.
   14. Study a person's responses. A "yes" does not necessarily indicate that a person understands the message or is willing to do what is being discussed. The person may simply be showing respect for the healthcare professional.
   15. Choose/modify written materials to meet literacy needs.
   16. Provide written information in patient's preferred language.

E. CKD and vegetarianism.
   1. The main reasons patients follow vegetarian diets are religious, ethnic/cultural, health reasons, concern for animals, and lack of taste for meat (Schatz, 2004).
   2. Types of vegetarian diets.
      a. Vegan: eliminates all meat, fish, poultry, eggs, dairy, and their derivatives.
      b. Lacto-ovo: eliminates animal flesh but permits use of eggs and dairy.
      c. Lacto-vegetarian: vegan diet plus dairy.
      d. Ovo-vegetarian: vegan diet plus eggs.
      e. Pesco-vegetarian or pescatarian: lacto-ovo vegetarian diet plus fish.
      f. Semi-vegetarian: excludes only red meat or includes less meat than usual.
   3. Vegetarian health practices, beliefs, and attitudes.
      a. Vegetarians more commonly take vitamins as well as mineral and other supplements.
         (1) Brewer's yeast related to belief that mega-vitamin therapy could cure certain diseases.
         (2) Seaweed is believed to benefit thyroid and protect from radiation.
         (3) Many vegetarians believe that disease is caused by an imbalance of nutrients.
      b. Common belief is that diseases can be cured by fasting and avoidance of certain foods.
      c. Common belief is that mind, body, and soul are all interconnected.
      d. Ayurvedic therapy is used to achieve balance. Ayur means "longevity" and veda means "science or knowledge."
         (1) Uses diet, herbal remedies, and meditation

to reestablish equilibrium between the sick person and the universe.
(2) Diet is considered the most significant part of the therapy.
(3) Foods are classified as "yin and yang" (hot and cold) depending on their effect on the body.
(4) Herbal infusions are prevalent.
  (a) Some herbal remedies are nephrotoxic due to aristolochic acid.
  (b) The use of herbal remedies is not recommended in patients with CKD (KDIGO, 2013a).
4. Benefits of a vegetarian diet.
   a. Plant protein sources have demonstrated a positive effect on GFR and renal blood flow.
   b. Milder renal histologic damage.
   c. Decreases proteinuria.
   d. Improved lipid profile.
5. Renal diet considerations.
   a. Sodium content of some vegetarian foods can be high. The use of meat analogs, salted nuts, miso, frozen entrees, and marinated tofu products will need to be limited.
   b. Phosphorus management is difficult since the lowest quantity of phosphorus (mg) per gram of protein comes from animal products. Consumption of a vegetarian diet will likely require an increase in the number of phosphate binders for patients on dialysis.
   c. Potassium control requires selection of lower potassium-containing fruits and vegetables to allow the use of some dairy products, legumes, nuts, and seeds, which are higher in potassium. Use of herbal supplements, roots, juices, and leaves will also contribute to potassium intake.
   d. Protein content of plant sources can provide adequate amounts of essential amino acids if a variety of plant foods are consumed and energy needs are met.

VI. Importance of controlling sodium.

A. Dietary sodium intake of adults in the United States exceeds physiologic need (IOM, 2013).
   1. Average sodium intake: 3,400 mg/day.
   2. Federal guideline Dietary Reference Intake (DRI) for sodium: less than 2,300 mg/day and 1500 mg/day for at risk individuals, including CKD.

B. Renal salt handling and blood pressure in CKD.
   1. Alterations in renal salt handling are likely to be a significant contributor to elevated blood pressure levels in patients with CKD (KDIGO, 2012).
   2. Recommended sodium intake is less than 2000 mg sodium/day to improve blood pressure, unless contraindicated (KDIGO, 2012).

3. Benefits of reducing sodium intake in patients with mild to moderate CKD.
   a. Could have a greater capacity to lower blood pressure in patients with CKD who have sodium and water retention (KDIGO, 2012).
   b. Reduces blood pressure in patients with CKD independent of hypertensive medication (de Brito-Ashurst et al., 2013).
   c. Reduces blood pressure, extracellular fluid volume, albuminuria, and proteinuria. May reduce cardiovascular risk (McMahon et al., 2013).
   d. May be considered for those with high blood pressure who have a poor response to angiotensin-converting enzyme (ACE) inhibitors or ARBs (KDIGO, 2012).

C. Sodium excess and adverse effects on target-organs; may cause severe structural and functional problems (Frohlich & Susic, 2011; Kotchen et al., 2013; Susic & Frohlich, 2011).
   1. Kidney.
      a. Increased renal vascular resistance and decreased renal blood flow.
      b. Increased glomerular arterial resistance.
      c. Changes in microcirculation favor progression of kidney injury.
      d. May stimulate local renin-angiotensin-aldosterone systems (RAAS) in the kidney (as well as heart and vessels) independent of the classical system.
   2. Heart.
      a. Cardiac hypertrophy.
      b. Diastolic dysfunction with normal systolic function.
      c. Systolic dysfunction.
   3. Blood vessels.
      a. Oxidative stress.
      b. Endothelial dysfunction.
      c. Decreased vascular elasticity and decreased pulse wave velocity.
      d. Fibrosis.

D. Caution regarding salt wasting (KDIGO, 2012).
   1. Some forms of CKD (such as tubular disease) may be associated with salt wasting from the kidney. Affected individuals may be at higher than usual risk of volume depletion and electrolyte disturbances potentiated by salt restriction.
   2. Volume and electrolyte status should be carefully monitored in patients with CKD undergoing salt restriction.

E. Salt intake and hemodialysis.
   1. In oligo-anuric hemodialysis subjects, renal sodium excretion is severely impaired; therefore, hemodialysis must remove sodium and water (McCausland et al., 2010).

2. Benefits associated with dietary salt restriction for patients on hemodialysis (Kayikcioglu et al., 2009; Maduell & Navarro, 2001; Ozkahya et al., 2006).
   a. Reduced interdialytic weight gain (IDWG).
   b. Lesser requirement for antihypertensive medication.
   c. Ameliorative effects on left ventricular hypertrophy.
3. Risks associated with greater sodium intake by patients on hemodialysis (McCausland et al., 2010).
   a. Increased risk of death.
   b. Modestly greater ultrafiltration (UF) requirement.

F. Measurement of salt intake in CKD (McMahon et al., 2012).
   1. Urinary sodium.
      a. 24-hour urinary sodium.
      b. Spot urinary sodium.
   2. Dietary assessment.
      a. Diet history.
      b. 24-hour diet recall.
      c. Food records (diaries).
      d. Food frequency questionnaire.

SECTION D
Nutrition Intervention
Louise Clement, Pamela S. Kent

I. Nutrients important in the management of kidney disease.

A. Protein and amino acids.
   1. Protein is a structural component of all living cells, found in muscles, nerves, bone, teeth, skin, hair, nails, blood, and glands. Almost all body fluids contain protein with the exception of urine, sweat, and bile.
   2. Protein is a regulator of blood pH, osmotic pressure, and water balance. It forms antibodies, aids in building resistance to infections, and transports other substances in the blood, such as drugs.
   3. Protein is stored in all lean tissues, but acute-critical or chronic illness or inadequate intake can lead to deficiency.
   4. As kidney function declines, nitrogenous wastes accumulate, plasma protein concentrations are altered, and protein catabolism is increased secondary to metabolic acidosis.
   5. In catabolic states or with inadequate protein intake, protein stores are broken down and can contribute to the accumulation of nitrogenous wastes.
   6. Amino acids and peptides are lost with each hemodialysis treatment. Protein losses that occur with peritoneal dialysis can double with peritonitis. The catabolic effect of high-dose steroids can increase protein requirements in kidney transplant patients.
   7. Essential amino acids must be provided by the diet. Nonessential amino acids can be synthesized by the body. Tyrosine, histidine, and serine are conditionally essential amino acids in kidney failure.
   8. As a source of energy, protein yields 4 calories per gram. This function should be spared by fat and carbohydrate so that protein is used for building and repairing tissues.
   9. An adjusted body weight is needed to calculate protein needs with underweight or overweight conditions.

B. Carbohydrate.
   1. Carbohydrate is the primary source of heat and energy. It has a protein-sparing effect and serves as the carbon skeleton for the synthesis of nonessential amino acids.
   2. Glucose is the major energy source of the brain and other nervous tissues. Carbohydrate occurs in the body chiefly as glucose, and is stored as glycogen in liver and muscle.
   3. Carbohydrate metabolism is altered in chronic kidney disease. Two major defects frequently noted are peripheral resistance to the action of insulin and impaired insulin secretion by the pancreas.
   4. Elevated parathyroid hormone (PTH) levels/secondary hyperparathyroidism can also contribute to glucose intolerance by inhibiting insulin secretion.
   5. Hypoglycemia may be noted in patients with and without diabetes when GFR falls below 40 mL/min. Insulin is metabolized and cleared by the kidney. Therefore, the half-life is increased as kidney disease progresses.
   6. Carbohydrate yields 4 calories per gram and provides 45–50% of the calories in the typical American diet.

C. Fats.
   1. Fat is a carrier of fat-soluble vitamins, is part of the essential structure of cells, adds palatability and satiety value to the diet, and has a protein-sparing effect.
   2. Fat is stored as adipose tissue, found mainly in

subcutaneous tissue and around visceral organs, and insulates the body against heat loss.

3. Fat provides the most concentrated source of calories, yielding 9 calories per gram. Fat stores are filled up or depleted depending on the balance between energy intake from food and energy expenditure.

4. Impaired kidney function and uremia are both associated with lipid abnormalities. These dyslipidemias are a contributing factor to the high incidence of cardiovascular events in CKD (KDIGO, 2013b).

5. In the nephrotic syndrome, increased cholesterol production and decreased clearance of lipids result in hypercholesterolemia and hypertriglyceridemia.

6. Hemodialysis patients frequently have elevated serum triglyderides and very low-density lipoprotein (VLDL) cholesterol, and low serum levels of high-density lipoprotein (HDL) cholesterol.

7. Peritoneal dialysis patients tend to have higher serum cholesterol, triglyceride, and low density lipoprotein (LDL) cholesterol levels than hemodialysis patients, possibly secondary to loss of proteins into the peritoneal dialysate and excessive absorption of glucose from the dialysate.

8. After kidney transplant, immunosuppressive therapy can lead to elevated serum cholesterol and triglycerides (KDIGO, 2009b).

9. The Dietary Reference Intake (DRI) suggests that 20–35% of daily caloric needs should be provided by fat (National Research Council [NRC], 2011).

10. When Therapeutic Lifestyle Changes (TLC) are implemented to lower elevated lipid levels, total fat should be 25% to 35% of calories, and saturated fat should be less than 7% of calories (National Cholesterol Education Program [NCEP], 2001).

11. The use of omega-3 fatty acids has not been extensively investigated in CKD, but they may be beneficial due to their ability to lower blood pressure, serum triglycerides, and inflammatory compounds (Chang & Kramer, 2013).

12. Supplementation with omega-3 fatty acids has been shown to decrease urinary protein excretion but not significantly improve eGFR (Miller et al., 2009).

D. Energy.
1. Actual energy requirements vary, based on age, growth, medical condition, activity, and amount of lean body tissue compared to total edema-free weight.
   a. An adjusted body weight should be calculated to account for these variables.

b. The widespread acceptance of one formula that accounts for these multiple contributing factors is still elusive.

2. Persons on peritoneal dialysis are exposed to a high glucose load, both on CAPD and APD, due to the peritoneal absorption of dextrose (see nutrition care for the patient receiving peritoneal dialysis, Section B. II. C. 9, to estimate calories absorbed from PD dialysate).

E. Alcohol.
1. Alcohol is metabolized primarily in the liver. Excessive consumption may lead to elevated levels of ketones, triglycerides, uric acid, lactic acid, acidosis, blood pressure, and stroke risk.

2. Alcohol should be avoided in pregnancy, pancreatitis, alcohol abuse, advanced neuropathy, and severely elevated triglyceride levels.

3. Light to moderate intake of alcohol may provide benefits for specific populations. Alcohol use raises HDL cholesterol, lowers LDL cholesterol, decreases the oxidation of LDL, and exerts anticlotting actions; all of these decrease the risk of coronary heart disease (Klatsky, 2003).

4. The consumption of alcohol along with certain medications is contraindicated due to the potential of alcohol as a stomach mucosal irritant, hepatotoxic agent, and as an agent that may produce additive toxicity during drug metabolism.

5. The fluid content of alcoholic beverages should be considered, along with other nutrients. The potassium content of wine ranges from 115 to 164 mg/5 oz serving. Mixed drinks may contain moderate to high potassium ingredients, such as tomato juice, orange juice, pineapple juice, and coconut cream.

6. See diabetes and kidney disease, Section C. II. D., Alcohol, for considerations in diabetes.

F. Fiber.
1. Dietary fiber is either soluble or insoluble. Soluble fiber, found in many vegetables and oatmeal, can moderately lower serum total and LDL cholesterol.

2. Many high fiber foods are also high in potassium or phosphorus, such as prunes, dried beans and peas, bran, nuts, and certain fruits and vegetables, such as bananas, melons, and tomatoes. Safer choices within a potassium or phosphorus restriction include green beans, cabbage, carrots, cauliflower, corn, eggplant, onions, alfalfa sprouts, apple with skin, blueberries, raspberries, popcorn, brown rice, and oatmeal, among others.

3. Commercial fiber supplements, such as psyllium (Metamucil®) and cellulose (Unifiber®), contain 3 grams of fiber per tablespoon, and may be used

Table 4.3

Vitamin B Complex Recommendations and Suggestions in Kidney Disease*

Vitamin	RDA	CKD 3-5	HD and PD
B1 (Thiamin) mg/d	1.1-1.2	1.1-1.2	1.1-1.2
B2 (Riboflavin) mg/d	1.1-1.3	Supplement if restricted protein diet	1.1-1.3
B3 (Niacin) mg/d	14-16	up to RDA	14-16
B6 (Pyridoxine) mg/d	1.3-1.7	5	10
Folic Acid mg/d	0.400	up to RDA	1
B12 (Cobalamin) µg/d	2.4	2.4	2.4
Pantothenic acid mg/d	5	Up to AI	5
Biotin µg/d	30	Up to AI	30

*Ranges depend on age and gender
RDA = recommended dietary allowance; AI = adequate intake
Source of data: Chazot & Kopple, 2013

when dietary fiber intake is insufficient. *Note*: Sugar-free, orange-flavored effervescent Metamucil® is high in potassium.
   4. Recommended intake is 20 to 25 g per day for HD and PD (McCann, 2009), and 20 to 30 grams recommended for Therapeutic Lifestyle Changes (TLC) (NCEP, 2001).

G. Vitamins: general.
   1. The recommended daily intake of vitamins varies depending on gender, age, and other conditions, such as pregnancy, lactation, and health status.
   2. Chronic kidney disease alters vitamin status, and both deficiencies and abnormally high levels of vitamins have been reported with kidney disease (Handelman & Levin, 2011).
   3. The Dialysis Outcomes and Practice Patterns Study (DOPPS) demonstrated that mortality rates were improved in patients on dialysis who took vitamin supplements (Fissell et al., 2004).
   4. Renal-specific formulations, or "renal vitamins," are oral multivitamin supplements that contain B vitamins and vitamin C, and may contain vitamins D and E, zinc, iron, selenium, and/or copper (Greene & Gutekunst, 2013).
      a. Renal vitamins are recommended to ensure adequate vitamin replacement and are usually given once a day after dialysis.
      b. For patients dialyzing more frequently than three times per week, such as in nocturnal dialysis at home, vitamin requirements may be higher due to increased vitamin losses.

H. Vitamins: water-soluble. Most water-soluble vitamins are not stored so daily intake is required, although

vitamin B12 is the exception (Chazot & Kopple, 2013).
   1. Vitamin C.
      a. Vitamin C is necessary for the synthesis of collagen, for wound healing, and for the ability to withstand the stress of injury and infection. It also enhances the absorption of iron and influences cellular and humoral immune responses.
      b. Intake may be low in patients with CKD because of potassium restriction.
      c. Losses occur with HD (about 50 mg per HD treatment) and PD.
      d. Recommended supplementation (Beindorff & Ulerich, 2013; Chazot & Kopple, 2013; NRC, 2011).
         (1) CKD: 30 to 60 mg/day.
         (2) HD and PD: DRI.
         (3) Transplant: DRI.
         (4) Healthy adults: DRI is 75 to 90 mg/day, depending on age and gender.
   2. Vitamin B complex.
      a. B complex vitamins include eight vitamins: thiamin, riboflavin, niacin, B6 or pyridoxine, folic acid, B12 or cobalamin, pantothenic acid, and biotin.
      b. Vitamins in this complex serve as coenzymes in a variety of biochemical reactions, including the production of energy; metabolism of proteins, lipids, and carbohydrates; and synthesis of body tissues.
      c. Primary sources are protein foods, whole grains, and fortified grains and cereals. Many B vitamins tend to be present in the same foods. Therefore, a deficiency of one may point to a deficiency in another, with some exceptions.

d. Requirements increase when metabolism is accelerated by fever, stress, or injury.

e. See Table 4.3, Vitamin B Complex Recommendations and Suggestions in Kidney Disease. Also refer to Table 4.1, Nutrition Recommendations for Kidney Transplant Recipients.

I. Vitamins: fat soluble. Fat soluble vitamins are stored in the body. Deficiencies can occur in fat malabsorption secondary to GI disorders, or with inadequate intake (Chazot & Kopple, 2013).

1. Vitamin A.
   a. Vitamin A is necessary for photoreception in rod and cone cells of the retina, bone growth and development, epithelial tissue development and maintenance, and immunity.
   b. Increased plasma levels occur in kidney failure. The vitamin A carrier, retinol-binding protein, is catabolized in the tubules, and this process decreases as kidney function drops. Vitamin A toxicity has been reported with supplementation.
   c. No losses occur with HD. Very small losses have been reported in PD.
   d. Renal vitamins do not contain vitamin A (Greene & Gutekunst, 2013).
   e. Recommended supplementation (Beindorff & Ulerich, 2013; Chazot & Kopple, 2013; NRC, 2011).
      (1) CKD: up to the RDI.
      (2) HD and PD: none.
      (3) Transplant: RDI.
      (4) Healthy adults: RDI is 700 to 900 retinol equivalents (RE)/day, depending on age and gender.

2. Vitamin D.
   a. The functions of the active form include:
      (1) Stimulating active GI absorption of calcium and phosphorus.
      (2) Working in conjunction with PTH to mobilize calcium and phosphate from the bone to maintain serum calcium and phosphate levels.
   b. The ability to synthesize 1,25-dihydroxyvitamin D3 decreases as kidney function declines and fibroblast growth homone 23 (FGF-23) levels rise. Therefore, supplementation with calcitriol and vitamin D analogs is usually needed in CKD, HD, and PD.
   c. Besides issues related to bone metabolism, calcitriol is involved in metabolic processes affecting cardiovascular disease, such as congestive heart failure, hypertension, left ventricular hypotrophy, and certain cancers, such as prostate.
   d. The nonactive form of vitamin D is a required

nutrient, even in persons with CKD. Uremic kidneys can lose vitamin D-binding protein in the urine, potentially causing a vitamin D deficiency. The older adult, housebound patients and people living in northern climates are also at risk (due to limited sun exposure).
   e. In CKD stages 3 to 5D, the nonactive form of vitamin D (serum 25-hydroxyvitamin D) should be measured. Supplement with ergocalciferol or cholecalciferol to correct vitamin D deficiency and insufficiency (KDIGO, 2009a).

3. Vitamin E.
   a. Functions of vitamin E.
      (1) Antioxidant; used commercially to retard spoilage.
      (2) Preserves integrity of red blood cells.
      (3) May protect structure and function of muscle tissues.
      (4) Prevents oxidation of unsaturated fats and LDL.
   b. Vitamin E coated dialyzers may decrease oxidative stress, but their use is not widespread.
   c. Recommended supplementation (Beindorff & Ulerich, 2013; Chazot & Kopple, 2013; NRC, 2011).
      (1) CKD: up to the RDI.
      (2) HD and PD: up to the RDI.
      (3) Transplant: RDI.
      (4) Healthy adults: RDI is 22.5 IU/day, depending on age and gender.

4. Vitamin K.
   a. Vitamin K is essential for both prothrombin formation for blood coagulation and for bone formation.
   b. The main source is *E. coli* synthesis in the large intestine.
   c. Generally, supplementation is not indicated (Greene & Gutekunst, 2013), but hospitalized patients with poor intake and an extended course of antibiotics are at risk for developing a deficiency, and supplementation may be necessary, since body stores are small (Alperin, 1987).
   d. Patients who take warfarin (Coumadin) need to maintain a steady intake of vitamin K to prevent blood coagulation problems, and foods high in vitamin K are restricted.

J. Minerals.
   1. Sodium (23 mg = 1 mEq).
      a. Sodium is the major cation in extracellular fluid.
      b. Functions of sodium (see Special considerations in kidney disease, Section C. VI., Importance of controlling sodium).
         (1) Regulation of extracellular fluid volume.

(2) Conduction of nerve impulses.
(3) Control of muscle contraction.
(4) Acid-base regulation.
(5) Cell membrane permeability.
c. Recommended intake (Beindorff & Ulerich, 2013; Jiwakanon & Mehrotra, 2013; Kalantar-Zadeh & Kopple, 2013; KDIGO, 2013a; NRC, 2011).
(1) CKD: less than 2,000 mg/day.
(2) HD: 750 to 2,000 mg/day.
(3) PD: 750 to 2,000 mg/day, monitor fluid balance.
(4) Transplant: 2,000 to 4,000 mg/day, with hypertension and/or edema.
(5) Healthy adults: DRI 1,200 to 2,300 mg/day; depending on age, race, and comorbidities.
2. Potassium (39 mg = 1 mEq).
a. Potassium is the major cation of intracellular fluid. Potassium makes up 5% of the total mineral content of the body.
b. Major functions of potassium.
(1) Aids in maintaining normal water balance, osmotic equilibrium, and acid-base balance.
(2) Aids in regulation of neuromuscular activity, particularly in transmission of electrical impulses in the heart.
(3) Participates in the conversion of glucose to glycogen.
c. Normally 80–90% of ingested potassium is excreted in the urine, and 10–20% is lost in the feces.
d. Potassium can shift from intracellular to extracellular fluid in conditions of acidosis and hyperglycemia.
e. Recommended intake (Beindorff & Ulerich, 2013; Jiwakanon & Mehrotra, 2013; Kalantar-Zadeh & Kopple, 2013; NRC, 2011).
(1) CKD: usually not restricted unless serum levels are elevated.
(2) HD: up to 70 to 80 mEq (2730 to 3120 mg)/day.
(3) PD: adjust based on serum levels; may need potassium supplement to maintain serum levels.
(4) Transplant: unrestricted unless hyperkalemic.
(5) Healthy adults: DRI is 4,700 mg/day.
3. Calcium (20 mg = 1 mEq).
a. Calcium is the most abundant mineral found in the body, with 99% located in hard tissues, bone, and teeth.
b. Functions of calcium.
(1) Build and maintain bones and teeth.
(2) Activation of enzymes for metabolic functions.
(3) Blood coagulation.
(4) Permeability of cell membrane.

(5) Transmission of nerve impulses.
(6) Contraction of skeletal, cardiac, and smooth muscle fibers.
c. Only 10–30% of ingested calcium is absorbed.
(1) Absorption is increased by activated vitamin D, acidic medium, lactose, and increased body need.
(2) Absorption is decreased by vitamin D deficiency, oxalic acid, phytic acid, fiber, alkaline medium, immobilizations, and trauma.
d. Recommended intake (Beindorff & Ulerich, 2013; Jiwakanon & Mehrotra, 2013; Kalantar-Zadeh & Kopple, 2013; NRC, 2011).
(1) Correct lab-reported serum calcium level for low serum albumin level, to prevent overadministration or underadministration of calcium supplements.

Corrected serum calcium =
Total calcium mg/dL + [0.8 x (4.0 – serum albumin (g/dL)]

(2) CKD: DRI of 1,000 to 1,200 mg/day: maintain serum levels WNL.
(3) HD: less than 1,000 mg/day, avoid excess intake.
(4) PD: 800 mg/day.
(5) Transplant: DRI.
(6) Healthy adult: DRI is 1,000 to 1,200 mg/day, depending on age and gender.
4. Phosphorus (31 mg = 1 mEq).
a. Phosphorus is the second most abundant mineral in the body. Approximately 80% is located in the bones and teeth.
b. Functions of phosphorus.
(1) Building and maintaining bones and teeth.
(2) Transfer of energy within cells.
(3) Activation of vitamin D.
(4) Normal nerve and muscle function.
(5) Fat transportation as phospholipids.
(6) Acid-base regulation.
c. Sources of dietary phosphorus (Uribarri & Calvo, 2003).
(1) Plant food, mostly as phytate; ~40% absorption.
(2) Animal based protein food; ~60% absorption.
(3) Phosphorus containing food additives; greater than 90% absorption. May increase the phosphorus intake by as a much as 1 g/day.
d. Phosphate binders are needed to decrease phosphate absorption in the GI tract in acute or chronic kidney failure to maintain acceptable serum levels.
e. Recommended intake (Beindorff & Ulerich, 2013; Jiwakanon & Mehrotra, 2013; Kalantar-

Zadeh & Kopple, 2013; NRC, 2011).
  (1) CKD: 800 to 1,000 mg/day. Maintain serum phosphorus and PTH within normal levels.
  (2) HD: 10 to 17 mg/kg/day.
  (3) PD: 800 mg/day.
  (4) Transplant: DRI.
  (5) Healthy adult: DRI is 700 mg/day.
5. Iron.
  a. Iron is an essential component of hemoglobin and myoglobin. It is important in oxygen transport and cellular oxidation.
  b. Between 60% and 70% of iron is in the functional form as transferrin, while 30–40% is stored as ferritin.
  c. Absorption is dependent on the amount of body stores, other medications, inflammation status, form of iron, and presence or absence of other meal components, such as vitamin C or phytic acid. Generally, 5–15% of iron intake is absorbed.
  d. Recommended intake (Beindorff & Ulerich, 2013; Jiwakanon & Mehrotra, 2013; Kalantar-Zadeh & Kopple, 2013; NRC, 2011).
    (1) CKD: individualize.
    (2) HD: individualize; IV iron is usually required to maintain acceptable stores.
    (3) PD: 10 to 15 mg/day; IV iron is sometimes required to maintain acceptable stores.
    (4) Transplant: DRI.
    (5) Healthy adult: DRI is 8–18 mg/day, depending on age and gender.
6. Zinc.
  a. The most important function of zinc is in the metabolic activity of cells. It is required for the activity of over 300 enzymes. Zinc is especially important in protein synthesis and taste and smell acuity.
  b. A zinc deficiency leads to extreme undernutrition and delayed wound healing.
  c. Zinc is primarily transported by albumin in plasma. Conditions which cause protein loss can also contribute to a loss of zinc.
  d. Zinc absorption is decreased with calcium-based binders and oral iron use.
  e. Recommended intake (Beindorff & Ulerich, 2013; Jiwakanon & Mehrotra, 2013; Kalantar-Zadeh & Kopple, 2013; NRC, 2011).
    (1) CKD: individualize.
    (2) HD: 15 mg/day.
    (3) PD: 12 to 15 mg/day.
    (4) Transplant: DRI.
    (5) Healthy adult: DRI is 8 to 11 mg/day, depending on age and gender.
7. Magnesium.
  a. Magnesium is the second most prevalent intracellular cation in humans, after potassium. About 60% is found in bones, 26% in muscle,

and the rest in soft tissue and body fluid. It is required for the metabolism of ATP.
  b. Elevated serum levels typically result from renal insufficiency, especially when GFR is less than 15 mL/min.
  c. Mild elevations are usually asymptomatic, but levels greater than 4 mEq/L may lead to loss of deep tendon reflexes, respiratory paralysis, and heart block.
  d. Positive magnesium balance in CKD 5 is partially treated with low magnesium dialysate for both hemodialysis and peritoneal dialysis, although serum levels are usually within normal limits if intake does not exceed the RDI (Haddad et al., 2013).

K. Fluid.
  1. Water is an essential component of all living matter.
    a. Water is the largest single component of the body, making up 60% of body weight.
    b. The proportion of body water as a percentage of total body weight decreases with age.
    c. Intracellular water makes up 40% of body weight.
    d. Extracellular fluids, made up of interstitial fluid, plasma, lymph, spinal fluid, and secretions, make up 20% of body weight.
  2. Functions.
    a. Water provides an aqueous environment necessary for all metabolism.
    b. It gives structure and form to the body.
    c. Water acts as a transport medium for nutrients and wastes.
  3. Recommended daily intake (Beindorff & Ulerich, 2013; Jiwakanon & Mehrotra, 2013; Kalantar-Zadeh & Kopple, 2013; NRC, 2011).
    a. CKD: usually no restriction.
    b. HD: usually 750 to 1,500 mL/day.
    c. PD: restrict to maintain fluid balance.
    d. Transplant: limited only by graft function; generally unrestricted.
    e. Healthy adults: intake to maintain fluid balance.

II. Health literacy and educational strategies.

A. Health literacy is the ability to obtain, process, and understand basic health information and services to make appropriate healthcare decisions (Benjamin, 2010).
  1. According to the National Assessment of Adult Literacy, only 12% of the U.S. population has a proficient health literacy level or can process challenging health information (Kutner et al., 2006).
  2. Limited health literacy in patients with CKD

results in poor management of chronic health conditions, inability to understand and adhere to medication and diet regimens, increased hospitalizations, and poor health outcomes (Norris & Nissenson, 2008).

3. To obtain optimal health outcomes, individuals need healthcare access, health knowledge, and behavior change.

B. Why is health literacy important? DeWalt and colleagues (2010) contribute this:
   1. Approximately 40–80% of medical information provided by healthcare providers is forgotten immediately by patients.
   2. Nearly 50% of the information that is remembered is incorrect.
   3. Health information tools are usually written at the tenth grade level or above.
   4. Medically underserved patients may have difficulty communicating with their healthcare providers.

C. High risk populations.
   1. Elderly.
   2. Minorities.
   3. Immigrants.
   4. Poverty-stricken.
   5. Persons with limited education.

D. Possible indicators of low health literacy.
   1. Excuses: "I forgot my glasses."
   2. Excessive paperwork folded up in purse or bag.
   3. Lack of follow-through with medical tests and appointments.
   4. Seldom asks questions.
   5. Questions are basic in nature.
   6. Difficulty explaining medical concerns or how to take medications.
   7. There may be no red flags.

E. Right to understand.
   1. Patients have the right to understand healthcare information that is necessary for them to manage a health condition.
   2. Healthcare providers have a duty to provide information in simple, clear, plain language that patients understand before ending the conversation.

F. Universal precautions refer to treating all patients as being health illiterate to minimize risk for everyone when it is unclear which patients may be affected (DeWalt et al., 2010). Clear communication practices and removing literacy-related barriers will improve care for all patients regardless of their health literacy.
   1. Key communication strategies.
      a. Welcome patients with a smile and a positive attitude.
      b. Respond effectively to the health literacy needs of populations served.
         (1) Bilingual staff.
         (2) Foreign language interpretation services.
         (3) Multilingual telecommunication systems.
         (4) Telecommunications for the deaf (TTY).
         (5) Assistive technology devices.
      c. Make appropriate eye contact throughout the interaction if culturally appropriate.
      d. Speak clearly and at a moderate pace.
      e. Prioritize what needs to be discussed and limit information to 3 to 5 key points.
      f. Use print materials in easy-to-read, low literacy picture and symbol formats.
      g. Provide materials in alternative formats (e.g., audiotape, Braille, enlarged print, or preferred language).
      h. Encourage patients to ask questions and be proactive in their health care. Use "Ask Me 3" (National Patient Safety Foundation, 2013).
         (1) What is my main problem?
         (2) What do I need to do?
         (3) Why is it important for me to do this?
      i. Teach-back confirms you have explained to the patient what they need to know in a manner that the patient understands.
      j. Keep instructions simple. Teach the smallest amount possible to accomplish goals.
      k. Use simple language and avoid technical or medical jargon.
   2. Self-management complements traditional patient education in supporting the patient to live the best possible quality of life with their medical condition (Bodenheimer et al., 2002).
      a. Self-management education teaches problem-solving skills.
      b. A central concept in self-management is self-efficacy — confidence to carry out a behavior necessary to reach a desired goal.
      c. Self-efficacy is enhanced when patients succeed in solving patient-identified problems.
      d. Self-management skills are more effective than information-only patient education in improving clinical outcomes.
      e. Self-management education is an integral part of quality care.
   3. Supportive services like community organizations and government agencies can assist patients with medications, transportation, and nutrition issues. Some patients will not achieve their health goals unless you assist them to obtain such services.

G. Tailoring education messages to patients' psychological readiness to make dietary changes may be helpful in planning the approach to patient education. The transtheoretical or stages of change

model suggests that health-related behavior occurs through five stages (Baldwin & Falciglia, 1995).
1. Precontemplation.
   a. Validate lack of readiness.
   b. Clarify it is their decision.
   c. Encourage reevaluation of current behavior.
   d. Encourage self-exploration, not action.
   e. Explain and personalize the risk.
2. Contemplation.
   a. Validate lack of readiness.
   b. Encourage evaluation of pros and cons of behavior change.
   c. Identify and promote new, positive outcome expectations.
3. Preparation.
   a. Identify and assist in problem solving.
   b. Verify that the patient has underlying skills for behavior change.
   c. Encourage small initial steps.
4. Action.
   a. Focus on restructuring cues and social support.
   b. Praise self-efficacy for dealing with obstacles.
   c. Combat feelings of loss and reiterate long-term benefits.
5. Maintenance.
   a. Plan for follow-up support.
   b. Reinforce internal rewards.
   c. Discuss coping with relapse.
6. Relapse.
   a. Evaluate trigger for relapse.
   b. Reassess motivation and barriers and coping strategies.

References

Academy of Nutrition and Dietetics (AND). (2006). Evidence Analysis Library. *Adult weight management evidence-based nutrition practice guideline.* Retrieved from http://www.adaevidencelibrary.com/topic.cfm?cat=2798

Academy of Nutrition and Dietetics (AND). (2008). Position of the American Dietetic Association: Nutrition and lifestyle for a healthy pregnancy outcome. *Journal of the American Dietetic Association, 108*(3), 553-561.

Academy of Nutrition and Dietetics (AND). (2009). Evidence Analysis Library. *Unintended weight loss in older adults evidenced-based nutrition practice guideline.* Retrieved from http://www.adaevidencelibrary.com/topic.cfm?cat=3651

Academy of Nutrition and Dietetics (AND). (2010). Evidence Analysis Library. *Chronic kidney disease evidence-based nutrition practice guideline.* Retrieved from http://www.adaevidencelibrary.com/topic.cfm?cat=3927

Academy of Nutrition and Dietetics (AND). (2013) *International Dietetics & Nutrition Terminology (IDNT) reference manual* (4th ed.). Chicago, IL: Academy of Nutrition and Dietetics.

Alperin, J.B. (1987). Coagulopathy caused by vitamin K deficiency in critically ill, hospitalized patients. *Journal of the American Medical Association, 258*(14), 1916-1919.

American Diabetes Association (ADA). (2012). Standards of medical care in diabetes – 2012. *Diabetes Care, 35*(S1), S11-S63.

Baldwin, T.T., & Falciglia, G.A. (1995). Application of cognitive behavioral theories to dietary change in clients. *Journal of the American Dietetic Association, 95*(11), 1315-1317.

Barbagallo, C.M., Cefalu, A.B., Gallo, S., Rizzo, M., Noto, D., Cavera, G., ... Averna, M.R. (1999). Effect of Mediterranean diet on lipid levels and cardiovascular risk in renal transplant recipients. *Nephron, 82*(3), 199-204.

Barboza, J. (2008). The aging adult. In L.D. Byham-Gray, J.D. Burrowes, & G.M. Chertow (Eds.), *Nutrition in kidney disease* (pp. 469-484). Totowa, NJ: Humana Press.

Beindorff, M.E., & Ulerich, L.M. (2013). Nutrition management of the adult renal transplant patient. In L. Byham-Gray, J. Stover, & K. Wiesen (Eds.), *A clinical guide to nutrition care in kidney disease* (2nd ed.). Chicago, IL: The Academy of Nutrition and Dietetics.

Benjamin, R.M. (2010) Improving health by improving health literacy. *Public Health Reports, 125*(6), 784-785.

Bethke, P.C., & Jansky, S.H. (2008). The effects of boiling and leaching on the content of potassium and other minerals in potatoes. *Journal of Food Science, 73*(5), H80-85.

Beto, J. (1992). Hyperkalemia: Evaluation of dietary and non-dietary etiology. *Journal of Renal Nutrition, 2*(1), 28-29.

Bodenheimer, T., Lorig, K., Holman, H., & Grumbach, K. (2002). Patient self-management of chronic disease in primary care. *Journal of the American Medical Association, 288*(19), 2469-2475.

Bostom, A., Carpenter, M., Kusek, J., Levey, A.S., Hunsicker, L., Pfeffer, M.A., ... Weir, M. (2011). Homocysteine-lowering and cardiovascular disease outcomes in kidney transplant recipients. *Circulation, 123*(16), 1763-1770.

Burrowes, J.D., & Ramer, N.J. (2008) Changes in potassium content of different potato varieties after cooking. *Journal of Renal Nutrition, 18*(6), 530-534.

Carrero, J.J., Stenvinkel, P., Cuppari, L., Ikizler, T.A., Kalantar-Zadeh, K., Kaysen, G., ... Franch, H.A. (2013). Etiology of the protein–energy wasting syndrome in chronic kidney disease: A consensus statement from the International Society of Renal Nutrition and Metabolism (ISRNM). *Journal of Renal Nutrition, 23*(2), 77-90. doi:10.1053/j.jrn.2013.01.001

Centers for Medicaid and Medicare Services (CMS). (2014). *Conditions of participation for transplant centers.* Retrieved from http://www.cms.gov/Medicare/Provider-Enrollment-and-Certification/CertificationandComplianc/Transplant.html

Chang, A., & Kramer H. (2013). Effect of obesity and the metabolic syndrome on incident kidney disease and the progression to chronic kidney failure. In J.D. Kopple, S.G. Massry, & K. Kalantar-Zadeh (Eds.), *Nutritional management of renal disease* (3rd ed., pp. 445-456). New York: Elsevier Academic Press.

Chang, H., Miller, M.A., & Bruns, F.J. (2002). Tidal peritoneal dialysis during pregnancy improves clearance and abdominal symptoms. *Peritoneal Dialysis International, 22*(2), 272-274.

Charney, P., & Marian, M. (2008) Nutrition screening and assessment. *ADA pocket guide to nutrition assessment* (2nd ed., pp. 1-19). Academy of Nutrition and Dietetics.

Chatzikyrkou, C., Menne, J., Gwinner, W., Schmidt, B.M., Lehner, F., Blume, C., ... Schiffer, M. (2011). Pathogenesis and management of hypertension after kidney transplant. *Hypertension, 29*(12), 2283-2294.

Chauveau, P., Combe, C., Laville, M., Foque, D., Azar, R., Cano, N., & Canaud, B. (2001). Factors influencing survival in hemodialysis patients aged older than 75 years: 2.5 year outcome study. *American Journal of Kidney Disease, 35*(5), 997-1003.

Chazot, C., & Kopple, J.D. (2013) Vitamin metabolism and requirements in renal disease and renal failure. In J.D. Kopple, S.G. Massry, & K. Kalantar-Zadeh (Eds.), *Nutritional management of renal disease* (3rd ed., pp 351-382). New York: Elsevier Academic Press.

Cooke, J. (2004). Practical aspects of herbal supplement use in chronic kidney disease. *Journal of Renal Nutrition, 14*(1), e1-e4.

Davidson, J., Wilkinson, A., Dantal, J, Dotta, F, Haller, H., Hernandez, D., ... Wheeler, D.C. (2003). New-onset diabetes after transplantation: 2003 International consensus guidelines. *Transplantation, 75*(Suppl. 10), SS3-SS24.

de Brito-Ashurst, I., Perry, L., Sanders, T.A., Thomas, J.E., Dobbie, H., Varagunam, M., & Yaqoob, M.M. (2013). The role of salt intake and salt sensitivity in the management of hypertension in South Asian people with chronic kidney disease: A randomized controlled trial. *Heart, 99*(17), 1256-1260.

DeWalt, D.A., Callahan, L.F., Hawk, V.H., Broucksou, K.A., Hink, A., Rudd, R., & Brach, C. (2010). *Health literacy universal precautions toolkit.* (Prepared by North Carolina Network Consortium, The Cecil G. Sheps Center for Health Services Research, The University of North Carolina at Chapel Hill, under Contract No. HHSA290200710014.) AHRQ Publication No. 10-0046-EF). Rockville, MD: Agency for Healthcare Research and Quality.

Diabetes Control and Complications Trial (DCCT) Research Group. (1993). The effect of intensive treatment of diabetes on the development and progression of long-term complications in insulin-dependent diabetes mellitus. *New England Journal of Medicine, 329*(14), 977-986.

DiBenedetto, P., & Brommage, D. (2013). Nutrition assessment in chronic kidney disease. In L. Byham-Gray, J. Stover, & K. Wiesen (Eds.), *A clinical guide to nutrition care in kidney disease* (2nd ed., pp. 7-24). Chicago: Academy of Nutrition and Dietetics.

DiCecco, S.R. (2007). Medical weight loss treatment options in obese solid-organ transplant candidates. *Nutrition in Clinical Practice, 22*(5), 505-511.

Evert, A.B., Boucher, J.L., Cypress, M., Dunbar, S.A., Franz, M.J., Mayer-Davis, E.J., ... Yancy, W.S. (2013). Nutrition therapy recommendations for the management of adults with diabetes. *Diabetes Care, 36*(11), 3821-3842.

Filipowicz, R., & Beddhu, S. (2013). Optimal nutrition for predialysis chronic kidney disease. *Advances in Chronic Kidney Disease, 20*(2), 175-179.

Fissell, R.B., Bragg-Gresham, J.L., Gillespie, B.W., Goodkin, D.A., Bommer, J., Saito, A., ... Young, E.W. (2004). International variation in vitamin prescription and association with mortality in the Dialysis Outcomes and Practice Patterns Study (DOPPS). *American Journal of Kidney Disease, 44*(2), 293-299.

Fouque, D., Kalantar-Zadeh, K., Kopple, J., Cano, N., Chauveau, P., Cuppari, L., ... Wanner, C. (ISRNM) (2008). A proposed nomenclature and diagnostic criteria for protein–energy wasting in acute and chronic kidney disease. *Kidney International, 73*(4), 391-398.

Fredericksen, M.C. (2001). Physiologic changes in pregnancy and their effect on drug disposition. *Seminars in Perinatology, 23*(3), 120-123.

Frohlich, E.D., & Susic, D. (2011). Sodium and its multiorgan targets. *Circulation, 124*(17), 1882-1885.

Fuhrman, M.P., & Charney, P. (2004). Hepatic proteins and nutrition assessment. *Journal of the American Dietetic Association, 104*(8), 1258-1264.

Gerich, J.E., Meyer, C., Woerle, H.J., & Stumvoll, M. (2001). Renal gluconeogenesis: Its importance in human glucose homeostasis. *Diabetes Care, 24*(2), 382-391.

Goody, C.M., & Drago, L.D. (2010). Introduction: Cultural competence and nutrition counseling. In C.M. Goody & L.D. Drago (Eds.), *Cultural food practices* (pp.1-17). Chicago: Academy of Nutrition and Dietetics.

Graves, D.E., & Suitor, C.W. (1998). Celebrating diversity: Approaching families through their food. Retrieved from http://www.mchlibrary.info/pubs/pdfs/CelebratingDiversity.pdf

Greene, J.H., & Gutekunst, L. (2013). Medications commonly prescribed in chronic kidney disease. In L. Byham-Gray, J. Stover, & K. Wiesen (Eds.), *A clinical guide to nutrition care in kidney disease* (2nd ed., pp. 217-238). Chicago: Academy of Nutrition and Dietetics.

Haddad, N., Hebert, L.A., & Shim, R. (2013). Nutritional management of water, sodium, potassium, chloride, and magnesium in kidney disease and kidney failure. In J.D. Kopple, S.G. Massry, & K. Kalantar-Zadeh (Eds.), *Nutritional management of renal disease* (3rd ed., pp. 323-338). New York: Elsevier Academic Press.

Hammond, K. (1997). Physical assessment: A nutritional perspective. *Nursing Clinics of North America, 32*(4), 779-790.

Hammond, K. (1999). The nutritional dimension of physical assessment. *Nutrition, 15*(5), 411-419.

Handelman, G.J., & Levin, N.W. (2011). Guidelines for vitamin supplements in chronic kidney disease patients: What is the evidence? *Journal of Renal Nutrition, 21*(1), 117-119.

Hasse, J.M., & Matarese, L.E. (2012). Solid organ transplantation. In M.M. Gottschlick (Ed.), *The A.S.P.E.N. nutrition support core curriculum.* Dubuque, IA: ASPEN.

Hou, S. (2008). Pregnancy and renal disease. In A.K. Singh (Ed.), *Educational review manual in nephrology* (2nd ed., pp. 251-278). New York: Castle Connolly Graduate Medical Publishing.

Hou, S. (2010). Pregnancy in women treated with dialysis: Lessons from a large series over 20 years. *American Journal of Kidney Disease, 56*(1), 5-6.

Hou, S., & Grossman, S. (2014). Obstetrics and gynecology in dialysis patients. In J.T. Daugirdas, P.G. Blake,. & T.S. Ing. (Eds.), *Handbook of dialysis* (5th ed, pp. 736-753). Baltimore: Lippincott Williams & Wilkins.

Hutson, B., & Stuart, N. (2013). Nutrition management of the adult hemodialysis patient. In L. Byham-Gray, J. Stover, & K. Wiesen (Eds.), *A clinical guide to nutrition care in kidney disease* (2nd ed., pp. 53-68), Chicago: Academy of Nutrition and Dietetics.

Institute of Medicine (IOM). (2010). *Dietary reference intake tables.* Retrieved from http://iom.edu/Activities/Nutrition/SummaryDRIs/DRI-Tables.aspx

Institute of Medicine (IOM). (2013). *Sodium intake of populations: Assessment of evidence.* Retrieved from http://www.iom.edu/~/media/files/report%20files/2013/sodium-intake-populations/sodiumintakeinpopulations_rb.pdf

Jiwakanon, S., & Mehrotra, R. (2013). Nutritional management of end-stage renal disease patients treated with peritoneal dialysis. In J.D. Kopple, S.G. Massry, & K. Kalantar-Zadeh (Eds.), *Nutritional management of renal disease* (3rd ed., pp. 539-561). New York: Elsevier Academic Press.

Johansson, L., Hickson, M., & Brown, E.A. (2013). Influence of psychosocial factors on the energy and protein intake of older people on dialysis. *Journal of Renal Nutrition, 23*(5), 348-355.

Kalantar-Zadeh, K., & Kopple, J.D. (2013) In J.D. Kopple, S.G. Massry, & K. Kalantar-Zadeh (Eds.), *Nutritional management of renal disease* (3rd ed., pp. 503-529). New York: Elsevier Academic Press.

Karosanidze, T. (2014). Kidney and pancreas transplantation: Nutrition challenges and management. *Renal Nutrition Forum, 33*(1), 15-19.

Kayikcioglu, M., Tumuklu, M., Ozkahya, M., Ozdogan, O., Asci, G., Duman, S., ... Ok, E. (2009). The benefit of salt restriction in the treatment of end-stage renal disease by haemodialysis. *Nephrology Dialysis Transplantation, 24*(3), 956-962.

Kidney Disease: Improving Global Outcomes (KDIGO). (2009a) Clinical practice guideline for the diagnosis, evaluation, prevention and treatment of chronic kidney disease-mineral and bone disorder. *Kidney International, 76*(Suppl. 113), S1-S130.

Kidney Disease: Improving Global Outcomes (KDIGO). (2009b). Transplant Work Group. KDIGO clinical practice guideline for the care of kidney transplant recipients. *American Journal of Transplantation 9*(Suppl. 3), S1-S157.

Kidney Disease: Improving Global Outcomes (KDIGO). (2012). KDIGO clinical practice guideline for the management of blood pressure in chronic kidney disease. *Kidney International Supplement, 2*(5), 337-414.

Kidney Disease: Improving Global Outcomes (KDIGO). (2013a). KDIGO clinical practice guideline for the evaluation and management of chronic kidney disease. *Kidney International Supplement, 3*(1), S1-S150.

Kidney Disease: Improving Global Outcomes (KDIGO). (2013b). KDIGO clinical practice guideline for lipid management in chronic kidney disease. *Kidney International, 3*(3), 1-305.

Klahr, S., Levey, A.S, Beck, G.J., Caggiula, A.W., Hunsicker, L., Kusek, J.W., & Striker, G., for the Modification of Diet in Renal Disease Study Group. (1994). The effects of dietary protein restriction and blood-pressure control on the progression of chronic renal disease. *New England Journal of Medicine, 330*(13), 877-884.

Klatsky, A.L. (2003). Drink to your health? *Scientific American, 288*(2), 74-81.

Knowler, W., Barrett-Connor, E., Fowler, S., Hamman, R., Lachin, J., Walker, E., & Nathan, D. (2002). Reduction in the incidence of type 2 diabetes with lifestyle intervention or Metformin. *New England Journal of Medicine, 346*(6), 393-403.

Kotchen, T.A., Cowley, A.W., Jr., & Frohlich, E.D. (2013). Salt in health and disease – A delicate balance. *New England Journal of Medicine, 368*(13), 1229-1237.

Kutner, M., Greenberg, E., Jin,Y., & Paulsen, C. (2006). *The health literacy of America's adults: Results from the 2003 National Assessment of Adult Literacy* (p. 483). U.S. Department of Education. Washington, DC: National Center for Education Statistics.

Maduell, F., & Navarro, V. (2001). Assessment of salt intake in hemodialysis. *Nefrologia, 21*(1), 71-77.

McCann, L. (2009). *Pocket guide to nutritional assessment of the renal patient* (4th ed.). New York: National Kidney Foundation.

McCann, L. (2013). Nutrition management of the adult peritoneal dialysis patient. In L. Byham-Gray, J. Stover, & K. Wiesen (Eds.), *A clinical guide to nutrition care in kidney disease* (2nd ed., pp. 69-85). Chicago: Academy of Nutrition and Dietetics.

McCausland, F.R., Waikar, S.S., & Brunelli, S.M. (2013). The relevance of dietary sodium in hemodialysis. *Nephrology Dialysis & Transplantation, 28*(4), 797-802.

McMahon, E.J., Bauer, J.D., Hawley, C.M., Isbel, N.M., Stowasser, M., Johnson, D.W., & Campbell, K.L. (2013). A randomized trial of dietary sodium restriction in CKD. *Journal American Society of Nephrology, 24*(12), 2096-2103.

McMahon, E.J., Campbell, K.L., Mudge, D.W., & Bauer, J.D. (2012). Achieving salt restriction in chronic kidney disease. *International Journal of Nephrology, 2012*, Article ID 720429. doi:10.1155/2012/720429

McMurray, S., Johnson, G., Davis, S., & McDougall, K. (2002). Diabetes education care management significantly improves patient outcomes in the dialysis unit. *American Journal of Kidney Diseases, 40*(3), 566-575.

McPartland, K.J., & Pomposelli, J.J. (2007). Update on immunosuppressive drugs used in solid-organ transplantation and their nutrition implications. *Nutrition in Clinical Practice, 22*(5), 467-473.

McPhatter, L. (2013). Nocturnal home hemodialysis. In L. Byhan-Gray, J. Stover, & K. Wiesen (Eds.), *A clinical guide to nutrition care in kidney disease* (2nd ed., pp 279-283). Chicago: Academy of Nutrition and Dietetics.

Meier-Kriesche, H., Andorfer, J.A., & Kaplan, B. (2002). The impact of body mass index on renal transplant outcomes: A significant independent risk factor for graft failure and patient death. *Transplantation, 73*(1), 70-74.

Miller, E.R., III, Juraschek, S.P., Appel, L.J., Madala, M., Anderson, C.A., Bleys, J., & Guallar, E. (2009). The effect of n-3 long-chain polyunsaturated fatty acid supplementation on urine protein excretion and kidney function: Meta-analysis of clinical trials. *American Journal of Clinical Nutrition, 89*(6), 1937-1945.

Modanlou, K.A., Muthyala, U., Xiao, H., Schnitzler, M.A., Salvalaggio, P.R., Brennan, D.C., … Lentine, K.L. (2009). Bariatric surgery among kidney transplant candidates and recipients: Analysis of the United States Renal Data System and literature review. *Transplantation, 87*(8), 1167-1173.

Molnar, M.Z., Streja, E., Kovesdy, C.P., Bunnapradist, S., Sampaio, M.S., Jing, J., … Kalantar-Zadeh, K. (2011). Associations of body mass index and weight loss with mortality in transplant-waitlisted maintenance hemodialysis patients. *American Journal of Transplantation, 11*(4), 725-736.

Nadeau-Fredette, A.C., Hladunewich, M., Hui, D., Keunen, J., & Chan, C.T. (2013). End-stage renal disease and pregnancy. *Advances in Chronic Kidney Disease, 20*(3), 246-252.

National Institute of Health (NIH) (2014). *Assessing your weight and health risk.* Retrieved from http://www.nhlbi.nih.gov/guidelines/obesity/e_txtbk/txgd/4142.htm

National Kidney Foundation (NKF). (2000). Kidney Disease Outcomes Quality Initiative (K/DOQI) clinical practice guidelines for nutrition in chronic renal failure. *American Journal of Kidney Disease, 35*(6 Suppl. 2), S1-S104.

National Kidney Foundation (NKF). (2012). Kidney Disease Outcomes Quality Initiative (K/DOQI) clinical practice guidelines for diabetes and CKD: 2012 Update. *American Journal of Kidney Disease, 60*(5), S60-S105.

National Cholesterol Education Program (NCEP). (2001). Expert panel on detection, evaluation, and treatment of high blood cholesterol in adults (Adult Treatment Panel III). *Journal of the American Medical Association, 285*(19), 2486-2497.

National Patient Safety Foundation. (2013) Ask Me 3. Retrieved from http://www.npsf.org/for-healthcare-professionals/programs/ask-me-3/

National Research Council (NRC). (2011). Food and Nutrition Board. *Dietary reference intakes.* Washington, DC: National Academy of Sciences. Retrieved from http://www.iom.edu/about-iom/leadership-staff/boards/food-and-nutrition-board.aspx

Norris, K., & Nissenson, A.R. (2008). Race, gender, and socioeconomic disparities in CKD in the United States. *Journal of the American Society of Nephrology, 19*(7), 1261-1270.

Nowack, R. (2008). Review article: Cytochrome P450 enzyme, and transport protein mediated herb-drug interactions in renal transplant patients: grapefruit juice, St John's Wort – and beyond. *Nephrology, 13*(4), 337-347.

Obayashi, P.A. (2012). Food safety for the solid organ transplant patient: Preventing foodborne illness while on chronic immunosuppressive drugs. *Nutrition in Clinical Practice, 27*(6), 758-766.

Ozkahya, M., Ok, E., Toz, H., Asci, G., Duman, S., Basci, A., … Dorhout Mees, E.J. (2006). Long-term survival rates in haemodialysis patients treated with strict volume control. *Nephrology Dialysis Transplantation, 21*(12), 3506-3513.

Phillips, S., & Heuberger, R. (2012). Metabolic disorders following kidney transplantation. *Journal of Renal Nutrition, 22*(5), 451-460.

Postorino, M., Marino, C., & Tripepe, G. (2009). Abdominal obesity and all-cause cardiovascular mortality in end-stage renal disease.

Journal of the American College of Cardiology, 53(15), 1265-1272.

Potluri, K., & Hou, S. (2010). Obesity in kidney transplant recipients and candidates. *American Journal of Kidney Diseases, 56*(1), 143-156.

Reddy, S.S., & Holley, J. (2007). Management of the pregnant dialysis patient. *Advances in Chronic Kidney Disease, 14*(2), 246-255.

Renal Dietitians Practice Group (RPG). (2013). *RPG patient education handouts: Treatment for low blood sugar (hypoglycemia).* Retrieved from http://renalnutrition.org/files/uploads/RPG_Hypoglycemia.pdf

Rodrigo, E., Fernandez-Fresnedo, G., Valero, R., Ruiz, J.C., Pinera, C., Palomar, R., … Arias, M. (2006). New-onset diabetes after kidney transplantation: risk factors. *Journal of the American Society of Nephrology, 17*(12)(Suppl. 3), S291-S295.

Schatz, S., & Pagenkemper, J. (2013). Nutrition management of diabetes in chronic kidney disease. In L. Byhan-Gray, J. Stover, & K. Wiesen (Eds.), *A clinical guide to nutrition care in kidney disease* (2nd ed., pp. 117-121). Chicago: Academy of Nutrition and Dietetics.

Schatz, S.R. (2004). Helpful hints for common problems. In L. Byhan-Gray, J. Stover, & K. Wiesen (Eds.), *A clinical guide to nutrition care in kidney disease* (2nd ed., pp. 230-231). Chicago: Academy of Nutrition and Dietetics.

Schlenker, E.D. (2011). The food environment and food safety. In E.D. Schlenker & S.L. Roth (Eds.), *Williams' essentials of nutrition and diet therapy* (pp.190-192). St. Louis: Elsevier.

Seidel, H.M., Ball, J.W., Dains, J.E., Flynn, J.A, Solomon, B.S., & Sewart, R.W. (2011). *Mosby's guide to physical examination* (7th ed.). St. Louis: Mosby.

Sucher, K.P., & Kittler, P.G. (2007). *Food and culture.* Belmont, CA: Wadsworth.

Susic, D., & Frohlich, E.D. (2011) Hypertensive cardiovascular and renal disease and target organ damage: Lessons from animal models. *Cardiorenal Medicine, 1*(3), 139-146.

United Kingdom Prospective Diabetes Study Group. (1998). Intensive blood-glucose control with sulphonylureas or insulin compared with conventional treatment and risk of complications in patients with type 2 diabetes (UKPDS 33). *Lancet, 352*(9131), 854-865.

United States Department of Agriculture-Food and Drug Administration (USDA-FDA). (2011). *Food safety for transplant recipients.* Retrieved from http://www.fda.gov/downloads/Food/ResourcesForYou/Consumers/SelectedHealthTopics/UCM312793.pdf

United States Renal Data System (USRDS). (2013). *Annual data report: Atlas of chronic kidney disease and end-stage renal disease in the United States* (pp. 215-228). Bethesda, MD: National Institutes of Health, National Institute of Diabetes and Digestive and Kidney Diseases.

Uribarri, J., & Calvo, M.S. (2003). Hidden sources of phosphorus in the typical American diet: does it matter in nephrology? *Seminars in Dialysis, 16*(3), 186-188.

Ward, H.J. (2009). Nutritional and metabolic issues in solid organ transplantation: Targets for future research. *Journal of Renal Nutrition, 19*(1), 111-122.

Ward, P., & Kutner, N.G. (1999.) Reported pica behavior in a sample of incident dialysis patients. *Journal of Renal Nutrition, 9*(1), 14-20.

White, J.V., Guenter, P., Jensen, G., Malone, A., & Schofield, M. (2012). Academy of Nutrition and Dietetics Malnutrition Work Group; A.S.P.E.N. Malnutrition Task Force; A.S.P.E.N. Board of Directors. Consensus statement of the Academy of Nutrition and Dietetics/American Society for parenteral and enteral nutrition: Characteristics recommended for the identification and documentation of adult malnutrition (undernutrition). *Journal of the Academy of Nutrition and Dietetics, 112*(5), 730-738.

World Health Organization (WHO) (2008).*Waist circumference and waist–hip ratio: Report of a WHO expert consultation.* Geneva, December 8-11. Retrieved from http://www.who.int/nutrition/publications/obesity/WHO_report_waistcircumference_and_waisthip_ratio/en/

Core Curriculum for Nephrology Nursing, Sixth Edition © 2015 American Nephrology Nurses' Association

Foundations in Pharmacology and Clinical Applications in Nephrology Nursing

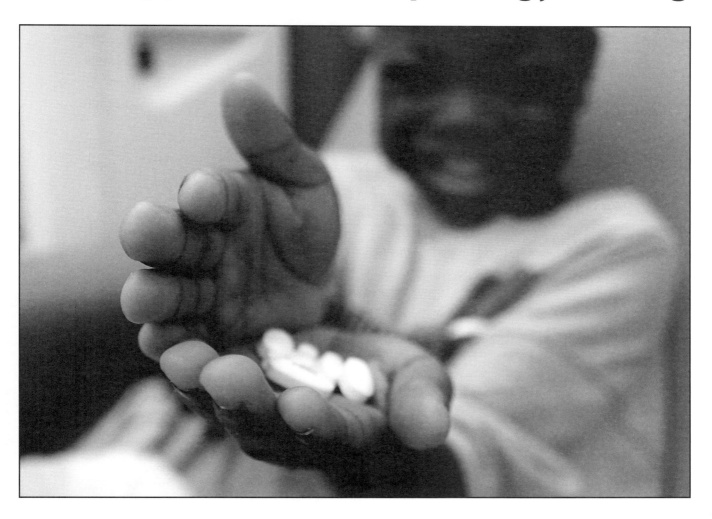

Chapter Editor
Elizabeth Wilpula, PharmD, BCPS

Authors
Elizabeth Wilpula, PharmD, BCPS
Francine D. Salinitri, PharmD

CHAPTER **5**

Foundations in Pharmacology and Clinical Applications in Nephrology Nursing

This offering for **1.6 contact hours with 1.6 contact hours of pharmacology content** is provided by the American Nephrology Nurses' Association (ANNA).

American Nephrology Nurses' Association is accredited as a provider of continuing nursing education by the American Nurses Credentialing Center Commission on Accreditation.

ANNA is a provider approved by the California Board of Registered Nursing, provider number CEP 00910.

This CNE offering meets the continuing nursing education requirements for certification and recertification by the Nephrology Nursing Certification Commission (NNCC).

To be awarded contact hours for this activity, read this chapter in its entirety. Then complete the CNE evaluation found at **www.annanurse.org/corecne** and submit it; or print it, complete it, and mail it in. Contact hours are not awarded until the evaluation for the activity is complete.

Example of reference in APA style for Chapter 5 Two authors for entire chapter.

Wilpula, E., & Salinitri, F.D. (2015). Foundations in pharmacology and clinical applications in nephrology nursing. In C.S. Counts (Ed.), *Core curriculum for nephrology nursing: Module 2. Physiologic and psychosocial basis for nephrology nursing practice* (6th ed., pp. 291-330). Pitman, NJ: American Nephrology Nurses' Association.

Interpreted: Chapter authors. (Date). Title of chapter. In ...

Cover photo by Robin Davis, BS, CCLS, Child Life Specialist, Texas Children's Hospital.

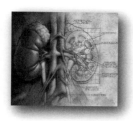

CHAPTER 5

Foundations in Pharmacology and Clinical Applications in Nephrology Nursing

Purpose

Patients with chronic kidney disease (CKD) are often prescribed numerous medications. As kidney function declines, comorbidities develop, and the number of medications prescribed usually increases. The average dialysis patient takes approximately 12 medications per day (Manley et al., 2004). As CKD progresses, drug disposition in the body is altered.

The large number of medications and changes in pharmacokinetic parameters may lead to an increased risk of toxicity, adverse drug reactions, and drug interactions. In addition, hemodialysis and peritoneal dialysis may have an effect on drug elimination and drug dosing.

All of these factors contribute to the need for drug dosage adjustments and/or increased monitoring in this patient population. Healthcare providers must be aware of the effects of kidney disease on medications in order to avoid adverse effects, provide education, and promote medication adherence.

The purpose of this chapter is to assist the clinician in meeting the challenges involved in the pharmacologic management of patients with CKD. To provide such assistance, the following topics are included:
1. An introduction to basic pharmacokinetic and pharmacodynamic principles.
2. The effect of chronic kidney disease on pharmacokinetics and pharmacodynamics.
3. Drugs commonly used with patients with CKD, including the purpose, goals of therapy, drug classification, and important nursing considerations.
4. An approach to drug dosing in patients with CKD.
5. The impact of dialysis on drug therapy.
6. The clinical significance for nursing, including monitoring and administering medications, educating the patient, and fostering adherence.

Objectives

Upon completion of this chapter, the learner will be able to:
1. Define the following pharmacokinetic concepts: half-life, steady state, protein binding, and concentration-time curve.
2. Describe pharmacokinetic changes that occur as kidney function declines.
3. Describe the goals of therapy for each of the common drug categories used in patients with CKD.
4. Differentiate and apply important nursing considerations for drugs within each category.
5. Compare and contrast a general approach for medication dosage adjustment for a patient with CKD who is receiving dialysis to one who is not.
6. Apply clinical concepts relating to pharmacology, medication administration, education, and adherence to the care of a patient with CKD.

Section A
Interactions Between Drugs and the Body

Interactions between drugs and the body are described by two terms: *pharmacokinetics* and *pharmacodynamics*. Pharmacokinetics refers to the way the body handles the drug while pharmacodynamics refers to the effects of the drug on the body.

I. Pharmacokinetics is the study of drug absorption, distribution, metabolism, and elimination. The pharmacokinetics of a drug will determine its plasma concentration levels at any given time. Other important concepts related to pharmacokinetics include bioavailability, half-life, and steady state.

A. Absorption.
1. Definition. Absorption is the process by which drugs pass from extravascular space (e.g., the skin, lungs, or GI tract) into the systemic circulation.
2. Rate of absorption. The rate of absorption is influenced by the following factors:
   a. The physiochemical properties of the drug.
   b. The concentration of the drug.
   c. The dosage form.
   d. The route of administration.
   e. The perfusion rate at the site of absorption.
   f. The surface area of the absorption site.
   g. The pH at the absorption site.
   h. First-pass metabolism. Table 5.1 summarizes these factors, their specific properties, and their effect on the rate of absorption.
3. Extent of absorption: bioavailability. The bioavailability is the extent or concentration of a

Table 5.1
Factors Affecting the Rate of Absorption

Factor	Specific Properties	Effect on Absorption Rate
Physicochemical properties	Molecular size	
	Large	Decreased
	Small	Increased
	Degree of ionization	
	Ionized	Decreased
	Nonionized	Increased
	Lipid solubility	
	High	Increased
	Low	Decreased
Concentration	High	Increased
	Low	Decreased
Dosage form	Liquid	
	Aqueous solution	Increased
	Oily solution	Increased over solid forms
	Suspension	Increased over some solid forms
	Solid	Decreased in comparison to many liquids
Route of administration	Intravenous	Circumvented – may have immediate effects
	Intramuscular	Rapid
	Subcutaneous	Rapid from aqueous solutions
	Pulmonary (gases, vapors, and aerosols)	Rapid
	Oral	Variable – drug dependent
	Sublingual/buccal	Rapid
	Rectal	Variable and often incomplete
	Topical	
	Mucous membranes	Semi-rapid
	Skin	Slow
Perfusion rate at absorption site	High flow rate	Increased
	Low flow rate	Decreased
Surface area of absorption site	Large surface area	Increased
	Small surface area	Decreased
pH at absorption site	Acidic pH	Increased for acidic compounds
	Basic pH	Decreased for acidic compounds
First-pass metabolism	High	Decreased
	Low	Increased

drug that reaches the systemic circulation once it has been absorbed. The absolute bioavailability is the amount of drug that has been absorbed by a certain route of administration (e.g., oral, subcutaneous, intraperitoneal) into systemic circulation. It is expressed as a fraction or percentage. For example, if 85% of an orally administered dose of a drug reaches systemic circulation, the bioavailability would be described as 0.85 or 85%.

    a. Clinical significance. The bioavailability is an important factor to determine the concentration of the drug at the site of action and the potential therapeutic or adverse effects. It is important to note, however, that the bioavailability of drugs is most often studied using healthy volunteers and may not always be extrapolated to patients with chronic kidney disease.

    b. First-pass metabolism. The bioavailability of an orally administered drug may be decreased by first-pass metabolism. First-pass metabolism is when a drug is metabolized by the gastro-intestinal tract or liver before it reaches systemic circulation. For example, if a drug is 100% absorbed through the gastrointestinal tract, but then 75% is eliminated during first-pass metabolism, then the bioavailability is 0.25, or 25%.

B. Distribution.
  1. Definition. Distribution is the movement of an absorbed drug from the site of administration to other locations in the body. The distribution of a drug will continue until the intravascular and extravascular concentrations reach equilibrium.
  2. Extent of distribution. The extent of distribution of a drug is dependent upon the factors listed below. Table 5.2 summarizes these factors, their specific properties, and their effects on drug distribution.
    a. Protein binding.
    b. Tissue binding.
    c. Lipid solubility.
    d. Polarity.
    e. The capillary permeability of various organs.
    f. The volume of body water.
    g. Perfusion rates.
    h. Redistribution.

C. Metabolism.
  1. Definition. Metabolism is the biochemical conversion of a drug to another chemical form via the processes of oxidation, reduction, hydrolysis, glucuronidation, and/or conjugation.
  2. Metabolism occurs primarily in the liver using the microsomal enzyme system, but it can also take

Table 5.2

Factors Affecting Drug Distribution

Factor	Specific Properties	Effect on Distribution
Protein binding	High percentage Low percentage	Decreased Increased
Tissue binding	High percentage Low percentage	Increased Decreased
Lipid solubility	High degree Low degree	Increased Decreased
Polarity	Polar Nonpolar	Decreased Increased
Capillary permeability	Increased Decreased	Increased Decreased
Volume of body water	Increased Decreased	Increased Decreased
Perfusion rates	Increased Decreased	Increased Decreased
Redistribution	Increased Decreased	Increased Decreased

place in the kidney, and to a lesser degree, in the lungs, plasma, and gastrointestinal tract.
  3. The result of metabolism is the production of drug metabolites that are usually more water soluble, less lipid soluble, more ionized at a normal pH, less protein bound, and less likely to be stored than the original drug.
  4. Drug metabolites are often excreted by the kidneys.

D. Elimination.
  1. Definition.
    a. Elimination is the process of removing drugs from the body in either their unaltered state or as metabolites.
    b. The kidneys perform their excretory function through the processes of glomerular filtration, tubular secretion, and tubular reabsorption.
  2. Influencing factors.
    a. The amount of drug that is filtered by the glomerulus and enters the tubules is dependent upon the concentration of the drug, its degree of plasma protein binding, perfusion rates, and the glomerular filtration rate (GFR).
    b. The renal clearance of a drug is determined by dividing the amount of the drug that is excreted over time by the plasma concentration of the drug.

3. Other systems involved in excreting drugs and their metabolites include the biliary, gastro-intestinal, pulmonary, integumentary, and glandular secretory systems.

E. Pharmacokinetic concepts and terms. The two pharmacokinetic parameters that affect all drugs include volume of distribution and clearance.

1. Volume of distribution (Vd). The volume of distribution is a term that relates the amount of drug distributed throughout the body to the amount of drug in the blood or intravascular space. It is an apparent volume that may exceed an individual's actual volume. The volume of distribution is used to determine necessary drug dose. The larger the volume of distribution, the more the drug distributes outside of the blood, and the greater the dose requirement would be.

   a. Clinical significance.
      (1) The volume of distribution is important to describe drug disposition and can give an indication of which compartment of the body (i.e., intravascular or extravascular) the drug has been distributed into. Drugs with a high volume of distribution generally have higher concentrations in the extravascular compartment. On the other hand, drugs with a volume of distribution similar to the volume of blood (i.e., 0.04 L/kg of body weight) are found primarily in the intravascular compartment.
      (2) The volume of distribution of a drug influences the half-life of a drug. The larger the volume of distribution, the longer the elimination half-life will be.
      (3) The volume of distribution of a drug determines the loading dose needed to reach a drug's intended systemic concentration.
   b. Plasma protein binding.
      (1) Definition. Drugs are often carried to the site of action by a carrier. Examples of carriers include:
         (a) Albumin.
         (b) Alpha-1-acid glycoprotein.
         (c) Other blood cells, such as erythrocytes.
      (2) Clinical significance. Drugs that are protein bound or bound to other cells are not active to exert the intended effect. The drug must be released from the protein (free drug) to exert its effect at the site of action. Only the free drug is active. Increases or decreases in plasma protein binding can have an effect on volume of distribution. As protein binding decreases, free drug increases and more drug is active and available to distribute throughout the body

(i.e., increased volume of distribution). The opposite is also true: as protein binding increases, there is less free drug to distribute and the volume of distribution is decreased. Dissolution from protein binding sites generally occurs passively from areas of higher concentration to lower concentration.
      (3) Principles of protein binding.
         (a) Serum blood concentrations for many drugs are a measure of the total concentration of drug in the body, including free drug and protein-bound drug. These are often referred to as total serum concentration.
         (b) The therapeutic effect of a given drug that corresponds to a total serum blood concentration will vary depending on the amount of drug that is bound to protein. At the same total serum concentration, a drug that is bound to more protein in the bloodstream will have less effect than if more drug is in the free state.
         (c) Metabolism and excretion are also dependent on protein binding. If more drug is bound to protein, less drug will be extracted by the liver for metabolism or by the kidney for excretion.
         (d) A drug can be displaced from protein binding sites by other drugs with a greater affinity for the protein. This will increase the amount of free drug in the bloodstream and increase the therapeutic or adverse effects of the drug.

2. Clearance.
   a. Definition. Clearance is the removal of active drug from the bloodstream. Clearance involves one or two processes: metabolism and/or elimination. Metabolism transforms the active drug into metabolites, which may be active or inactive. Elimination involves the removal of the active drug and/or metabolites from the bloodstream, usually by the kidney or biliary tract.
   b. Clinical significance.
      (1) The clearance of a drug is critical in determining the drug's half-life.
      (2) The clearance of a drug determines the maintenance dose of a drug.

3. Half-life (t ½).
   a. Definition. The half-life is the amount of time that it takes the body to decrease the concentration of the drug in the blood by one-half. As time continues to elapse in increments

equal to the half-life of the drug, exponential elimination of the drug will also continue.

b. Clinical significance. The half-life of a drug is a crucial element in determining the appropriate dosing intervals necessary for a drug to maintain therapeutic concentration levels in the body. Establishing time intervals for repeated dosages of a drug that are shorter than the amount of time required for elimination of the drug will result in accumulation of the drug and elevated serum concentrations. This could lead to toxicity and/or significant adverse effects for the patient.

4. Steady state.
   a. Definition. When a drug is administered repeatedly at a constant dosage and interval, it accumulates and the concentration in the blood reaches a plateau. The level of the concentration plateau is a function of the actual drug dosage and the dosage intervals. The time that is required for the concentration to reach the plateau is directly dependent upon the half-life of the drug. Once a plateau is reached, it will be maintained as long as the dosage and frequency of administration remain constant. Fluctuations in concentration will occur during the interim periods between dosage administrations; however, these fluctuations

occur around the plateau mean at identical intervals. Once steady state is achieved, the rate of drug going into the body equals the rate of drug being cleared from the body.

   b. Clinical significance. The steady state concept illustrates the importance of maintaining constant dosages and dosage intervals in achieving the specific, predictable, pharma-cologic action of a drug.

   c. Principles of steady state.
      (1) A loading dose is a bolus dose that can be administered to reach the desired concentration faster. A maintenance dose is then administered to maintain that concentration.
      (2) Often, loading doses are administered intravenously, but they can also be administered via other routes of administration.
      (3) If a loading dose is not administered, the time to reach steady state concentrations is generally equal to 4 to 5 half-lives of most drugs.

5. Concentration-time curve. Figure 5.1 illustrates a concentration-time curve. This is a generic representation of a drug concentration over time. The time and concentration designations are specific for each drug and patient, and are

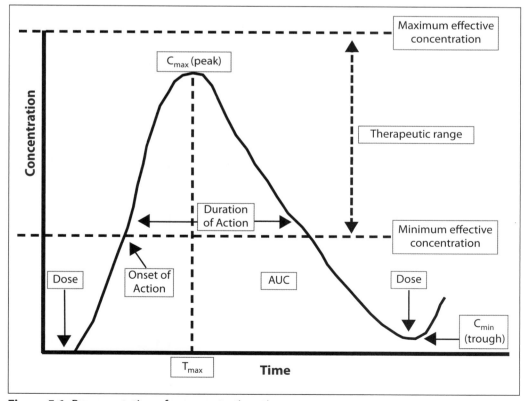

Figure 5.1. Representation of a concentration–time curve.

dependent upon the pharmacokinetic properties of the drug.

  a. Time designations.

    (1) Time of dose administration.

    (2) Time of maximum concentration (T_{max}). It is the time the drug reaches the maximum concentration.

    (3) The duration of action is the time that the drug exerts its intended effects. Generally, it is the time the drug concentration is above the minimum effective concentration.

    (4) Onset of action is the time that elapses between the time of administration and time to reach the minimum effective concentration.

  b. Concentration designations.

    (1) Maximum concentration (C_{max}). This is also called the *peak* concentration.

    (2) Minimum concentration (C_{min}). This is also called the *trough* concentration.

    (3) Maximum effective concentration.

    (4) Minimum effective concentration.

    (5) The area under the curve (AUC) illustrates the total amount of drug exposure over time.

    (6) The therapeutic range is the concentration range that the drug will have its intended effects with minimal toxicity.

II. Pharmacodynamics is the study of how a drug acts on the body. It refers to the biochemical effects and mechanisms of action of a drug in relation to specific dosages. The specific aspects of the drug that are important to pharmacodynamics are the drug effects, mechanisms of action, dosage-response curve of the drug, and therapeutic index.

A. Drug effects.

  1. Definition. Drug effects are those events that occur subsequent to the action of a drug. The action of a drug is the initial result of the interaction between a drug and a cell. During the interaction of a drug and a cell, cell function alters and begins a series of biochemical and physiologic changes that are characteristic of the drug. The initial result is the action of the drug, and all subsequent events constitute the effect of the drug.

  2. Example. The action of heparin is that it binds to a protein in the blood and inactivates clotting factors, while its effect is that it alters coagulation.

B. Mechanisms of action.

  1. Sites of action. In general, drugs act at one of three different sites within the body.

    a. Extracellularly.

    b. At the cellular membrane.

    c. Intracellularly.

  2. Mechanisms of action. Drugs act in different ways.

    a. Altering the chemical properties of a body fluid.

    b. Nonspecifically interacting with cell membranes.

    c. Selectively and specifically interacting with receptors.

C. Dose-response curve. The dose-response curve of a drug displays the observed patient response. A dose-response curve illustrates the threshold and maximal efficacy levels of a drug. Figure 5.2 presents an example of a generic dose-response curve.

D. Therapeutic index. The therapeutic index of a drug is an approximate quantification of its relative safety as it relates the minimum effective dose to the maximum tolerated dose.

  1. The therapeutic index of a drug is expressed as a ratio of the median toxic or lethal dose to the median therapeutic dose.

  2. As the therapeutic index of a drug becomes higher (expressed by increasingly wide ratios), the relative safety of the drug increases.

  3. As the therapeutic index of a drug narrows, the margin of safety becomes smaller, and the chances of toxicity or other adverse reactions increase.

  4. Drugs with a narrow therapeutic index are usually monitored by periodically checking serum concentrations. This is called "therapeutic drug monitoring." It helps to assure the drug concentrations are within a desired range to avoid toxicity and maintain efficacy.

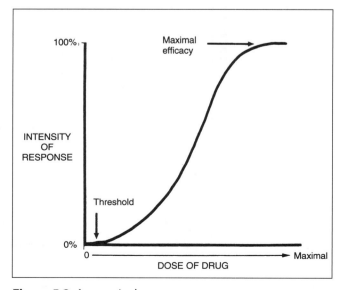

Figure 5.2. A generic dose-response curve.

E. Drug interactions.
1. Previously, concurrently, or subsequently administered drugs can modify the effects of another drug, often by altering the pharmacokinetics or pharmacodynamics of the drug.
2. Drug interactions may enhance or detract from the original therapeutic intent of the drug.
3. Drug interactions may lead to loss of efficacy or toxicity.

SECTION B
Effects of Chronic Kidney Disease on Drug Activity

As kidney function declines, the normal pharmacokinetics of drugs may be altered. As a result, some drugs may be contraindicated in patients with kidney disease or require dosage adjustment to avoid toxicity.

I. **Pharmacokinetics. The influence of CKD on the pharmacokinetics of drug activity is most obvious in the distribution and elimination processes.** However, absorption and metabolism are also somewhat altered.

A. Absorption. Factors affecting absorption.
1. Increased gastric pH. Some oral medications require an acidic environment for maximal absorption; increased gastric pH will result in decreased bioavailability.
   a. Increased gastric ammonia production.
   b. Antacids.
2. Altered gastrointestinal transit time. Altered transit time may affect the time of drug absorption but may not always affect the extent of absorption.
   a. Diarrhea.
   b. Vomiting.
   c. Diabetic gastroparesis.
3. Multiple medications and potential drug–drug interactions.
4. Alterations in first-pass metabolism can vary.

B. Distribution. The effect of CKD on the distribution of a drug is primarily related to the increased fluid volume and decreased amount of protein binding that occurs in uremic patients.
1. Alterations in fluid volume.
   a. Increased fluid volume increases the volume of distribution of water-soluble drugs because the drug distributes into the fluid, resulting in decreased plasma levels.
   b. Intravascular volume depletion and muscle wasting can decrease the volume of distribution, resulting in higher plasma levels.
2. Alterations in protein binding.
   a. Decreased serum albumin.
      (1) Serum albumin levels may be decreased in CKD due to malnutrition or chronic disease.
      (2) Decreased albumin results in decreased protein binding for acidic drugs, increasing free drug concentrations and volume of distribution.
   b. Uremia.
      (1) Uremia alters the structural orientation, decreases the number of binding sites on plasma proteins, and changes the binding affinity of drugs, resulting in higher free drug concentrations and increased volume of distribution.
      (2) Endogenous substances may accumulate in CKD and compete with binding sites on plasma proteins, resulting in increased free drug concentrations and volume of distribution.
   c. Increased alpha-1-acid glycoprotein.
      (1) Serum levels of alpha-1-acid glycoprotein may be increased.
      (2) Increased alpha-1-acid glycoprotein results in increased protein binding for basic drugs, decreasing free drug concentrations and possibly decreasing volume of distribution.

C. Metabolism. The kidney is a site for metabolism of some drugs. Consequently, renal metabolism is impaired when kidney function declines. Interestingly, CKD also has an effect on nonrenal metabolism as well. These effects are not well understood. However, the accumulation of specific uremic toxins may alter hepatic microsomal enzyme function (Yeung et al., 2013).

D. Elimination. The extent to which CKD influences drug excretion is a function of the percent of drug that is cleared unchanged by the kidney and by the pharmacologic activity of the drug's metabolites.
1. Drugs that are dependent upon the kidneys for elimination will have a decreased clearance and prolonged half-life in the presence of CKD.
2. The half-life of a drug increases gradually as the kidney function declines until the GFR falls below approximately 30 mL/minute. From that point, the half-life increases rapidly as the GFR continues to decrease. Figure 5.3 illustrates this relationship.
3. If the metabolites of a drug are dependent upon the kidney for elimination, the accumulation will occur. These metabolites may exhibit no effect, the desired effect of the parent drug (active metabolites), or possibly toxic adverse reactions.

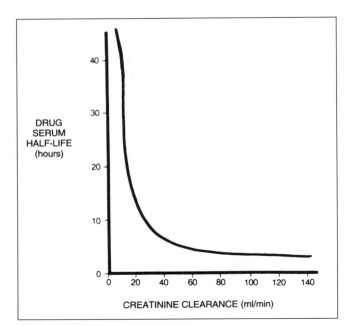

Figure 5.3. The relationship between drug half-life and creatinine clearance.

Examples:
  a. Toxic metabolite: normeperidine. Patients with kidney disease are at risk for central nervous system (CNS) toxicity and seizures due to the accumulation of meperidine's (Demerol®) renally eliminated metabolite, normeperidine.
  b. Active metabolite: morphine-6-glucuronide. Morphine-6-glucuronide is a major metabolite of morphine. It is a renally eliminated, active metabolite, and it can cause CNS toxicity and respiratory depression.

E. Concentration-time curve, half-life, and steady state. The concentration-time curve, half-life, and steady state of a drug will be altered by CKD.
  1. The concentration-time curve of a drug may be altered by CKD because of the effects on the pharmacokinetics of the drug.
  2. The half-life of a drug will be prolonged if the clearance or volume of distribution is altered by CKD.
  3. The steady state is reflective of the half-life and dosing schedule of a drug. If the half-life of a drug is extended, the time to reach steady state will be longer. In patients with CKD, the steady state concentration may also be higher than in individuals with normal kidney function. Meticulous monitoring and altering drug dosage schedules accordingly will help maintain a steady state that more closely approximates the normal range for a given drug.

Commonly prescribed drugs used in patients with CKD include the following: analgesics, acid suppressive therapy, alkalinizing agents, antianemics, antidiarrheals, antihypertensives, antimicrobials, calcimimetics, cation-exchange resins, cholesterol-lowering agents, diuretics, heavy metal chelating agents, H1 receptor antagonists, immunosuppressive agents, phosphate binders, prokinetics, and vitamin D. For each drug class, the use in CKD, goals of therapy, common agents, adverse effects, monitoring, and nursing considerations are listed.

I. Analgesics.

A. Use in CKD. Analgesics, both opioid and nonopioid, are used to control pain in patients with CKD when other types of interventions either do not work or are not appropriate.

B. Goals of therapy.
  1. Optimize pain control.
  2. Improve quality of life.
  3. Avoid analgesic induced complications. (American Society of Anesthesiologists Task Force on Chronic Pain Management & American Society of Regional Anesthesia and Pain Medicine, 2010).

C. Classification.
  1. Opioid analgesics (Chou et al., 2009).
    a. Agents.
      (1) Codeine.
      (2) Hydrocodone.
      (3) Hydromorphone (Dilaudid®).
      (4) Fentanyl (Duragesic®).
      (5) Meperidine (Demerol®).
      (6) Methadone (Dolopine®).
      (7) Morphine.
      (8) Oxycodone.
      (9) Tramadol (Ultram®).
    b. Mechanism of action. Opioid analgesics act on opioid receptors to alter the perception of pain, alter the pain threshold, or interfere with the conduction and response to pain in the central and peripheral nervous systems.
    c. Adverse effects and monitoring.
      (1) The most common adverse effect of opioid analgesics is constipation, so bowel regimens are routinely recommended with use of these agents. All vital signs must be monitored before administration and after the peak effect has been reached.

(2) Nausea, vomiting, sedation, altered mentation, pruritus, rash, and respiratory depression may occur.

(3) The use of these agents can lead to dependence, tolerance, and overdose.

d. Considerations.

(1) The smallest effective doses for alleviating pain should be administered.

(2) Many opioid analgesics are available in combination with nonopioid analgesics (e.g., hydrocodone/acetaminophen such as Vicodin®, Norco®, or Lortab®).

(3) Tramadol is often used over nonopioid analgesics for moderate pain in the CKD population because it is not associated with nephrotoxicity. Dose adjustments are required because the active metabolite of tramadol is renally eliminated and can accumulate in kidney disease.

(4) Morphine and codeine have an active metabolite that is eliminated by the kidney and may accumulate in patients with kidney disease. Although they are not contraindicated, repetitive doses should be avoided, and patients with CKD should be closely monitored for adverse effects.

(5) Normeperidine, a toxic metabolite of meperidine, is eliminated by the kidney and can accumulate in kidney disease, causing seizures. Use of this drug is contraindicated in patients with CKD.

(6) Patients taking opioids should avoid driving and dangerous work.

2. Nonopioid analgesics.

a. Agents.

(1) Acetaminophen (Tylenol®).

(2) Nonsteroidal antiinflammatory drugs (NSAIDs).

(a) Diclofenac (Voltaren®).

(b) Fenoprofen (Nalfon®).

(c) Ibuprofen (Advil®, Motrin®).

(d) Indomethacin (Indocin®).

(e) Ketoprofen (Orudis®).

(f) Ketorolac (Toradol®).

(g) Meloxicam (Mobic®).

(h) Naproxen (Naprosyn®).

(i) Celecoxib (Celebrex®).

(3) Salicylates.

(a) Aspirin.

(b) Diflunisal (Dolobid®).

(c) Salsalate.

b. Mechanism of action. Nonopioid analgesics decrease the production of prostaglandins, resulting in decreased sensitization of pain receptors and response to pain by the central nervous system.

c. Adverse effects and monitoring.

(1) NSAIDs and aspirin may cause gastrointestinal ulcers and bleeding. Celecoxib may have a lower incidence of this adverse effect.

(2) Prolonged use and high doses of NSAIDs can cause kidney damage and should be avoided in patients with CKD.

(3) The inhibition of cyclooxygenase (COX) impedes platelet function and may prolong bleeding or increase the risk of bleeding. Therefore NSAIDs and aspirin should be held prior to surgery.

d. Considerations.

(1) Nonopioid analgesics are preferred for mild to moderate pain.

(2) The smallest effective dose should be administered for the shortest amount of time.

(3) Acetaminophen is considered to be safe in patients with CKD and can be successfully used alone or in combination with low-dose opioids. High doses should also be avoided in severe kidney disease.

(4) Aspirin should be avoided in high doses in patients with CKD because the antiplatelet effects of aspirin and the effects of uremia on platelets increase the risk of bleeding. It can also lead to direct nephrotoxicity. However, low-dose aspirin (e.g., 81 to 325 mg/day) is often used for its cardioprotective effects.

(5) NSAIDs are used for their anti-inflammatory and analgesic properties; however, prostaglandin inhibition may compromise renal blood flow and result in direct nephrotoxic damage, particularly in individuals with preexisting kidney disease. These agents should be avoided in patients with CKD.

(6) Due to selective COX-2 enzyme inhibition, celecoxib has less gastrointestinal bleeding risk but a similar risk of nephrotoxicity as other NSAIDs.

(7) NSAIDs are associated with an increased risk of cardiovascular events (U.S. Food and Drug Administration [FDA], 2005). This risk may be increased with prolonged use and in patients with cardiovascular disease.

3. Anticonvulsants.

a. Agents.

(1) Gabapentin (Neurontin®).

(2) Pregabalin (Lyrica®).

b. Mechanism of action. Gabapentin and pregabalin have antinociceptive properties by inhibiting excitatory neurotransmitter release and are used specifically for neuropathic pain.

c. Adverse effect and monitoring (Zand et al., 2010).
   (1) Common adverse effects of these agents are dizziness, headache, somnolence, dry mouth, edema, blurred vision, weight gain, and difficulty concentrating.
   (2) Toxic adverse effects of gabapentin include dizziness, drowsiness, confusion, mental sluggishness, ataxia, myoclonus, and asterixis.
d. Considerations.
   (1) Gabapentin and pregabalin are primarily eliminated by the kidney and require dosage adjustment in patients with kidney disease.
   (2) These agents can be used as adjuncts to opioid analgesics to reduce opioid requirements (American Academy of Pain Medicine, 2013).

II. Acid suppressive therapy.

A. Use in CKD. Acid suppressive therapy is used to prevent or treat gastric irritation, ulceration, and bleeding.

B. Goals of therapy.
   1. Relieve symptoms of heartburn, reflux, esophagitis, and ulcers.
   2. Decrease recurrence of disease.
   3. Promote healing of esophagitis and ulcers.

C. Classification.
   1. H2 receptor antagonists.
      a. Agents.
         (1) Cimetidine (Tagamet®).
         (2) Famotidine (Pepcid®).
         (3) Ranitidine (Zantac®).
         (4) Nizatidine (Axid®).
      b. Mechanism of action. These agents competitively inhibit the action of histamine at the H2 receptor sites of the gastric parietal cells. As a result, the volume and hydrogen ion concentration of gastric acid secretions are decreased.
      c. Adverse events and monitoring.
         (1) These agents may cause hematologic abnormalities such as thrombocytopenia, leukopenia, and pancytopenia.
         (2) H2 receptor antagonists have been associated with the development of acute interstitial nephritis.
      d. Considerations.
         (1) Dosage adjustment is recommended for patients with hepatic and kidney disease.
         (2) Cimetidine inhibits tubular secretion of creatinine and may cause an increase in

serum creatinine without altering kidney function.
   2. Proton pump inhibitors.
      a. Agents.
         (1) Esomeprazole (Nexium®).
         (2) Lansoprazole (Prevacid®).
         (3) Omeprazole (Prilosec®).
         (4) Pantoprazole (Protonix®).
         (5) Rabeprazole (Aciphex®).
      b. Mechanism of action. These agents inhibit the H+-K+-ATPase pump in the gastric parietal cells. This results in dose-related decrease in gastric acid secretion.
      c. Adverse effects and monitoring.
         (1) These agents may cause nausea, vomiting, diarrhea, abdominal pain, headache, or dizziness.
         (2) Proton pump inhibitors, similar to H2 receptor antagonists, have been associated with the development of acute interstitial nephritis.
      d. Considerations.
         (1) These agents are metabolized in the liver and do not require dosage adjustments in patients with kidney disease.
         (2) These agents increase the gastric pH and can decrease the absorption of many drugs including iron salts and ketoconazole.
         (3) Safety with long-term use has not been fully elucidated. However, proton pump inhibitors may be associated with an increased risk of pneumonia, *Clostridium difficile* infection, and bone fractures.

III. Alkalinizing agents.

A. Use in CKD. Systemic alkalinizing agents are used in patients with CKD to prevent or treat metabolic acidosis.

B. Goals of therapy.
   1. Maintain systemic pH in the normal range (7.35 to 7.45).
   2. Maintain serum bicarbonate within the normal range (22 to 26 mEq/L) (National Kidney Foundation [NKF], 2000).

C. Classification.
   1. Systemic antacid.
      a. Agents.
         (1) Sodium bicarbonate.
         (2) Citrate/citric acid preparations (Shohl's solution and Bicitra®).
      b. Mechanism of action. Bicarbonate neutralizes hydrogen ions, causing increased systemic and urinary pH.
      c. Adverse effects and monitoring. These agents

can cause metabolic alkalosis, fluid retention, nausea, vomiting, and diarrhea.
  d. Considerations.
    (1) Use with caution in patients with heart failure.
    (2) Medications containing citrate should not be used with aluminum-containing agents because citrate significantly increases aluminum absorption. Aluminum accumulation can lead to encephalopathy and/or osteomalacia.
    (3) Alkalinizing agents may be discontinued once dialysis is initiated.

IV. Antianemics.

A. Use in CKD. Antianemic therapies are used to treat anemia associated with CKD. Patients with CKD develop a normochromic, normocytic anemia due to the lack of erythropoietin production by the diseased kidney. The Anemia Work Group of the National Kidney Foundation's (NKF) Kidney Disease Outcomes Quality Initiative (KDOQI) Project and more recently the Kidney Disease: Improving Global Outcomes (KDIGO) Anemia Work Group developed Clinical Practice Guidelines to assist the clinician with the management of anemia associated with CKD (Kliger et al., 2012; Kidney Disease: Improving Global Outcomes [KDIGO], 2012a).

B. Goals of therapy.
  1. Increase the quality of life of patients with CKD and prevent complications related to anemia.
  2. Maintain hemoglobin (Hgb) that does not exceed 11.5 mg/dL.
  3. Minimize the need for blood transfusion and the use of erythropoiesis-stimulating agents, and decrease anemia-related symptoms.
  4. Avoid or minimize risks associated with treatment (KDIGO, 2012a).

C. Classification.
  1. Erythropoiesis-stimulating agents (ESAs).
    a. Agents.
      (1) Darbepoetin alfa (Aranesp®).
      (2) Epoetin alfa (Epogen®, Procrit®).
    b. Mechanism of action. These agents are glycoproteins that are biologically similar to endogenous erythropoietin. They act on erythroid tissues within the bone marrow to stimulate differentiation of erythroid progenitor and early precursor cells to increase red blood cell production.
    c. Adverse effects and monitoring.
      (1) ESAs can increase blood pressure. Caution should be used when administering ESAs to patients with uncontrolled hypertension.
      (2) Other rare but serious adverse effects are thrombosis, seizure, and stroke.
    d. Considerations.
      (1) Use of ESAs to target hemoglobin above 11 mg/dL in patients with CKD has been associated with increased risk of death, serious cardiovascular events, stroke, and thrombosis (Drüeke et al., 2006; Pfeffer et al., 2009; Singh et al., 2006).
      (2) In patients with CKD not on dialysis, initiating ESA therapy when Hgb is >10 mg/dL is not recommended (KDIGO, 2012a).
      (3) In patients with CKD receiving hemodialysis, it is recommended to initiate ESA therapy when Hgb is between 9 mg/dL and 10 mg/dL to prevent the need for blood transfusions.
      (4) If there is an intent to cure, then due to disease progression and decreased survival, ESAs should be avoided in patients with breast, cervical, head and neck, lymphoid, and nonsmall-cell lung cancers.
  2. Iron supplementation.
    a. Agents.
      (1) Oral iron supplements.
        (a) Ferrous salts (ferrous sulfate, ferrous gluconate).
        (b) Polysaccharide iron complex (Niferex®).
      (2) Intravenous (IV) iron supplements.
        (a) Ferric carboxymaltose (Injectafer®).
        (b) Ferumoxytol (Feraheme®).
        (c) Iron dextran (INFeD®, DexFerrum®).
        (d) Iron sucrose (Venofer®).
        (e) Sodium ferric gluconate (Ferrlecit®).
    b. Mechanism of action. Iron deficiency is a common cause of anemia in patients with CKD. Iron supplementation replaces iron stores to ensure adequate erythropoiesis. Iron deficiency results in a microcytic, hypochromic anemia. In circulation, iron is bound to transferrin and can be released for incorporation into red blood cells. Excess iron is stored in the form of ferritin.
    c. Adverse effects and monitoring.
      (1) Oral formulations can cause gastrointestinal intolerances such as constipation, irritation, bloating, and dark stools.
      (2) IV iron formulations can cause hypotension, flushing, nausea, and injection site reactions.
      (3) Anaphylactoid reactions have been seen with the use of iron dextran, and rarely with the newer formulations (ferumoxytol, ferric carboxymaltose). All patients receiving intravenous iron should be

monitored closely. Iron dextran exhibits the highest risk of anaphylaxis; therefore, a test dose is recommended prior to its use.

    (4) Ferumoxytol can alter MRI results for up to 3 months after administration. Patients should be educated to notify their physicians if they are scheduled to undergo an MRI.

  d. Considerations.

    (1) Oral iron preparations are best absorbed in a fasting state.

    (2) Oral iron preparations can be given after meals to decrease gastric irritation and still provide adequate absorption.

    (3) Administering antacids or phosphate binders and iron preparations together significantly decreases iron bioavailability.

    (4) Oral iron preparations can decrease the absorption of drugs such as tetracycline and fluoroquinolone antibiotics.

    (5) Iron stores must be adequate to support bone marrow formation of new red blood cells before initiating therapy with ESAs.

    (6) It is recommended to trial iron therapy in patients naive to treatment prior to initiating ESAs when transferrin saturation (TSAT) is ≤ 30% and ferritin is ≤ 500 ng/mL (KDIGO, 2012a).

    (7) IV iron is preferred in hemodialysis patients, while oral or IV iron may be used in peritoneal dialysis or patients with CKD not receiving dialysis (KDIGO, 2012a).

    (8) If the iron stores become depleted during ESA therapy, replacement iron should be initiated.

    (9) Avoid giving IV iron to patients with active infection.

  3. B vitamins.

    a. Agents.

      (1) Cyanocobalamin (vitamin B12).

      (2) Folic acid (Folvite®).

      (3) Pyridoxine (vitamin B6).

      (4) Combination products (Nephrocap®, Nephrovite®, Rena-vite®).

    b. Mechanism of action. Deficiencies in B vitamins are often associated with distinct types of megaloblastic anemias. Supplements can replace lost or deficient stores in patients with CKD. The B vitamins are important in DNA synthesis and RBC proliferation.

    c. Adverse effects and monitoring. Minimal adverse effects are associated with B vitamin supplementation.

    d. Considerations.

      (1) B vitamins are water soluble and removed by hemodialysis and peritoneal dialysis.

      (2) Combination products are commonly prescribed to patients to replace B vitamins removed during hemodialysis.

      (3) B vitamins must be present in sufficient quantities for a patient to respond appropriately to ESA therapy.

V. Antidiarrheals.

A. Use in CKD. Antidiarrheals are used to treat persistent diarrhea resulting from intestinal irritation, medications, and other factors.

B. Goals of therapy.
  1. Prevent adverse effects related to dehydration and loss of electrolytes.
  2. Relieve symptoms.

C. Classification.
  1. Antimotility.
    a. Agents.
      (1) Loperamide (Immodium®).
      (2) Diphenoxylate/atropine (Lomotil®).
    b. Mechanism of action. Loperamide and diphenoxylate are opioid derivatives. They act on the intestine through the opioid receptor inhibiting GI motility.
    c. Adverse effects and monitoring.
      (1) Both agents may cause drowsiness or dizziness.
      (2) Diphenoxylate preparations contain atropine to discourage abuse. However, this may cause flushing, dry skin and mucous membranes, hyperthermia, tachycardia, and urinary retention.
    d. Considerations.
      (1) The underlying cause of diarrhea should be evaluated prior to initiating these therapies.
      (2) Diarrhea with an infectious etiology should be treated with antibiotics.
      (3) Diphenoxylate interacts with monoamine oxidase inhibitors and can precipitate a hypertensive crisis.

VI. Antihypertensives.

A. Use in CKD. Hypertension is the second leading cause of kidney disease requiring hemodialysis and is associated with significant cardiovascular morbidity and mortality (United States Renal Data System [USRDS], 2013). Hypertension is also a complication of CKD, and treatment often requires the use of two or more concurrently administered antihypertensive agents. All of these agents should be initiated at low doses and titrated to optimal effect (NKF, 2004).

B. Goals of therapy.
  1. Prevent the onset of kidney disease.
  2. Slow the progression of kidney disease.
  3. Reduce the risk of cardiovascular disease.
  4. Achieve a blood pressure goal of ≤ 140/90 mmHg in those who have normal urinary albumin excretion and ≤ 130/80 mmHg in those with evidence of moderately or severely increased albumin excretion (KDIGO, 2012b).

C. Classification.
  1. Alpha-1 adrenergic blockers.
    a. Agents.
      (1) Doxazosin (Cardura®).
      (2) Prazosin (Minipres®).
      (3) Terazosin (Hytrin®).
    b. Mechanism of action. These drugs decrease blood pressure by occupying the alpha-1 receptors of the sympathetic nervous system and blocking the effects of epinephrine and norepinephrine at those sites. This results in vasodilation, decreased peripheral resistance, and decreased plasma renin activity.
    c. Adverse effects.
      (1) All of these agents produce significant orthostatic hypotension and first-dose syncope as well as tachycardia and headache.
      (2) As a result of vasodilation, these agents may cause peripheral edema.
    d. Considerations.
      (1) These agents can be used as adjunct therapy in those patients with hypertension already treated with or who have failed on angiotensin-converting enzyme inhibitor or angiotensin receptor blocker, diuretic, calcium channel blocker, or beta-blocker (KDIGO, 2012b; James et al., 2014).
      (2) They improve maximal urine flow in males with benign prostatic hypertrophy.
  2. Alpha and beta adrenergic blockers.
    a. Agents.
      (1) Carvedilol (Coreg®).
      (2) Labetalol (Trandate®).
    b. Mechanism of action. These agents decrease blood pressure by blocking alpha and beta 1 and 2 adrenergic receptors. As a result, they decrease peripheral resistance, plasma renin levels, aldosterone levels, renal vascular resistance, and cardiac output. They also may increase plasma volume, renal blood flow, and GFR.
    c. Adverse effects.
      (1) These agents are known to cause broncho-spasms due to nonselective beta-blockade.
      (2) Mixed adrenergic blockers can mask the signs and symptoms of hypoglycemia in patients with diabetes.

    d. Considerations.
      (1) These agents should also be used with caution in patients with pulmonary disease and decompensated heart failure. In these patients, a B1-selective agent would be more appropriate if a beta-blocker is the drug of choice.
      (2) These agents should be avoided in patients with second- and third-degree heart block.
      (3) Beta-blockers should be used in patients with compelling indications such as history of heart failure, postmyocardial infarction, or cardiovascular disease (Yancy et al., 2013).
      (4) Carvedilol has demonstrated decreased mortality in patients with heart failure (Packer et al., 2002).
      (5) Labetolol is a short-acting beta-blocker and offers advantages for flexibility of dosing in patients receiving hemodialysis.
  3. Beta adrenergic blockers.
    a. Agents.
      (1) Selective B1 antagonists.
        (a) Atenolol (Tenormin®).
        (b) Bisoprolol (Zebeta®).
        (c) Metoprolol (Lopressor®, Toprol XL®).
      (2) Nonselective B1 + B2 antagonists.
        (a) Nadolol (Corgard®).
        (b) Pindolol (Visken®).
        (c) Propranolol (Inderal®).
        (d) Timolol (Blocadren®).
    b. Mechanism of action. Beta-blockers differ in their mechanisms of action based upon their selectivity for beta adrenergic receptors. B1 selective agents inhibit B1-receptors in the heart, causing a decrease in AV node conduction, heart rate, and contractility, which results in lowering blood pressure. B1 selective agents also lower blood pressure by inhibiting B1-receptors at the site of the juxtaglomerular apparatus where renin is released in the kidneys. Nonselective beta-blockers can also inhibit B2-receptors in the vasculature to decrease peripheral resistance and compete with norepinephrine for beta receptor sites, antagonizing the membrane effect of norepinephrine and epinephrine and blocking sympathetic stimulation.
      (1) These pharmacologic effects lead to decreased sympathetic outflow from vasomotor centers in the brain and thus reduce cardiac output and blood pressure.
      (2) They are also used to treat patients after a myocardial infarction (MI) and those with chronic heart failure.
    c. Adverse effects and monitoring.
      (1) These agents can cause fatigue, decreased

exercise tolerance, insomnia, bradycardia, and hypotension.

(2) Bradycardia is a common effect of beta-blockers, and heart rate should be monitored.

(3) Nonselective beta-blockers can cause bronchospasms.

(4) These agents can mask the signs and symptoms of hypoglycemia in patients with diabetes.

(5) All of these agents can precipitate or worsen depression.

d. Considerations.

(1) Beta-blockers should be used with caution in patients with pulmonary disease and decompensated heart failure. In these patients, a B1 selective agent would be preferred.

(2) These agents should be avoided in patients with second- and third-degree heart block.

(3) Beta-blockers should be used in patients with compelling indications such as history of heart failure, post-MI, or cardiovascular disease (Yancy et al., 2013).

(4) Bisoprolol and metoprolol succinate have demonstrated decreased mortality in patients with heart failure (Metoprolol CR/XL Randomised Intervention Trial in Congestive Heart Failure Study Group, [MERIT-HF], 1999; The Cardiac Insufficiency Bisoprolol Study Investigators and Committees [CIBIS], 1994, 1999).

4. Calcium channel blockers.

a. Agents.

(1) Nondihydropyridines.

(a) Diltiazem (Cardizem®, Cartia XT®, Tiazac®).

(b) Verapamil (Isoptin®, Calan®, Covera-HS®).

(2) Dihydropyridines.

(a) Amlodipine (Norvasc®).

(b) Felodipine (Plendil®).

(c) Isradipine (DynaCirc®).

(d) Nicardipine (Cardene®).

(e) Nifedipine (Procardia XL®, Adalat CC®).

(f) Nisoldipine (Sular®).

b. Mechanism of action. There are two main classes of calcium channel blockers: nondihydropyridines and dihydropyridines. All calcium channel blockers decrease blood pressure by preventing the entry of calcium into the cell and reducing the contraction of vascular smooth muscle. Nondihydropyridine calcium channel blockers preferentially decrease SA and AV conduction, heart rate, myocardial contractility, and peripheral

vascular resistance. The dihydropyridines decrease peripheral resistance by selectively causing vasodilatation and have fewer cardiac effects. In the kidney, nondihydropyridines dilate the afferent and efferent arterioles, reducing glomerular pressure, and cause decreased urine albumin excretion. Older dihydropyridines may cause an increase in urinary albumin excretion; however, this has not been shown with newer agents (Bakris et al., 2004; KDIGO, 2012b).

c. Adverse effects and monitoring.

(1) Nondihydropyridines can cause bradycardia, hypotension, headache, and constipation.

(2) Dihydropyridines have been associated with flushing, headache, dizziness, and peripheral edema.

d. Considerations.

(1) Nondihydropyridines have negative cardiac inotropic effects and must be used with caution in patients who have left ventricular dysfunction and systolic heart failure. These agents should also be avoided in patients with second- and third-degree heart block.

(2) Nondihydropyridines decrease urinary albumin excretion (KDIGO, 2012b). New dihydropyridine agents may also have this effect.

(3) Long-acting dihydrophyridines are often used in patients with angina because they may also decrease coronary vasospasm.

(4) Short-acting dihydropyridines produce significant vascular side effects, blood pressure swings, and concurrent increases in adrenergic responses such that they are not frequently used in treating hypertension in patients with CKD or in the general population.

5. Central acting.

a. Agents.

(1) Clonidine (Catapres®).

(2) Methyldopa (Aldomet®).

b. Mechanism of action. These agents decrease blood pressure by reducing sympathetic activity and subsequently decreasing arteriolar vasoconstriction. Clonidine stimulates inhibitory alpha-2 adrenergic receptors in the medulla to decrease sympathetic tone, peripheral resistance, heart rate, and cardiac output. Methyldopa forms a false neurotransmitter that stimulates the alpha adrenergic receptors and decreases sympathetic tone in the peripheral and renal vasculature.

c. Adverse effects and monitoring (KDIGO, 2012b).

(1) Both agents can cause dry mouth,

drowsiness, and sedation and sexual dysfunction.

   (2) Sudden discontinuation of these agents may result in a rebound hypertension.

d. Considerations.

   (1) Clonidine is available in topical patches for patients who are unable to take or are nonadherent to oral therapy.

   (2) Clonidine can be very effective for refractory hypertension in patients already receiving angiotensin-converting enzyme inhibitors, beta-blockers, and calcium channel blockers.

   (3) Clonidine should be avoided in patients with bradycardia and heart block, as well as when overt heart failure is present.

   (4) Methyldopa is commonly prescribed to treat hypertension in pregnancy.

6. Direct vasodilators.

a. Agents.

   (1) Hydralazine (Apresoline®).

   (2) Minoxidil (Loniten®).

   (3) Nitroprusside (Nipride®).

b. Mechanism of action. These drugs decrease blood pressure by relaxing arteriolar smooth muscle and producing vasodilation. Hydralazine and minoxidil also alter cellular calcium metabolism and inhibit calcium movement within the vascular smooth muscle. All of these agents decrease peripheral resistance and increase plasma volume, plasma renin activity, and heart rate. They all increase cardiac output.

c. Adverse effects.

   (1) All of these agents may produce fluid retention, reflex tachycardia, palpitations, peripheral edema, and headaches.

   (2) Minoxidil causes hirsutism.

   (3) Minoxidil has been reported to cause pericardial effusion and cardiac tamponade.

d. Considerations.

   (1) Beta-blockers are often given concurrently with these drugs to decrease the reflex tachycardia.

   (2) The adverse effects of minoxidil limit its use, especially in women, and thus it is primarily prescribed in patients with refractory hypertension.

   (3) Nitroprusside is available only in intravenous form and is primarily used in patients with hypertensive emergency.

   (4) Nitroprusside does not require dose adjustments in patients with kidney disease; however, accumulation of thiocyanate may occur with subsequent toxicity. Prolonged use of this agent should be avoided in this population.

7. Renin-angiotensin-aldosterone system antagonists.

a. Agents.

   (1) Angiotensin-converting enzyme (ACE) inhibitors.

     (a) Benazepril (Lotensin®).

     (b) Captopril (Capoten®).

     (c) Enalapril (Vasotec®).

     (d) Fosinopril (Monopril®).

     (e) Lisinopril (Prinivil®, Zestril®).

     (f) Moexipril (Univasc®).

     (g) Quinapril (Accupril®).

     (h) Rampril (Altace®).

   (2) Angiotensin II receptor blockers (ARBs).

     (a) Candesartan (Atacand®).

     (b) Irbesartan (Avapro®).

     (c) Losartan (Cozaar®).

     (d) Telmisartan (Micardis®).

     (e) Valsartan (Diovan®).

   (3) Renin inhibitor. Aliskiren (Tekturna®).

b. Mechanism of action. ACE inhibitors block the angiotensin-converting enzyme that converts angiotensin I to angiotensin II, while ARBs block angiotensin II receptors on target tissues. Through preventing the production or blocking the action of angiotensin II, these agents cause vasodilation and systemically lower blood pressure. They also decrease sodium and water retention and peripheral resistance, and increase cardiac output. In the kidney, they preferentially dilate the efferent arterioles, decreasing intraglomerular pressure and reducing urinary protein excretion. Renin inhibitors bind directly to renin, which prevents the conversion of angiotensinogen to angiotensin I. The decreased formation of angiotensin I results in decreased production of angiotensin II, systemically lowering blood pressure.

c. Adverse effects and monitoring.

   (1) Adverse effects associated with ACE inhibitors and ARBs include anemia, hyperkalemia, and orthostatic hypotension.

   (2) ACE inhibitors and ARBs may cause hyperkalemia. The risk of this adverse effect is increased in patients who are elderly or volume depleted; have diabetes, kidney disease, or heart failure; or in those receiving concomitant agents that cause potassium retention.

   (3) Angioedema is a rare but life-threatening adverse effect of ACE inhibitors and ARBs and is a contraindication for continued use. The risk is lower with ARBs than ACE inhibitors.

   (4) ACE inhibitors can cause chronic cough. Patients who develop this adverse effect should be switched to an ARB.

(5) ACE inhibitors and ARBs may cause acute kidney injury, particularly in patients with bilateral renal artery stenosis or patients who are volume depleted. Kidney function should be assessed at baseline and monitored within 1 month of initiation, during titration, and then annually or as indicated.

(6) In patients experiencing acute kidney injury, these agents should be held and be restarted when kidney function has recovered.

(7) A decrease in GFR of less than 30% or increase in serum creatinine of 30% is expected, and therapy should continue unless the decrease in GFR worsens.

d. Considerations.

(1) In patients with hypertension and CKD, ACE inhibitors or ARBs should be used as first-line therapy or add-on therapy (James et al., 2014).

(2) It is recommended that patients with diabetes and CKD not receiving hemodialysis and urine albumin excretion > 300 mg per day receive ACE inhibitors or ARBs to decrease the progression of kidney disease. These agents should also be considered in those patients who have a urine albumin excretion of 30 to 300 mg per day (KDIGO, 2012b).

(3) It is recommend that patients with CKD not receiving hemodialysis, without diabetes, who have a urine albumin excretion > 300 mg per day, and require blood pressure lowering agents, receive ACE inhibitors or ARBs to decrease the progression of kidney disease. These agents should also be considered in patients who have a urine albumin excretion of 30 to 300 mg per day (KDIGO, 2012b).

(4) ACE inhibitors decrease mortality and should be used in patients with systolic heart failure, with CAD, or post-MI. If a patient cannot tolerate an ACE inhibitor, an ARB may be used (Pfeffer et al., 2003; The Results of the Cooperative North Scandinavian Enalapril Survival Study [CONSENSUS] Group, 1987; The SOLVD Investigators, 1992; Yancy et al., 2013).

(5) Direct renin inhibitors should not be used in combination with ACE inhibitors or ARBs due to the potential risk of increased adverse events (KDIGO, 2012b).

VII. Antimicrobials.

A. Use in CKD. Chronic kidney disease and dialysis increase the risk of infection. As a result, these patients frequently require treatment with antimicrobial agents. Many antimicrobial agents require dosage adjustments when being administered to patients with CKD. Table 5.3 lists selected antimicrobial agents that require varying levels of dosage adjustments for use in these patients.

B. Goals of therapy: optimize clinical outcomes associated with infections.

C. Classification.
   1. Antifungals.
      a. Azole antifungals.
         (1) Agents.
            (a) Fluconazole (Diflucan®).

Table 5.3

Selected Antimicrobial Agents Requiring Dosage or Interval Adjustment in Patients with CKD

No Adjustment	Adjustment
Amphotericin B*	Acyclovir*
Azithromycin	Amikacin*
Caspofungin	Amoxicillin
Chloramphenicol	Ampicillin
Clindamycin	Aztreonam
Doxycycline	Carbenicillin
Erythromycin	Cefepime
Ketoconazole	Cefazolin
Linezolid	Ceftaroline
Metronidazole	Ceftazidime
Micafungin	Cefotetan
Moxifloxacin	Cefoxitin
Nafcillin	Ciprofloxacin
Rifampin	Daptomycin
Tigecycline	Ertapenem
	Fluconazole
	Foscarnet*
	Ganciclovir
	Gentamicin*
	Imipenem/Cilastin
	Kanamycin*
	Levofloxacin
	Meropenem
	Neomycin*
	Penicillin G
	Piperacillin/tazobactam
	Streptomycin*
	Sulfamethoxazole/Trimethoprim
	Ticarcilllin
	Tobramycin*
	Vancomycin

* Can be nephrotoxic.

(b) Itraconazole (Sporanox®).
(c) Ketoconazole (Nizoral®).
(d) Miconazole (Monistat®).
(e) Posaconazole (Noxafil®).
(f) Voriconazole (Vfend®).
(2) Mechanism of action. Azole antifungals inhibit the enzyme responsible for the formation of ergosterol, which results in the inhibition of the fungal cell membrane.
(3) Adverse effects and monitoring.
  (a) Hepatotoxicity has been reported with all azole antifungals. Monitoring of liver function tests is recommended.
  (b) Recent ketoconazole product labeling changes include a warning about severe liver toxicity, QT prolongation, and adrenal insufficiency (FDA, 2013).
  (c) Visual disturbances, neurologic toxicity, and rash are adverse reactions associated with voriconazole.
(4) Considerations.
  (a) Drug interactions are common with azole antifungals because they are substrates and inhibitors of some CYP450 enzymes.
  (b) The absorption of posaconazole is increased when taken with high-fat foods.
  (c) Itraconazole and ketoconazole require an acidic environment for absorption. H2 receptor antagonists and PPI may decrease their absorption.
  (d) While the pharmacokinetics of posaconazole and voriconazole are not altered in kidney disease, the intravenous formulations contain a vehicle (sulfobutyl ether beta-cyclodextrin sodium) that may accumulate. The intravenous formulations should be used with caution or avoided in these patients.
  (e) The dose of fluconazole should be decreased in patients with kidney disease.
b. Echinocandins.
  (1) Agents.
    (a) Caspogungin (Cancidas®).
    (b) Micafungin (Mycamine®).
  (2) Mechanism of action. Inhibit the synthesis of β-(1,3)-D-glycan, which is essential in the cell wall formation of some species of fungi.
  (3) Adverse effects and monitoring. These agents are well tolerated; however, may rarely cause hepatotoxicity or mild gastrointestinal effects such as nausea, vomiting, and diarrhea.

(4) Considerations. These agents are available in intravenous form only.
c. Amphotericin B.
  (1) Agents.
    (a) Amphotericin B deoxycholate (Fungizone®).
    (b) Amphotericin B lipid complex (Abelcet®).
    (c) Liposomal amphotericin B (Ambisome®).
  (2) Mechanism of action. Amphotericin B binds to ergosterol and alters fungal cell wall permeability. This leads to cell death.
  (3) Adverse effects and monitoring.
    (a) Amphotericin is a nephrotoxic agent. Nephrotoxicity may occur in up to 50% of patients on the conventional formulation (amphotericin B deoxycholate) (Pappas et al., 2009). Serum creatinine and urine output should be monitored closely and its use should be avoided with other nephrotoxic drugs. The incidence of nephrotoxicity with the lipid formulations is less than the conventional formulation.
    (b) Nephrotoxicity caused by amphotericin B has been associated with an increased risk of death (Bates et al., 2001).
    (c) Premedications may be administered to some patients to prevent infusion reactions. Patients should be monitored closely during the infusion for fever, chills, nausea, vomiting, hypotension, bronchospasm, and anaphylaxis. They often occur 1 to 2 hours after the start of the infusion.
    (d) Electrolyte abnormalities, including hypomagnesemia and hypokalemia, are common.
  (4) Considerations.
    (a) Patients receiving other nephrotoxic agents or longer durations of therapy have an increased risk of nephrotoxicity.
    (b) Adequate hydration can decrease the risk of nephrotoxicity.
2. Antibacterial agents.
  a. Aminoglycosides.
    (1) Agents.
      (a) Amikacin (Amikin®).
      (b) Gentamicin (Garamycin®).
      (c) Kanamycin (Kentrex®).
      (d) Tobramycin (Tobrex®).
    (2) Mechanism of action. Aminoglycosides interfere with bacterial protein synthesis by binding to the 30s and 50s ribosomal subunits.

(3) Adverse effects and monitoring.
  (a) Aminoglycosides are nephrotoxic agents. Close monitoring of serum creatinine and urine output is required throughout therapy.
  (b) Aminoglycosides can cause vestibular toxicity. This risk is increased with prolonged use and may be irreversible.
  (c) Serum peak and trough levels are monitored to evaluate efficacy and decrease the risk of toxicity.
(4) Considerations.
  (a) Aminoglycosides are primarily eliminated by the kidney. Dosage adjustment is necessary if they are used in patients with CKD.
  (b) Preexisting CKD is a risk factor for the development of nephrotoxicity, and their use is often avoided in this population.
  (c) Aminoglycosides and penicillins should not be administered within 2 hours of one another.
b. Cephalosporins.
  (1) Agents.
    (a) First generation.
      i. Cefazolin (Ancef®).
      ii. Cephalexin (Keflex®).
    (b) Second generation.
      i. Cefotetan (Cefotan®).
      ii. Cefoxitin (Mefoxitin®).
      iii. Cefuroxime (Ceftin®).
    (c) Third generation.
      i. Cefotaxime (Claforan®).
      ii. Ceftazidime (Fortaz®).
      iii. Ceftriaxone (Rocephin®).
    (d) Fourth generation: cefepime (Maxipime®).
    (e) Fifth generation: ceftaroline (Teflaro®).
  (2) Mechanism of action. These agents are beta-lactam antibiotics that inhibit bacterial cell wall synthesis.
  (3) Adverse effects and monitoring.
    (a) These antibiotics are generally well tolerated.
    (b) High doses and accumulation may cause mental status changes and seizures.
    (c) Cephalosporins are associated with the development of acute interstitial nephritis.
  (4) Considerations.
    (a) These agents are classified into five groups (referred to as generations) based on their spectrum of activity.
    (b) Patients with penicillin allergy may have cross-reactivity with

cephalosporins; thus, these drugs should be avoided in those with a history of a severe reaction.
    (c) Most cephalosporins require dosage adjustment in kidney disease.
c. Penicillins and penicillin/B-lactamase inhibitors.
  (1) Agents.
    (a) Penicillins.
      i. Amoxicillin (Amoxil®).
      ii. Dicloxacillin (Dynapen®).
      iii. Nafcillin (Unipen®).
      iv. Penicillin G, penicillin VK.
      v. Piperacillin (Pipracil®).
    (b) Penicillin/B-lactamase inhibitors.
      i. Amoxicillin/clavulanate (Augmentin®).
      ii. Ampicillin/sulbactam (Unasyn®).
      iii. Piperacillin/tazobactam (Zosyn®).
      iv. Ticarcillin/clavulanate (Timentin®).
  (2) Mechanism of action. Penicillins inhibit bacterial cell wall synthesis, resulting in bactericidal activity. The addition of B-lactamase inhibitor (clavulanate, sulbactam, tazobactam) extends the activity of the penicillin to organisms, which produce a B-lactamase.
  (3) Adverse effects and monitoring.
    (a) Penicillins may cause rash, hypersensitivity reactions, or anaphylaxis.
    (b) These agents may cause neurotoxicity. This is usually associated with large doses.
    (c) Nafcillin may case pain, phlebitis, and tissue necrosis if extravasation occurs.
    (d) Penicillin antibiotics are associated with the development of acute interstitial nephritis.
  (4) Considerations.
    (a) Intravenous infusions of penicillin antibiotics should be separated from aminoglycosides by 2 hours.
    (b) Ticarcillin/clavulanate contains a significant amount of sodium and should be used with caution in patients with severe kidney disease or heart failure.
    (c) Most penicillins require dosage adjustments in patients with kidney disease or acute kidney injury.
d. Tetracyclines.
  (1) Agents.
    (a) Doxycycline (Vibramycin®).
    (b) Minocycline (Minocin®).
    (c) Tetracycline (Acromycin®, Sumycin®).
    (d) Tigecycline (Tygacil®).
  (2) Mechanism of action. Tetracyclines inhibit

bacterial protein synthesis by binding to the 30s ribosomal subunit.
  (3) Adverse effects and monitoring.
    (a) Tetracyclines cause photosensitivity. Patients should be warned to avoid excessive sunlight while taking these agents.
    (b) Tetracyclines are rarely associated with life-threatening skin reactions including Stevens-Johnson syndrome and toxic epidermal necrolysis.
    (c) These agents may cause discoloration of teeth.
  (4) Considerations. Tetracyclines can chelate with divalent cations such as calcium, magnesium, and iron in the gastrointestinal tract, causing decreased antibiotic absorption. To avoid this interaction, tetracyclines should be separated by several hours from food, milk, or drugs containing divalent cations.
e. Macrolides.
  (1) Agents.
    (a) Azithromycin (Zithromax®).
    (b) Clarithromycin (Biaxin®).
    (c) Erythromycin (E-Mycin®).
  (2) Mechanism of action. Macrolides interfere with bacterial protein synthesis by binding to the 50s ribosomal subunit.
  (3) Adverse effects and monitoring.
    (a) Macrolides can prolong QTc interval. Use should be avoided in patients taking other medications known to prolong QTc.
    (b) Nausea and diarrhea are common adverse effects associated with macrolides.
    (c) Clarithromycin may cause taste disturbances.
  (4) Considerations.
    (a) Clarithromycin and erythromycin have many drug interactions because they are strong inhibitors of CYP450 enzymes.
    (b) Erythromycin is sometimes used to increase gastrointestinal motility in patients with gastroparesis.
f. Carbapenems.
  (1) Agents.
    (a) Ertapenem (Invanz®).
    (b) Imipenem/cilastatin (Primaxin®).
    (c) Meropenem (Merrem®).
  (2) Mechanism of action. Carbapenems are B-lactam antibiotics that inhibit bacterial cell wall synthesis.
  (3) Adverse effects and monitoring. Carbapenems may cause seizures and

should be used with extreme caution in patients with a history of seizures.
  (4) Considerations.
    (a) Allergic cross-reactivity may occur in patients who have penicillin allergies. These drugs may be avoided in patients with a history of severe penicillin and/or cephalosporin allergy.
    (b) All carbapenems require dosage adjustment in patients with CKD or acute kidney injury.
g. Fluoroquinolones.
  (1) Agents.
    (a) Ciprofloxacin (Cipro®).
    (b) Levofloxacin (Levaquin®).
    (c) Moxifloxacin (Avelox®).
    (d) Norfloxacin (Noroxin®).
    (e) Ofloxacin (Floxin®).
  (2) Mechanism of action. Fluoroquinolone antibiotics inhibit DNA gyrase, an enzyme responsible for bacterial DNA synthesis.
  (3) Adverse effects and monitoring.
    (a) Fluoroquinolones can prolong QTc interval. Use should be avoided in patients taking other medications known to prolong QTc.
    (b) Peripheral neuropathy, photosensitivity, hepatotoxicity, hypoglycemia and tendon rupture are other adverse effects associated with fluoroquinolones.
    (c) These agents have been associated with the development of acute interstitial nephritis.
  (4) Considerations.
    (a) Fluoroquinolones chelate with divalent cations such as calcium, magnesium and iron in the gastrointestinal tract, causing decreased antibiotic absorption. To avoid this interaction, they should be separated by several hours from food, milk, or drugs containing divalent cations.
    (b) Most fluoroquinolones require dosage adjustment in patients with kidney dysfunction.
h. Others.
  (1) Agents.
    (a) Clindamycin (Cleocin®).
    (b) Daptomycin (Cubicin®).
    (c) Linezolid (Zyvox®).
    (d) Metronidazole (Flagyl®).
    (e) Sulfamethoxazole/trimethoprim (Bactrim®).
    (f) Vancomycin (Vancocin®).
  (2) Mechanism of action. The mechanism of action of these unrelated antibiotics vary. Clindamycin, linezolid, and metronidazole

inhibit bacterial protein synthesis. Vancomycin inhibits bacterial cell wall synthesis. Daptomycin inhibits bacterial DNA synthesis. Sulfamethoxazole/trimethoprim inhibits the bacterial folic acid pathway.
  (3) Adverse effects and monitoring.
    (a) Sulfamethoxazole/trimethoprim is associated with life-threatening skin reactions, including Stevens-Johnson syndrome and toxic epidermal necrolysis.
    (b) Vancomycin is nephrotoxic and kidney function should be monitored regularly throughout therapy.
    (c) Vancomycin trough levels are monitored to evaluate efficacy and prevent toxicity.
    (d) Linezolid is associated with myelosuppression and rarely serotonin syndrome.
    (e) Daptomycin may cause myopathy and rhabdomyolysis. Creatine phosphokinase (CPK) and symptoms of muscle pain or weakness should be monitored during therapy.
    (f) Sulfamethoxazole/trimethoprim is associated with the development of acute interstitial nephritis.
  (4) Considerations. Trimethoprim inhibits the tubular secretion of creatinine and may cause an increase in serum creatinine without altering kidney function.
3. Antiviral agents.
  a. Agents.
    (1) Acyclovir (Zovirax®), valacyclovir (Valtrex®).
    (2) Cidofovir (Vistide®).
    (3) Famciclovir (Famvir®).
    (4) Foscarnet (Foscavir®).
    (5) Ganciclovir (Cytovene®), valganciclovir (Valcyte®).
  b. Mechanism of action. These agents inhibit DNA polymerase, an enzyme involved in viral DNA synthesis, thus preventing viral replication. Valacyclovir is an oral prodrug and is converted to acyclovir, and valganciclovir is an oral prodrug that is converted to ganciclovir. These prodrugs result in enhanced bioavailability.
  c. Adverse effects and monitoring.
    (1) Acyclovir can cause crystal-induced acute kidney injury.
    (2) Adverse effects associated with ganciclovir include leukopenia, anemia, and thrombocytopenia.
    (3) Patients receiving foscarnet or cidofovir must be monitored for nephrotoxicity.

    (4) Foscarnet may cause electrolyte abnormalities including hypokalemia, hypocalcemia, and hypomagnesemia.
  d. Considerations.
    (1) To minimize the risk of nephrotoxicity associated with acyclovir, foscarnet or cidofovir, patients should be well hydrated and avoid concomitant nephrotoxic drugs.
    (2) These agents require a dosage adjustment in patients with kidney dysfunction.
    (3) Valganciclovir should be taken with food to maximize oral bioavailability.

VIII. Calcimimetics.

A. Use in CKD. This agent is used to treat secondary hyperparathyroidism associated with CKD.

B. Goals of therapy.
  1. Maintain intact parathyroid hormone (PTH) level 2 to 9 times the laboratory normal (KDIGO, 2009).
  2. Prevent complications associated with CKD-mineral bone disorder.

C. Classification.
  1. Calcimimetics.
    a. Agent: cinacalcet (Sensipar®).
    b. Mechanism of action. This agent acts by increasing the sensitivity of the calcium receptors on the parathyroid gland to reduce the production and secretion of PTH, thereby reducing GI absorption and bone resorption of calcium.
    c. Adverse effects and monitoring.
      (1) Gastrointestinal side effects, including nausea and vomiting, are commonly associated with cinacalcet.
      (2) Monitor serum calcium levels for hypocalcemia. Cinacalcet use is contraindicated in patients with hypocalcemia.
    d. Considerations.
      (1) Cinacalcet is used in patients with CKD who have hyperparathyroidism in conjunction with hypercalcemia.
      (2) This agent is commonly used in addition to vitamin D therapy for the treatment of hyperparathyroidism.

IX. Cation-exchange resin.

A. Use in CKD. Patients with CKD may develop hyperkalemia due to the kidney's inability to eliminate potassium effectively.

B. Goals of therapy.
1. Decrease serum potassium levels.
2. Decrease the risk of complications associated with high serum potassium levels.

C. Classification.
1. Agent: Sodium polystyrene sulfonate (Kayexalate®).
2. Mechanism of action. Sodium polystyrene sulfonate is a cation-exchange resin. It functions primarily in the large intestine where sodium ions are exchanged for potassium ions. The potassium ions are then excreted in the feces resulting in decreased serum potassium.
3. Adverse effects and monitoring.
   a. The patient must be monitored for hypokalemia, hypocalcemia, hypomagnesemia, and hypernatremia.
   b. Formulations containing sorbitol have been associated with colonic necrosis.
4. Considerations.
   a. Sodium polystyrene sulfonate may be given orally or as an enema.
   b. When given by enema, the drug must be retained in the intestine 30 to 45 minutes to be effective.
   c. When given orally, the concurrent administration of an osmotic laxative, such as sorbitol, facilitates the exchange process by promoting the movement of extracellular fluid into the lumen of the gut and also helps to prevent fecal impaction.
   d. This drug is not appropriate for use in acute hyperkalemia.

X. Cholesterol-lowering agents.

A. Use in CKD. These agents are used for lowering blood cholesterol, and for primary and secondary prevention of atherosclerotic cardiovascular disease (Stone et al., 2013).

B. Goals of therapy (Stone et al., 2013).
1. Lower blood cholesterol levels.
2. Decrease atherosclerotic cardiovascular disease risk (ASCVD) with the use of HMG CoA reductase inhibitors (i.e., statins).

C. Classification.
1. Bile-acid sequestrants.
   a. Agents.
      (1) Cholestyramine (Questran®).
      (2) Colesevelam (Welchol®).
      (3) Colestipol (Colestid®).
   b. Mechanism of action. These agents combine with the bile acids in the GI tract to form insoluble complexes. This decreases the bile acid level in the gallbladder and triggers the liver to synthesize more bile acids from their precursor, cholesterol. The overall effect is to decrease the serum cholesterol levels.
   c. Adverse effects and monitoring. The most common adverse effects associated with these agents are GI-related effects, including constipation, diarrhea, flatulence, abdominal pain, and bloating.
   d. Considerations. Bile-acid sequestrants may bind to drugs in the GI tract and decrease their absorption. Thus, administration of these agents should be separated by at least 2 hours before or 4 hours after other medications.
2. Fibric acid derivatives.
   a. Agents.
      (1) Fenofibrate (Lofibra®, Tricor®).
      (2) Gemfibrozil (Lopid®).
   b. Mechanism of action. These agents are thought to decrease cholesterol formation, mobilize cholesterol from the tissues, increase sterol excretion, decrease lipoprotein synthesis and secretion, and decrease triglyceride synthesis.
   c. Adverse effects and monitoring.
      (1) Adverse effects associated with fibric acid derivatives include myopathies and rhabdomyolysis. Patients should be advised to notify their healthcare provider if they experience muscle pain or discomfort.
      (2) These agents can also increase liver enzymes. Liver function tests should be monitored routinely.
   d. Considerations.
      (1) These agents are effective in decreasing triglyceride levels.
      (2) Gemfibrozil is not recommended to be used in combination with statin therapy due to the risk of rhabdomyolysis.
      (3) Fenofibrate requires dose adjustments in patients with kidney disease; kidney function should be monitored while on therapy.
3. Cholesterol synthesis inhibitors (HMG CoA reductase inhibitors, statins).
   a. Agents.
      (1) Atorvastatin (Lipitor®).
      (2) Fluvastatin (Lescol®).
      (3) Lovastatin (Mevacor®).
      (4) Pravastatin (Pravachol®).
      (5) Rosuvastatin (Crestor®).
      (6) Simvastatin (Zocor®).
   b. Mechanism of action. These agents inhibit the biochemical conversion of the precursor of cholesterol by inhibiting hydroxymethylglutaryl-coenzyme A (HMG CoA) reductase. This increases the expression of low-density lipoprotein (LDL) receptors on the surface of various cells, which increases the clearance of

LDL from the bloodstream, reducing LDL concentrations.

c. Adverse effects and monitoring.
   (1) These agents may cause myopathies and rhabdomyolysis. Patients should be advised to notify their healthcare provider if they experience muscle pain. The risk of rhabdomyolysis increases if patients are taking drugs that inhibit the oxidative metabolism of statins.
   (2) These agents can also increase liver enzymes. Liver function tests should be monitored routinely in patients receiving HMG CoA reductase inhibitors.
   (3) Initiation of simvastatin at a dose of 80 mg is no longer recommended due to the increased risk of development of rhabdomyolysis (FDA, 2011).

d. Considerations.
   (1) The 2013 American College of Cardiology/American Heart Association guideline on the treatment of blood cholesterol to reduce atherosclerotic cardiovascular risk in adults (Stone et al., 2013) recommends use of moderate to high intensity statin therapy in four patient populations:
      (a) Individuals with ASCVD without heart failure or receiving hemodialysis.
      (b) Individuals with LDL cholesterol ≥ 190 mg/dL.
      (c) Individuals 40 to 75 years of age with diabetes and LDL cholesterol 70 to 189 mg/dL without ASCVD.
      (d) Individuals without ASCVD or diabetes who are 40 to 75 years of age with LDL cholesterol 70 to 189 mg/dL and 10-year estimated ASCVD risk of ≥ 7.5%.
   (2) The current guideline does not recommend using statins to treat to a specific LDL cholesterol goal.
   (3) For patients requiring high-intensity statin therapy to decrease ASCVD, a reduction of LDL cholesterol by ≥ 50% is recommended.
   (4) For patients requiring moderate-intensity statin therapy to decrease ASCVD, a reduction of LDL cholesterol by 30–50% is recommended.
   (5) There are currently no recommendations regarding the use of statins in the hemodialysis patient population due to the lack of evidence demonstrating cardiovascular benefit (Fellström et al., 2009; Wanner et al., 2005).

4. Cholesterol absorption inhibitors.
   a. Agents: ezetimibe (Zetia®).
   b. Mechanism of action. These agents block the absorption of cholesterol, reducing the uptake of cholesterol from the intestines into the liver. This decreases the amount of cholesterol stored in the liver and increases the clearance of cholesterol from the bloodstream.
   c. Adverse effects and monitoring. The most common side effects associated with ezetimibe are GI related, including abdominal pain and diarrhea.
   d. Considerations.
      (1) Ezetimibe is available in combination with simvastatin (Vytorin®) and atorvastatin (Liptruzet®).
      (2) In patients with kidney disease, combination simvastatin 20 mg and ezetimibe was demonstrated to be safe. Higher doses of statins in this combination have not been studied (Baigent et al., 2011).

5. Nicotinic acid.
   a. Agents: Niacin (Niaspan®).
   b. Mechanism of action. This agent inhibits lipolysis in adipose tissue, decreases esterification of triglycerides in the liver, increases lipoprotein lipase activity, and decreases the liver's production of very low-density lipoproteins (VLDL) and LDL.
   c. Adverse effects and monitoring.
      (1) The most common side effect of niacin is flushing that results from vasodilation of peripheral blood vessels. Aspirin can be administered 30 minutes before the dose, or gradual increases in doses can reduce the incidence of flushing (Stone et al., 2013).
      (2) Niacin can increase liver enzymes. LFTs should be monitored routinely in patients receiving niacin.
   d. Considerations.
      (1) Niacin is useful to reduce cholesterol, triglyceride, and LDL cholesterol levels, and increase HDL cholesterol levels.
      (2) Niacin has been shown to increase blood glucose and can impact glucose control in patients with diabetes.

XI. Diuretics.

A. Use in CKD. Diuretics are used in patients experiencing fluid retention caused by various disease states. Some of these agents may also be used for their antihypertensive effects.

B. Goals of therapy.
   1. Relieve symptoms of fluid retention.
   2. Lower blood pressure.

C. Classification.
   1. Carbonic anhydrase inhibitors.
      a. Agent: acetazolamide (Diamox®).
      b. Mechanism of action. These agents inhibit carbonic anhydrase in the proximal tubule to increase hydrogen ion secretion and decrease sodium and bicarbonate reabsorption.
      c. Adverse effects and monitoring. Acetazolamide can cause somnolence and paresthesias.
      d. Considerations.
         (1) Cross-reactivity can occur in patients with a known sulfa allergy.
         (2) Carbonic anhydrase inhibitors may be used in patients with edema and metabolic alkalosis.
         (3) Use this agent with caution in patients with diabetes or hepatic disease.
         (4) Carbonic anhydrase inhibitors can be used to treat open angle glaucoma.
   2. Aldosterone antagonists.
      a. Agents.
         (1) Eplerenone (Inspra®).
         (2) Spironolactone (Aldactone®).
      b. Mechanism of action. These agents competitively inhibit the binding of aldosterone to mineralocorticoid receptors in the distal tubule and collecting duct. This mechanism increases excretion of salt and water and decreases the excretion of potassium and hydrogen.
      c. Adverse effects and monitoring.
         (1) Hyperkalemia is an adverse effect that limits their use in patients with CKD. Potassium levels should be monitored on initiation of therapy and throughout treatment.
         (2) Spironolactone use has been associated with adverse effects such as gynecomastia and menstrual disturbances, which may lead to discontinuation of this agent. These effects are not seen with eplerenone.
      d. Considerations.
         (1) When used in combination with ACE inhibitors or ARBs in patients with CKD and hypertension, these agents have been shown to reduce urine albumin excretion (Bianchi et al., 2006; Epstein et al., 2006; Mehdi et al., 2009).
         (2) Spironolactone and eplerenone have been shown to decrease mortality in heart failure (Pitt et al., 1999; Zannad et al., 2011) and after myocardial infarction with systolic dysfunction (Pitt et al., 2003).
         (3) Spironolactone is often used in patients with hepatic cirrhosis.
   3. Loop diuretics.
      a. Agents.
         (1) Bumetanide (Bumex®).
         (2) Ethacrynic acid (Edecrin®).
         (3) Furosemide (Lasix®).
         (4) Torsemide (Demadex®).
      b. Mechanism of action. Loop diuretics alter sodium and water reabsorption from the ascending limb of the loop of Henle, where 20–25% of filtered sodium is normally reabsorbed.
      c. Adverse effects and monitoring.
         (1) In patients receiving these diuretics, daily weights are used to monitor efficacy and adjust doses.
         (2) Ototoxicity may occur with rapid intravenous administration.
         (3) Loop diuretics cause electrolyte abnormalities such as hypokalemia, hypomagnesemia, hypocalcemia, and hyperuricemia.
         (4) Loop diuretics are associated with acute interstitial nephritis.
      d. Considerations.
         (1) In patients with a known sulfa allergy, cross-reactivity can occur.
         (2) Ethacrynic acid is the only loop diuretic without a sulfonamide group allowing it to be safe to use in patients with a sulfa allergy.
         (3) In patients with CKD stages 4 and 5, loop diuretics can maintain their saluretic effects and are predominantly used over other diuretics in this population.
         (4) Loop diuretics are recommended in patients with heart failure and fluid retention to improve symptoms (Yancy et al., 2013).
         (5) Patients with nephrotic range proteinuria may be diuretic resistant and require higher doses.
         (6) These agents can promote the nephrotoxicity of drugs by altering the hydration state.
   4. Potassium-sparing.
      a. Agents.
         (1) Amiloride (Midamor®).
         (2) Triamterene (Dyrenium®).
      b. Mechanism of action. Potassium-sparing diuretics promote the excretion of sodium and water through the increased reabsorption of potassium in the distal tubule and collecting duct.
      c. Adverse effects and monitoring.
         (1) These agents provoke hyperkalemia and are not recommended for use in patients with CKD.
         (2) Potassium-sparing diuretics can also cause metabolic alkalosis and hyponatremia.

d. Considerations.
  (1) These agents have less of a diuretic effect then loop and thiazides.
  (2) Are generally used for their potassium sparing effects.
5. Thiazides and thiazide-like.
  a. Agents.
    (1) Thiazide.
      (a) Chlorothiazide (Diuril®).
      (b) Chlorthalidone (Thalitone®).
      (c) Hydrochlorothiazide (Esidrix®, HydroDiuril®).
    (2) Thiazide-like.
      (a) Indapamide (Lozol®).
      (b) Metolazone (Zaroxolyn®).
  b. Mechanism of action. These diuretics inhibit the reabsorption of sodium and water in the distal convoluted tubule causing diuresis. They can also decrease plasma volume, stroke volume, and cardiac output. Chronically, these agents decrease peripheral vascular resistance lending to their hypotensive effect.
  c. Adverse effects and monitoring.
    (1) Thiazide diuretics can cause hypokalemia, hypomagnesemia, hypercalcemia, hyperuricemia, hyperglycemia, and hyperlipidemia.
    (2) These agents are associated with the development of acute interstitial nephritis.
  d. Considerations.
    (1) These agents lose their saluretic effect in patients with CKD stages 4 and 5, and thus are generally not used in this population.
    (2) Metolazone may retain efficacy in patients with CKD stages 4 and 5 and is often used as an adjunct to loop diuretics in these patients.
    (3) Thiazides can potentiate the antihypertensive effects of ACE inhibitors and ARBs in additional to other agents. This has led to a number of combination products becoming available.
    (4) Current guidelines recommend that in patients with CKD, initial antihypertensive therapy should include thiazide diuretics (James et al., 2014).
    (5) These agents can promote the nephrotoxicity of drugs by altering the hydration state.

XII. Heavy metal chelating agents.

A. Use in CKD. Heavy metal chelating agents are used to treat aluminum and iron toxicity.

B. Goals of therapy.
  1. Treat or prevent adverse outcomes associated with iron overload, such as cardiovascular, hepatic, and renal complications.
  2. Diagnose aluminum toxicity (KDOQI, 2003).
  3. Treat or prevent complications associated with aluminum toxicity, such as aluminum bone disease (NKF, 2003).

C. Classification.
  1. Agent: deferoxamine mesylate (Desferal®).
  2. Mechanism of action. Deferoxamine complexes with heavy metals, preventing free radical tissue damage. These complexes are then eliminated by the kidney or by dialysis.
  3. Adverse effects and monitoring.
    a. Neurologic toxicities such as ototoxicity and visual disturbances have been reported (Olivieri et al., 1986).
    b. Patients must be frequently monitored for urticaria, hypotension, and flushing following administration.
    c. Deferoxamine has been associated with an increased risk of infection.
  4. Considerations.
    a. It gives the urine a reddish coloration.
    b. If given intravenously, administer slowly to decrease the risk of infusion reactions. In patients on dialysis, it is given at the end of a dialysis treatment.

XIII. H1 receptor antagonists.

A. Use in CKD. Pruritus is a common problem in patients with CKD and uremia. This may be associated with inadequate dialysis, dry skin, or abnormal calcium and phosphorus metabolism. H1-receptor antagonists, commonly called anti-histamines, are prescribed to decrease this symptom.

B. Goal of therapy: relieve symptoms of pruritus.

C. Classification.
  1. Agents.
    a. First-generation H1 receptor antagonists.
      (1) Diphenhydramine (Benadryl®).
      (2) Hydroxyzine (Atarax®).
    b. Second-generation H1 receptor antagonists.
      (1) Cetirizine (Zyrtec®).
      (2) Fexofenadine (Allegra®).
      (3) Loratadine (Claritin®).
  2. Mechanism of action. These agents inhibit the H1 receptors in the gastrointestinal tract, respiratory tract and vasculature, blocking the effects of histamine.
  3. Adverse effects and monitoring.
    a. The most common adverse effects of the first-generation H1 receptor antagonists are sedation and somnolence. Higher doses of the

second-generation agents may cause similar effects.

b. First-generation antihistamines may have anticholinergic effects, such as dry mouth, urinary retention or frequency, and dysuria. The second-generation agents have minimal anticholinergic effects.

4. Considerations. Patients should avoid driving when taking antihistamines.

XIV. Immunosuppressive agents.

A. Use in CKD. Immunosuppressive agents may be used to treat certain glomerular diseases. Some of these agents are also used in patients with a kidney transplant to prevent or treat organ rejection.

B. Goals of therapy.
   1. Prevent the progression of kidney disease.
   2. Achieve remission of the underlying glomerular disease state.
   3. Maximize efficacy while minimizing the risk of infection and malignancy.

C. Classification.
   1. Alkylating agents.
      a. Agents: cyclophosphamide (Cytoxan®).
      b. Mechanism of action. This agent possesses cytotoxic effects by preventing DNA synthesis and cell replication. Cyclophosphamide suppresses T-cell and B-cell function.
      c. Adverse effects and monitoring.
         (1) Adverse effects associated with cyclophosphamide include bone marrow suppression, nausea/vomiting, impaired fertility, and hemorrhagic cystitis.
         (2) These effects are generally dose dependent.
      d. Considerations.
         (1) It is recommended to administer antiemetics prior to intravenous cyclophosphamide.
         (2) Cyclophosphamide may cause infertility in women and men; therefore, patients of child-bearing age should be informed prior to initiation of therapy.
         (3) Increased intravenous and/or oral fluid intake is recommended to prevent bladder complications.
         (4) Mesna may be given in conjunction with cyclophosphamide to inactivate the toxic metabolites which cause hemorrhagic cystitis.
         (5) Cyclophosphamide is often used in combination with glucocorticoids for the treatment of certain causes of glomerulonephritis (KDIGO, 2012c).
   2. Aminoquinolines.
      a. Agents: hydroxychloroquine (Plaquenil®).
      b. Mechanism of action. Hydroxychloroquine's immunosupressive effects may be due to its ability to alter lysosome stability, prevent antigen presentation and inhibit cytokine production (Lee et al., 2011).
      c. Adverse effects and monitoring.
         (1) Hydroxychloroquine has been associated with ocular effects such as blurred vision, abnormal pigmentation and color vision, and photophobia. An ophthalmologic examination should be performed before initiation and with prolonged use of this agent (Lee et al., 2011).
         (2) This agent may cause dermatologic effects, myopathy, polyneuropathy, and cardiac toxicity.
      d. Considerations.
         (1) KDIGO guidelines suggest that all patients with lupus nephritis should be treated with this agent unless contraindicated (KDIGO, 2012c).
         (2) This agent may have a beneficial effect on blood cholesterol levels.
         (3) This agent should not be used in patients with G6PD deficiency.
   3. Calcineurin inhibitors.
      a. Agents.
         (1) Cyclosporine (Sandimmune®, Neoral®).
         (2) Tacrolimus (Prograf®, Astagraf®).
      b. Mechanism of action. Calcineurin inhibitors prevent the production of interleukin-2 and the activation of T-lymphocytes.
      c. Adverse effects and monitoring.
         (1) Cyclosporine and tacrolimus are nephrotoxic agents. Close monitoring of kidney function is required.
         (2) Electrolyte abnormalities are associated with calcineurin inhibitors. Potassium and magnesium should be monitored regularly.
         (3) Cyclosporine may cause hypertension, hyperlipidemia, gingival hyperplasia, and hirsutism.
         (4) Adverse effects associated with tacrolimus include neurotoxicity, hypertension, glucose intolerance and diabetes, and alopecia.
         (5) Calcineurin inhibitors have a narrow therapeutic index and require trough monitoring to maintain efficacy and prevent toxicity.
      d. Considerations.
         (1) The use of other nephrotoxic agents should be avoided in patients taking cyclosporine and tacrolimus.
         (2) These drugs are metabolized by the CYP enzyme system and are associated with many drug interactions.

(3) Diarrhea may increase the bioavailability of these drugs and patients may require dosage adjustment until it subsides.

(4) These agents may be used as first- or second-line treatment depending on the etiology of the glomerulonephritis (KDIGO, 2012c).

4. Glucocorticoids.
   a. Agents.
      (1) Methylprednisolone (Medrol®, Solu-Medrol®).
      (2) Prednisone (Deltasone®).
   b. Mechanism of action. The mechanism of action of systemic glucocorticoids is not well understood. They appear to suppress hypersensitivity and immune response by preventing cell-mediated immune reactions, decreasing the binding of antibodies to cell surface receptors, and inhibiting interleukin synthesis.
   c. Adverse effects and monitoring.
      (1) Long-term administration may result in Cushing's syndrome.
      (2) These agents increase catabolism, blood glucose levels, potassium excretion, sodium and water retention, and decrease wound healing.
      (3) These agents can cause GI ulcerations.
      (4) Long-term use will suppress the hypothalamic-pituitary-adrenal (HPA) axis. Discontinuation should occur slowly.
      (5) Glucocorticoids may cause glaucoma, muscle weakness, myopathy, osteoporosis, and femoral avascular necrosis.
   d. Considerations.
      (1) Administer these agents with milk or food.
      (2) These agents are often used alone or in combination with other immuno-suppressive agents for certain glomerular diseases (KDIGO, 2012c).

5. Monoclonal antibody.
   a. Agent: rituximab (Rituxan®).
   b. Mechanism of action. Rituximab is a monoclonal antibody targeting CD20 on B-lymphocytes, leading to cell death.
   c. Adverse effects and monitoring.
      (1) Rituximab is associated with severe infusion reactions including hypotension, fever, bronchospasm, and angioedema. Patients should be monitored closely during the infusion.
      (2) Rituximab may cause pancytopenia.
      (3) Reactivation of hepatitis B infection has been reported with rituximab use.
   d. Considerations.
      (1) It is recommended to administer antihistamines and acetaminophen to prevent or minimize infusion reactions.

(2) The infusion must be titrated slowly.
(3) This agent may be used to treat some forms of resistant glomerulonephritis (KDIGO, 2012c).

6. Mycophenolic acid.
   a. Agents.
      (1) Mycophenolate mofetil (Cellcept®).
      (2) Enteric-coated mycophenolic acid (Myfortic®).
   b. Mechanism of action. Mycohenolate mofetil is a prodrug and is converted to mycophenolic acid. Mycophenolic acid inhibits T and B-lymphocyte proliferation by inhibiting IMPDH, the enzyme involved in guanosine nucleotide synthesis.
   c. Adverse effects and monitoring.
      (1) Nausea, vomiting, and diarrhea are commonly associated with these drugs.
      (2) Mycophenolic acid may cause leukopenia, anemia, and thrombocytopenia.
   d. Considerations.
      (1) Enteric-coated mycophenolic acid may have fewer upper gastrointestinal effects than mycophenolate mofetil.
      (2) Mycophenolic acid is teratogenic; female patients of child-bearing age should be instructed to use two forms of contraception while taking these drugs.
      (3) These agents may be used in combination with glucocorticoids in patients with most classes of lupus nephritis and other glomerular diseases (KDIGO, 2012c).

XV. Phosphate binders.

A. Use in CKD. Calcium products, aluminum-based products, phosphate binding polymers, and lanthanum are administered to assist in managing the hyperphosphatemia that is associated with CKD.

B. Goals of therapy (KDIGO, 2009; NKF, 2010).
   1. Maintain a serum phosphorus level within the reference range in patients with CKD not receiving dialysis.
   2. Maintain a serum phosphorus level toward the reference range in dialysis patients.
   3. Maintain a serum calcium in the reference range for all patients with CKD.
   4. Prevent complications associated with CKD-mineral bone disorder.

C. Classification.
   1. Agents.
      a. Aluminum-based phosphate binders. Aluminum hydroxide gel (Amphojel®, Alternagel®).
      b. Calcium-based phosphate binders.

(1) Calcium acetate (PhosLo®, Phoslyra®).
(2) Calcium carbonate (Os-Cal®, Tums®).
c. Noncalcium, nonaluminum-based phosphate binders.
(1) Ferric citrate.
(2) Lanthanum carbonate (Fosrenol®).
(3) Sevelamer carbonate (Renvela®).
(4) Sevelamer hydrochloride (Renagel®).
(5) Sucroferric oxyhydroxide (Velphoro®).
2. Mechanism of action. These agents act by binding phosphate in the GI tract and facilitate the excretion of phosphate in the feces.
3. Adverse effects and monitoring.
a. Aluminum accumulation can result in bone disease, anemia, and encephalopathy. These binders are reserved for short-term use in patients with persistently high serum phosphorus levels.
b. The administration of calcium-based phosphate binders can result in hypercalcemia. It is important to monitor serum calcium levels closely.
c. Phosphate binders can cause gastrointestinal adverse effects such as nausea, bloating, and constipation.
4. Considerations.
a. Hypercalcemia may lead to vascular and/or soft tissue calcification.
b. Dietary phosphate should be restricted during the therapy.
c. These agents are administered with meals to bind to phosphate in the GI tract.
d. Aluminum-based phosphate binders and lanthanum have the most potency, followed by calcium acetate and sevelamer, and calcium carbonate.
e. Phosphate binders may decrease absorption of certain drugs when given concomitantly and therefore should be separated by 2 to 4 hours.
f. Lanthanum is a chewable phosphate binder and should not be swallowed whole.
g. Calcium acetate and calcium carbonate are available in liquid formulations.
h. Sevelamer carbonate is available in a powder formulation and should be mixed with water.
i. The iron-based phosphate binders, ferric citrate and sucroferric oxyhydroxide, may cause discoloration of the stool.
j. Ferric citrate has been associated with increasing serum iron, TSAT, and serum ferritin due to systemic iron absorption. Sucroferric oxyhydroxide has minimal effect on iron parameters.

XVI. Prokinetic agents.

A. Use in CKD. These agents are used to treat patients who experience hypomotility of the GI tract, or gastroparesis, and thus have a delayed emptying of the stomach resulting in clinical signs and symptoms, such as nausea, vomiting, indigestion, or gastroesophageal reflux.

B. Goals of therapy.
1. Treat the symptoms of gastroparesis.
2. Decrease adverse outcomes associated with gastroparesis (Camilleri et al., 2013).

C. Classification.
1. Agent: metoclopramide (Reglan®).
2. Mechanism of action. This agent acts as a dopamine antagonist resulting in accelerated gastric emptying and enhanced transit in the small intestine.
3. Adverse effects and monitoring. Metoclopramide can result in restlessness, drowsiness, fatigue, depression, extrapyrimidal symptoms, and tardive dyskinesia.
4. Considerations.
a. Metoclopramide should not be used with patients for whom an increased GI motility might be hazardous, such as those with GI bleeding or obstruction.
b. The dose of metoclopramide should be reduced in patients with moderate to severe kidney dysfunction.
c. Patients should be monitored closely for early signs of tardive dyskinesia. To minimize the risk, the smallest possible dose should be used and drug holidays can be considered. Discontinue therapy if signs or symptoms become apparent (Camilleri et al., 2013).

XVII. Vitamin D and vitamin D analogs.

A. Use in CKD. As kidney function declines, the conversion of inactive vitamin D (25-hydroxy-vitamin D) to the active form (1,25-dihydroxy-vitamin D) decreases. This decrease in active vitamin D, along with other factors, results in decreased serum calcium and elevated parathyroid hormone (PTH) levels.

B. Goals of therapy.
1. Prevent and treat vitamin D deficiency.
2. Decrease serum PTH levels and maintain the PTH level 2 to 9 times the laboratory normal.
3. Promote calcium and phosphorus homeostasis.
4. Prevent complications associated with CKD-mineral bone disorder (KDIGO, 2009).

C. Classification.
1. Agents.
   a. Inactive vitamin D.
      (1) Cholecalciferol.
      (2) Ergocalciferol.
   b. Active vitamin D.
      (1) Calcitriol (Calcijex®, Rocaltrol®).
      (2) Doxercalciferol (Hectorol®).
      (3) Paricalcitol (Zemplar®).
2. Mechanism of action. Inactive vitamin D is converted to the active form by the liver and kidney. Active vitamin D binds to vitamin D receptors in the kidney, bone, intestine, and parathyroid gland to increase serum calcium levels and provide negative feedback to the parathyroid gland to reduce PTH secretion.
3. Adverse effects and monitoring.
   a. Calcitriol, doxercalciferol, and to a lesser extent, paricalcitol, can increase serum calcium and phosphate levels by increasing the absorption from the GI tract and resorption from the bones.
   b. Serum calcium and phosphorus levels must be monitored before initiating and during vitamin D therapy.
   c. Phosphorus levels must be toward the normal range before initiating therapy with these agents to minimize further elevations.
   d. These agents should not be initiated in patients with hypercalcemia, and their doses should be held or decreased if a patient becomes hypercalcemic during therapy.
4. Considerations.
   a. Oral vitamin D can be administered daily or three times weekly.
   b. Intravenous vitamin D is generally administered three times weekly with dialysis therapy.
   c. The dosage of vitamin D is adjusted based on serum calcium and PTH levels.
   d. Some patients may receive inactive and active vitamin D concurrently.

SECTION D
Assessment of Kidney Function and Medication Dosing in Patients with CKD

The kidney is a major site for drug and drug metabolite elimination. Therefore, when kidney function is abnormal, it may be necessary to decrease the dose and/or dosing interval to avoid or minimize a drug's toxic effects. Assessment of kidney function and review of medication dosages should be done routinely by healthcare providers caring for patients with kidney disease.

I. **Assessment of kidney function. The most accurate method to assess kidney function is to determine the glomerular filtration rate (GFR).** However, glomerular filtration rate is not routinely measured in everyday practice, so kidney function is often assessed by using serum creatinine levels. Serum creatinine is easily measured and it is produced endogenously. But, serum creatinine alone does not always give a clear indication of kidney function. Therefore, other methods using serum creatinine can improve accuracy when measuring or estimating kidney function.

A. Limitations of using creatinine as a marker of kidney function.
   1. Creatinine is not solely eliminated by glomerular filtration. There is some tubular secretion of creatinine.
   2. Creatinine is generated from muscle mass, so a "normal" serum creatinine may vary depending on the muscle mass of the patient.
   3. The assay used to measure creatinine may detect other noncreatinine substances in the serum.

B. Methods for measuring or estimating kidney function.
   1. Measured GFR. To measure GFR, a substance must be used that is completely eliminated by glomerular filtration, with no tubular secretion or reabsorption. Examples of ideal substances include inulin, iothalamate, and iohexol. These substances are not endogenously produced. To determine the measured GFR, these agents are administered intravenously or subcutaneously and the patient's urine is subsequently collected over a period of time. A measured GFR is not performed routinely in clinical practice; however, it may be done in special circumstances or study protocols (Stevens & Levey, 2009).
   2. Measured creatinine clearance. The clearance of creatinine can be used as an estimate of GFR, but

due to the tubular secretion of creatinine, it will always overestimate filtration (e.g., GFR). A timed urine collection is a way to measure creatinine clearance and determine kidney function. A 24-hour collection is preferred over a shorter time interval because it accounts for diurnal variations in the production and excretion of creatinine throughout the day. It is important to note that error in the collection technique may compromise the results of the study. Therefore, the patient should be carefully instructed in the following key elements of a timed urine collection to obtain the most accurate result:

a. Completely void before starting the timed urine collection. Discard the urine from this void.
b. Accurately record the time of the complete void as the start time of the urine collection.
c. Collect the urine from each void during the timed collection.
d. Ensure proper storage of the urine collection during and after the time collection.
e. At the end of the time collection period, completely void and collect the final urine void.
f. Accurately record the time of the final urine void as the end time of the urine collection.

3. Estimating equations. Estimating equations have been found to be comparable to measured creatinine clearance or GFR. They are commonly used in clinical practice for stratifying CKD and dosing medications. These formulas have limitations and have not been validated in all patient populations. They should only be used in patients with stable kidney function and cannot be used in patients receiving hemodialysis or peritoneal dialysis.

a. Cockcroft and Gault equation. Cockcroft and Gault (1976) developed a formula for estimating creatinine clearance. This formula is based on the fact that creatinine clearance is proportional to body mass and inversely proportional to age. The formula is:

$$\text{CrCl (mL/min)} = \frac{(140 - \text{age}) \times (\text{body weight in kg})}{(72) \times (\text{serum creatinine in mg/dL})}$$

This formula is an accurate method for estimating creatinine clearance. When it is used in female patients, the result should be decreased by 10–15% to account for lower average muscle mass; thus, the calculated creatinine clearance is multiplied by 0.85. The Cockcroft and Gault equation is often used to determine the degree of kidney dysfunction when dosing medications in patients with CKD.

b. MDRD equation. The Modification of Diet in Renal Disease (MDRD) Study data was used to develop an equation to estimate glomerular filtration rate (eGFR) in patients with CKD (Levey et al., 2006). The original formula included six parameters: age, sex, ethnicity, serum creatinine, BUN, and serum albumin level. An abbreviated version provides similar accuracy in estimating GFR using four of those parameters: age, gender, ethnicity, and serum creatinine concentration. The formula is:

$$\text{GFR (mL/min/1.73m}^2) = 175 \times (\text{SCr})^{-1.154} \times (\text{Age})^{-0.203} \times (0.742 \text{ if female}) \times (1.21 \text{ if African American})$$

c. CKD-EPI equation (Levey et al., 2009). This formula is the most recent formula developed for estimating GFR. It is the most accurate formula when evaluating kidney function in patients with normal kidney function. The equation is currently not used in everyday clinical practice. The formula is:

$$\text{eGFR (mL/min/1.73m}^2) = 141 \times \min(\text{Scr}/k, 1)^a \times \max(\text{Scr}/k, 1)^{-1.209} \times 0.993^{\text{Age}} \times 1.018 \text{ [if female]} \times 1.159 \text{ (if African American)}$$

Scr = standardized serum creatinine
k = 0.7 for females and 0.9 for males
a = –0.329 for females and –0.411 for males
min indicates the minimum of Scr/k or 1
max indicates the maximum of Scr/k or 1

II. Alterations in medication dosage and frequency.

A. General approach to determine dosing adjustments. Most drugs have dosing recommendations in the package labeling based upon creatinine clearance ranges. An estimated creatinine clearance should always be used in conjunction with patient specific factors including indication for treatment, potential for toxicity and consequences of underdosing. The following is a general approach to determine the appropriate dosing adjustment in patients with CKD.

1. Obtain the history and relevant clinical information from the patient.
2. Estimate the creatinine clearance to determine kidney function.
3. Identify medications requiring dosage adjustments.
4. Determine treatment goals.
5. Calculate and/or review dosing recommendations.
6. Monitor for drug response and toxicity.
7. Adjust the drug regimen based on drug response or change in patient status.

B. Specific considerations to determine dosage adjustments in patients with CKD.
1. Serum levels. Monitoring serum drug levels is commonly done to maximize efficacy or prevent toxicity for drugs with a narrow therapeutic index.

The timing of the drug level may be important depending on the drug's pharmacokinetics and/or pharmacodynamics. Some drugs require monitoring peak and/or trough levels. A peak level is the maximum concentration during the dosing interval and is usually reached shortly after the drug's administration. A trough level is the minimum concentration during the dosing interval, which is right before the next dose is administered.

  a. Monitor and maintain peak levels (maximum serum concentration) for drugs whose effect or toxicity is correlated with the peak level. *Dosing adjustment strategy*: increasing the dosing interval will maintain similar peak levels.

  b. Monitor and maintain trough levels for most drugs whose effect or toxicity is dependent on a minimum concentration. *Dosing adjustment strategy*: decreasing the dose will maintain similar trough levels for drugs with a short half-life.

  c. Maintain average steady state drug levels for drugs that have no specific target peak or trough levels.

  (1) Dosing adjustment strategies.

    (a) Decreasing the dose will maintain adequate drug levels for most drugs.

    (b) A combination of decreasing the dose and increasing the dosing interval may be required for some drugs, particularly as kidney function worsens and for patients receiving dialysis.

  d. Monitoring free drug concentrations for the drug whenever possible will allow a more accurate determination of the necessary dosing adjustment.

  e. Serum levels of drugs that are removed by hemodialysis should generally not be drawn immediately after dialysis. Drug is removed during hemodialysis from the vasculature. After hemodialysis is completed, redistribution of drug from the tissue will occur and therefore the serum level will slightly increase.

2. Pharmacodynamics. Decreasing the dosage or interval for some drugs may be dependent on a pharmacodynamic effect. For example, B-lactam antibiotics (e.g., penicillins, cephalosporins) exhibit time-dependent killing. This means that the amount of time the concentration of the drug is above the minimum inhibitory concentration (MIC) for a certain bacteria is the most important factor for bacterial killing (Lodise et al., 2006). Therefore, when adjusting the dose of a B-lactam antibiotic in a patient with CKD, it would be preferred to decrease the dose rather than extend the dosing interval.

3. Supplemental dosing.
  a. Principles of supplemental dosing in patients receiving hemodialysis.
    (1) If the concentration of a drug decreases because of dialysis, a supplemental dose may need to be given to reestablish or maintain therapeutic levels.
    (2) Supplemental dosing after hemodialysis is based on the amount of drug removed, half-life of the drug, the dosage interval in relation to the hemodialysis schedule, and the amount of drug rebound or redistribution that occurs after dialysis.
    (3) The key to supplemental dosing is to replace the amount of the drug that was actually removed during hemodialysis.
  b. Examples. Table 5.4 summarizes the dialyzability of selected drugs that are frequently used in treating patients with CKD.

III. Drug dialyzability. Dialysis therapy significantly influences the pharmacologic management of patients with CKD.

A. Definition. A drug is considered to be dialyzable if the serum concentration can be significantly decreased during dialysis.

B. Influencing factors.
  1. Hemodialysis.
    a. Dialysis-dependent factors.
      (1) Blood flow rates.
      (2) Dialysate flow rate.
      (3) Dialysis membrane.
        (a) Surface area.
        (b) Pore size.
      (4) Length of dialysis.
      (5) Type of dialysis.
    b. Drug dependent factors.
      (1) Molecular weight. Drugs with a high molecular weight are not able to pass through the dialysis membrane. High-flux dialyzers will be able to remove substances with larger molecular weight than traditional low-flux dialyzers.
      (2) Plasma protein binding. Drugs that are highly plasma protein bound are not significantly removed by dialysis because the drug–protein complex is too large to pass through the dialysis membrane. Only unbound drug can be removed by dialysis.
      (3) Volume of distribution. Dialysis can remove substances from the intravascular space. If a drug has a large volume of distribution, most of the drug is located extravascular, in the tissues. In contrast, drugs with a small volume of distribution

Table 5.4

The Dialyzability of Selected Pharmacologic Agents

Drug	Removed by hemodialysis (Differences noted for high permeability dialysis when applicable)	Removed by peritoneal dialysis	Supplemental dose required (hemodialysis)	Drug	Removed by hemodialysis (Differences noted for high permeability dialysis when applicable)	Removed by peritoneal dialysis	Supplemental dose required (hemodialysis)
Analgesics				**Antihyperlipidemics**			
Acetaminophen	Yes	No	Yes	Fibric acid derivatives	No	No	No
Aspirin	Yes	Yes	Yes	Niacin	No	No	No
Codeine	No	?	No	Statins	No	?	No
Fentanyl	?	?	?	**Antihypertensives**			
Meperidine	No	No	No	Acebutolol	Yes	No	Yes
Methadone	No	No	No	Amlodipine	No	No	No
Morphine	No (Yes)	?	No	Atenolol	Yes	No	Yes
Pentazocine	Yes	?	Yes	Benzapril	No	?	No
Propoxyphene	No	No	No	Candesartan	No	?	No
Salsalate	Yes	No	Yes	Captopril	Yes	No	Yes
Antiarrhythmics				Clonidine	No	No	No
Amiodarone	No	No	No	Diltiazem	No	No	No
Bretylium	Yes	?	Yes	Doxazosin	No	No	No
Disopyramide	No	?	No	Enalapril	Yes	Yes	Yes
Flecanide	No	?	No	Esmolol	Yes	Yes	Yes
Lidocaine	No	?	No	Felodipine	No	?	No
Mexiletine	Yes	No	Yes	Hydralazine	No	No	No
N-Acetylprocainamide	Yes	No	Yes	Irbesartan	No	?	No
Procainamide	Yes	No	Yes	Labetalol	No	No	No
Propafenone	No	No	No	Lisinopril	Yes	?	Yes
Sotalol	Yes	?	Yes	Losartan	No	No	No
Tocainide	Yes	?	Yes	Methyldopa	Yes	Yes	Yes
Anticoagulants				Metoprolol	Yes	?	Yes
Dalteparin	No	No	No	Minoxidil	Yes	Yes	Yes
Enoxaparin	No	No	No	Nadolol	Yes	?	Yes
Fondaparinux	No	No	No	Nicardipine	No	?	No
Heparin	No	No	No	Nifedipine	No	No	No
Tinzaparin	No	No	No	Nimodipine	No	No	No
Warfarin	No	No	No	Nitrendipine	No	?	No
Anticonvulsants				Nitroprusside	Yes	Yes	Yes
Carbamazepine	No	No	No	Quinapril	No	No	No
Ethosuximide	Yes	?	Yes	Penbutolol	No	No	No
Lamotrigine	No	No	No	Prazosin	No	No	No
Phenobarbital	Yes	Yes	Yes	Propranolol	No	No	No
Phenytoin	No (Yes)	No	No	Ramipril	Yes	?	Yes
Primidone	Yes	?	Yes	Reserpine	No	No	No
Topiramate	Yes	?	Yes	Terazosin	No	No	No
Valproic acid	No	No	No	Timolol	No	No	No
Antidepressants				Valsartan	No	No	No
Amitriptyline	No	No	No	Verapamil	No	No	No
Buproprion	No	No	No	**Antiinflammatories**			
Citalopram	No	No	No	Celecoxib	?	?	?
Desipramine	No	No	No	Cortisone	No	No	No
Doxepin	No	No	No	Dexamethasone	No	No	No
Escitalopram	?	?	?	Fenoprofen	No	?	No
Fluoxetine	No	No	No	Ibuprofen	No	?	No
Imipramine	No	No	No	Indomethacin	No	?	No
Nortriptyline	No	No	No	Mefenamic acid	No	?	No
Paroxetine	No	No	No	Methylprednisolone	Yes	?	Yes
Sertraline	No	No	No	Naproxen	No	?	No
Antihistamines				Prednisolone	No	No	No
Cetirizine	No	No	No	Prednisone	No	No	No
Chlorpheniramine	Yes	No	Yes				
Fexofenadine	No	No	No				
Hydroxyzine	No	No	No				
Loratidine	No	No	No	*Table continues on next page*			

Table 5.4 (continued)

The Dialyzability of Selected Pharmacologic Agents

Drug	Removed by hemodialysis (Differences noted for high permeability dialysis when applicable)	Removed by peritoneal dialysis	Supplemental dose required (hemodialysis)	Drug	Removed by hemodialysis (Differences noted for high permeability dialysis when applicable)	Removed by peritoneal dialysis	Supplemental dose required (hemodialysis)
Antimicrobials				**Antineoplastics**			
Amikacin	Yes	Yes	Yes	Bleomycin	No	No	No
Amoxicillin	Yes	No	Yes	Carboplatin	Yes	?	Yes
Ampicillin	Yes	No	Yes	Carmustine	No	?	No
Azithromycin	No	No	No	Chlorabucil	No	No	No
Aztreonam	Yes	?	Yes	Cyclophosphamide	Yes	?	Yes
Carbenicillin	Yes	No	Yes	Doxorubicin	No	?	No
Cefaclor	Yes	Yes	Yes	Etoposide	No	No	No
Cefadroxil	Yes	No	Yes	Fluorouracil	Yes	?	Yes
Cefamandole	Yes	?	Yes	Hydroxyurea	No	?	No
Cefazolin	Yes	Yes	Yes	Lomustine	No	?	No
Cefepime	No	No	No	Mercaptopurine	Yes	?	Yes
Cefixime	No	No	No	Methotrexate	Yes	No	Yes
Cefoperazone	No	No	No				
Cefotaxime	Yes	No	Yes	**Antipsychotics**			
Cefotetan	Yes	Yes	Yes	Buspirone	Yes	?	Yes
Cefoxitin	Yes	No	Yes	Chlorpromazine	No	No	No
Ceftazidime	Yes	Yes	Yes	Haloperidol	No	No	No
Ceftriaxone	No	No	No	Mirtazapine	No	No	No
Cephalexin	Yes	No	Yes	Olanzapine	No	No	No
Cephalothin	Yes	No	Yes	Trifluoperazine	No	No	No
Cephadrine	Yes	Yes	Yes				
Chloramphenicol	Yes	No	Yes	**Antituberculosis**			
Cilastatin	Yes	?	Yes	Aminosalicylic acid	Yes	?	Yes
Ciprofloxacin	No	No	No	Ethambutol	No	?	No
Clarithromycin	?	?	?	Isoniazid	No	No	No
Clindamycin	No	No	No	Pyrazinamide	Yes	No	Yes
Cloxacillin	No	No	No				
Dicloxacillin	No	No	No	**Antivirals**			
Doxycycline	No	No	No	Acyclovir	Yes	No	Yes
Erythromycin	No	No	No	Adefovir	No	No	No
Gentamicin	Yes	Yes	Yes	Amantadine	No	No	No
Imipenem	Yes	Yes	Yes	Foscarnet	Yes	?	Yes
Kanamycin	Yes	Yes	Yes	Ganciclovir	Yes	?	Yes
Lincomycin	No	No	No	Lamivudine	No	No	No
Methicilin	No	No	No	Valacyclovir	Yes	?	Yes
Nafcillin	No	No	No	Valganciclovir	Yes	?	Yes
Norfloxacin	No	?	No				
Oxacillin	No	No	Yes	**Cardiotonics**			
Penicillin G	Yes	No	Yes	Digitoxin	No	No	No
Pentamidine	No	No	No	Digoxin	No	No	No
Piperacillin	Yes	No	Yes				
Rifampin	No	No	No	**Diuretics**			
Streptomycin	Yes	Yes	Yes	Bumetanide	No	?	No
Sulbactam	Yes	No	Yes	Chlorthalidone	No	?	No
Sulfamethoxazole	Yes	No	Yes	Ethacrynic acid	No	No	No
Sulfisoxazole	Yes	Yes	Yes	Furosemide	No	?	No
Tetracycline	No	No	No	Hydrochlorothiazide	No	?	No
Ticarcillin	Yes	No	Yes	Indapamide	No	?	No
Tobramycin	Yes	Yes	Yes	Metolazone	No	?	No
Trimethoprim	Yes	?	Yes	Spironolactone	No	No	No
Vancomycin	No (Yes)	No	No	Torsemide	No	No	No
Antimycotics							
Amphotericin B	No	No	No				
Caspofungin	No	No	No				
Fluconazole	Yes	No	Yes				
Flucytosine	Yes	Yes	Yes				
Ketoconazole	No	No	No				
Miconazole	No	No	No				
Voriconazole	No	No	No	*Table continues on next page*			

Table 5.4 (continued)

The Dialyzability of Selected Pharmacologic Agents

Drug	Removed by hemodialysis (Differences noted for high permeability dialysis when applicable)	Removed by peritoneal dialysis	Supplemental dose required (hemodialysis)	Drug	Removed by hemodialysis (Differences noted for high permeability dialysis when applicable)	Removed by peritoneal dialysis	Supplemental dose required (hemodialysis)
Gastrointestinal agents				**Miscellaneous agents, continued**			
Cimetidine	Yes	No	Yes	Filgrastim	No	No	No
Famotidine	No	No	No	Fludrocortisone	?	?	?
Granisetron	?	?	?	Gabapentin	Yes	?	Yes
Lansoprazole	No	No	No	Gold Na Thiomalate	No	?	No
Metoclopramide	No	No	No	Interferon	No	?	No
Nizatidine	No	No	No	Iron dextran	No	No	No
Omeprazole	?	?	?	Iron sucrose	No	No	No
Ondansetron	?	?	?	Penicillamine	Yes	?	Yes
Raniditine	No	No	No	Quinidine	No	No	No
Sucralfate	No	No	No	Theophylline	Yes	?	Yes
				Tolbutamide	No	?	No
Hypoglycemic agents							
Glipizide	No	No	No	**Sedatives-Hypnotics**			
Glyburide	No	?	No	Alprazolam	No	?	No
Insulin (all types)	No	No	No	Chloral hydrate	Yes	Yes	Yes
Metformin	Yes	?	Yes	Chlordiazepoxide	No	?	No
Nateglinide	No	No	No	Clonazepam	No	?	No
Pioglitazone	No	No	No	Clorazepate	No	?	No
Rosiglitazone	No	No	No	Diazepam	No	?	No
				Flurazepam	No	?	No
Immunosuppressants				Meprobamate	Yes	Yes	Yes
Azathioprine	Yes	?	Yes	Midazolam	No	?	No
Cyclosporine	No	No	No	Oxazepam	No	?	No
Mycophenolate	No	No	No	Pentobarbital	No	?	No
Sirolimus	No	No	No	Secobarbital	No	No	No
Tacrolimus	No	?	No	Temazepam	No	?	No
				Triazolam	No	?	No
Miscellaneous agents				Zaleplon	?	?	?
Allopurinol	Yes	?	Yes	Zolpidem	No	No	No
Calcitriol	No	No	No				
Darbepoetin	No	No	No	**Vasodilators**			
Doxercalciferol	No	No	No	Isosorbide dinitrate	No	No	No
Epoetin (EPO)	No	No	No	Isosorbide mononitrate	Yes	No	Yes
Ferric gluconate	No	No	No	Nitroglycerin	No	No	No
Ferrous salts	No	No	No				

Misc. agents continued at top of next column

are contained primarily in the vascular space and therefore are more likely to be removed by dialysis.
2. Peritoneal dialysis.
   a. Dialysis-dependent factors.
      (1) Surface area of peritoneum.
      (2) Blood flow rates to the peritoneum.
      (3) Type of dialysis.
   b. Drug-dependent factors.
      (1) Molecular weight. Drugs with a high molecular weight or a large particle size are not able to pass through the peritoneal membrane.

   (2) Plasma protein binding. Drugs that are largely protein bound are not removed by dialysis because the protein is too large to pass through the peritoneal membrane.
   (3) Volume of distribution. Similar to hemodialysis, drugs with a low volume of distribution are contained primarily in the vascular space and therefore are more likely to be removed by peritoneal dialysis.
   (4) Drug ionization at physiologic pH. Drugs that are ionized at physiologic pH cannot be removed by peritoneal dialysis.

SECTION E
The Clinical Significance for Nursing

From a nursing perspective, understanding pharmacology and how it relates to CKD is important for three essential areas of patient care: administering and monitoring medications, providing education, and fostering patient adherence.

I. **Administering and monitoring medications. Adverse effects can be avoided or minimized when the nurse appropriately administers and monitors pharmacologic agents.**

A. Be aware of all of the patient's medications.
   1. Refer to the prescriber's orders and medication record.
   2. Perform a medication reconciliation. A medication reconciliation should be performed any time a patient is transitioned from one healthcare setting to another (e.g., from an outpatient dialysis center to an inpatient hospital setting or from an intensive care unit within the hospital to an acute care unit within the hospital). This is done by comparing the medications that a patient was taking in his/her previous setting to the medications that are currently ordered. It will help to prevent any drug-related problems including medication omissions, duplications, or dosing errors. Healthcare organizations such as the Joint Commission (JC) and the Institute for Safe Medication Practices (ISMP) have recognized the importance of medication reconciliation as a safety tool (Greenwald et al., 2010). A thorough medication history can be obtained from the patient and/or caregiver. It is also important to specifically ask for any over-the-counter drugs, herbal supplement, or vitamin use. If the patient or caregiver is unable to give a complete history, the prescribed medications can be verified by the physician's office, hemodialysis center, or the patient's pharmacy.

B. Understand the pharmacokinetic and pharmaco-dynamic parameters of medications and if they are affected by CKD. This can be accomplished by considering the following questions in relation to each medication:
   1. Is the drug readily absorbed?
   2. Will the absorption be altered by CKD?
   3. Will the distribution be altered by CKD?
   4. Is the drug excreted unchanged or does it undergo significant metabolism?
   5. What is the primary route of excretion?
   6. Does CKD influence the excretion of the drug or its metabolites?
   7. What are the major characteristics of its metabolites?
   8. Is the drug nephrotoxic, and, if so, at what levels?
   9. What is the onset and duration of the pharmacologic effect?
   10. What is the influence of CKD on the half-life of the drug?
   11. Are dosage and frequency interval adjustments required in patients with CKD?
   12. Is the drug dialyzable?
   13. Will alterations in the normal administration schedule be necessary on dialysis days?
   14. Is supplemental dosing necessary after dialysis?
   15. What are the potential side effects of the drug?
   16. How is the drug likely to interact with other medications that the patient is taking?

C. Evaluation of serum electrolytes and drug levels. Serum electrolytes may become dangerously high or low in patients with abnormal kidney function, and monitoring regularly is necessary. Drug levels may also be monitored when a patient is on a drug with a narrow therapeutic window. This is done to ensure there is an optimal concentration in the body to have the intended effects and avoid toxic effects. The timing of serum drug levels may be particularly important for some drugs. All of these values are significant in the management of the patient with CKD.

D. Assessment of kidney function. Drug elimination by the kidney varies depending on the drug's chemical and pharmacokinetic properties. The clearance and half-life of many drugs and drug metabolites are altered as kidney function declines. Therefore, many drugs will require a drug dosage adjustment in patients with chronic or acute kidney disease. The degree of dosage adjustment depends on the degree of kidney dysfunction. Kidney function may change due to progression of chronic disease or acute injury, so an assessment should be performed regularly.

E. Improve patient safety.
   1. Medication errors. According to the FDA, medication errors cause at least one death every day and injure approximately 1.3 million people annually in the United States (FDA, 2009). Medication errors can occur at any time during medication ordering, transcribing, dispensing and/or preparing, or administration. Common causes of errors include similar product names or packaging, poor communication, and misinterpreting abbreviations or handwriting. Other errors may occur due to medication

omissions or duplications. These errors can be prevented by performing a medication reconciliation.

2. Five "rights" of medication administration. Prior to the administration of any medication, the five "rights" should be verified: right patient, right medication, right dose, right time, and right route.

   a. Right patient. Before administering any medication, it should be verified that the medication is being given to the correct patient. Using at least two patient identifiers, such as name, birthdate, or medical record number, will help to avoid this error. Many hospitals have implemented bar coding systems on patient wristbands to prevent a medication being administered to the wrong patient during hospitalization.

   b. Right medication. Factors that may contribute to administering the wrong medication include similar color or writing on medications or medication packaging, sound-alike medications (example Zantac®/Zyrtec®, dopamine/dobutamine), and transcribing orders. If it's necessary to take a verbal order from a prescriber, write down the order immediately and read it back to the prescriber aloud to verify. Always clarify orders if they are incomplete or illegible. Do not assume any part of an order.

   c. Right dose. Administering the correct dose of medication is very important. Always use leading zeros and avoid using trailing zeros (see "Error-Prone Abbreviations" below) when transcribing to avoid tenfold errors in dosing. Any unfamiliar doses should be verified by a reference and/or with the prescriber. Dosing calculations should always be double checked before administration.

   d. Right time. Timing of medication administration is sometimes important. Some drugs need to be separated by a given amount of time to avoid drug–drug interactions. For example, certain antibiotics must be separated from calcium, magnesium, and iron to ensure proper absorption. Drug–food interactions can also be significant, and some medications should be given on an empty stomach or full stomach depending on their pharmacokinetic properties. Timing of medications is also especially important in patients who are on dialysis. Some medications should be held until after dialysis or supplemented after dialysis because a significant proportion is removed during the hemodialysis procedure.

   e. Right route. Many drugs can be given by multiple routes of administration, such as intravenous, oral, intramuscular, subcutaneous, rectal, transdermal, and/or intraperitoneal. The dosage prescribed often depends on the bioavailability of the drug for the specific route of administration. For example, many medications require higher oral dosages than intravenous dosages. An oral dosage given intravenously could result in toxic adverse effects.

3. Error-prone abbreviations. Organizations such as the FDA and ISMP support avoiding error-prone abbreviations when ordering medications. There are many abbreviations that have routinely resulted in harmful errors. A few examples of abbreviations to avoid include:

   a. q.d or QD. Although the usual intended meaning of this abbreviation is once daily, it has been mistaken as q.i.d (4 times daily) or q.o.d. (every other day). It is recommended to use the word "daily" instead.

   b. q.o.d. or QOD. This may be interpreted as q.d. or QD. Use "every other day" instead.

   c. U or u. This abbreviation commonly used for "unit" has resulted in insulin errors because U may be read as 0 or 4. For example 2U may be read as 20. Using the word "unit" instead of U or u will help to avoid these errors. IU, an abbreviation for international unit, should also not be used.

   d. Leading and trailing zeros. Avoiding trailing zeros will help to prevent dosing errors. 2.0 mg may be seen as 20 mg if the decimal point is not seen. In addition, using a leading zero is recommended when ordering dosages less than 1 mg. Avoid potential errors by using 0.1 mg rather than .1 mg.

II. Providing education. When educating the patient about medications, the following information must be included.

A. The prescribed drug.

B. The purpose and actions of the drug.

C. The frequency, dosage, and route of administration of the drug.

D. The major side effects of the drug.

III. Fostering adherence.

Patient adherence with a prescribed healthcare regimen is a primary component that directly influences drug activity. The World Health Organization (WHO) has recognized that 30–50% of all patients are not adherent with their medication regimens. They have published evidence-based guidelines on improving patient adherence to improve outcomes and decrease healthcare costs (Sabate, 2003). Some of the most common reasons for not adhering to medication regimens include forgetfulness, fear of side effects, lack of noticeable effect, and cost. Striving to improve adherence should be a multidisciplinary approach. Nurses can be particularly influential in promoting medication adherence because of their prolonged and involved contact with the patient. Some examples of how nurses can help to foster adherence to medications include:

A. Helping the patient understand the rationale for treatment.

B. Encouraging the patient to become an active participant in the therapy.

C. Simplifying the medication regimen to fit the patient's daily routine.

D. Providing consistent continuity of care and supervision for the patient when he or she is assuming responsibility for the medication regimen.

E. Providing adequate, liberal amounts of feedback, and positive reinforcement.

F. Encouraging the family to become involved in the therapy so they can act as a support system for the patient.

G. Providing written as well as verbal instructions and information regarding the medications.

H. Establishing contacts with the patient to help in modifying behavior.

References

American Academy of Pain Medicine. (2013). Use of opioids for the treatment of chronic Pain. A statement from the American Academy of Pain Medicine. Retrieved from http://www.painmed.org/files/use-of-opioids-for-the-treatment-of-chronic-pain.pdf

American Society of Anesthesiologists Task Force on Chronic Pain Management & American Society of Regional Anesthesia and Pain Medicine. (2010). Practice guidelines for chronic pain management: An updated report by the American Society of Anesthesiologists Task Force on Chronic Pain Management and the American Society of Regional Anesthesia and Pain Medicine. *Anesthesiology, 112*(4), 810-833.

Bakris, G.L., Weir, M.R., Secic, M., Campbell, B., & Weis-McNulty, A. (2004). Differential effects of calcium antagonist subclasses on markers of nephropathy progression. *Kidney International, 65*, 1991–2002.

Baigent, C., Landray, M.J., Reith, C., Emberson, J., Wheeler, D.C., Tomson, C., … Collins, R., SHARP Investigators. (2011). The effects of lowering LDL cholesterol with simvastatin plus ezetimibe in patients with chronic kidney disease (Study of Heart and Renal Protection): A randomized placebo-controlled trial. *Lancet, 377*(9784), 2181-2192.

Bates, D.W., Su, L., Yu, D.T., Chertow, G.M., Seger, D.L., Gomes, D.R., … Platt, R. (2001). Mortality and costs of acute renal failure associated with amphotericin B therapy. *Clinical Infectious Diseases, 32*(5), 686-93.

Bianchi, S., Bigazzi, R., & Campese, V.M. (2006). Long-term effects of spironolactone on proteinuria and kidney function in patients with chronic kidney disease. *Kidney International, 70*, 2116–2123.

Camilleri, M. Parkman, H.P., Shafi, M.A., Abell, T.L., & Gerson, L. (2013). Clinical guideline: Management of gastroparesis. *American Journal of Gastroenterology, 108*(1), 18-38.

Chou, R., Fanciullo, G.J., Alder, J.A., Ballantyne, J.C., Davies, P., Donovan, M.I., … Miaskowski, C. (2009). American Pain Society-American Academy of Pain Medicine Opioids Guidelines Panel. Clinical guidelines for the use of chronic opioid therapy in chronic noncancer pain. *Journal of Pain, 10*(2), 113-130.

Cockcroft, D.W., & Gault, M.H. (1976). Prediction of creatinine clearance from serum creatinine. *Nephron, 16*(1) 31-41.

Drüeke, T.B., Locatelli, F., Clyne, N., Eckardt, K.U., Macdougall, I.C., Tsakiris, D., … Scherhag, A., CREATE Investigators. (2006). Normalization of hemoglobin level in patients with chronic kidney disease and anemia. *New England Journal of Medicine, 355*(20), 2071-2084.

Epstein, M., Williams, G.H., Weinberger, M., Lewin, A., Krause, S., Mukherjee, R., … Beckerman, B. (2006). Selective aldosterone blockade with eplerenone reduces albuminuria in patients with type 2 diabetes. *Clinical Journal of the American Society of Nephrology, 1*, 940–951.

Fellström, B.C., Jardine, A.G., Schmieder, R.E., Holdaas, H., Bannister, K., Beutler, J., … Zannad, F. (2009). Rosuvastatin and cardiovascular events in patients undergoing hemodialysis. AURORA Study Group. *New England Journal of Medicine, 360*(14), 1395- 1407.

Greenwald, J.L., Halasyamani, L.K., Greene, J., LaCivita, C., Stucky, E., Benjamin, B., …Williams, M.V. (2010). Making inpatient medication reconciliation patient centered, clinically relevant, and implementable: A consensus statement on key principles and necessary first steps. *Journal of Hospital Medicine, 5*(8), 477-485.

James, P.A., Oparil, S., Carter, B.L., Cushman, W.C., Dennison-Himmelfarb, C., Handler, J., … Ortiz, E. (2014). Evidence-based guideline for the management of high blood pressure in adults:

Report from the panel members appointed to the Eighth Joint National Committee (JNC 8). *The Journal of the American Medical Association, 311*(5), 507-520.

Kidney Disease: Improving Global Outcomes (KDIGO) CKD–MBD Work Group. (2009). KDIGO clinical practice guideline for the diagnosis, evaluation, prevention, and treatment of chronic kidney disease–mineral and bone disorder (CKD–MBD). *Kidney International, 76*(Suppl 113), S1–S130.

Kidney Disease: Improving Global Outcomes (KDIGO) Anemia Work Group. (2012a). KDIGO clinical practice guideline for anemia in chronic kidney disease. *Kidney International, 2*(4, Suppl. 2), 279–335.

Kidney Disease: Improving Global Outcomes (KDIGO) Blood Pressure Work Group. (2012b). KDIGO clinical practice guideline for the management of blood pressure in chronic kidney disease. *Kidney International, 2*(5, Suppl. 2), 337-414.

Kidney Disease: Improving Global Outcomes (KDIGO) Glomerulonephritis Work Group. (2012c). KDIGO clinical practice guideline for glomerulonephritis. *Kidney International, 2*(Suppl 2), 139–274.

Kliger, A.S., Foley R.N., Goldfarb, D.S., Goldstein S.L., Johansen, K., Ajay Singh, A., … Szczech, L. (2012). K/DOQI US commentary on the 2012 KDIGO clinical practice guideline for anemia in CKD. *American Journal of Kidney Disease, 62*(5), 849-859.

Lee, S.J., Silverman, E., & Bargman, M. (2011). The role of antimalarial agents in the treatment of SLE and lupus nephritis. Nature Reviews. *Nephrology, 7*(12), 718- 729.

Levey, A.S., Coresh, J., Greene, T., Stevens, L.A., Zhang, Y.L., Hendriksen, S., ... Van Lente, F. (2006). Using standardized serum creatinine values in the modification of diet in renal disease study equation for estimating glomerular filtration rate. *Annals of Internal Medicine, 145*(4), 247-254.

Levey, A.S., Stevens, L.A., Schmid, C.H., Zhang, Y.L., Castro, A.F., Feldman, H.I., ... Coresh, J. (2009). A new equation to estimate glomerular filtration rate. *Annals of Internal Medicine, 150*(9), 604-612.

Lodise, T.P., Lomaestro, B.M., & Drusano, G.L. (2006). Application of antimicrobial pharmacodynamic concepts into clinical practice: Focus on beta-lactam antibiotics: Insights from the society of infectious diseases pharmacists. *Pharmacotherapy, 26*(9), 1320-1332.

Manley, H.J., Garvin, C.G., Drayer, D.K., Reid, G.M., Bender, W.L., Neufeld, T.K., ... Muther, R.S. (2004). Medication prescribing patterns in ambulatory haemodialysis patients: Comparisons of USRDS to a large not-for-profit dialysis provider. *Nephrology Dialysis Transplantation, 19*, 1842-1848.

Mehdi, U.F., Adams-Huet, B., Raskin, P., Vega, G.L., & Toto, R.D. (2006). Addition of angiotensin receptor blockade or mineralocorticoid antagonism to maximal angiotensin-converting enzyme inhibition in diabetic nephropathy. *Journal of the American Society of Nephrology, 20*(12), 2641-2650.

Metoprolol CR/XL Randomised Intervention Trial in Congestive Heart Failure (MERIT-HF) Study Group. (1999). Effect of metoprolol CR/XL in chronic heart failure; Metoprolol CR/XL Randomised Intervention Trial in Congestive Heart Failure (MERIT-HF). *Lancet, 353*(9169), 2001-2007.

National Kidney Foundation (NKF). (2000). K/DOQI clinical practice guidelines on nutrition in renal failure. *American Journal of Kidney Disease, 35*(6, Suppl. 2), S1-S140.

National Kidney Foundation (NKF). (2003). K/DOQI clinical practice guidelines for bone metabolism and disease in chronic kidney disease. *American Journal of Kidney Disease, 43*(Suppl. 3), S1-S202.

National Kidney Foundation (NKF). (2004). K/DOQI clinical practice guidelines on hypertension and antihypertensive agents in chronic kidney disease. *American Journal of Kidney Disease, 43*(5, Suppl. 1), S1-S209.

National Kidney Foundation (NKF). (2010). KDOQI US commentary on the 2009 KDIGO clinical practice guidelines for the diagnosis, evaluation, and treatment of CKD-mineral and bone disorder (CKD-MDB). *American Journal of Kidney Disease, 55*(5), 773-799.

Olivieri, N.F., Buncic, J.R., Chew, E., Gallant, T., Harrison, R.V., Keenan, N., … Freedman, M.H. (1986). Visual and auditory neurotoxicity in patients receiving subcutaneous deferoxamine infusions. *New England Journal of Medicine, 314*(14), 869-873.

Packer, M., Fowler, M.B., Roecker, E.B., Coats, A.J., Katus, H.A., Krum, H., … DeMets, D.L. (2002). Effect of carvedilol on the morbidity of patients with severe chronic heart failure: Results of the carvedilol prospective randomized cumulative survival (COPERNICUS) study. *Circulation, 6*(17), 2194-9.

Pappas, P.G., Kauffman, C.A., Andes, D., Benjamin, D.K., Calandra, T.F., Edwards, J.E., … Sobel, J.D. (2009). Clinical practice guidelines for the management of candidiasis: 2009 update by the Infectious Diseases Society of America. *Clinical Infectious Diseases, 48*(5), 503-535.

Pfeffer, M.A., McMurray, J.J., Velazquez, E.J., Rouleau, J.L., Køber. L., Maggioni, A.P., … Califf, R.M. (2003). Valsartan, captopril, or both in myocardial infarction complicated by heart failure, left ventricular dysfunction, or both. *New England Journal of Medicine, 349*(20), 1893-906.

Pfeffer, M.A., Burdmann, E.A., Chen, C.Y., Cooper, M.E., de Zeeuw, D., Eckardt, K.U., … Toto, R. TREAT Investigations. (2009). A trial of darbepoetin alfa in type 2 diabetes and chronic kidney disease. *New England Journal of Medicine, 361*(21), 2019-2032.

Pitt, B., Zannad, F., Remme, W.J., Cody, R., Castaigne, A., Perez, A., … Wittes, J. (1999). The effect of spironolactone on morbidity and mortality in patients with severe heart failure. Randomized Aldactone Evaluation Study Investigators. *New England Journal of Medicine, 341*(10), 709-717.

Pitt, B., Remme ,W., Zannad, F., Neaton, J., Martinez, F., Roniker, B., … Gatlin, M., Eplerenone Post-Acute Myocardial Infarction Heart Failure Efficacy and Survival Study Investigators. (2003). Eplerenone, a selective aldosterone blocker, in patients with left ventricular dysfunction after myocardial infarction. *New England Journal of Medicine, 348*(14), 1309–21.

Sabate, E. (Ed.). (2003). *Adherence to long-term therapies: Evidence for action.* Geneva, Switzerland: World Health Organization. Retrieved from http://whqlibdoc.who.int/publications/2003/9241545992.pdf

Singh, A.K., Szczech, L., Tang, K.L., Barnhart, H., Sapp, S., Wolfson, M., … Reddan, D., CHOIR Investigators. (2006). Correction of anemia with epoetin alfa in chronic kidney disease. *New England Journal of Medicine, 355*(20), 2085-2098.

Stevens, L.A., & Levey, A.S. (2009). Measured GFR as a confirmatory test for estimated GFR. *Journal of the American Society of Nephrology, 20*, 2305-2313.

Stone, N.J., Robinson, J., Lichtenstein, A.H., Bairey Merz, C.N., Lloyd-Jones, D.M., Blum, C.B., …. Wilson, P.W. (2013). 2013 ACC/AHA guideline on the treatment of blood cholesterol to reduce atherosclerotic cardiovascular risk in adults: A report of the American College of Cardiology/American Heart Association Task Force on Practice Guidelines. *Circulation*, 1-84. Retrieved from http://circ.ahajournals.org/content/early/2013/11/11/01.cir.0000437738.63853.7a.long

The Cardiac Insufficiency Bisoprolol Study (CIBIS) Investigators and Committees. (1994). A randomized trial of beta-blockade in heart failure. The Cardiac Insufficiency Bisoprolol Study (CIBIS). *Circulation, 90*(4), 1765-1773.

The Cardiac Insufficiency Bisoprolol Study (CIBIS) Investigators and

Committees. (1999). The Cardiac Insufficiency Bisoprolol Study II (CIBIS-II): A randomised trial. *Lancet, 353*(9146), 9-13.

The Results of the Cooperative North Scandinavian Enalapril Survival Study (CONSENSUS) Group. (1987). Effects of enalapril on mortality in severe congestive heart failure. *New England Journal of Medicine, 316*(23), 1429-1435.

The SOLVD Investigators. (1992). Effect of enalapril on mortality and the development of heart failure in asymptomatic patients with reduced left ventricular ejection fractions. *New England Journal of Medicine, 327*(10), 685-691.

U.S. Food and Drug Administration (FDA). (2005). *Public heath advisory – FDA announces important changes and additional warnings for COX-2 selective and nonselective nonsteroidal antiinflammatory drugs (NSAIDS)*. Retrieved from http://www.fda.gov/Drugs/DrugSafety/PostmarketDrug SafetyInformationforPatientsandProviders/ucm150314.htm

U.S. Food and Drug Administration (FDA). (2009). *Medication error reports*. Retrieved from http://www.fda.gov/Drugs/DrugSafety/MedicationErrors/ucm080 629.htm

U.S. Food and Drug Administration (FDA). (2011). *FDA drug safety communication: New restrictions, contraindications, and dose limitations for Zocor (simvastatin) to reduce the risk of muscle injury*. Retrieved from http://www.fda.gov/drugs/drugsafety/ucm256581.htm

U.S. Food and Drug Administration (FDA). (2013). *FDA drug safety communication: FDA limits usage of Nizoral (ketoconazole) oral tablets due to potentially fatal liver injury and risk of drug interactions and adrenal gland problems*. Retrieved from http://www.fda.gov/drugs/drugsafety/ucm362415.htm

U.S. Renal Data System (USRDS).(2013). *Annual data report: Atlas of chronic kidney disease and end-stage renal disease in the United States*. National Institutes of Health, National Institute of Diabetes and Digestive and Kidney Diseases. Bethesda, MD. Retrieved from http://www.usrds.org/atlas.aspx

Wanner. C., Krane, V., März, W., Olschewski, M., Mann, J.F., Ruf. G., … Ritz. E., German Diabetes and Dialysis Study Investigators. (2005). Atorvastatin in patients with type 2 diabetes mellitus undergoing hemodialysis. *New England Journal of Medicine, 353*(3), 238-248.

Yancy, C.W., Jessup, M., Bozkurt, B., Butler, J., Casey, D.E., Drazner, M.H., … Wilkoff, B.L., American College of Cardiology Foundation; American Heart Association Task Force on Practice Guidelines. (2013). 2013 ACCF/AHA guideline for the management of heart failure: A report of the American College of Cardiology Foundation/American Heart Association Task Force on Practice Guidelines. *Journal of American College of Cardiology, 62*(16), e147-239.

Yeung, C.K., Shen, D.D., Thummel, K.E., & Himmelfarb, J. (2014). Effects of chronic kidney disease and uremia on hepatic drug metabolism and transport. *Kidney International, 85*, 522-528.

Zand, L., McKian, K.P., & Qian, Q. (2010). Gabapentin toxicity in patients with chronic kidney disease: A preventable cause of morbidity. The *American Journal of Medicine, 123*, 367-373.

Zannad, F., McMurray, J.J., Krum, H., van Veldhuisen, D.J., Swedberg, K., Shi, H., … Pitt, B., M.D. EMPHASIS-HF Study Group. (2011). Elperenone in patients with systolic heart failure and mild symptoms. *New England Journal of Medicine, 364*, 11-21.

Foundations in Infection Prevention, Control, and Clinical Applications in Nephrology Nursing

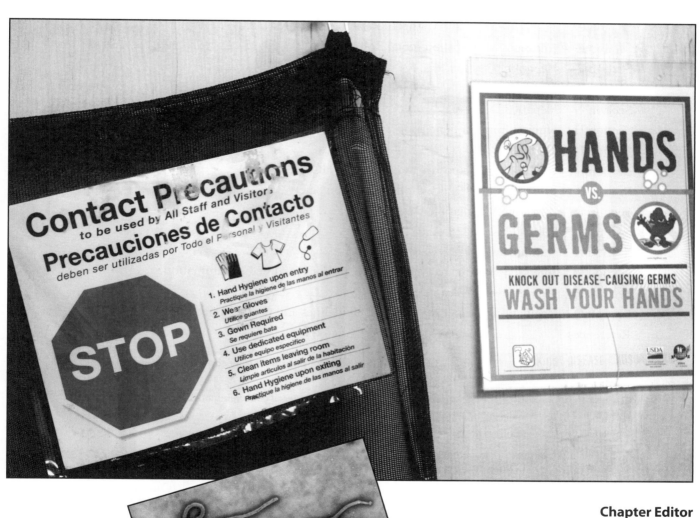

Chapter Editor
Eileen J. Peacock, MSN, RN, CNN,
CIC, CPHQ, CLNC

Authors
Eileen J. Peacock, MSN, RN, CNN,
CIC, CPHQ, CLNC
Caroline S. Counts, MSN, RN, CNN
Silvia German, RN, CNN
Kerri Holloway, RN, CNN
Liz Howard, RN, CNN
Karen Wiseman, MSN, RN, CNN

CHAPTER **6**

Foundations in Infection Prevention, Control, and Clinical Applications in Nephrology Nursing

This offering for **2.1 contact hours with 1.25 contact hours of pharmacology content** is provided by the American Nephrology Nurses' Association (ANNA).

American Nephrology Nurses' Association is accredited as a provider of continuing nursing education by the American Nurses Credentialing Center Commission on Accreditation.

ANNA is a provider approved by the California Board of Registered Nursing, provider number CEP 00910.

This CNE offering meets the continuing nursing education requirements for certification and recertification by the Nephrology Nursing Certification Commission (NNCC).

To be awarded contact hours for this activity, read this chapter in its entirety. Then complete the CNE evaluation found at **www.annanurse.org/corecne** and submit it; or print it, complete it, and mail it in. Contact hours are not awarded until the evaluation for the activity is complete.

Example of reference in APA style for Chapter 6.

Peacock, E.J., Counts, C.S., German, S., Holloway, K., Howard, L., & Wiseman, K. (2015). Foundations in infection prevention, control, and clinical applications in nephrology nursing. In C.S. Counts (Ed.), *Core curriculum for nephrology nursing: Module 2. Physiologic and psychosocial basis for nephrology nursing practice* (6th ed., pp. 331-396). Pitman, NJ: American Nephrology Nurses' Association.

Interpreted: Chapter authors. (Date). Title of chapter. In ...

Cover photo by Counts/Morganello.

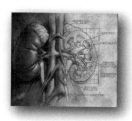

CHAPTER 6

Foundations in Infection Prevention, Control, and Clinical Applications in Nephrology Nursing

Purpose

The purpose of this chapter is to provide a cognitive understanding of current concepts in infectious diseases and their implications for practice in hemodialysis centers. Bear in mind that information pertaining to infectious diseases continually changes and that it is wise to monitor sources of reliable information, such as the Centers for Disease Control and Prevention (CDC).

Objectives

Upon completion of this chapter, the learner will be able to:
1. List methods that decrease the risk of infections in the vascular access.
2. Describe factors that contribute to development of drug resistance.
3. Describe the specific infection control requirements for patients with viral infectious diseases.
4. Discuss methods to prevent occupational exposure in a healthcare facility.
5. Describe the difference between latent TB infection and active disease.
6. Outline current recommendations for immunizations in patients with chronic kidney disease.
7. Identify how contamination of the delivery system fluid pathway can contribute to patient infections.
8. Define how the CQI process may be used to address infection control issues in the dialysis unit.

SECTION A
Overview

I. Patients with chronic kidney disease, stage 5, are at risk of infection for a number of reasons.

A. Impaired immune function.

B. Presence of a vascular access to perform kidney replacement therapy.

C. Presence of one or more additional chronic illnesses.

D. Frequent hospitalizations, surgeries, and/or medical procedures.

E. Provision of care in a setting where multiple patients are treated at the same time by multiple caregivers.

F. Use of immunosuppressive medications.

II. In patients with chronic kidney disease, stage 5, infections are the second most common cause of death. A large number of hospitalizations of dialysis patients and transplant patients are due to infections.

III. In healthy individuals, inflammation is a protective mechanism that assists in removing the antigen and facilitates the healing process. Patients with CKD are known to have ongoing micro-inflammation. Inflammation in patients with CKD is due to multiple factors.

A. Infection.

B. Use of bioincompatible dialyzer membranes.

C. Backfiltration of nonsterile dialysate during the hemodialysis treatment.

D. Periodontal disease.

E. Ongoing uremic environment.

F. Malnutrition.

G. Hemolysis.

H. Surgery.

IV. When inflammation becomes excessive or continuous, inflammatory processes no longer contribute to healing. Growth factors are inhibited and wound healing cells do not function normally. Healing is impaired and a vicious cycle of ongoing injury begins. Ongoing inflammation leads to:

A. Loss of muscle mass and hypoalbuminemia.

B. Cardiovascular disease.

C. Erythropoietin resistance.

V. Recent studies imply that cardiovascular events (such as myocardial infarction and congestive heart failure) may be influenced by infections because of increased inflammatory mediators that accompany the infections.

Section B
Bacteremia

I. Overview.

A. Bloodstream infections remain a significant cause of morbidity and mortality in the hemodialysis patient.

B. Per the CDC, hospitalization rates related to bloodstream infections among hemodialysis patients have increased 47% since 1993.

II. Kidney failure and bacteremia risk factors.

A. Chronic hemodialysis requiring vascular access for prolonged periods.

B. The hemodialysis environment, which provides opportunities for transmission of infectious agents.

C. Patients with kidney failure have higher incidence of bloodstream infections (bacteremia).
   1. Altered immune response due to kidney failure.
   2. Impaired neutrophil function.
   3. Frequent hospitalizations.

D. Patient factors.
   1. Extremes of age; older adults at greatest risk.
   2. Chronic health problems and comorbid conditions.
      a. Diabetes mellitus.
      b. Disorders of the kidney.
      c. Malnutrition.
      d. Debilitation.
      e. Splenectomy.
      f. Wounds.
   3. Immunosuppression due to:
      a. Suppressed inflammatory response.
      b. High level of circulating uremic toxins.
      c. Abnormal intake of nutrients necessary for white blood cell (WBC) growth and function.

E. Treatment factors.
   1. Hospitalization.
   2. Invasive procedures.

3. Instrumentation or artificial devices that penetrate the body (e.g., central venous catheter).
   a. Frequency of manipulation.
   b. Site of insertion.
   c. Contamination of dialysis catheter at time of insertion or contamination of hub at the time of use.
   d. Portals of entry by which the infectious agent can enter the human body include disruption of the skin, the body's first line of defense. A susceptible host is one which lacks effective resistance to the infectious agent. Risk factors include:
      (1) Age of host and general health, including comorbidities.
      (2) Nutritional status.
      (3) Absent or abnormal immunoglobulins/ability of hematopoietic system to function.
   e. Nasal and skin colonization (O'Grady et al., 2011).
      (1) Number of organisms present at exposure.
      (2) Duration of exposure.
4. Catheters.
   a. Associated with a high prevalence of catheter-related bacteremia (O'Grady et al., 2011).
   b. Catheter location.
   c. Catheter colonization.
   d. Duration of catheterization.
   e. Dialysis catheters are associated with significant risk of bacteremia compared to arteriovenous fistulas.
5. Immunosuppression.
   a. Suppressed inflammatory response.
   b. High level of circulating uremic toxins.
   c. Abnormal intake of nutrients necessary for WBC growth and function.

III. Causes. Presence of bacteria within the bloodstream. Bacteria more commonly associated with catheter-related bacteremia include the following:

A. Coagulase-negative staphylococci (CNS).
   1. Example: *Staphylococcus epidermidis*.
   2. Commonly found on skin and mucosal surfaces.
   3. Frequent cause of infection of vascular access devices.
   4. Infection can result from invasion from a person's endogenous strain.
   5. Foreign bodies such as intravascular catheters or prosthetic heart valves are predisposed to infection with CNS.

B. *Staphylococcus aureus*.
   1. Considered part of normal human skin flora.
   2. Colonization common in anterior nares and moist body areas.

3. Causes a wide variety of infections, ranging from localized (e.g., wound infection) to disseminated disease (e.g., septicemia).
4. Foreign bodies, such as intravascular catheters, commonly lead to infection with *S. aureus*.

C. Gram-negative bacilli. Examples:
   1. *Pseudomonas.*
   2. *Escherichia coli.*
   3. *Klebsiella pneumoniae.*
   4. *Serratia.*
   5. *Enterobacter.*

IV. Physiologic response to infection.

A. Bacteremia does not always result in systemic inflammatory response syndrome or sepsis.

B. Systemic inflammatory response syndrome (SIRS).
   1. Widespread, systemic inflammatory activation to bodily insult, such as invading organism(s), ischemia, inflammation, or trauma.
   2. SIRS may be due to more than one factor and is not always related to infection.
   3. SIRS criteria. Presence of two or more of the following:
      a. Temperature alteration.
      b. Heart rate > 90/min.
      c. Respiratory rate > 20/min.
      d. White blood cell count alteration.
   4. Causes of SIRS may be infectious or noninfectious. Examples:
      a. Trauma/tissue injury.
      b. Pancreatitis.
      c. Infective endocarditis.
      d. Thermal injury.
      e. Drug reactions.
      f. Surgical procedures.
      g. Candidiasis.
      h. Bacterial infection.

C. Sepsis = infection plus SIRS.
   1. Sepsis criteria.
      a. Hypotension (functional hypovolemia).
      b. Hypoperfusion of tissues and organs.
      c. Organ dysfunction.
         (1) Oliguria.
         (2) Mental changes.
         (3) Hyperdynamic state.
            (a) Increased cardiac output.
            (b) Peripheral vasodilatation.
            (c) Decreased systemic vascular response (SVR).
   2. Sepsis is a systemic response to infection, resulting in:
      a. Activation of the inflammatory cascade with ability to damage organ systems.

b. Activation of both the cellular and humoral immune systems (Silva et al., 2008).
c. Damage to the vascular endothelium.
d. Microcapillary leakage occurs toward the third space.
e. Cardiac dysfunction secondary to toxins and inflammatory mediators; diminished ejection fraction.
   3. Increasing incidence of sepsis is due to:
      a. Immunocompromised patients (including those with kidney disease).
      b. Resistant microorganisms.
      c. Increasing elderly population.
      d. Increased use of invasive procedures/lines.
      e. Increasing population with comorbid conditions.
   4. Sepsis has been identified as one of the most common causes of death in the intensive care unit (ICU).
   5. Compared to the general population, patients on dialysis have a higher annual mortality rate due to sepsis.

V. Management of sepsis.

A. Management of sepsis includes (Society of Critical Care Medicine, 2013):
   1. Eliminate cause of sepsis/eradication of the causative organism.
      a. Empirical intravenous antibiotics to cover both gram positive and gram negative organisms.
      b. Adjustment of antibiotics based on culture and sensitivity results.
      c. Removing potentially infecting device.
         (1) Catheter removal.
         (2) Catheter exchange.
      d. Surgical management of septic source when appropriate (e.g., debridement of infected or necrotic tissue, graft excision or total removal).
   2. Hemodynamic support consists of:
      a. Administration of fluids.
      b. Use of vasoactive drugs.
   3. Respiratory support.

B. Criteria for septic shock.
   1. Sepsis hypodynamic phase or late phase when heart can no longer compensate.
      a. Hypotension despite fluid resuscitation.
      b. Decreased cardiac output.
      c. Peripheral vasoconstriction.
      d. Increased systemic vascular resistance.
      e. Hypoperfusion; tissue hypoxia.
      f. Multiple organ dysfunction results in:
         (1) Oliguria.
         (2) Hepatic failure.
         (3) Mental changes.
         (4) Respiratory failure.

(5) Disseminated intravascular coagulation (DIC).

2. Septic shock occurs as result of bacteria and/or toxins released by bacteria circulating in the blood.

a. Proinflammatory cytokines and other metabolites (prostaglandins) cause an increase in endothelial-derived nitric oxide.

b. Nitric oxide causes changes in cell wall transport mechanisms.

c. Decreases in intracellular calcium lead to vasodilatation and resistance to vasopressor agents.

d. A primary cause of the shock is systemic vasoactive mediators released by gram-negative bacteria associated with vasodilatation, affecting almost every physiologic system.

e. Some vessels (arterioles) remain vasoconstricted due to various inflammatory mediators (e.g., tumor necrosis factor), leading to maldistribution of blood flow.

VI. Laboratory test and interpretation.

A. Interpretation/evaluation of culture and sensitivity, CBC with differential.

1. Identify causative agent.

a. Blood cultures should be obtained whenever antibiotics are started for a suspected bloodstream infection.

b. Collected prior to administration of antibiotic.

c. Bacterial growth is identified and classified by shape and size.

d. Organisms undergo gram staining procedure.
(1) Rapid test to characterize microorganisms.
(2) Organisms are identified as gram-positive or gram-negative prior to final identification of the microorganism(s).
(3) Shape of organism is determined – rods vs. cocci.
(4) Fungi may be seen on gram stain.
    (a) Single cell with buds (yeast).
    (b) Presence of hyphae or plant-like filamentous branches (mold).
(5) Gram stain results should be promptly reported to help guide treatment.

2. Organism identification by isolation from culture.

a. Common pathogens such as *Staphylococci, Streptococci*, and *Enterococci* can be identified within 48 hours.

b. Fungal organisms may take 10–14 days for identification.

c. Organism identification should be promptly reported.

3. Sensitivity reports are obtained on clinically significant isolates (Baron et al., 2013) and based on:

a. Minimum inhibitory concentration that will inhibit growth of an organism.

b. Agar diffusion tests reported as resistant if growth is not altered or sensitive if growth is inhibited.

4. Resolution of infection, minimizing the use of broad spectrum antibiotics by targeting antibiotic therapy, and preventing the emergence of drug resistant organisms, requires prompt reporting of the gram stain, the preliminary and final organism identification, and antibiotic sensitivities to the physician, advanced practice registered nurse (APRN), or physician assistant (PA).

5. Avoid administration of antibiotics for organisms that may not be the causative agent of the infection. For example, if a single blood culture is positive for CNS, and other blood cultures are negative, consider the possibility that the culture was contaminated with skin flora (*S. epidermidis*).

6. Complete blood count (CBC) provides:

a. White blood cell count (WBC).
(1) Total number of circulating leukocytes.
(2) Differential.
(3) Provides important information concerning the inflammatory response of the patient, as well as the response to therapy.
(4) Total number of circulating leukocytes and the differential change during bacterial or viral infection.
(5) Acute bacterial infection causes a rise in the white blood cell neutrophils and increased bands (immature neutrophils).

b. Red blood cell count (RBC): hematocrit/hemoglobin levels.

c. Platelets: presence of thrombocytopenia.

VII. Blood culture collection.

A. Two sets of blood cultures should be drawn. Each set includes a bottle for aerobic and a bottle for anaerobic medium.

B. Proper collection and handling of specimens is imperative for the causative organism to be correctly identified.

C. Avoid potential contamination of the specimen. Aseptic technique is mandatory to avoid contaminating the specimen with organisms that colonize the skin or are present on the central venous catheter hub or port.

D. When possible, obtain blood specimen by peripheral venipuncture.

1. Cultures drawn from central venous catheters may reflect organisms that have colonized the catheter

and may not accurately reflect organisms freely circulating in the patient's bloodstream.

2. Evaluate results drawn from central venous catheters carefully. If bacterial growth is present only in the sample obtained from the central venous catheter and not from peripheral cultures, the bacteria from the central venous catheter may not be the cause of the infection and may not require treatment with antibiotics.

E. Centers for Disease Control and Prevention (CDC) recommend treatment only for demonstrated bacteremia, and not for results obtained from catheter tips.

VIII. CDC Dialysis Bloodstream Infection (BSI) Prevention Collaborative.

A. Preventing bloodstream infections among dialysis patients has been identified as a national priority by the U.S. Department of Health and Human Services.

B. Package or bundle of interventions shown to prevent bloodstream infections were collaboratively developed (CDC, 2012c; Patel et al., 2013).

C. Several interventions have been recommended particularly for hemodialysis patients with central lines.

D. The CDC (2014h) has published the interventions/recommendations as *Core Interventions for Dialysis Bloodstream Infection (BSI) Prevention* and are available at http://www.cdc.gov/dialysis/prevention-tools/core-interventions.html

E. Conducting monthly surveillance of bloodstream infections using the National Healthcare Safety Network (NHSN) surveillance system allows dialysis facilities to track infections and have access to different analysis options that can be used to make informed decisions about quality improvement initiatives.

F. Audit tool and checklist are available as part of the CDC Dialysis BSI Prevention Collaborative aimed at preventing bloodstream infections (BSIs) in hemodialysis patients. Available audit tools include hand hygiene observations and access-related observations. The audit tools are available at http://www.cdc.gov/dialysis/PDFs/collaborative/audit-tools-Portfolio2.pdf

SECTION C
Vascular Access and Catheter-Related Infections

I. Overview.

A. Infection is the second leading cause of death in dialysis patients. Among hemodialysis patients, infections may account for 15% of deaths (Arduino & Tokars, 2005).

B. Access-related infections are the leading cause of infection in CKD stage 5 patients (KDOQI, 2006).

C. Access infections may vary from minor infections at the needle insertion site to severe infections of the entire access, which may require graft or catheter removal.

D. Disseminated bacteremia and sepsis and life-threatening complications increase morbidity and mortality in these patients.

E. Infection can occur from movement of the patient's normal skin flora on or into the vascular access during cannulation or when accessing the hemodialysis catheter.

F. Patient infection can result from failure to follow established vascular access care procedures and meticulous aseptic technique or strict infection control practices.

G. Access infection is a preventable complication.

II. Risk factors.

A. The primary risk factor for access infection is the type of access.
   1. AV fistulas have a lower incidence of infection compared to AV grafts or catheters (KDOQI, 2006).
   2. Catheters have the highest incidence of infection.
      a. Permanent catheters should be reserved for patients who are not candidates for an AVF or AVG.
      b. NKF/DOQI guidelines recommend no more than 10% of patients be maintained with a permanent catheter and that 40% of prevalent patients who initiate hemodialysis have a native AV fistula constructed.

B. Other potential risk factors include the following.
   1. Location of vascular access in the lower extremity.
   2. Trauma to the access site or arm.

3. Recent access surgery.
4. Hematoma.
5. Dermatitis.
6. Poor patient hygiene.
7. Iron overload.
8. Diabetes (Arduino & Tokars, 2005).

III. Infection type, signs and symptoms, and infecting organisms.

A. Immunosuppression and manifestations of infection.
1. Patients with chronic kidney disease stage 5 may not demonstrate signs and symptoms of infection normally seen in immune competent patients. For example, a low-grade temperature can be significant and a serious infection can exist with few signs or symptoms (such as little to no redness or swelling).
2. As part of the pretreatment assessment, the patient should be asked about any unusual occurrences involving the access or possible signs of infection that may have been experienced since the last dialysis treatment.

B. Local infection.
1. Local involving blood vessel, graft, or surrounding tissue.
2. Signs and symptoms.
   a. Fever or chills.
   b. Pain or tenderness of access or exit site.
   c. Redness or erythema.
   d. Loculated fluid or purulent drainage from access, exit site, or catheter insertion site.
   e. Induration within 2 cm of exit site.
   f. Swelling and inflammation.
   g. Warmth or hot to touch.
   h. Localized area of cellulitis or breakdown of skin at access site (Arduino & Tokars, 2005).

C. Systemic infection.
1. Systemic: sepsis from infection spilling into the bloodstream.
2. Signs and symptoms may include the following.
   a. Malaise.
   b. Fever and chills.
   c. Presence of local infection symptoms.
   d. Altered mental status or confusion.
   e. Hypotension.
   f. Septicemia.

D. Infecting organisms.
1. Gram-positive organisms (*Staphylococcus aureus*, coagulase negative staphylococci [CNS], *Staphylococcus epidermidis*).
   a. Most common causes of vascular access-related infections are staphylococci. Infections from staphylococci are associated with high rates of

recurrence, metastatic complications, and mortality (Nassar & Avus, 2001).
   b. The number of infections caused by *S. aureus* is higher among patients with fistulas or grafts.
   c. The number of infections caused by CNS is higher among patients dialyzed with catheters.
2. Gram negative organisms, enterococci, and fungi (Arduino & Tokars, 2005; CDC, 2001a).

IV. Catheter-related infections.

A. Infection is the leading cause of catheter loss. Infection in central venous catheters may occur at the exit site, at the tunnel track, or systemically.

B. Intravascular catheter-related bloodstream infections lead to increased morbidity, prolonged hospital stays, and increased medical costs.

C. Bacteria can spread from the patient's skin to the catheter exit site, along the exterior catheter surface or internally from external contamination of the catheter lumen, or from colonization of bacteria from other infected areas.

D. Inappropriate catheter care guidelines, failure to access central venous catheter using aseptic technique, and inadequate hand hygiene can result in infection.

E. Prevention.
1. Recommendations for preventing vascular access infection have been developed by the Vascular Access Workgroup of the National Kidney Foundation – Dialysis Outcomes Quality Initiative (NKF-DOQI) in 1998. The Clinical Practice Guidelines for Vascular Access were updated in 2006.
2. Selected recommendations for preventing hemodialysis catheter-related infections (Arduino & Tokars, 2005; KDOQI, 2006).
   a. Use sterile technique during catheter insertion.
   b. Limit the use of noncuffed catheters to 3 to 4 weeks.
   c. Use the catheter solely for dialysis unless there is no other alternative.
   d. The catheter exit site should be examined for signs and symptoms of infection by experienced trained dialysis staff at each dialysis treatment and before opening and accessing the catheter.
   e. Restrict catheter manipulation and dressing changes to trained personnel.
   f. Replace catheter-site dressing at each dialysis treatment or if damp, loose, or soiled.
   g. Disinfect skin before catheter insertion and dressing changes.
   h. CDC recommends using povidone iodine

ointment or bacitracin/gramicidin/polymyxin B ointment at the hemodialysis catheter exit site after catheter insertion and at each hemodialysis session. The CDC recognizes concerns exist about development of antimicrobial resistance (CDC, 2014h).

    i. Ensure that catheter-site care products and ointments are compatible with the catheter material. *Note*: Ingredients in antibiotic and povidone-iodine ointments may interact with the chemical composition of certain catheters.

    j. Wear a surgical mask or face shield (both patient and caregiver) during connect and disconnect procedures.

    k. Use strict aseptic technique when accessing catheters or performing catheter dressing changes.

    l. Teach patient and staff early identification of signs and symptoms of infection.

    m. Track and trend infections to identify source and allow corrective action.

F. Treatment.
1. Treat catheter infections with antibiotic therapy based on the organism isolated.
2. Antimicrobials at infected access site.
3. Catheter lock solutions containing antimicrobial agents.
4. Catheter removal recommended for noncuffed catheters.
5. Catheter removal for cuffed catheters if not responsive to treatment.
6. Infected catheters should be exchanged as soon as possible and within 72 hours of initiating antibiotic therapy in most instances.

V. AV fistula and graft infections.

A. Inappropriate access site preparation, poor cannulation technique, and inadequate hand hygiene can result in patient infection.

B. Prevention.
1. Teach patient proper personal hygiene.
2. Strict aseptic cannulation technique.
3. Access care and protection.
4. Train dialysis staff in infection control procedures.
5. Proper hand washing.
6. Teach patient and staff early identification of signs and symptoms of infection.
7. Track and trend infections to identify source and allow corrective action.
8. Early referral for fistula/graft access placement to minimize catheter use.
9. Improve cannulation skills (i.e., cannulation camp, mentorship program).

C. Treatment.
1. Appropriate antibiotics based on culture and sensitivity as ordered.
2. Antimicrobials at infected access site.
3. Graft or fistula removal if indicated.
4. Avoid cannulation of infected access.

VI. Approach to BSI prevention in dialysis facilities – Core Interventions for Dialysis Bloodstream Infection (BSI) Prevention.

A. The CDC (2014h) has published recommendations to prevent bloodstream infections in hemodialysis patients. These recommendations, *The Core Interventions for Dialysis Bloodstream Infection (BSI) Prevention* are available at http://www.cdc.gov/dialysis/prevention-tools/core-interventions.html

B. These CDC recommendations include the following.
1. Conducting monthly infection event surveillance using CDC's National Healthcare Safety Network (NHSN).
2. Observing dialysis staff hand hygiene practices monthly.
3. Observing dialysis staff vascular access care and catheter connection and disconnection technique as well as dressing change technique quarterly.
4. Training staff on infection control topics, including access care and aseptic technique.
5. Performing vascular access-related skills competency check upon hire and every 6 to12 months.
6. Providing standardized education to all patients on infection prevention topics including vascular access care, hand hygiene, risks related to catheter use, signs of infection, and directions for access management when away from the dialysis unit.
7. Reducing the use of catheters.
8. Using alcohol-based chlorhexidine solution as the skin antiseptic agent for central line insertion and during dressing changes. Alternatives include povidone-iodine with alcohol or 70% alcohol.
9. Performing catheter hub scrub with an appropriate antiseptic after cap is removed and before accessing the catheter.
10. Using an antibiotic ointment or povidone-iodine ointment at catheter exit site.

C. Audit tool and checklist are available as part of the CDC Dialysis BSI Prevention Collaborative, a partnership aimed at preventing bloodstream infections (BSIs) in hemodialysis patients: http://www.cdc.gov/dialysis/PDFs/collaborative/checklist-Portfolio.pdf. A hand hygiene checklist is available. Specific checklists for preventing vascular access related infections include the following.

1. Hemodialysis catheter exit site care.
2. Hemodialysis catheter connection.
3. Hemodialysis catheter disconnection.
4. Arteriovenous fistula/ graft cannulation.
5. Arteriovenous fistula/ graft decannulation.

SECTION D
Antibiotic and Antimicrobial Resistance

I. Overview.

A. "Antimicrobial resistance is one of our most serious health threats. Infections from resistant bacteria are now too common, and some pathogens have even become resistant to multiple types or classes of antibiotics" (CDC, 2013a).
   1. In the United States alone, at least 2 million people acquire an infection with antibiotic-resistant bacteria, and at least 23,000 people die each year as a direct result (CDC, 2013a).
   2. More die from related conditions that were complicated by an antibiotic-resistant infection (Ingham, 2014), increasing the number of deaths to approximately 90,000 per year (Collins, 2008; FDA, 2014b).
   3. Greater than 70% of bacteria that cause hospital-associated infections are resistant to one or more of the antibiotics used as treatment (Collins, 2008; FDA, 2014b; Muto, 2005).
   4. According to the CDC, almost all significant bacterial infections are becoming resistant to the antibiotic used as the treatment of choice (CDC, 2013a; FDA, 2014a; Laxminarayan et al., 2013).

B. Antibiotic resistance is the lack of effect of an antibiotic. Simply stated, it is when an antibiotic is no longer able to effectively control or kill bacterial growth (APUA, 2013).
   1. Antibiotic-resistant bacteria continue to multiply in the presence of what should be therapeutic levels of an antibiotic.
   2. Resistance develops when bacteria find new ways to disarm the drug.
   3. Some bacteria have natural resistance and other bacteria have acquired resistance.
   4. It is not unusual for more than one mechanism to work together to confer resistance to an antibiotic (AMRLS, 2014; Boozer et al., 2014).

C. In the CDC report, *Antibiotic Resistance Threats in the United States, 2013*, the loss of effective antibiotics to fight infections is seen as a significant public health threat.
   1. Antibiotic resistance hinders the ability to manage the infectious complications common in vulnerable populations, such as patients receiving dialysis and organ transplantation.
   2. Antibiotic-resistant infections may result in longer duration of illness, higher mortality, and higher costs of treatment.
   3. Antibiotic resistance may even result in the inability to perform necessary medical procedures that rely on antibiotics to prevent infection (CDC, 2013a; Laxminarayan et al., 2013; WHO, 2014a).

II. Resistance mechanisms.

A. Natural or intrinsic resistance of bacteria.
   1. Intrinsic or innate ability to resist a given antibiotic's therapeutic effects.
   2. Due to functional or structural qualities of the bacteria.
      a. Lack of transport system for the antibiotic into the bacteria.
      b. Lack of a target for the antibiotic within the bacteria.
      c. The antibiotic's inability to penetrate the outer membrane or cell wall of the bacteria. An example of this type of intrinsic resistance is the structure of the complex cell wall of gram-negative bacteria that does not allow the antibiotic vancomycin to diffuse into the bacteria through the narrow cell wall channels (AMRLS, 2014; ASM, 2005; Neu & Gootz, 1996).
      d. Innate production of enzymes that destroy the drug.
      e. Spontaneous mutation or bacterial errors when copying their DNA (ASM, 2005; Boozer et al., 2014; Holmes & Jobling, 1996; Rice & Bonomo, 2007).

B. Acquired resistance refers to bacteria that have been sensitive to an antibiotic but subsequently develop resistance by mutations in chromosomes, or by acquiring resistance genes carried on mobile genetic elements (plasmids, transposons, integrons) through different mechanisms such as horizontal gene transfer (HGT) via transformation, transduction or conjugation. HGT has been responsible for the antimicrobial-resistance determinants found in many different species of bacteria (AMRLS, 2014; ASM, 2005; Barlow, 2009; Boozer et al., 2014; Holmes & Jobling, 1996; Rao, 2006). An example of resistance due to HGT is *Staphylococcus aureus* resistance to methicillin (MRSA) by acquisition of mecA genes responsible for the resistance.
   1. *Transformation* – uptake of short fragments of DNA found in the bacteria's external environment. These fragments are from the death and dissolution of other bacteria.
   2. *Transduction*– bacteriophages (viruses that infect

bacteria) carry that bacterium's DNA into closely related bacteria and, with it, transfer resistance genes.

3. *Conjugation* – transfer of DNA via bacteria's sexual pilus, which attaches to the recipient bacteria, bringing the two cells together and allowing for the exchange of genetic material (AMRLS, 2014; ASM, 2005; Boozer et al., 2014; Holmes & Jobling, 1996; Rao, 2006; Rice & Bonomo, 2007).

III. Factors contributing to the development of resistance.

A. Development of resistance once a new antibiotic is introduced into clinical practice is common and is found all over the world (Davies & Davies, 2010).
   1. Appropriate use and misuse of antibiotics contributes to resistance (FDA, 2014a). Many antibiotics are thought to be used unnecessarily or not prudently.
   2. Antibiotics are widely used in food animal production to prevent infection and promote growth of the animal (APUA, 2013).
   3. Use of antibiotics causes selective pressure on bacteria, killing the susceptible bacteria while resistant bacteria survive and multiply (Davies & Davies, 2010).

B. The World Health Organization (WHO) sees antibiotic resistance as a threat to global health security and has proposed measures necessary to stem the dramatic increase in the number of drug resistant bacteria worldwide.
   1. The problem is multifaceted and a comprehensive and coordinated response is required.
   2. Education to address resistance in various settings, such as programs for the community, healthcare providers, laboratory staff, veterinarians, and food animal producers are considered essential (Laxminarayan et al., 2013).
   3. Policies addressing prudent antibiotic use in human and in animal husbandry, established infection prevention and control standards, antibiotic stewardship programs, as well as global antibiotic resistance surveillance and monitoring systems, are considered by experts an essential part of a comprehensive global strategy (Laxminarayan et al., 2013; WHO, 2014c).

IV. Trends in drug resistance.

A. The discovery of antibiotics was considered one of the most significant achievements of modern time.
   1. However, the use of antibiotics has been accompanied by the rapid emergence of bacteria with resistance.

2. For example, penicillin was discovered in 1928, and although the antibiotic did not have widespread use until 1943, penicillin-resistant *Staphyloccocus* had already been identified a few years earlier. This resistant strain of the gram-positive bacteria *Staphylococcus* produced penicillinase, an enzyme capable of breaking down the antibiotic structure and rendering the drug ineffective (Aminov, 2010; Ayliffe, 1997; Davies & Davies, 2010; Martinez, 2012).

B. In 1960, a semisynthetic penicillin, considered to be protective against the destructive penicillinase enzymes, was introduced.
   1. This antibiotic, methicillin, was not affected by the bacterial enzymes that inactivated penicillin and soon became common treatment for *Staphylococcus aureus* (*S. aureus*) infections.
   2. The appearance of methicillin-resistant *S. aureus* (MRSA) in 1962 was followed by the first U.S. hospital outbreak of MRSA in 1968 (Ayliffe, 1997).
   3. Vancomycin became common treatment for serious infections caused by methicillin-resistant *S. aureus*. MRSA is now resistant to multiple antibiotics.
   4. Today, MRSA continues to cause life-threatening bloodstream infections, pneumonia, and surgical site infections. It continues to be a significant threat that requires ongoing public health monitoring and prevention activities (CDC, 2013a).

C. By 2002, the emergence of vancomycin-resistant *S. aureus* strains was seen in the United States. Fortunately, as of October 2010, all vancomycin-intermediate *Staphylococcus aureus* (VISA) and vancomycin-resistant *Staphylococcus aureus* (VRSA) isolates have been susceptible to several FDA-approved antibiotics (CDC, 2013a).

D. Widespread use of antibiotics has led to a rapid emergence and spread of infectious organisms that have developed resistance to available antibiotics, making these drugs ineffective.
   1. Bacterial resistance ranges from resistance to a single antibiotic or related class of antibiotics to development of resistance to several antibiotic agents or classes (Davies & Davies, 2010; FDA, 2014b).
   2. Resistance is emerging among some fungi, such as those responsible for infections in transplant patients with weakened immune systems (CDC, 2013a; FDA, 2014b).

V. Common antibiotic resistant pathogens.

A. MRSA (Methicillin/oxacillin-resistant *S. aureus*) may be healthcare-associated (HA-MRSA) or community-associated (CA-MRSA) (CDC, 2014g).
  1. HA-MRSA occurs most frequently among patients who undergo invasive procedures, have weakened immune systems, and are being cared for in a hospital or other healthcare facility.
     a. Hemodialysis patients are 100 times more likely to acquire an invasive MRSA bloodstream infection compared to the general population (CDC, 2007; CDC, 2011b).
     b. CDC analysis of surveillance data from the Active Bacterial Core surveillance (ABCs) system revealed approximately 85% of dialysis patients had an invasive device or catheter in place at the time of MRSA infection (CDC, 2007).
     c. Two in 100 people carry MRSA. Nasal carriage/colonization with MRSA is a recognized risk factor in patients on hemodialysis for developing vascular access-associated infections and worse outcomes (Lai et al., 2011; Schmid et al., 2013).
  2. CA-MRSA refers to infection with MRSA in persons with no healthcare contact or healthcare-associated risk factors.
     a. Microbiologically and epidemiologically distinct from HA-MRSA (Nair et al., 2014).
     b. Usually cause skin infections, such as abscesses, boils, and other pus-filled lesions.
     c. Most infections are not invasive or fatal, but severe invasive disease, necrotizing fasciitis, and sepsis have been reported.
     d. Associated with skin-to-skin contact, compromised skin integrity, sharing of contaminated items, and poor hygienic practices.
     e. Outbreaks have been reported among military recruits, prison inmates, athletes, and in persons who use intravenous drugs (Malcolm, 2011; Turabelidze, 2006).

B. MRSE (methicillin/oxacillin-resistant *S. epidermidis*, coagulase-negative staphylococcus (CNS).
  1. Infections may occur after major medical procedures such as total hip replacement and valve replacement.
  2. Risk factors for infection include foreign bodies such as indwelling prosthetic devices or intravascular catheters.
  3. Pathogenicity is related to the ability of the bacteria to form biofilm.
  4. CNS peritonitis is a common complication of peritoneal dialysis, and methicillin resistance is not uncommon.

C. VRE (vancomycin-resistant *Enterococci*).
  1. *Enterococci* are gram-positive bacteria naturally present in the human intestinal tract and aid in the breakdown of complex carbohydrates. The bacteria can survive and grow in many environments. *Enterococcus faecalis* and *Enterococcus faecium* account for more than 90% of the clinical isolates of enterococci (Fraser et al., 2014).
  2. Some strains of enterococci have become resistant to the glycopeptide antibiotic vancomycin and are referred to as VRE (CDC, 2013a).
  3. Most VRE, particularly *Enterococcus faecium* strains, are also resistant to antibiotics previously used to treat infections caused by common disease-causing bacteria (e.g., aminoglycosides and ampicillin).
  4. An increased risk for VRE infection and colonization has been associated with certain risk factors including the following.
     a. Previous vancomycin use.
     b. Multiple antibiotic therapies.
     c. Severe underlying disease.
     d. Immunosuppression.
     e. Intraabdominal surgery.
  5. VRE is usually spread by direct and indirect contact.
     a. Hands of healthcare workers.
     b. Contaminated environmental surfaces.
     c. Contaminated medical equipment.

D. VISA/VRSA (vancomycin-intermediate and vancomycin-resistant *Staphylococcus aureus*).
  1. Antibiotic resistant bacteria demonstrate an increase in the minimum inhibitory concentration (MIC). The MIC is the concentration of an antibiotic that will inhibit the growth of the isolated bacteria.
     a. *Staphylococcus* bacteria are classified as VISA if the MIC for vancomycin is 4 to 8 µg/ml.
     b. *Staphylococcus* bacteria are classified as VRSA if the vancomycin MIC is ≥ 16 µg/ml.
  2. For some time researchers had been concerned that vancomycin-resistant genes present in VRE could be transferred to other gram-positive bacteria, such as *Staphylococcus aureus*, through horizontal gene transfer. The vanA gene is usually found in enterococci and confers a high level of vancomycin resistance. This occurrence of gene transfer would leave very limited treatment options for the patient with an infection due to vancomycin-resistant *Staphylococcus aureus* (VRSA).
  3. In the year 2002, the first case of VRSA was identified and the infection found in a U.S. patient on chronic hemodialysis. Testing indicated the VRSA isolate contained the vanA resistance gene present in VRE and the methicillin resistance mecA gene from MRSA. It is believed the vanA

gene was acquired through exchange of genetic material from VRE to *S. aureus* (CDC, 2002).

4. Risk factors include underlying health conditions, indwelling devices, previous infections with MRSA, and recent exposure to vancomycin and other antibiotics (CDC, 2013a).

5. Most isolates of *S. aureus* are susceptible to vancomycin (CDC, 2013a).

E. *Clostridium difficile* (*C. diff*).
1. Anaerobic, large, gram-positive, spore-forming rod.
2. Common cause of antibiotic-associated diarrhea (AAD) and accounts for 15% to 25% of all episodes of AAD (CDC, 2012a).
3. Linked to 14,000 deaths each year in the United States (CDC, 2013a).
4. Natural bowel colonization with *C. difficile* overgrows in the presence of antibiotic therapy, which destroys competing bacteria (Johnson et al., 2007).
5. Incubation period may be 5 to 10 days or 2 to 10 weeks following antibiotic treatment.
6. The bacteria attaches to the bowel producing at least two different toxins (A and B).
   a. Certain strains produce greater quantities of toxins A and B and are resistant to the fluoroquinolone antibiotics, such as cipro-floxacin and levofloxacin (Oldfield et al., 2014).
   b. Responsible for watery diarrhea and local inflammation of the bowel.
   c. Toxins produce foul-smelling stools containing mucus.
   d. Other symptoms include abdominal pain and distention, loss of appetite, nausea, and fever.
   e. Toxic megacolon (dilation of the colon), perforation, sepsis, and death may result (CDC, 2012a).
7. Colonization is more common than infection.
   a. Those colonized exhibit no clinical symptoms, but test positive for the organisms and/or its toxin.
   b. Risk for infection may last for up to 3 months or more following the discontinuation of antibiotics.
8. Shed in feces and the period of communicability continues until diarrhea subsides (Cohen et al., 2010).
   a. Spores can survive in the environment for several months.
   b. Surfaces in the environment may become contaminated and serve as reservoir for transmission.
   c. Patients with existing infection are thought to be the main source of infections for other patients.
   d. Fecal-oral route of transmission. The bacteria

enter the body through ingestion of the spores, often following the touching of contaminated surfaces or items (Cohen et al., 2010).
   e. Transmission-based precautions, glove use, strict adherence to hand hygiene, contact precautions until diarrhea resolves, "deep" cleaning of areas used by patients. Restriction of patient movements in facility by treating in designated area are all used to halt spread of the organism (APIC, 2013).
   f. Use of soap and water is more efficacious than alcohol-based hand rubs because spores are resistant to alcohol.

VI. Emerging MDRGNB (multidrug-resistant gram negative bacteria).

A. Multidrug-resistant gram-negative bacteria (MDRGNB) are a rapidly emerging threat due to their resistance to multiple antibiotics. They have become increasingly resistant to most available antibiotics, and infections have occurred for which there are no adequate treatment options (CDC, 2013a; Giske et al., 2008).

MDRGNB have developed ways of achieving drug resistance and can pass along genetic materials that allow other bacteria to become drug-resistant. CDC's National Healthcare Safety Network (NHSN) collects data on antibiotic-resistance patterns in gram-negative bacteria in healthcare settings. In 2008, based on NHSN data, 13% of *Escherichia coli* and *Klebsiella*, 17% of *Pseudomonas aeruginosa* and 74% of *Acinetobacter baumannii* in intensive-care units were multidrug-resistant. *Acinetobacter baumannii*, *Pseudomonas aeruginosa*, and *Klebsiella pneumoniae* are often extensively drug resistant.

B. ESBL-producing bacteria (extended spectrum beta lactamase producing bacteria).
1. Produce enzymes (beta lactamases) that hydrolyze or break down the beta-lactam ring, which is part of the core structure of multiple beta-lactam antibiotics, including penicillins and the third generation cephalosporins (ASM, 2005). These enzymes do not affect the cephamycins or carbapenem classes of antibiotics. The carbapenem antibiotics are typically used to treat infections caused by ESBL-producing bacteria.
2. The genes encoding these enzymes are carried in plasmids and are passed on via conjugation. Most of these plasmids also carry genes that confer resistance to other classes of antibiotics, such as the aminoglycosides (Paterson & Bonomo, 2005).
3. ESBL-producing strains have been found throughout the *Enterobacteriaceae*, a large family of gram-negative, rod-shaped bacteria that

includes well-known bacteria such as *Escherichia coli* and *Klebsiella pneumoniae* that are part of the normal flora of the GI tract.
4. Prevalence of ESBL infections is increasing worldwide and is associated with increased hospital costs, prolonged length of stay, possible treatment failure, and patient mortality.
5. Strains have been isolated from abscesses, blood, catheter tips, peritoneal fluid, sputum, and respiratory cultures.
6. ESBL-producing bacteria have been assigned a CDC threat level of "serious," meaning the bacteria are a serious concern and require prompt and sustained action to ensure the problem does not grow (CDC, 2013a).

C. CRE (carbapenem-resistant Enterobacteriaceae).
1. The carbapenem class of antibiotics is often considered the treatment of last resort for serious infections caused by multidrug-resistant bacteria. Some bacteria are now able to produce enzymes called carbapenemnases, a form of the beta-lactamase enzyme. The carbapenemnase enzymes are able to hydrolyze the beta-lactam ring, an essential chemical structure of carbapenem antibiotics, making them ineffective (CDC, 2012d).
2. Types of CRE are sometimes known by the enzyme produced by the bacteria. Some examples are as follows.
   a. KPC (Klebsiella pneumoniae carbapenemase).
   b. Imipenemase Metallo-beta-lactamase (IMP).
   c. NDM (New Delhi Metallo-beta-lactamase).
3. KPC-producing bacteria have a resistance trait encoded by a highly transmissible plasmid which has enabled it to spread widely across the United States since first being isolated in 2001 in the state of North Carolina (Arnold et al., 2011; CDC 2013i). KPCs have since been found in many gram-negative bacteria (Lee, 2012). Some examples include the following.
   a. *Escherichia coli.*
   b. *Pseudomonas* species.
   c. *Acinetobacter baumannii.*
   d. *Serratia* species.
4. CRE infections most commonly occur among patients in healthcare settings who are receiving treatment for other conditions and whose care requires invasive devices such as intravenous catheters and central lines.
5. CRE can contribute to death in up to 50% of patients who become infected and has been assigned a CDC threat level of "urgent" and considered an immediate public health threat that requires urgent and aggressive action (CDC, 2013a).

D. Acinetobacter.
1. Gram-negative bacteria commonly found in the soil and water.
2. Can colonize most areas of the human body.
3. Among the different species, *A. baumannii* accounts for about 80% of reported infections.
4. Cause of ventilator-associated pneumonia (VAP), endocarditis, wound infections, urinary tract infections, and septicemia.
5. Outbreaks of *Acinetobacter* infections typically occur in intensive care units and healthcare settings housing very ill immunocompromised patients.
6. Known to frequently contaminate the healthcare environment and can survive for an extended period of time on surfaces (APIC, 2010).
7. Frequently resistant to aminoglycosides, fluoroquinolones, and all beta-lactam antibiotics, with the exception of the carbapenems. However, the emergence of carbapenem-resistant acinetobacter (CRAB) has dramatically limited available treatment options (Evans et al., 2013).
8. Multidrug-resistant *A. baumannii* has been assigned a CDC threat level of "serious," meaning the bacterium is a serious concern and requires prompt and sustained action to ensure the problem does not grow (CDC, 2013a).

VII. Colonization vs. infection.

A. Colonization.
1. Microbial colonization often precedes infection.
2. Colonized patient does not exhibit signs/symptoms of active infection.
3. Colonized bacteria adhere to and multiply on surfaces or host tissues.
4. Bacteria may colonize work surfaces, medical devices, indwelling catheters, and central lines.
5. Bacterial biofilm can form within 24 hours and provide protection for bacteria fostering growth.
6. Resistance to antimicrobial agents is an important feature of biofilm.
7. Biofilm is difficult to eliminate without removal of the device.
8. Strict attention to infection control practices must be followed to prevent transmission of bacteria that can result in colonization and subsequent infection.

B. Infection.
1. Once pathogens have successfully invaded and are multiplying within body tissues, signs and symptoms of an infection are present.
2. An infection may remain localized or become systemic.
3. Culture bacteria from source.

C. Preventing colonization and infection will reduce the burden of antibiotic resistance in healthcare settings.

VIII. Management of patients with drug resistant organisms.

A. Patients infected or colonized with drug resistant organisms (CDC, 2001a).
   1. CDC *Recommendations for Preventing Transmissions of Infections among Chronic Hemodialysis Patients* are adequate for most outpatients infected with pathogenic bacteria, including drug resistant strains.
   2. Consistent hand hygiene and glove use.
   3. Staff education.
   4. Thorough environmental cleaning.
   5. Improvements in communication about patients with drug-resistant infections within and between healthcare facilities are vital.

B. Patients at increased risk for transmitting pathogenic bacteria require additional or enhanced precautions.
   1. Patient characteristics include but not limited to the following.
      a. Has infected wound with drainage that is not contained by dressing.
      b. Diapered or incontinent.
      c. Has diarrhea not contained by personal hygiene measures.
      d. Unable to perform self-care activities consistent with good personal hygiene.
      e. Previously associated with transmission.
   2. Additional precautions.
      a. Wear a separate, long-sleeved, fluid resistant/fluid impervious barrier garment that is removed and discarded after caring for the patient.
      b. Dialyze the patient at a station with as few adjacent stations as possible, e.g., at the end or corner of the treatment area.
      c. Patients should have their own supplies, including stethoscope and blood pressure cuff.
      d. Use dedicated equipment if possible.
      e. Attention to cleaning all frequently touched surfaces, equipment, nondisposable items, and bathrooms is required.
      f. Perform consistent hand hygiene and hand washing.
      g. When caring for a patient with active *C. difficile* infection, hand hygiene using alcohol-based hand gels or foam is not recommended because spores are resistant to alcohol.

C. Hospital setting: use contact precautions, gloving, gowning, hand hygiene, private room, cohorting.

IX. National surveillance systems.
Together with other participating agencies, the CDC facilitates numerous surveillance systems that collect data on antibiotic resistance. Surveillance goals generally center on improving the detection, monitoring, and characterization of drug-resistant infections to foster a better understanding of the impact of antibiotic use and develop effective strategies to prevent drug resistance. Examples of national surveillance programs are listed below.

A. Emerging Infections Program (EIP) Network was established in 1995 and is a national resource for the surveillance, prevention, and control of emerging infectious diseases. Activities conducted through the EIP Network include the following examples.
   1. Active Bacterial Core Surveillance (ABC) which involves population-based laboratory surveillance for invasive bacterial disease. Pathogens for surveillance include groups A and B streptococcus, *Haemophilus influenzae*, *Neisseria meningitidis*, *Streptococcus pneumoniae*, and MRSA.
   2. Healthcare Associated Infections Community Interface (HAIC) is an active population-based surveillance for *C. difficile* infection and other healthcare-associated infections caused by pathogens such as MRSA, Candida, and multidrug-resistant, gram-negative bacteria. Participating sites also use the National Healthcare Safety Network (NHSN) to perform time-limited analysis of data among NHSN facilities participating in the EIP NHSN network.

B. National Antimicrobial Resistance Monitoring System for Enteric Bacteria (NARMS).
   1. Collaborates with the CDC, FDA, USDA, and state and local health departments to monitor antibiotic resistance in enteric bacteria isolated from humans, retail meat, and food animals.
   2. Helps protect public health by providing information about emerging bacterial resistance, the ways in which resistance is spread, and how resistant infections differ from susceptible infections.

C. National Healthcare Safety Network (NHSN).
   1. Nation's most widely used healthcare-associated infection tracking system.
   2. Provides healthcare facilities a method to track, analyze, and interpret data on healthcare-associated infections (HAIs), including those caused by antibiotic-resistant strains.
   3. Provides facilities, states, regions, and the nation with data to identify problem areas, measure progress of interventions, and eliminate healthcare-associated infections.

X. Antibiotic stewardship.

A. Antimicrobial stewardship programs (ASP) are interventions designed to ensure that patients in any healthcare setting receive the right antibiotic, at the right dose, at the right time, and for the right duration. The number of U.S. healthcare institutions reporting implementation of an ASP over the past 10 years has increased (Johannsson et al., 2011).

B. Appropriate use of antibiotics.
   1. Maximizing therapeutic impact while minimizing development of resistance.
   2. Prescribing antimicrobial therapy only when beneficial.
   3. Targeting the therapy to the pathogens.

C. Improved outcomes through antibiotic stewardship programs include the following (Ohl & Luther, 2011).
   1. Reduced mortality.
   2. Reduced risks of *C. diff*-associated diarrhea.
   3. Shorter hospital stays.
   4. Reduced overall antibiotic resistance within an institution.
   5. Cost savings.

D. CDC materials that can be used to implement antimicrobial stewardship interventions include the following.
   1. "Get Smart for Healthcare" slide deck.
   2. Implementing and improving stewardship efforts.
      a. Keys for success, getting started.
      b. Tools.
      c. Resources.
   3. Antibiotic Stewardship Drivers and Change Package.

XI. Education campaigns.

A. Together with its partners, the CDC developed several education campaigns to address issue of antimicrobial resistance in various settings. Educational materials can be downloaded from the individual sites.
   1. Get Smart: Know When Antibiotics Work.
      a. Targets patients and providers through distribution of educational materials.
      b. Promotes adherence to appropriate prescribing guidelines.
      c. Educates to decrease demand for antibiotics for viral upper respiratory infections.
      d. Educates to increase adherence to prescribed antibiotics for upper respiratory infections caused by bacteria.
      e. Provides funding and technical assistance for local campaigns.
   2. Get Smart for Healthcare: Know When Antibiotics Work.
      a. CDC campaign focused on improving antibiotic use in inpatient healthcare facilities, starting with hospitals and then expanding to long-term care facilities.
      b. Goal is to preserve antibiotic effectiveness and combat resistance.
      c. Promotes "antimicrobial stewardship" through implementation of interventions and programs designed to improve antibiotic use.
   3. Get Smart: Know When Antibiotics Work on the Farm.
      a. Promotes appropriate antibiotic use in veterinary medicine and animal agriculture.
      b. Serves as a liaison among the public health community, veterinarians, and food animal producers.
   4. National MRSA Education Initiative. Prevention of MRSA skin infections through education.
   5. Hand Hygiene Saves Lives. Campaigns include material to promote hand hygiene in schools, during emergencies, before and after daily activities.
      a. Hand hygiene basics.
      b. Interactive hand hygiene training.
      c. CDC hand hygiene guidelines.
      d. Measuring hand hygiene adherence.
      e. Educational materials for patients and healthcare providers.

B. Additional information on antibiotic resistance can be found on the websiteswebpages listed in Table 6.1.

SECTION E
Hepatitis B

I. Characteristics and epidemiology.

A. Humans are the only known host.

B. As shown in Figure 6.1, the hepatitis B virus (HBV) is a small, double-shelled DNA virus and member of the family Hepadnoviridae.

C. Replicates within infected hepatocytes.

D. Infectious Dane particle consists of an inner core and an outer shell or surface coat.

E. Contains numerous antigenic components, including hepatitis B surface antigen (HBsAg), hepatitis B core antigen (HBcAg), and hepatitis B e antigen (HBeAg).

Table 6.1

Antibiotic-Resistance-Associated Websites

Website/Webpage	URL
Alliance for the Prudent Use of Antibiotics (APUA)	http://www.tufts.edu/med/apua/about_issue/multi_drug.shtml
Bacterial Resistance Strategies – Michigan State University	http://amrls.cvm.msu.edu/microbiology/bacterial-resistance-strategies/introduction
Centers for Disease Control and Prevention (CDC) Antibiotic/Antimicrobial Resistance	www.cdc.gov/drugresistance
Centers for Disease Control and Prevention (CDC) Get Smart: Know When Antibiotics Work	http://www.cdc.gov/getsmart/antibiotic-use/antibiotic-resistance-faqs.html
Centers for Disease Control and Prevention (CDC) Methicillin-resistant Staphylococcus aureus (MRSA) Infections	http://www.cdc.gov/mrsa/
Centers for Disease Control and Prevention (CDC) Healthcare-associated Infections (HAI) – VISA/VRSA	http://www.cdc.gov/HAI/organisms/visa_vrsa/visa_vrsa.html
Infectious Diseases Society of America Antimicrobial Resistance	http://www.idsociety.org/AR_Policy/
National Antimicrobial Resistance Monitoring System (NARMS)	http://www.cdc.gov/narms/
National Institute of Allergy and Infectious Diseases – Antimicrobial (Drug) Resistance	http://www.niaid.nih.gov/topics/antimicrobialresistance/Pages/default.aspx
World Health Organization (WHO) Antimicrobial Resistance	www.who.int/drugresistance

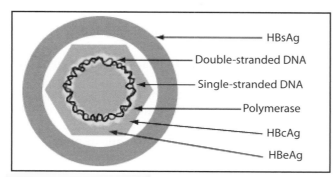

Figure 6.1. Structure of HBV.

Source: Parker, J., Dickenson, L., Wiseman, K.C., Alexander, D., & Peacock, E. (1998). Control of infectious diseases in the renal patient. In J. Parker (Ed.), *Contemporary nephrology nursing* (1st ed., p. 354). Pitman, NJ: American Nephrology Nurses' Association. Used with permission.

F. Acute HBV infection is one of the most commonly reported vaccine-preventable diseases, yet approximately 2 billion persons worldwide have been infected with HBV, and more than 350 million persons have chronic infections (CDC, 2012b).

G. Rate of new infections in the United States has decreased approximately 82% since 1991, when a national strategy to eliminate HBV infection was implemented and routine vaccination of children was first recommended. The decline has been greatest among children and adolescents reflective of effective immunization practices. Figure 6.2. demonstrates the reported number of acute HBV cases from 2000 to 2012.

H. Rates of infection are highest among adults, particularly males aged 25 to 44 years.

I. In the United States, approximately 800,000 to 1.4 million persons have chronic HBV infection.

J. Approximately 620,000 person's worldwide die from HBV related liver disease every year.

II. Risk factors. Per the CDC, the following populations are at increased risk of becoming infected with HBV (CDC, 2014a):

A. Infants born to an infected mother.

B. Sexual partners of an infected person.

C. Sexually active persons who are not in a long-term, mutually monogamous relationship.

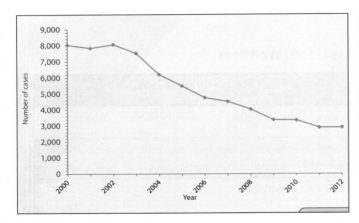

Figure 6.2. Reported number of acute hepatitis B cases — United States, 2000-2012.

Source: CDC (2014e). Viral hepatitis statistics and surveillance –Surveillance for Viral Hepatitis – United States, 2012.

D. Men who have sex with men.

E. Injecting drug users.

F. Household contacts of a chronically infected person.

G. Healthcare and public safety workers who may come in contact with blood or body fluids.

H. Hemodialysis patients.

I. Residents and staff of facilities that care for persons with developmental disabilities.

J. Travelers to countries with intermediate or high rates of hepatitis B infection.

III. Transmission – HBV is the microbe that is most efficiently transmitted in the dialysis setting.

A. Percutaneous (i.e., puncture through the skin) or permucosal (i.e., direct contact with mucous membranes) exposure to infectious blood or to body fluids that contain blood.

B. Patients who are chronically infected are central to the epidemiology of HBV transmission in dialysis.

C. All patients who are HBsAg-positive are infectious and able to transmit the virus, although HBsAg itself is not infectious. Only the complete virus (Dane particle) is infectious. When HBsAg is present in the blood, the complete virus is also present and the patient is able to transmit infection (CDC, 2012b).

D. Healthcare workers with acute or chronic hepatitis rarely infect patients. They may continue to work when infection control measures are followed.

E. HBV can be present on environmental surfaces in

the absence of any visible blood and still result in transmission.

F. Blood-contaminated surfaces not routinely or adequately cleaned and disinfected are a reservoir for HBV transmission.

G. HBV has been detected in dialysis centers on clamps, scissors, dialysis machine control knobs, and doorknobs.

H. The virus is stable in the environment and remains viable for at least 7 days on environmental surfaces at room temperature.

I. Outbreaks of HBV infection among hemodialysis patients have been caused by cross-contamination to patients through the following.
 1. Environmental surfaces, supplies (e.g., hemostats, clamps).
 2. Equipment not routinely disinfected after each use.
 3. Multiple-dose medication vials and intravenous solutions not used exclusively for one patient.
 4. Medications for injection prepared in areas adjacent to areas where blood samples were handled.
 5. Staff members who simultaneously cared for both HBV-infected and susceptible patients (CDC, 2001a).

IV. Clinical features.

A. Causes both acute and chronic hepatitis.

B. Incubation period 45 to 160 days (average 120 days).

C. Immunosuppressed adults with newly acquired infection are usually asymptomatic.

D. Acute infection may be asymptomatic or present as mild disease; rarely fulminant hepatitis results.

E. Disease is more severe among adults aged > 60 years.

F. Symptoms, if present, usually last for several weeks.

G. Clinical symptoms are often insidious and include the following.
 1. Anorexia.
 2. Malaise.
 3. Nausea.
 4. Vomiting.
 5. Abdominal pain.
 6. Jaundice.

Table 6.2

Interpretation of Serologic Test Results for Hepatitis B Virus Infection

Serologic Markers				Interpretation
HBsAg*	Total Anti-HBc†	IgM§ Anti-HBc	Anti-HBs¶ –*Confers immunity*	
–	–	–	–	Susceptible, never infected
+	–	–	–	Acute infection, early incubation**
+	+	+	–	Acute infection
–	+	+	–	Acute resolving infection
–	+	–	–	Past infection, recovered and immune
+	+	–	–	Chronic infection
–	+	–	–	False positive (i.e., susceptible), past infection, or "low-level" chronic infection
–	–	–	+	Immune if titer is ≥ 10 mLU/mL

* Hepatitis B surface antigen.

†Antibody to hepatitis B core antigen.

§Immunoglobulin M.

¶Antibody to hepatitis B surface antigen.

** Transient HBsAg positivity (lasting ≤ 18 days) might be detected in some patients during vaccination.

Source: Centers for Disease Control and Prevention (CDC). (2001a). Recommendations for preventing transmission of infections among chronic hemodialysis patients. *MMWR, 50*(RR05), 1-43 (Available from http://www.cdc.gov/mmwr/preview/mmwrhtml/rr5005a1.htm).

V. Disease outcomes.

A. Acute HBV infection.
1. 15% to 20% of acute infections are acquired from a known infected contact and could have been prevented by timely preexposure or postexposure prophylaxis.
2. Up to 98% of adults with normal immune status recover completely, eliminating virus from the blood.
3. Hemodialysis patients with newly acquired HBV infections are less likely to have symptomatic illness, are more likely to become chronic carriers, and represent an ongoing source of HBV transmission (Einollahi, 2012).

B. Chronic HBV infection.
1. Up to two thirds of Americans living with chronic HBV infection do not know they are infected.
2. Asians and Pacific Islanders account for more than 50% of Americans living with chronic HBV infection.
3. Chronically infected persons are at increased risk for persistent liver disease, cirrhosis, and hepatocellular carcinoma.
4. Liver disease develops in two thirds of chronic carriers.

5. Approximately 15% to 25% die prematurely from cirrhosis or liver cancer.
6. In the United States, chronic HBV infection results in estimated 2,000 to 4,000 deaths per year.

VI. Serologic test/markers – One or more of these markers are present during different phases of infection (see Table 6.2).

A. HBsAg.
1. The hepatitis B virus has an outer covering consisting of a lipoprotein known as the surface antigen or HBsAg.
2. Detected in the blood 30 to 60 days after exposure.
3. Presence in the blood indicates current infection and transmissibility.
4. Transient positive HBsAg may be detected in some patients during vaccination with the hepatitis B vaccine.
5. HBsAg present for more than 6 months typically indicates chronic infection.
6. In persons who recover from infection, HBsAg is eliminated from the blood in 2 to 3 months.
7. Susceptible or nonimmune patients must be screened for HBsAg monthly, including those who:
   a. Have not yet received the hepatitis B vaccine.
   b. Are in the process of being vaccinated.

c. Have not adequately responded to the vaccine series.

B. HBeAg and HBeAb.
1. Hepatitis B e antigen (HBeAg) is part of the interior core antigen or HBcAg.
2. It appears simultaneously with the HBsAg and denotes viral replication.
3. Can be detected in the blood of persons with acute or chronic infection.
4. Presence of HBeAg correlates with viral replication and higher level of virus; it is thought to indicate a highly contagious state.
5. The antibody to HBeAg or the anti-HBe (HBeAb) indicates low viral replication, but does not confer immunity.
6. All HBsAg positive patients are considered potentially infectious regardless of HBeAg or HBeAb status.
7. Not used as a routine screening test.

C. Total anti-HBc (hepatitis B total core antibody).
1. Antibodies produced in response to the hepatitis B interior core antigen (HBcAg).
2. The interior core antigen (HBcAg) can be detected in liver tissue taken from a liver biopsy but cannot be detected in serum.
3. Antibodies to the core antigen (anti-HBc) develop in all HBV infections appearing at the onset of symptoms.
4. Antibodies to the core antigen appear together as immunoglobulin M (IgM) class and immunoglobulin G (IgG) class.
5. During the course of infection and recovery, the IgM class antibody will decline and can no longer be detected, but the IgG class antibody will persist for life.
6. Anti-HBc does not neutralize the virus and does not confer immunity.
7. A positive anti-HBc may indicate acute, chronic, or a past hepatitis B infection; additional markers must be considered when evaluating a positive test result.

D. IgM anti-HBc (hepatitis B core IgM antibody).
1. Presence indicates acute or acute resolving infection.
2. Present within 4 to 6 weeks following initial infection.
3. May persist for approximately 6 months.
4. May be the only marker during the window period with acute resolving infection when the HBsAg is no longer detected and before the appearance of the surface antibody (anti-HBs).

E. Anti-HBs.
1. Hepatitis B surface antibodies (anti-HBs or HBsAb) can neutralize the hepatitis B virus.
2. HBV surface antibodies (anti-HBs) appear 2 to 3 months after the onset of symptoms.
3. Confers immunity.

F. HBV DNA.
1. Can be detected in the serum very early on following initial infection.
2. May be used to monitor progression of disease and response to antiviral therapy.
3. Qualitative and quantitative testing available.

VII. Screening and vaccination of staff.

A. Screening for HBV infection among staff is no longer considered necessary.

B. Testing for HBV markers not recommended except when required to document response to vaccination.

C. Hepatitis B vaccination recommended for all susceptible staff.

D. OSHA mandates that each facility offer and provide HBV vaccine to all susceptible staff members.

E. Recombinant vaccines currently available in the U.S. are Recombivax HB® and Engerix-B®.

F. Test all vaccinated staff for anti-HBs 1 to 2 months after the last dose of the primary vaccine series.

G. A second series of the HBV vaccine is indicated for those who do not respond with protective levels of anti-HBs following the primary series.
1. Retesting for anti-HBs response is also indicated 1 to 2 months after the last vaccine dose of the second series.
2. No additional doses are warranted for those who do not respond with protective HBsAb levels after two full series.

H. Staff not responding to the second full series of the HBV vaccine should be evaluated for HBsAg positivity and follow-up with medical evaluation and counseling.

VIII. Routine screening and vaccination of patients.

A. Routine serologic testing; the schedule can be found in Table 6.3.
1. Outbreaks of HBV infection among hemodialysis patients have resulted from failure to routinely screen for hepatitis B infection and failure to routinely review the results to identify infected patients (CDC, 2001a).

Table 6.3

Schedule for Routine Testing for Hepatitis B Virus (HBV) and Heptatitis C Virus (HCV) Infections

Patient Status	On Admission	Monthly	Semiannual	Annual
All patients	HBsAg*			
	Anti-HBc* (total)			
	Anti-HBs*			
	Anti-HCV, ALT**			
HBV-susceptible, including nonresponders to vaccine		HBsAg		
Anti-HBs positive (≥ 10 mIU/mL), anti-HBc negative				Anti-HBs
Anti-HBs and anti-HBc positive	No additional HBV testing needed			
Anti-HCV negative		ALT	Anti-HCV	

*Results of HBV testing should be known before the patient begins dialysis.

**HBsAg = hepatitis B surface antigen; Anti-HBc = antibody to hepatitis B core antigen; Anti-HBs = antibody to hepatitis B surface antigen; Anti-HCV = antibody to hepatitis C virus; ALT = alanine aminotransferase.

Source: Centers for Disease Control and Prevention (CDC). (2001a). Recommendations for preventing transmission of infections among chronic hemodialysis patients. *MMWR, 50*(RR05), 1-43 (Available from http://www.cdc.gov/mmwr/preview/mmwrhtml/rr5005a1.htm).

2. Routine serologic testing for markers of HBV infection and prompt review of the result is vital to the prevention of HBV transmission.
3. Patients should be screened prior to or at entry to the dialysis.
4. If results are not known prior to admission because of an emergency situation, test patient immediately upon intake; results should be known within 7 days of admission.
   a. HBsAg.
   b. HBsAb or Anti-HBs.
   c. Anti-HBc (total).
5. Hepatitis B vaccination is recommended for all susceptible patients and should be offered immediately upon admission (see Table 6.4).
6. Higher doses of the vaccine are recommended for patients on hemodialysis due to their immune-compromised state. Doses and schedules can be found in Table 6.5.

B. HBV-susceptible patients (negative HBsAg and HBsAb or anti-HBs, anti-HBc).
   1. Vaccinate all susceptible patients with a full series of the HBV vaccine.
      a. Test for anti-HBs 1 to 2 months after last dose.
      b. If anti-HBs is < 10 mIU/mL, revaccinate with

an additional vaccine series and retest for anti-HBs.
   c. No additional doses are warranted for those who do not respond. Primary vaccine nonresponders are considered susceptible and must be tested for HBsAg monthly.
   2. If anti-HBs is ≥ 10 mIU/mL, consider patient immune and retest annually for anti-HBs.

Table 6.4

Hepatitis B Vaccination for Susceptible Patients

- Vaccinate all susceptible patients against hepatitis B.
- Test for anti-HBs 1 to 2 months after last dose.
  - If anti-HBs is < 10 ml/mL, consider patient susceptible, revaccinate with a second series, and retest for anti-HBs.
  - If anti-HBs is ≥ 10 ml/mL, consider patient immune, and retest annually for anti-HBs to determine need for booster dose.
    - Give booster dose of vaccine if anti-HBs declines to <10 ml/mL and continue to retest annually.

Source: Centers for Disease Control and Prevention (CDC). (2001a). Recommendations for preventing transmission of infections among chronic hemodialysis patients. *MMWR, 50*(RR05), 1-43 (Available from http://www.cdc.gov/mmwr/preview/mmwrhtml/rr5005a1.htm).

Table 6.5

Doses and Schedules of Licensed Hepatitis B Vaccines for Hemodialysis Patients and Staff Members

Group	Recombivax HB™ *			Engerix-B®†		
	Dose	Volume	Schedule	Dose	Volume	Schedule
Patients aged ≥ 20 years Predialysis§	10μg	1.0 mL	0, 1, and 6 months	20 μg	1.0 mL	0, 1, and 6 months
Dialysis-dependent	40 μg	1.0 mL¶	0, 1, and 6 months	40 μg	2-1.0 mL doses at one site	0, 1, 2, and 6 months
Patients aged < 20 years**	5 μg	0.5 mL	0, 1, and 6 months	10 μg	0.5 mL	0, 1, and 6 months
Staff members aged ≥ 20 years	10 μg	1.0 mL	0, 1, and 6 months	20 μg	1.0 mL	0, 1, and 6 months

* Merck & Company, Inc., West Point, Pennsylvania.
† SmithKline Beecham Biologicals, Philadelphia, Pennsylvania.
§ Immunogenicity might depend on degree of renal insufficiency.
¶ Special formulation.
** Doses for all persons aged < 20 years approved by the U.S. Food and Drug Administration; for hemodialysis.
Note: All doses should be administered in the deltoid by the intramuscular route.

Source: Centers for Disease Control and Prevention (CDC). (2001a). Recommendations for preventing transmission of infections among chronic hemodialysis patients. *MMWR, 50*(RR05), 1-43 (Available from http://www.cdc.gov/mmwr/preview/mmwrhtml/rr5005a1.htm).

a. Administer booster dose if anti-HBs decline to < 10 mIU/mL on annual testing and continue to test annually for antibodies.
b. Follow-up testing after the booster dose is not recommended.
c. Patients who require a booster dose of the vaccine should not be assigned to a staff member concurrently caring for the HBsAg positive patient.
3. The CDC defines an adequate response to vaccination as a laboratory result of ≥ 10 mIU/mL anti-HBs.
a. The laboratory performing the testing for anti-HBs must be able to define a 10 mIU/mL concentration. Results should be reported as a numeric value; a result of "positive" or "negative" is not sufficient.
b. Some manufacturers of anti-HBs assays consider a level of anti-HBs that is greater than 10 mIU/mL to be protective. For these assays, the higher level of titer considered to be protective by the manufacturer of the kit should be used to determine whether or not the person is immune.

C. Patients who are HBV-immune.
1. Annual anti-HBs testing of patients who are

positive for anti-HBs ≥ 10 mIU/mL, and negative for HBsAg and negative for anti-HBc, determines the need for booster doses of vaccine. These patients have vaccine induced immunity and require annual anti-HBs testing.
2. No routine follow-up testing is indicated for patients who are positive for both anti-HBs and anti-HBc. These patients have recovered from past infection with hepatitis B and do not need to be vaccinated.

D. HBV infected patients are able to transmit the virus and require additional precautions to prevent transmission.
1. Patients who are chronically infected (i.e., those who are HBsAg positive, total anti-HBc positive, and IgM anti-HBc negative) do not require additional HBV testing. Annual testing for HBsAg is reasonable to detect the small percentage of HBV infected patients who might lose their HBsAg.
2. A positive HBsAg test result may be the only routine serologic marker initially detected in patients newly infected. Following confirmed conversion to a positive HBsAg status, perform the following.
a. Repeat HBsAg testing and test for anti-HBc

(including IgM anti-HBc) 1 to 2 months later.
  b. Repeat HBsAg testing and test for anti-HBs 6 months later to determine clinical outcome and need for counseling, medical evaluation, and vaccination of contacts.
  3. Patients who become HBsAg negative are no longer infectious.

E. Isolated anti-HBc positive patients.
  1. Patients who test positive for isolated anti-HBc (i.e., those who are anti-HBc positive, HBsAg negative, and anti-HBs negative) should be retested for total anti-HBc, and if positive, test for IgM anti-HBc.
  2. If total anti-HBc is negative, the patient is considered susceptible and should be provide hepatitis B vaccination.
  3. If total anti-HBc is positive and IgM anti-HBc is negative, follow recommendations for hepatitis B vaccination.
    a. If anti-HBs is < 10 mIU/mL even after revaccination, test for HBV DNA. If HBV DNA is negative, consider patient susceptible and test monthly for HBsAg.
    b. If HBV DNA is positive, consider patient as having past infection or "low-level" chronic infection. Isolation is not necessary because HBsAg is not detectable.
    c. If both total and IgM anti-HBc are positive, consider patient recently infected and test for anti-HBs in 4 to 6 months. No further routine testing is necessary and isolation is not necessary because HBsAg is not detectable.

IX. Hepatitis B isolation precautions.

A. Preventing transmission of HBV from an infected hemodialysis patient requires infection control precautions recommended for all hemodialysis patients, routine serologic testing for markers of HBV infection, and isolation of HBsAg-positive patients during treatment.

B. Incidence of HBV infection is substantially lower in hemodialysis units where HBV infected patients are isolated.

C. Isolation practices have resulted in a 70 to 80% reduction in the incidence of HBV infection.

D. Isolation requires a designated separate room for treatment, a dedicated machine and equipment.

E. Dedicated supplies and equipment, including blood glucose monitors, and all supplies used in the isolation room/area, such as clamps, blood pressure cuffs, testing reagents, etc., should be labeled "isolation" and not routinely removed from the isolation room/area.

F. Staff members who are caring for HBsAg-positive patients should not care for susceptible patients at the same time.

G. If a separate room is not possible, and the dialysis facility is able to establish an isolation area in compliance with the Conditions for Coverage for ESRD Facilities, the area used for the HBsAg-positive patient must be separated from other stations by a space at least equivalent to the width of one dialysis station in an area removed from the mainstream of activity to decrease the number of adjacent stations. The patient should undergo dialysis on dedicated machines, using dedicated supplies.

H. Refillable concentrate containers must be surface disinfected at the completion of each treatment.

I. Refillable concentrate containers may be kept in the isolation area and refilled at the door or removed for cleaning and disinfection. If the container is removed from the room, the exterior must be cleaned and disinfected prior to removal.

J. When there are no longer any patients who are HBsAg-positive on the census, the isolation room/area must be cleaned and disinfected prior to being used as a nonisolation room/area.

K. When the isolation machine is no longer dedicated to a patient who is HBsAg positive, the internal pathways of the machine can be disinfected using conventional protocols; external surfaces should be cleaned and disinfected and the machine returned to general use.

L. Separate gowns must be used in the isolation area and removed before leaving the isolation room/area. Anyone entering the isolation room/area during the patient's treatment must wear a protective gown.

M. Patients who are HBsAg-positive should not participate in dialyzer reprocessing programs (CDC, 2001a; CMS, 2008). Other considerations in the care of these patients can be found in Table 6.6.

X. Treatment.

A. Several antiviral nucleoside analogue drugs are available for treating chronic HBV infection including entecavir, which may be administrated as a first-line oral therapy.

B. Interferons are not recommended in dialysis patients with HBV infection.

Table 6.6

Management of HBsAg Positive Patients

Follow infection control practices for hemodialysis units for all patients.
Dialyze HBsAg positive patients in a separate room using separate machines, equipment, instruments, and supplies.
Staff members caring for HBsAg positive patients should not care for HBV susceptible patients at the same time (e.g., during the same shift or during patient changeover).

Source: Centers for Disease Control and Prevention (CDC). (2001a). Recommendations for preventing transmission of infections among chronic hemodialysis patients. *MMWR, 50*(RR05), 1-43. (Available from http://www.cdc.gov/mmwr/preview/mmwrhtml/rr5005a1.htm).

C. Persons with chronic HBV infection receiving antiviral therapy require medical evaluation and regular monitoring.

D. Laboratory monitoring may include serum alanine aminotransferase (ALT), HBV DNA PCR, HBeAg and HBeAb, and alpha-fetoprotein levels.

E. Goal of therapy is to prevent the development of irreversible chronic hepatitis B complications such as cirrhosis, liver failure, and hepatic cancer (Einollahi, 2012).

SECTION F
Hepatitis C (HCV)

I. Characteristics and epidemiology.

A. Single-stranded RNA virus classified as a separate genus in the Flaviridae family.

B. Six known genotypes and more than 90 subtypes.

C. Multiple quasispecies may co-exist in a single infected individual. Infection with one genotype or subtype does not protect against reinfection or superinfection with other strains (CDC, 2001a).

D. Different genotypes and subtypes have different geographic distributions. Predominant genotypes in the United States are 1a and 1b.

E. Approximately 150 to 170 million people worldwide are infected with HCV and more than 350,000 people die every year from HCV-related liver disease (Esforzado & Campistol, 2012; WHO, 2014e).

F. Most common chronic bloodborne infection in the United States.

G. Most common cause of liver damage in patients with chronic kidney disease.

H. From 2007 through 2010, the acute hepatitis C rate in the United States remained stable at 0.3 cases per 100,000 population, but increased to 0.4 cases per 100,000 population in 2011. Figure 6.3 shows the reported number of acute hepatitis C cases in the United States from 2000 to 2012.

I. Among the 3.2 million chronically infected in the United States, infection is most prevalent among those born during 1945 to 1965. These individuals were likely infected when rates were the highest during the 1970s and 1980s. CDC recommends that everyone in the United States born from 1945 through 1965 be tested for HCV infection (CDC, 2014c).

J. Transfusion-related infections account for less than one per million units of blood.

K Many infections are due to illegal intravenous drug use.

L. Approximately 40% to 60% of chronic liver disease is attributable to HCV.

M. Limited incidence and prevalence data in the chronic hemodialysis population as not all dialysis units perform routine HCV testing.

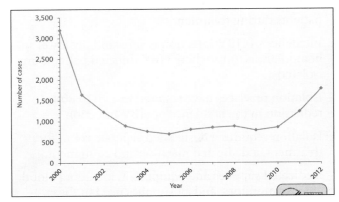

Figure 6.3. Reported number of acute hepatitis C cases — United States, 2000-2012

Source: CDC (2014e). Viral hepatitis statistics and surveillance –Surveillance for Viral Hepatitis – United States, 2012.

II. Risk factors. CDC recommends HCV testing for persons with risks for HCV infection.

A. Current or former injection drug users.

B. Recipients of clotting factor concentrates made before 1987.

C. Recipients of blood transfusions or solid organ transplants before July 1992. Blood transfusion was a leading cause of HCV transmission before screening of blood for HCV became available in 1992.

D. Chronic hemodialysis patients.

E. Persons with known exposures to HCV, such as healthcare workers following needlesticks involving HCV-positive blood and recipients of organs or blood from a positive donor.

F. Persons with human immunodeficiency virus (HIV) infection.

G. Children born to HCV-positive mothers.

III. Transmission.

A. Most efficiently transmitted by direct percutaneous exposure to infectious blood.

B. The chronically infected person is central to the epidemiology of transmission in the dialysis setting.

C. Number of years on dialysis is major risk factor independently associated with higher rates of HCV infection.

D. Inadequate infection control practices are associated with outbreaks of HCV in dialysis units.
   1. Use of common medication carts to prepare and distribute medications at patients' stations.
   2. Supply carts moved from one station to another.
   3. Sharing of multiple-dose medication vials, which were placed at patients' stations on top of hemodialysis machines.
   4. Contaminated priming buckets that were not routinely changed or cleaned and disinfected between patients.
   5. Machine surfaces not routinely cleaned and disinfected between patients.
   6. Blood spills not cleaned up promptly (CDC, 2001a).

IV. Clinical features.

A. Causes both acute and chronic hepatitis.

B. Natural history of infection is difficult to establish, but the disease often extends over decades (Esforzado & Campistol, 2012).

C. Incubation period ranges from 14 to 180 days (average 6 to 7 weeks).

D. Those with newly acquired infection are asymptomatic or have a mild clinical illness.

E. In those persons who do develop symptoms, the average time from exposure to symptoms is 4 to 12 weeks.

F. Most hemodialysis patients with newly acquired HCV infection have elevated serum ALT levels. Aspartate aminotransferase (AST) is a less specific indicator of HCV-related liver disease (CDC, 2001a).

V. Disease outcomes.

A. Acute HCV infection.
   1. Course is often variable.
   2. Approximately 20% to 30% of those newly infected experience fatigue, abdominal pain, poor appetite, or jaundice.
   3. Symptoms typically go unnoticed.

B. Chronic HCV infection.
   1. Up to 85% of newly infected persons develop chronic infection with viremia persisting over time (Esforzado & Campistol, 2012).
   2. Approximately 60% to 70% of those infected experience persistent fluctuating ALT elevations indicating liver disease while progression to cirrhosis is often silent.
   3. Chronic infection is associated with hepatitis inflammation and progression to fibrosis (Pol et al., 2012).
   4. Cirrhosis develops in 10% to 20% of persons who have chronic infection and hepatocellular carcinoma develops in 1% to 5%.
   5. Liver failure from chronic hepatitis C is one of the most common causes of liver transplants in the United States.

VI. Serologic test/markers.

See Figure 6.4 for the CDC's recommended testing sequence for identifying current HCV infection and Table 6.7 for help with interpreting results of tests for HCV infection.

A. Anti-HCV (hepatitis C antibody) can be detected 4 to 10 weeks after infection. Anti-HCV can be detected in > 97% of persons by 6 months after exposure.

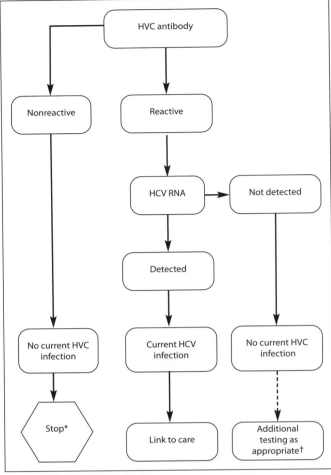

* For persons who might have been exposed to HCV within the past 6 months, testing for HCV RNA or follow-up testing for HCV antibody is recommended. For persons who are immunocompromised, testing for HCV RNA can be considered.

† To differentiate past, resolved HCV infection from biologic false positivity for HCV antibody, testing with another HCV antibody assay can be considered. Repeat HCV RNA testing if the person tested is suspected to have had HCV exposure within the past 6 months or has clinical evidence of HCV disease, or if there is concern regarding the handling or storage of the test specimen.

Figure 6.4. Recommended testing sequence for identifying current hepatitis C virus (HCV) infection. Testing for HCV infection begins with either a rapid or a laboratory-conducted assay for HCV antibody in blood. A non-reactive HCV antibody result indicates no HCV antibody detected. A reactive result indicates one of the following: 1) current HCV infection, 2) past HCV infection that has resolved, or 3) false positivity. A reactive result should be followed by NAT for HCV RNA. If HCV RNA is detected, that indicates current HCV infection. If HCV RNA is not detected, that indicates either past, resolved HCV infection, or false HCV antibody positivity.

Source: Centers for Disease Control and Prevention (CDC). (2013g). Testing for HCV infection: An update of guidance for clinicians and laboratorians. *MMWR*, *62*(18). Available from http://www.cdc.gov/mmwr/preview/mmwrhtml/mm6218a5.htm?s_cid=mm6218a5_w

1. Initial screening tests for antibody to HCV (anti-HCV).
2. Two test methods are available; enzyme immunoassay (EIA) and enhanced chemiluminescence immunoassay (CIA).
3. Anti-HCV tests do not distinguish between acute, chronic, or resolved infection.
4. A nonreactive HCV antibody result indicates no HCV antibody detected.
5. A reactive result may indicate current HCV infection, past HCV infection that has resolved, or a false positive.
6. Anti-HCV usually persists indefinitely following infection but does not confer immunity.
7. CDC recommends a reactive anti-HCV result be followed by NAT for HCV RNA testing (CDC, 2013g).

B. HCV RNA can be detected as early as 2 to 3 weeks after infection and weeks before onset of ALT elevations. Nucleic acid test (NAT) used for detection of HCV RNA in serum or plasma from blood of patients who test reactive for HCV antibody.
   1. When HCV RNA is not detected in someone who has a reactive anti-HCV test, this indicates either past resolved HCV infection or false HCV antibody positivity.
   2. Detection of HCV RNA indicates current HCV infection.

C. Genotyping (genetic structure of the virus).
   1. Helpful in making recommendations regarding treatment options.
   2. Different genotypes and subtypes are associated with different rates of disease progression, severity, and response to treatment.
   3. Recommended duration of treatment depends on the genotype when using combination therapy.
   4. Patients with genotypes 2 and 3 are more likely to respond to therapy than patients with genotype 1.

D. ALT or alanine aminotransferase.
   1. Also known as serum glutamic pyruvic transaminase (SGPT).
   2. Useful in the diagnosis of viral hepatitis and cirrhosis.
   3. Elevated ALT often precedes anti-HCV seroconversion.
   4. CDC recommends monthly ALT testing of anti-HCV negative patients to facilitate detection of new infections and provide pattern from which to determine when exposure may have occurred.

Table 6.7

Interpretation of results of tests for hepatitis C virus (HCV) infection and further actions

Test Outcome	Interpretation	Further Action
HCV antibody nonreactive	No HCV antibody detected	Sample can be reported as nonreactive for HCV antibody. No further action required.
		If recent HCV exposure in person tested is suspected, test for HCV RNA.*
HCV antibody reactive	Presumptive HCV infection	A repeatedly reactive result is consistent with current HCV infection, or past HCV infection that has resolved, or biologic false positivity for HCV antibody. Test for HCV RNA to identify current infection.
HCV antibody reactive, HCV RNA detected	Current HCV infection	Provide person tested with appropriate counseling and link person tested to medical care and treatment.†
HCV antibody reactive, HCV RNA not detected	No current HCV infection	No further action required in most cases.
		If distinction between true positivity and biologic false positivity for HCV antibody is desired, and if sample is repeatedly reactive in the initial test, test with another HCV antibody assay.
		In certain situations follow up with HCV RNA testing and appropriate counseling.§

* If HCV RNA testing is not feasible and person tested is not immunocompromised, do follow-up testing for HCV antibody to demonstrate seroconversion. If the person tested is immunocompromised, consider testing for HCV RNA.

† It is recommended before initiating antiviral therapy to retest for HCV RNA in a subsequent blood sample to confirm HCV RNA positivity.

§ If the person tested is suspected of having HCV exposure within the past 6 months, or has clinical evidence of HCV disease, or if there is concern regarding the handling or storage of the test specimen.

Source: Centers for Disease Control and Prevention (CDC). (2013g). Testing for HCV infection: An update of guidance for clinicians and laboratorians. *MMWR, 62*(18). (Available from http://www.ncbi.nlm.nih.gov/pubmed/23657112)

VII. Schedule for routine testing/screening.

A. Routine testing of dialysis staff members is not recommended.

B. Routine ALT and anti-HCV testing of hemodialysis patients is recommended for monitoring transmission within centers and ensuring appropriate dialysis precautions are being followed.

C. Test all patients at admission for anti-HCV and ALT level.
   1. In the absence of unexplained ALT elevations, anti-HCV testing every 6 months is recommended for those testing negative for anti-HCV.
   2. Repeat anti-HCV testing if unexplained ALT elevations are observed.
   3. Consider testing for HCV RNA if unexplained ALT elevations persist in patients who are repeatedly anti-HCV negative.

VIII. Precautions.

A. Strict adherence to infection control precautions recommended for all patients on hemodialysis.

B. Patients who are anti-HCV positive or HCV RNA positive do not have to be isolated or dialyzed separately on dedicated machines. They can participate in the dialyzer reprocessing programs.

IX. Anti-HCV seroconversion

A. In the event of a seroconversion, review all other patients' routine laboratory test results to identify additional cases.

B. Investigate potential sources for infection to determine if transmission might have occurred within the dialysis unit.

C. Increasing the frequency of anti-HCV testing in the facility may be considered for a limited time to detect additional new infections (CDC, 2001a).

X. Prevention.

A. Research into the development of a vaccine is underway.

B. Effective preexposure or postexposure prophylaxis (i.e., immune globulin) is not available.

XI. Treatment.

A. Significant advances have been made in the development of antiviral agents with improved efficacy against HCV.

B. Decreasing liver-related morbidity and mortality is the goal of HCV treatment.

C. Patients with CKD who have HCV infection should be encouraged to receive antiviral therapy (Liu & Kao, 2011).

SECTION G
Hepatitis D (Delta Hepatitis)

I. Characteristics and epidemiology.

A. Single-stranded circular defective RNA virus.

B. Replicates only in hepatocytes and has complex interaction with HBV.

C. Requires presence of HBV to replicate.

D. Structurally unrelated to the Hepatitis A, B, or C.

E. Genotypes and subtypes have been identified.

F. Certain genotypes may be associated with less severe disease.

G. High prevalence areas include the Mediterranean Basin, Middle East, Central Asia, West Africa, and the Amazon Basin of South America (WHO, 2014c).

H. There is a low prevalence of HDV infection in the United States.

I. Rates less than 1% of HBsAg-positive persons in the general population.

J. Rates greater than 10% in HBsAg-positive persons with repeated percutaneous exposures (e.g., injecting drug users).

K. Limited data on the prevalence among patients on chronic hemodialysis.

II. Transmission.

A. Only occurs in the presence of hepatitis B infection.

B. Transmitted by blood and blood products; percutaneous (i.e., injecting drug use) and permucosal exposure.

C. Risk factors for infection are similar to those for hepatitis B virus infection.

D. Sexual transmission of HDV is less efficient than for HBV.

E. Perinatal HDV transmission is rare.

III. Clinical features.

A. Co-infection.
   1. Occurs when someone is infected simultaneously with HBV and HDV.
   2. Co-infections are usually acute.
   3. Result in chronic HDV infections in less than 5% of co-infected individuals.

B. Superinfection (Hughes et al., 2011; Pascarella & Negro, 2011; Yurdaydın et al., 2010).
   1. Occurs when someone with existing chronic HBV infection becomes infected with HDV.
   2. Associated with severe hepatitis and progresses to chronic HDV infection in up to 80% of cases.
   3. Over 60% of patients with chronic infection will develop cirrhosis.

IV. Serologic testing and interpretation.

A. Blood assays used for diagnosis include the HDV antibody (anti-HD) and the HDV RNA.

B. HDV antibodies appear during the acute phase of infection and usually decline after infection to non-detectable levels.

C. HDV antibodies and HDV RNA persist with chronic infection.

D. HDV RNA is also used to monitor response of treatment with interferons.

E. Routine testing of patients on hemodialysis is not necessary or recommended (CDC, 2001a).

F. Screen for delta antibody if a patient is known to be infected with HDV, or if evidence exists of transmission of HDV in a dialysis unit.

V. Precautions for dialysis.

A. Prevention of HBV infection will prevent HDV infection in a person susceptible to HBV.

B. Patients who are known to be infected with HDV should be isolated from all other dialysis patients, especially those who are HBsAg-positive (CDC, 2001a).

SECTION H
Human Immunodeficiency Virus (HIV)

I. Epidemiology.

A. Human immunodeficiency virus (HIV) infection and acquired immunodeficiency syndrome (AIDS) remain a major global public health concern and are leading causes of morbidity and mortality in the United States.

B. In the U.S., approximately 50,000 people become infected with HIV each year.

C. Highly active antiretroviral therapy (HAART) has extended survival of those living with HIV/AIDS. It is estimated 1.2 million people in the United States are now living with HIV.

D. Approximately 16,000 persons with AIDS die each year in the United States (CDC, 2011c).

II. HIV and kidney disease.

A. Kidney disease is a common complication of HIV infection. Persons with HIV infection are at increased risk for chronic kidney disease, and up to 30% of people living with HIV have abnormal kidney function, which can lead to CKD stage 5 (AIDS.gov, 2013; Bickel et al., 2013).

B. Patients at time of HIV diagnosis should be assessed for existing kidney disease.

C. Focal segmental glomerulosclerosis (FSGS) is the predominant renal lesion of HIV-associated nephropathy (HIVAN). HIVAN is less prevalent in patients who have achieved sustained suppression of viral replication (AIDS.gov, 2013; Bickel et al., 2013).

D. Nephrotoxicity is a complication of long-term exposure to antiretroviral therapy, protease inhibitors, and nucleoside reverse transcriptase inhibitors (AIDS.gov, 2013; Bickel et al., 2013; Jao & Wyatt, 2010).

III. Serologic testing/screening.

A. The CDC estimates 18% of people infected with HIV in the United States are unaware of their infection.

B. Per the CDC, HIV testing is vital for preventing new infections and improving the health of people living with HIV.

C. The CDC has issued guidelines, recommendations, and fact sheets about the prevention, screening, diagnosis, treatment, and management of HIV infection and HIV-related diseases. These recommendations are available at http://www.cdc.gov/hiv/guidelines/index.html

D. The recommendations are intended for clinicians in all healthcare settings, public health professionals, program managers in clinical and nonclinical settings, persons at risk for HIV infection, and the general public.

E. Per the recommendations, diagnostic HIV testing should be a part of routine clinical care in all health care settings and should include:
   1. Adolescents and adults being tested at least once as a routine part of medical care.
   2. Annual testing for individuals at risk of infection.
   3. Testing women with each pregnancy.

F. Available HIV tests include:
   1. Antibody test.
      a. Detects the presence of antibodies against HIV.
      b. Can be conducted on a sample of blood or oral fluid.
   2. Combination antigen-antibody test.
      a. Detects both the antibody to HIV and the p24 antigen.
      b. The p24 antigen can be detected within 4 to 7 days before the appearance of antibodies.
      c. Combination test can be used to detect early infection.
   3. RNA test.
      a. Detects the presence of the virus in the blood.
      b. Can detect very early infection, within 10 to 15 days of exposure, before antibody tests are able to detect HIV.

G. Routine screening of patients on dialysis for HIV infection for infection control purposes is not necessary or recommended by the CDC (CDC, 2001).

IV. General infection control measures.

A. Patients infected with HIV can be dialyzed by either hemodialysis or peritoneal dialysis.

B. Infection control precautions recommended for all patients on hemodialysis are sufficient to prevent HIV transmission between patients.

C. Patients who are HIV-positive do not have to be isolated or dialyzed separately on dedicated machines.

D. Patients who are HIV positive can participate in a dialyzer reuse program.

1. There is no epidemiologic evidence that dialyzer reuse in the United States has led to either an occupational or healthcare-acquired infection with HIV.
2. Because HIV is not transmitted efficiently through occupational exposures, reprocessing dialyzers from patients who are HIV-positive should not place staff members at increased risk for infection (CDC, 2001a).
3. In addition, data from the CDC annual surveillance of dialysis-associated diseases does not suggest that reuse is a risk factor for HIV. Follow the AAMI recommended practices for reuse of hemodialyzers.

E. Infection control precautions apply for all patients on dialysis. There are no special precautions for patients with HIV or AIDS. There are several reasons why no special precautions are recommended for these patients receiving maintenance hemodialysis.
1. HIV is not efficiently transmitted in the dialysis setting.
2. Standard infection control precautions used for the care of all patients on hemodialysis are sufficient to prevent the transmission of the virus in the dialysis setting.
3. Transmission from the hemodialysis machine to the patient has not been observed.

SECTION I
The Ebola Virus

I. **Background information.** *Note*: The information in this section was obtained from the Centers for Disease Control and Prevention's (CDC's) website on November 1, 2014. Because the body of knowledge and subsequent recommendations regarding Ebola are evolving, the reader should visit the CDC website to obtain the most recent information (www.CDC.gov).

A. The Ebola virus disease (EVD).
1. Ebola, previously known as Ebola hemorrhagic fever, is a rare and deadly disease caused by infection with one of the five identified Ebola virus strains (see Figure 6.5). Ebola can cause disease in humans and nonhuman primates (monkeys, gorillas, and chimpanzees).
2. Ebola was first discovered in 1976 near the Ebola River in what is now the Democratic Republic of the Congo. Since then, outbreaks have appeared sporadically in Africa.
3. The natural reservoir host of Ebola virus remains unknown; researchers believe that the virus is animal-borne and that bats are the most likely reservoir. Four of the five virus strains occur in an animal host native to Africa.

B. Pathogenesis.
1. Ebola virus enters the patient through mucous membranes, breaks in the skin, or parenterally and infects many cell types, including monocytes, macrophages, dendritic cells, endothelial cells, fibroblasts, hepatocytes, adrenal cortical cells, and epithelial cells.
2. The incubation period may be related to the infection route (e.g., 6 days for injection versus 10 days for contact).
3. Ebola virus migrates from the initial infection site to regional lymph nodes and subsequently to the liver, spleen, and adrenal gland.
4. Although not infected by the Ebola virus, lymphocytes undergo apoptosis, resulting in decreased lymphocyte counts.
5. Hepatocellular necrosis occurs and is associated with dysregulation of clotting factors and subsequent coagulopathy.
6. Adrenocortical necrosis also can be found and is associated with hypotension and impaired steroid synthesis.
7. Ebola virus appears to trigger a release of pro-inflammatory cytokines with subsequent vascular leak and impairment of clotting ultimately resulting in multiorgan failure and shock.

C. Symptoms of Ebola may appear anywhere from 2 to 21 days after exposure, but the average is 8 to 10 days. Symptoms include:
1. Fever.
2. Severe headache.
3. Muscle pain.
4. Weakness.
5. Diarrhea.
6. Vomiting.
7. Abdominal (stomach) pain.
8. Unexplained hemorrhage (bleeding or bruising).

D. Recovery depends on good supportive clinical care and the patient's immune response. Patients who recover from Ebola infection develop antibodies that last for at least 10 years.

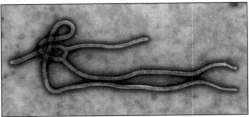

Figure 6.5. Transmission electron micrograph (TEM) of ebola virus virion.

Source: http://www.cdc.gov/vhf/ebola/

1. It isn't known if people who recover are immune for life or if they can become infected with a different species of Ebola.
2. Some people who have recovered from Ebola have developed long-term complications, such as joint and vision problems.

II. Transmission of the infection.

A. The way in which the virus first appears in a human at the start of an outbreak is unknown.
   1. Scientists believe that the first patient becomes infected through contact with an infected animal, such as a fruit bat or primate (apes and monkeys), called a *spillover event*.
   2. Person-to-person transmission follows and can lead to large numbers of affected people.

B. When an infection does occur in humans, the virus can be spread in several ways to others through direct contact (through broken skin or mucous membranes in, for example, the eyes, nose, or mouth) with:
   1. Blood or body fluids (including but not limited to urine, saliva, sweat, feces, vomit, breast milk, and semen) of a person who is sick with Ebola.
   2. Objects (like needles and syringes) that have been contaminated with the virus.
   3. Infected fruit bats or primates (apes and monkeys).

C. Ebola is not spread through the air, by water, or in general, by food.
   1. However, in Africa, Ebola may be spread as a result of handling bushmeat (wild animals hunted for food) and contact with infected bats.
   2. There is no evidence that mosquitos or other insects can transmit Ebola virus.
   3. Only a few species of mammals (for example, humans, bats, monkeys, and apes) have shown the ability to become infected with and spread Ebola virus.

D. Those at the highest risk of getting sick because they may come in contact with infected blood or body fluids of the sick patients include:
   1. Healthcare providers caring for patients with Ebola.
   2. The patient's family and friends who are in close contact.

E. During outbreaks of Ebola, the disease can spread quickly within healthcare settings (such as a clinic or hospital) where hospital staff are not wearing appropriate protective equipment, including masks, gowns, and gloves and eye protection.
   1. Dedicated medical equipment (preferable disposable, when possible) should be used. Proper cleaning and disposal of instruments, such as needles and syringes, is also important.

2. If instruments are not disposable, they must be sterilized before being used again. Without adequate sterilization, virus transmission can continue and amplify an outbreak.

III. Preventing the spread of the disease.

A. Healthcare workers who may be exposed to patients with Ebola should follow these steps:
   1. Wear appropriate personal protective equipment (PPE).
   2. Practice proper infection control and sterilization measures.
   3. Isolate patients with Ebola from other patients.
   4. Avoid direct contact with the bodies of people who have died from Ebola.
   5. Notify health officials if you have had direct contact with the blood or body fluids, such as but not limited to feces, saliva, urine, vomit, and semen of a person who is sick with Ebola.

B. Once someone recovers from Ebola, they can no longer spread the virus.
   1. However, the Ebola virus has been found in semen for up to 3 months.
   2. Abstinence from sex (including oral sex) is recommended for at least 3 months.
   3. If abstinence is not possible, condoms may help prevent the spread of disease.

IV. Clinical presentation and clinical course.

A. Patients with EVD generally have abrupt onset of fever and symptoms typically 8 to 12 days after exposure.

B. Initial signs and symptoms are nonspecific and may include elevated body temperature or subjective fever, chills, myalgias, and malaise.

C. Patients can progress from the initial nonspecific symptoms after about 5 days to develop gastrointestinal symptoms such as severe watery diarrhea, nausea, vomiting, and abdominal pain.
   1. Other symptoms such as chest pain, shortness of breath, headache, or confusion may also develop.
   2. Patients often have conjunctival infection.
   3. Hiccups have been reported.
   4. Seizures may occur, and cerebral edema has been reported.

D. Bleeding is not universally present but can manifest later in the course as petechiae, ecchymosis/bruising, or oozing from venipuncture sites and mucosal hemorrhage. Frank hemorrhage is less common.

E. Patients may develop a diffuse erythematous maculopapular rash by day 5 to 7 (usually involving the neck, trunk, and arms) that can desquamate.

Table 6.8

Laboratory Tests Used in the Diagnosis of Ebola Infection

Timeline of Infection	Diagnostic tests available
Within a few days after symptoms begin	Antigen-capture enzyme-linked immunosorbent assay (ELISA) testing IgM ELISA Polymerase chain reaction (PCR) Virus isolation
Later in disease course or after recovery	IgM and IgG antibodies
Retrospectively in deceased patients	Immunohistochemistry testing PCR Virus isolation

F. Pregnant women may experience spontaneous miscarriages.

G. Patients with fatal disease usually develop more severe clinical signs early during infection and die typically between days 6 and 16 of complications including multiorgan failure and septic shock.

H. In nonfatal cases, patients may have fever for several days and improve, typically around day 6. Patients that survive can have a prolonged convalescence.

V. Diagnosis.

A. Diagnosing Ebola in a person who has been infected for only a few days is difficult.

B. The early symptoms, such as fever, are nonspecific to Ebola infection and are seen often in patients with more commonly occurring diseases, such as malaria and typhoid fever.

C. If a person has the early symptoms of Ebola, he/she should be isolated and public health professionals notified, if the person had contact with:
1. The blood or body fluids of a person sick with Ebola.
2. Objects that have been contaminated with the blood or body fluids of a person sick with Ebola.
3. Contact with infected animals.

D. Samples from the patient can then be collected and tested to confirm infection. Laboratory tests used in diagnosis can be seen in Table 6.8.

E. Laboratory findings.
1. Laboratory findings at admission may include leukopenia frequently with lymphopenia followed later by elevated neutrophils and a left shift.
2. Platelet counts are often decreased in the 50,000 to 100,000 range.
3. Amylase may be elevated, reflecting pancreatic involvement (inflammation/infection).
4. Hepatic transaminases are elevated with aspartate aminotransferase (AST) exceeding alanine aminotransferase (ALT); these values may peak at more than 1,000 IU/L.
5. Proteinuria may be present.
6. Prothrombin (PT) and partial thromboplastin times (PTT) are prolonged and fibrin degradation products are elevated, consistent with disseminated intravascular coagulation (DIC).

VI. Treatment.

A. Standard, contact, and droplet precautions are recommended for management of hospitalized patients with known or suspected EVD. Additional infection control measures might be warranted if a patient with EVD has other conditions or illnesses for which other measures are indicated (e.g., tuberculosis, multidrug resistant organisms).

B. Symptoms of Ebola are treated as they appear.

C. The following basic interventions, when used early, can significantly improve the chances of survival:
1. Providing intravenous fluids (IV) and balancing electrolytes.
2. Maintaining oxygen status and blood pressure.
3. Treating other infections if they occur.

D. Clinical management should focus on supportive care of complications, such as hypovolemia, electrolyte abnormalities, hematologic abnormalities, refractory shock, hypoxia, hemorrhage, septic shock, multiorgan failure, and DIC. Recommended care includes:
1. Volume repletion.

2. Maintenance of blood pressure (with vasopressors if needed).
3. Maintenance of oxygenation.
4. Pain control.
5. Nutritional support.
6. Treating secondary bacterial infections and preexisting comorbidities.

E. Some patients develop profound third-spacing of fluids due to vascular leak.

F. Infection prevention and control measures are a critical part of clinical management; all bodily fluids and clinical specimens should be considered potentially infectious. The precautions are described in the document entitled *Infection Prevention and Control Recommendations for Hospitalized Patients with Known or Suspected Ebola Virus Disease in U.S. Hospitals.*

G. Recovery from Ebola depends on good supportive care and the patient's immune response.

VII. The CDC's recommendations for safely performing acute hemodialysis in patients with EVD in hospitals in the United States.

A. Acute kidney injury requiring kidney replacement therapy can occur in critically ill patients infected with Ebola virus.

B. Treatment decisions should be made by the clinical team caring for the patient. Infection control considerations may help to inform providers' decisions and should influence hospitals' planning processes.

C. Inpatient care of patients with Ebola should be provided in a hospital with capacity to perform continuous renal replacement therapy (CRRT). Efforts to minimize direct blood exposure to healthcare personnel and blood contamination of the environment are of principal importance due to the high concentration of Ebola virus that can be present in an infected patient's blood and the large volumes of blood involved in hemodialysis.

D. Hemodialysis/CRRT should only be performed in the patient's isolation room.

E. Patients with Ebola may have disseminated intravascular coagulation (DIC) and correction of coagulopathy is not always possible.

F. Designate a highly competent individual, who has also been trained to follow CDC guidelines for proper personal protective equipment (PPE) procedures, to perform catheter insertion.
1. Perform catheter insertion in the isolation room and use local strategies to minimize blood exposure during dialysis catheter placement.

2. The subclavian site for catheter insertion should be avoided because of the challenges with direct site compression if bleeding occurs.
3. Selection of the internal jugular vs. femoral vein for catheter insertion may depend on patient characteristics and operator proficiency.
4. Using a chest x-ray to confirm line placement will require availability of portable x-ray equipment within the isolation room. This and other factors should be considered in the planning stage before it becomes necessary.
5. Ultrasound guidance should be used (by an individual fully trained in this technique) to reduce cannulation attempts and mechanical complications, including arterial puncture. If used, the ultrasound machine should be dedicated to the isolation room until it can be terminally cleaned and disinfected. Read more on *Guidelines for the Prevention of Intravascular Catheter-Related Infections, 2011* (PDF - 83 pages).
6. Attach closed, needleless connector devices to the catheter hubs to reduce blood exposure during catheter connections and disconnections.

G. If possible, limit the number and different types of healthcare personnel involved in hemodialysis and CRRT procedures. For example, ICU nurses performing CRRT could eliminate need for dialysis unit nursing staff to also care for the patient.

H. All staff involved in providing dialysis should follow recommendations for appropriate PPE. Staff should wear a fluid-resistant or impermeable gown if they will be performing any circuit connection/disconnection procedures, handling used dialyzers or tubing, or handling or draining effluent.

I. A hemodialysis/CRRT machine should be dedicated for use on the patient and kept in the isolation room until terminal disinfection procedures are undertaken.

J. All other dialysis-related supplies, including the dialyzer, should be disposed of after use in accordance with local, state, and federal regulations. Read more on Ebola-Associated Waste Management.

K. Under no circumstances should a used dialyzer be reprocessed or reused.

L. The Ebola virus should not be able to cross an intact dialyzer membrane.
1. Because a small dialyzer leak might not be apparent, dialysis effluent should always be handled with care, and while wearing appropriate PPE, to avoid contact and splashes.
2. The effluent should be disposed of in the toilet or other dedicated drain in a manner that prevents splashes, and can be safely drained into the waste water sewer system.

M. Use a dialysis machine that is familiar to the staff that will perform dialysis.

N. Certain CRRT machines have features that make them easier to manage and decontaminate in the context of caring for a patient with Ebola than traditional hemodialysis machines, such as a completely closed system, lack of an internal pathway, and use of disposable dialysate and saline supplies.
 1. The possibility of blood contamination of internal machine components through pressure monitors is also much less likely with these machines than other hemodialysis machines.
 2. During CRRT, staff should pay close attention to pressure alarms and failures of pressure monitors, and look for and document any failure of the tubing or spillage of fluid outside of the tubing, as these may have implications for more extensive machine disinfection procedures.

O. Additional considerations:
 1. If clinically appropriate, consider regional citrate anticoagulation during CRRT to reduce episodes of filter clotting that require manipulation of the dialyzer and/or circuit. Regional citrate anticoagulation for CRRT should be used only if the hospital has a protocol in place and nurses who are trained in the protocol.
 2. Consider using the same CRRT machine for hemodialysis of the patient for as long as possible (while kidney replacement therapy is needed) to avoid introducing a second dialysis machine.

P. If use of an intermittent hemodialysis machine is warranted:
 1. Complete all priming of the circuit prior to connecting bloodlines to the patient's catheter.
 2. Use disposable accessory supplies, such as priming bucket and concentrate containers, if possible.
  a. Establish steps for handling accessory supplies that are not disposable, must be dedicated to the patient, and disinfected between uses.
  b. If an attached computer keyboard is needed, use a flat solid surface keyboard that can be easily disinfected or a keyboard cover that can be disinfected or disposed of.
 3. Pay close attention to pressure alarms and failures of the pressure monitor. Look for and document any flow of blood in the line approaching the external transducer protector, as these may signal internal contamination of the machine with blood.

Q. Machine decontamination/terminal disinfection.
 1. External machine surfaces. Cleaning and disinfection of external machine surfaces should be performed in accordance with CDC's *Interim*

Guidance for Environmental Infection Control in Hospitals for Ebola Virus and manufacturer's instructions.
 a. General principles include the following.
  (1) Use appropriate PPE.
  (2) Perform a cleaning step using a detergent.
  (3) Perform disinfection using an U.S. Environmental Protection Agency (EPA)-registered hospital disinfectant recommended for use against Ebola during the 2014 outbreak. The EPA-registered hospital disinfectant must have a label claim of potency at least equivalent to that for a nonenveloped virus (e.g., norovirus, rotavirus, adenovirus, poliovirus).
  (4) Ensure all surfaces are cleaned and disinfected (including accessory equipment such as IV poles), paying particular attention to high-touch surfaces, such as control panels.
  (5) Assure sufficient wet contact time of disinfectant according to label claims for inactivation of a nonenveloped virus.
 b. Additional considerations:
  (1) Vaporized hydrogen peroxide and ultraviolet (UV) light applications for decontamination of isolation room surfaces (during terminal disinfection) might serve to disinfect external surfaces of dialysis machines. If UV light is used, the importance of a direct line of sight for efficient disinfection should be considered.
  (2) CDC has been in contact with some machine manufacturers and may be able to assist in providing more specific guidance for machine terminal disinfection procedures (CDC Emergency Operations Center, 770-488-7100).
 2. Internal pathways.
 a. Standard heat or chemical disinfection procedures recommended by machine manufacturers and used routinely by dialysis providers are sufficient to inactivate Ebola virus.
 b. Internal machine disinfection of hemodialysis machines should be performed between treatments and conducted in the isolation room.
 c. Other internal machine components. If there is concern about the possibility of fluid contamination of internal machine components such as pressure monitors, contact the manufacturer for guidance and notify the appropriate local or state health department and CDC (CDC Emergency Operations Center, 770-488-7100).

VIII. Exposures.

A. High risk examples.
   1. Direct contact with body fluids, from a person sick with Ebola and showing symptoms, through:
      a. A needlestick.
      b. Splashes to eyes, nose, or mouth.
      c. Getting body fluids directly on skin.
   2. Touching a dead body while in a country with a large Ebola outbreak without wearing recommended personal protective equipment (PPE) or not wearing PPE correctly.
   3. Both living with and taking care of a person sick with Ebola.
B. Some risk of exposure examples.
   1. Close contact (within 3 feet) of a person sick with Ebola for a long time.
   2. Direct contact with a person sick with Ebola (such as in a hospital) in a country with a large Ebola outbreak even while wearing PPE correctly.
C. Examples of low (but not zero) risk of exposure.
   1. Having been in a country with a large Ebola outbreak within the past 21 days with no known exposure (such as NO direct contact with body fluids from a person sick with Ebola).
   2. Being in the same room for a brief period of time with a person sick with Ebola.
   3. Brief direct contact, like shaking hands, with someone sick with Ebola.
   4. Direct contact with a person sick with Ebola in the United States while wearing PPE correctly.
   5. Traveling on an airplane with a person sick with Ebola.

D. Examples of no risk of exposure assuming there are no other risk factors from previous categories.
   1. Having contact with a healthy person who had contact with a person sick with Ebola.
   2. Having contact with a person sick with Ebola before he or she had any symptoms.
   3. Someone who left a country with a large Ebola outbreak more than 21 days ago and has not been sick with Ebola since leaving that country.
   4. Having been in a country where there have been Ebola cases, but no large Ebola outbreak (for example, Spain).
Content source:
   • Centers for Disease Control and Prevention
   • National Center for Emerging and Zoonotic Infectious Diseases (NCEZID)
   • Division of High-Consequence Pathogens and Pathology (DHCPP)
   • Viral Special Pathogens Branch (VSPB)

SECTION J
Occupational Exposure to BBP (HBV, HCV, HIV)

I. Scope of problem and preventing exposure.

A. Healthcare workers are at risk for occupational exposure to bloodborne pathogens.

B. Infection with hepatitis B virus (HBV), hepatitis C virus (HCV), and human immunodeficiency virus (HIV) may result from parenteral, mucous membrane, and nonintact skin exposures to infectious blood and body fluids.

C. Measures to prevent exposures include adherence to OSHA's Bloodborne Pathogens Standard and the CDC recommended infection control practices and precautions, use of personal protective equipment, consistent use of sound work practices, and use of engineering controls, such as safety needles and needle-free IV line connectors to prevent needlestick injuries.

D. Estimates indicate that 600,000 to 800,000 needlestick injuries occur each year in the United States.

II. Infection risk.

A. Risk of HIV infection after a needlestick or cut exposure to HIV-infected blood is approximately 0.3%.

B. Risk of HCV infection after a needlestick or cut exposure to HCV-infected blood is approximately 1.8%.

C. Risk of HBV infection of a susceptible person, after a needlestick or cut exposure to HBV-infected blood is approximately 6% to 30% depending on the HBeAg status of the source individual. When the HBeAg is positive, indicating high HBV replication and viral load, the risk of infection is much greater.

III. Initial postexposure management.

A. Following an exposure, immediately wash needlestick site and cuts with soap and water.

B. The nose, mouth, and eyes should be flushed with water following an exposure to those areas.

C. Immediately report to ensure prompt exposure management follow-up, which should begin as soon as possible following exposure.

D. OSHA's Bloodborne Pathogens Standard defines employer requirements following possible occupational exposure of a healthcare worker to a bloodborne pathogen and includes referral for postexposure evaluation. The complete Bloodborne Pathogens Standard can be found in Title 29 of the Code of Federal Regulations at 29 CFR 1910.1030 (United States Department of Labor, Occupational Health & Safety, 2014).

IV. Postexposure management.

A. HBV.
1. The CDC provides guidance for evaluating healthcare workers for hepatitis B virus protection and for administering postexposure management. See Table 6.9. for detailed updated guidelines.
2. Postexposure follow-up and treatment should begin as soon as possible, including HBsAg testing of the source person.
3. Healthcare institutions' procedures should be followed for testing source persons, including obtaining informed consent in accordance with law.
4. When a source person is unknown, the exposed individual should be managed as if the source person were HBsAg-positive.
5. Regardless of the source person's HBsAg status, healthcare workers who have written documentation verifying they have received a complete hepatitis B vaccine series and have documented anti-HBs ≥ 10 mIU/mL, do not require postexposure management for HBV.
6. Healthcare workers who have anti-HBs < 10 mIU/mL, or who are unvaccinated or incompletely vaccinated, and sustain an exposure to an HBsAg-positive or an unknown HBsAg source, should undergo initial baseline testing for HBV infection as soon as possible after exposure and at 6 months postexposure.
7. Hepatitis B immune globulin (HBIG), which provides passive temporary protection, should be provided for the exposed individual who is a previously documented vaccine nonresponder after having received 6 doses of the vaccine.
8. HBIG and the hepatitis B vaccine should be provided for other exposed individuals who are susceptible (CDC, 2013d).

B. HCV.
1. There is no effective approved vaccine to protect against hepatitis C infection.
2. Postexposure immune globulin or postexposure antiviral therapy is not recommended.
3. For HCV postexposure management, the HCV status of the source and the exposed person should be determined.
4. If the source is hepatitis C antibody negative, no further testing is necessary and no additional testing beyond initial HCV testing is indicated for the exposed healthcare worker.
5. Healthcare workers exposed to an HCV-positive source should have follow-up testing to determine if infection develops.
6. The healthcare worker exposed to an HCV-positive source should have follow-up testing completed at 4 to 6 months after the exposure. Testing for HCV RNA may be performed at 4 to 6 weeks following exposure (CDC, 2001b).

C. HIV.
1. There is no effective approved vaccine to protect against human immunodeficiency virus (HIV).
2. U.S. Public Health Service recommendations for the management of healthcare personnel who experience occupational exposure to blood and/or body fluids that might contain human immunodeficiency virus (HIV) were recently updated. Updates were made to the recommended HIV postexposure prophylaxis (PEP) regimens and the duration of HIV follow-up testing for the exposed individual.
3. PEP with antiretroviral medication, to reduce the risk of transmission, is recommended for occupational exposures to a source person who has HIV, or when there is a reasonable suspicion of HIV infection in the source person.
4. When possible, the HIV status of the source person should be determined to guide the use of PEP.
5. FDA-approved rapid HIV tests provide results within 30 minutes, and the use of PEP should not be delayed waiting for results.
6. PEP should be initiated as soon as possible, preferably within hours, following occupational exposure to HIV, should include three or more antiretroviral drugs, and be continued for 4 weeks.
7. HIV testing should be completed at baseline, at 6 weeks, 12 weeks, and 6 months after exposure.
8. Following baseline testing, an alternative testing schedule may be used with testing completed at 6 weeks after exposure and 4 months after exposure, if a fourth-generation combination HIV p24 antigen–HIV antibody test is used.
9. It is recommended PEP be discontinued and no HIV follow-up testing of the exposed person if the test results indicate the source person is HIV-negative (Kuhar et al., 2013; Panlilio et al., 2005).

Table 6.9

Postexposure management of healthcare personnel after occupational percutaneous and mucosal exposure to blood and body fluids by healthcare personnel HepB vaccination and response status

Healthcare personnel status	Postexposure testing		Postexposure prophylaxis		Postvaccination serologic testing
	Source patient (HBsAg)	HCP testing (anti-HBs)	HBIG*	Vaccination	
Documented responder§ after complete series (≥ 3 doses)	No action needed				
Documented nonresponder¶ after 6 doses	Positive/unknown	—**	HBIG x2 separated by 1 month	—	No
	Negative	No action needed			
Response unknown after 3 doses	Positive/unknown	< 10mIU/mL**	HBIG x1	Initiate revaccination	Yes
	Negative	< 10mIU/mL	None		
	Any result	≥ 10mIU/mL	No action needed		
Unvaccinated/incompletely vaccinated or vaccine refusers	Positive/unknown	—**	HBIG x1	Complete vaccination	Yes
	Negative	—	None	Complete vaccination	Yes

Abbreviations: HCP = health-care personnel; HBsAg = hepatitis B surface antigen; anti-HBs = antibody to hepatitis B surface antigen; HBIG = hepatitis B immune globulin.

* HBIG should be administered intramuscularly as soon as possible after exposure when indicated. The effectiveness of HBIG when administered >7 days after percutaneous, mucosal, or nonintact skin exposures is unknown. HBIG dosage is 0.06 mL/kg.

† Should be performed 1–2 months after the last dose of the HepB vaccine series (and 4–6 months after administration of HBIG to avoid detection of passively administered anti-HBs) using a quantitative method that allows detection of the protective concentration of anti-HBs (≥10 mIU/mL).

§ A responder is defined as a person with anti-HBs ≥10 mIU/mL after ≥3 doses of HepB vaccine.

¶ A nonresponder is defined as a person with anti-HBs <10 mIU/mL after ≥6 doses of HepB vaccine.

** HCP who have anti-HBs <10mIU/mL, or who are unvaccinated or incompletely vaccinated, and sustain an exposure to a source patient who is HBsAg-positive or has unknown HBsAg status, should undergo baseline testing for HBV infection as soon as possible after exposure, and follow-up testing approximately 6 months later. Initial baseline tests consist of total anti-HBc; testing at approximately 6 months consists of HBsAg and total anti-HBc.

Source: Centers for Disease Control and Prevention (CDC). (2013d). Guidance for evaluating health-care personnel for hepatitis B virus protection and for administering postexposure management. *MMWR, 62*(rr10);1-19.

SECTION K
Safe Injection Practices and Medication Safety

I. Overview.

A. Unsafe injection practices have resulted in outbreaks of both hepatitis B and C in U.S. ambulatory care settings.

B. Outbreak investigation found inadequate infection control practices were related to:
   1. Using the same syringe to administer medication to more than one patient, even if the needle was changed or the injection was administered through an intervening length of IV tubing.
   2. Accessing a medication vial or bag with a syringe that was first used to administer medication to a patient and then reusing contents from that vial or bag for another patient.
   3. Using medications considered single-dose/single-use for more than one patient.
   4. Not using proper aseptic technique when preparing and administering injections.
   5. Reinserting used needles into a multiple-dose vial or solution containers such as a saline bag.
   6. Using saline solutions from a common source IV bag to flush IV lines and catheters.

C. Adherence to the principles of aseptic technique for the preparation and administration of parenteral medications is vital to prevent disease transmission. (CDC, 2013d, 2014a, 2014b; Pegues et al., 2011).

II. Fundamentals of safe injection practices.

A. Needles and syringes are single-use only.

B. Medications must be prepared in a clean area on a clean surface away from the dialysis stations and away from potentially contaminated items.

C. Use of aseptic technique to avoid contamination of sterile injection equipment (e.g., vials and syringes).

D. Proper hand hygiene must be performed before handling medications.

E. The rubber stopper or septum of medication vials must be disinfected prior to piercing it and drawing up the medication.

F. Multidose medication vials should be assigned to a single patient whenever possible.

G. Multiple-dose vials are only entered with a new, sterile syringe and needle.

H. Not administering medications from one syringe to multiple patients, even if the needle on the syringe is changed.

I. Not administering medications from single-dose vials or ampules to multiple patients or combining leftover contents for later use.

J. Not using intravenous solution bags as a common source of supply for multiple patients (e.g., drawing up flushes).

K. A syringe or needle must be considered contaminated once it has been used to enter or connect to an intravenous solution bag, administration set, or extracorporeal circuit.

L. A needle or other device should never be left inserted into a medication vial for multiple uses.

M. Not storing medication vials in the immediate patient treatment area.

N. The United States Pharmacopeia (USP) General Chapter 797 recommends if a multidose vial has been opened or accessed (e.g., needle-punctured), the vial should be dated and discarded within 28 days unless the manufacturer specifies a different (shorter or longer) date for that opened vial.

O. In addition, the CDC (2001a) *Recommended Infection Control Practices for Hemodialysis Units at a Glance* specifically includes the following.
   1. Unused medications (including multiple-dose vials containing diluents) or supplies (e.g., syringes, alcohol swabs) taken to the patient's station should be used only for that patient and not returned to a common clean area or used on other patients.
   2. When multiple-dose medication vials are used (including vials containing diluents), prepare individual patient doses in a clean (centralized) area away from dialysis stations and deliver separately to each patient.
   3. Not carrying multiple-dose medication vials from station to station.
   4. Not using common medication carts to deliver medications to patients.
   5. Not carrying medication vials, syringes, alcohol swabs, or supplies in pockets.
   6. If trays are used to deliver medications to individual patients, they must be cleaned between patients.
   7. Clean areas should be clearly designated for the preparation, handling, and storage of medications and unused supplies and equipment.
   8. Clean areas should be clearly separated from contaminated areas where used supplies and equipment are handled.
   9. Not handling and storing medications or clean supplies in the same or an adjacent area to where used equipment or blood samples are handled.

III. "One and Only" campaign.

A. Public health campaign led by the Centers for Disease Control and Prevention (CDC) and the Safe Injection Practices Coalition (SIPC).

B. Goal is to raise awareness about safe injection practices and eradicate outbreaks resulting from unsafe injection practices.

C. To prevent transmission of infections, the CDC National Campaign for Injection Safety calls for "one needle, one syringe, only one time" (CDC, 2014d).

SECTION L
Aerosol Transmissible Diseases

Aerosol transmissible diseases can be divided into two groups, airborne transmissible and droplet transmissible.

I.   Droplet transmissible.

A. Droplet transmission occurs when an infectious person generates respiratory droplets by coughing or sneezing and involves contact of the conjunctivae or the mucous membranes of the nose or mouth.

B. Once generated, the droplets do not remain suspended in the air and usually only travel short distances. Droplets are heavy and typically fall within 3 feet of the person. Droplet precautions are used for large droplets > 5 microns. An example of a droplet transmissible disease is seasonal influenza.

C. Organisms transmitted by the droplet route do not remain infectious over long distances, and do not require special air handling and ventilation as would an airborne transmissible disease.

D. In addition to the use of precautions recommended for all hemodialysis patients, individuals known to have or are suspected of having diseases spread by droplet transmission must be placed on droplet precautions until no longer considered potentially infectious.

E. The patient presenting with signs of symptoms of a droplet transmissible disease should be provided a surgical mask to wear, be assessed by a physician, and a determination made by the physician regarding the necessity for hospitalization.

F. Droplet precautions should include:
   1. Dialyzing the patient in a defined area away from other patients by at least 3 feet.
   2. Limiting contact between nonessential personnel and the patient.
   3. In addition to PPE required for providing the dialysis treatment, patient care providers must wear a surgical mask when working within 3 feet of the patient.
   4. Gloves, gown, mask, and face shield are used for contact with respiratory secretions and changed before caring for another patient.

G. Patients and staff must be familiar with respiratory hygiene/cough etiquette measures that include:
   1. Covering mouth and nose with a tissue when coughing or sneezing.
   2. Immediately disposing of the tissue after use in a waste receptacle.
   3. Performing hand hygiene after having contact with respiratory secretions and contaminated objects/materials.

II.   Airborne transmissible.

A. Airborne transmission occurs when the bacteria or virus causing the disease is small enough to remain suspended in the air and easily carried over long distances on normal room air current (e.g., pulmonary *M. tuberculosis*).

B. Airborne precautions prevent transmission of such infectious agents and include preferred placement of the patient in an airborne-infection isolation room (AIIR) (Siegel et al., 2007).

C. AIIR is a single-patient room equipped with special air handling, provides negative pressure relative to the surrounding area, and has a minimum number of air exchanges per hour usually recirculated through HEPA filtration before return.

D. Healthcare workers providing care to a patient in an AIIR must have been trained in respiratory protection including the use of N95 respirators and must have participated in fit-testing.

E. It is expected that patients with active TB disease or other airborne transmissible diseases will be dialyzed in the hospital setting where appropriate isolation is available. An airborne-infection isolation room is beyond the capacity of an outpatient dialysis facility and not required in the outpatient setting.

F. The patient suspected of having an airborne transmissible disease should be provided a mask to wear and promptly assessed by an MD/APRN/PA to determine if hospitalization is necessary.
   1. The receiving facility or hospital must be notified.
   2. While awaiting prompt transport to the hospital, the patient should be maintained in an area away from other patients by at least 6 feet. Precautions, including a surgical mask or respirator if available, should be used when coming within 6 feet of the patient.

G. Table 6.10 provides examples of airborne and droplet transmissible diseases.

Table 6.10

Aerosol Transmissible Diseases

Examples of Airborne Transmissible Diseases	Examples of Droplet Transmissible Diseases
Disseminated Herpes zoster (varicella-zoster) (shingles) or localized disease in immunocompromised patient until disseminated infection has been ruled out	Seasonal Influenza
Measles (rubeola)	Mumps (infectious parotitis)
Tuberculosis (*M. tuberculosis*) - Pulmonary or laryngeal disease; confirmed or suspected	Pertussis (whooping cough); single-patient room preferred.
Varicella Zoster (Chicken Pox)	Rhinovirus

Source: Siegel et al., 2007

SECTION M
Tuberculosis

I. Epidemiology.

A. Tuberculosis (TB) occurs in every part of the world.
   1. As reported by the World Health Organization, "TB is second only to HIV/AIDS as the greatest killer worldwide due to a single infectious agent" (WHO, 2014d).
   2. In 2012, 8.6 million people throughout the world were diagnosed with TB, and 1.3 million died from TB.

B. In the United States overall, TB cases have been steadily declining, but cases continue to be reported in almost every state throughout the country.

C. Per the CDC, 2013 was the 21st year of decline in the number of TB cases reported in the United States since the peak of a TB resurgence in 1992 (see Figure 6.6).

D. The national average for 2013 was 3.0 TB cases per 100,000 population. Forty-one states reported a rate less than the national average, and nine states and DC reported a rate above the national average. These nine states accounted for 62% of the national total in 2013 (see Figure 6.7.)

II. Etiology.

A. Tuberculosis is caused by the tubercle bacillus *Mycobacterium tuberculosis* (see Figure 6.8).
   1. TB is spread primarily through respiratory means and is not transmitted by surface contact.
   2. While this disease can involve any organ, the lungs remain the primary site of infection.

B. When respiratory droplets are released into the air, the smallest of the droplets (droplet nuclei) become airborne and may contain one to several mycobacteria.
   1. The droplet nuclei particles are about 1 to 5 microns in diameter and small enough to remain suspended in the air for up to several hours depending on the environment.
   2. When inhaled, the smaller droplet nuclei may reach the alveoli where infection can begin in the susceptible host (CDC, 2013c).

C. Infectiousness usually coincides with the number of infectious organisms in sputum, the extent of pulmonary disease, and the frequency of coughing.
   1. Patients with pulmonary TB disease generally expel a greater amount of tubercle bacilli if their cough produces a large amount of sputum.
   2. Children generally do not produce a significant amount of sputum when coughing and are less likely than adults to be infectious.

D. When *M. tuberculosis* is presented to a host with a functioning immune system, repeated prolonged exposure is usually necessary for infection to occur. When the immune system is defective, infection can progress to active disease after short exposure times to small numbers of organisms.

E. Approximately 30% to 40% of close contacts of an individual with infectious TB disease will become infected (CDC, 2013c).

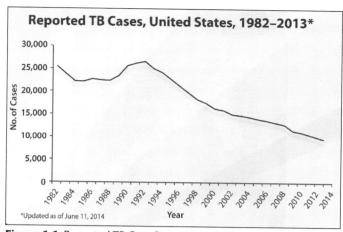

Figure 6.6. Reported TB Case Rates, United States, 1982–2013.

Source: Centers for Disease Control (CDC). (2013h). Trends in tuberculosis, 2012. http://www.cdc.gov/tb/publications/factsheets/statistics/Trends2013.pdf

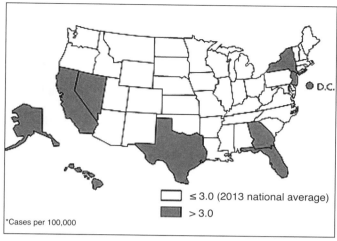

Figure 6.7. TB Case Rates, United States, 2013.

Source: Centers for Disease Control (CDC). (2013h). Trends in tuberculosis, 2012. http://www.cdc.gov/tb/publications/factsheets/statistics/Trends2013.pdf

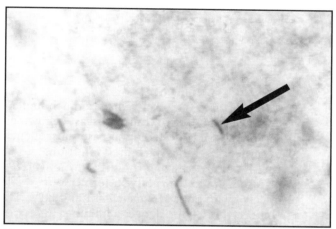

Figure 6.8. Acid fast bacteria seen on smear are tubercle bacilli.

Source: Centers for Disease Control and Prevention: Division of Tuberculosis Elimination. (2004). *Core curriculum on tuberculosis* (4th ed). Slide sets. Available from http://www.cdc.gov/ tb/pubs/slidesets/core/ html/trans5_slides.htm. Used with permission.

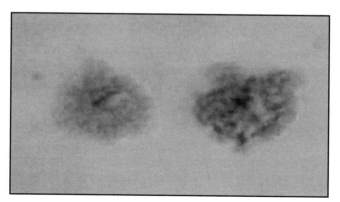

Figure 6.9. Colonies of *M. tuberculosis* growing on media.

Source: Centers for Disease Control and Prevention: Division of Tuberculosis Elimination. (2004). *Core curriculum on tuberculosis* (4th ed). Available from http://www.cdc.gov/tb/pubs/ slidesets/core/ html/trans5_slides.htm. Used with permission.

III. Pathophysiology.

A. While *M. tuberculosis* is similar in many ways to other bacteria, there are characteristics that are important to remember when caring for patients with TB.

1. *M. tuberculosis* is an acid-fast bacilli (AFB) with a mean doubling time of 12 to 24 hours. It may require weeks of growth to produce a visible colony on culture (see Figure 6.9).

a. This can delay identification of the organism.

b. In some cases (e.g., drug resistant strains), drug-susceptibility testing and drug therapy can be delayed.

2. The cell wall structure of *M. tuberculosis* contains an outer layer of fatty acids and waxes that are toxic to host cells and tissue.

a. This cell layer contributes to its slow growth rate and also protects the organism from antimicrobial agents contributing to its virulence.

b. The layer also prevents the body's macrophages from being able to completely destroy all the invading bacilli, contributing to the need for prolonged drug therapy.

B. Once an individual inhales the tubercle bacilli into the alveoli, how the body reacts to the bacilli depends in part on host susceptibility, the number of inhaled particles, and the virulence of the organisms.

1. The lung responds to the bacilli with inflammation.

2. Inflammation may lead to development of primary tubercle nodules.
3. Cells gather around the tubercle, the outer portion becomes fibrosed and the center becomes necrotic.
4. If the material is coughed up, it may leave a hollow space or cavity in the lung tissue.
   a. These cavities often occur in patients with severe pulmonary TB disease and may contain many tubercle bacilli.
   b. Large amounts of tubercle bacilli may be expelled when coughing, increasing potential infectiousness.
   c. On x-ray, these cavities are highly suggestive of TB disease and can be visualized in Figure 6.10.

C. If the host has a competent immune system, multiplication and spread of the organisms are halted, usually within 2 to 10 weeks.
   1. Alveolar macrophages ingest most of the bacilli, although some viable bacilli remain in the macrophages in a dormant state, and reactivation of the disease at a later time is possible.
   2. These people are considered to have TB infection or latent TB infection (LTBI). Even though they have TB, they have no signs or symptoms of the disease and are not capable of transmitting TB.
   3. These persons usually have a positive reaction to a tuberculin skin test (TST) or will be positive on testing with an interferon–gamma releasing assay (IGRA).
   4. Unless treated for latent TB infection, during their lifetime these persons have a 10% risk of developing active TB. The greatest risk is within 2 years after the original infection.
   5. If the host's immune system is deficient and unable to prevent spread of the bacillus, active TB disease develops. The individual will have clinical symptoms of TB and will be capable of spreading the disease to others.

D. From latent TB infection (LTBI) to TB (See Tables 6.11 and 6.12).
   1. A number of the new cases of TB are seen in older people who were remotely infected decades earlier (LTBI). The disease later emerges when the host's immune system is weakened.
   2. Rates of TB are also increased in racial and ethnic minorities who have other risk factors for TB, such as:
      a. Birth in a country with high prevalence rates of TB.
      b. HIV infection.
      c. Low socioeconomic status.
      d. Exposure in congregate settings (e.g., prisons, shelters, drug houses).

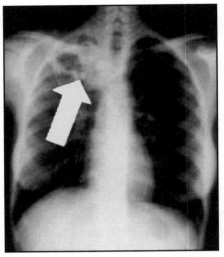

Figure 6.10. Chest x-ray of a patient with TB; arrow points to cavity in patient's right upper lobe.

Source: Centers for Disease Control and Prevention: Division of Tuberculosis Elimination. (2004). *Core curriculum on tuberculosis* (4th ed). Available from http://www.cdc.gov/tb/pubs/slidesets/core/ html/trans5_slides.htm. Used with permission.

3. Patients who are HIV positive have a much higher risk of developing active clinical disease following initial infection or developing disease subsequent to an earlier or remotely acquired infection.
   a. The risk of progressing from LTBI to active TB disease is 7% to 10% per year for persons infected with both *M. tuberculosis* and HIV.
   b. This is a very high risk over a lifetime (CDC, 2013c, 2013e).

IV. Multidrug-resistant TB (MDR-TB) and extensively drug-resistant TB (XDR-TB).

A. TB that is resistant to at least two of the first-line drugs, isoniazid and rifampin, continues to be isolated (CDC, 2013c).
   1. In the past, drug resistance was a result of inappropriate or inadequate treatment of TB, known as secondary or acquired drug resistance.
   2. Primary drug resistance occurs when only a few of the organisms present have an inherent resistance to one or more of the most commonly used antitubercular drugs.
   3. This type of MDR-TB has been transmitted by direct exposure, particularly in areas with large populations of HIV-infected patients.

B. Situations in which an exposed person is at increased risk of infection with drug-resistant TB include:
   1. Exposure to a person who has known drug-resistant tuberculosis.

Table 6.11

Latent TB Infection (LTBI) vs. TB Disease

Latent TB Infection (LTBI)	TB Disease (pulmonary)
Inactive tubercle bacilli in the body	Active tubercle bacilli in the body
Tuberculin skin test (TST) or Interferon-gamma releasing assay (QFT-G or T-Spot) results usually positive	Tuberculin skin test (TST) or Interferon-gamma releasing assay (QFT-G or T-Spot) results usually positive
Chest x-ray usually normal	Chest x-ray usually abnormal
Sputum smears and cultures negative	Sputum smears and cultures positive
No symptoms	Symptoms such as cough, fever, weight loss
Not infectious	Often infectious before treatment
Not a case of TB	A case of TB

Source: Centers for Disease Control (CDC). (2008). Self-Study Modules on tuberculosis (1-5).

2. Exposure to someone who has active tuberculosis following TB treatment.
3. Exposure took place in an area with a high prevalence of drug-resistant cases.
4. Exposure to someone who continues with sputum samples positive for AFB despite treatment.

C. To prevent emergence of drug-resistant strains of TB, appropriate drug regimens must contain several different drugs to which the organism is susceptible.
   1. The dosing schedule must maintain sufficient concentrations to inhibit or kill the organisms present.
   2. Drugs must be continued long enough to ensure all organisms are eliminated.
   3. When TB is resistant to isoniazid and rifampin, treatment can last 2 years or longer (CDC, 2013e).

D. Specific drug therapy for resistant strains of TB depend on whether the organism is resistant to one or more of the drugs commonly used to treat TB.
   1. Some organisms are resistant to only one drug, while others are resistant to multiple drugs.
   2. Extensively drug resistant TB (XDR-TB) is a rare type of MDR-TB.
      a. XDR-TB is resistant to isoniazid and rifampin and also resistant to any fluoroquinolone and at least one of the three injectable second line drugs.
      b. XDR-TB is uncommon in the United States.
         (1) Sixty-three cases of XDR-TB were reported to the CDC between 1993 and 2011.

Table 6.12

Medical Conditions that Increase the Risk of Developing TB Disease Once Infection Has Occurred

- HIV Infection
- Substance abuse (especially drug injection)
- Silicosis
- Recent infection with *M. tuberculosis* within the previous 2 years
- Persons with a history of untreated or inadequately treated TB disease, including persons with chest radiograph findings with previous TB disease
- Diabetes mellitus
- Prolonged corticosteroid therapy
- Other immunosuppressive treatments (including tumor necrosis factor-alpha antagonists)
- Organ transplants
- Hematologic disorders (for example, leukemia, Hodgkin's disease)
- Other malignancies (e.g., carcinoma of the head and neck, or lung)
- Chronic kidney disease
- Intestinal bypass or gastrectomy
- Chronic malabsorption syndromes
- Being > 10% below ideal body weight

Adapted from Centers for Disease Control and Prevention (CDC). (2005). Guidelines for preventing the transmission of *M. tuberculosis* in health-care settings. *MMWR, 54,* RR-17.

(2) Twelve XDR-TB cases reported from 2008 to 2011; 11 of the cases were among foreign-born persons (CDC, 2013f).

V. Signs and symptoms of TB.

A. Pulmonary TB should be suspected in people who complain of fever, chills, night sweats, fatigue, weight loss, decreased appetite, chest pain, prolonged and productive coughing (longer than 3 weeks), or hemoptysis.

B. Extrapulmonary TB occurs most often in people with HIV.
   1. Pulmonary TB is the most common form of TB, including those with HIV.
   2. Patients who are HIV-negative have a 10% rate of extrapulmonary TB, while those with full-blown AIDS have a 70% rate of TB at sites other than the lung.
   3. Patients with HIV and impaired immune systems have a 24% to 45% incidence of extrapulmonary TB.
   4. The presence of extrapulmonary disease does not exclude pulmonary TB disease.

C. Patients with HIV and extrapulmonary TB demonstrate lymphatitis and miliary disease (formation of tubercles) throughout the body organs from dissemination of bacillus through the bloodstream. Symptoms include tender lymph nodes, fever, fatigue, and weight loss.

D. People with extrapulmonary TB are usually not considered infectious unless they have an open abscess or draining lesion.

E. Anyone suspected of having TB disease must be placed in isolation and be referred for further evaluation consisting of a physical examination, a Mantoux tuberculin skin test, IGRA assay, chest x-ray, and sputum smears and cultures.

VI. Screening test.

A. Screening tests in the United States are used to identify infected people who need preventive therapy and as part of the workup for those with signs or symptoms of active disease.
   1. Screen groups with disease and infection rates in excess of those in the general population.
   2. Institutional screening for staff of all healthcare facilities and residents of long-term care facilities.
   3. The Centers for Disease Control and Prevention (CDC) recommend all healthcare facilities establish a TB screening program for healthcare workers. The Occupational Safety and Health Administration (OSHA) mandates that employers develop and follow TB screening and control programs for staff.
   4. To assess the risk for exposure to TB in the workplace, the risk factors associated with TB must be identified.
   5. While TB can occur in any population or group, certain subpopulations have been identified as having a higher-than-average risk for TB.
      a. Close contact with infectious tuberculosis cases.
      b. Medically underserved, low-income populations, including high risk racial and ethnic groups.
      c. Foreign-born persons from high-prevalence countries (Asia, Africa, Latin America).
      d. Older adults.

B. Tuberculin skin tests.
   1. Screening programs for TB usually consist of the Mantoux purified protein derivative tuberculin skin test (TST) or one of the interferon-gamma releasing assays. Included in the group of who should be screened are people who have medical conditions that increase their risk of clinical disease when exposed to TB.
      a. Close contacts of infectious TB cases.
      b. Persons with medical conditions that increase the risk of TB.
      c. Foreign-born persons from high-prevalence countries.
      d. Low-income populations, including high risk minorities.
      e. Alcoholics and intravenous drug users.
      f. Residents of long-term care facilities (including prisons).
      g. Populations identified locally as being at increased risk for TB such as healthcare workers in some settings.
   2. The depressed cell-mediated immunity that occurs with CKD makes *M. tuberculosis* infection more difficult to diagnose. CKD is also associated with an increased risk of progression of latent TB infection (LTBI) to active TB disease (CDC, 2000). Per the *Guidelines for Tuberculosis Screening and Treatment of Patients with Chronic Kidney Disease* published by the California Tuberculosis Controllers Association (CTCA), the risk of active TB in hemodialysis patients is 7 to 52 times higher than in the general population (CTCA, 2007).
   3. CKD may cause cutaneous anergy (inability to react to a skin test antigen) that can result in a false-negative TB test.
      a. Causes of anergy include medical conditions causing immunosupression such as HIV infection, poor nutrition, some medications, live virus vaccinations, and TB disease.

b. A negative test does not exclude a diagnosis of TB disease or infection with *M. tuberculosis*.

c. Anergy skin testing in conjunction with TST is no longer recommended for routine use.

4. The Mantoux skin test (TST) is the recommended skin test method. Using a tuberculin syringe with 0.1 mL (5 units) of purified protein derivative (PPD), inject intradermally forming a wheal just under the skin. Trained staff read the test in 48 to 72 hours, and only the area of induration is measured. Documentation of skin test results must include the exact measurement in millimeters of induration, even if considered nonreactive (see Table 6.13).

a. False-positive results to TST can be due to measuring the area of redness that extends beyond the area of induration, infections with mycobacterium other than *M. tuberculosis* or due to immunization with bacillus Calmette-Guérin (BCG).

(1) BCG is used in multiple countries where TB disease is endemic.

(2) A positive TST reaction as a result of BCG wanes after 5 to 10 years.

(3) Therefore, persons who had BCG vaccine will frequently have a negative TST.

(4) Because persons with a history of BCG are frequently from countries with a high prevalence of TB infection, the CDC recommends TB skin testing.

(5) If the TST is positive, the results are interpreted as indicating infection.

b. False-negative results can occur in people recently infected with TB. It may take 2 to 10 weeks after infection to mount an immune response.

c. Two-step testing is used in settings where periodic testing will occur, such as healthcare workers, nursing homes, and dialysis units.

(1) The first time the person is tested they are given an initial skin test.

(2) If the first test is considered negative, a second TST is given 1 to 3 weeks later.

(3) If the first and second tests are negative, then any subsequent positive skin test is more likely to be due to a recent TB infection (TB conversion).

C. Interferon-gamma releasing blood assays or IGRAs.

1. QuantiFERON-TB Gold test (QFT-G) and the T-Spot are FDA approved interferon-gamma releasing (IGRA) blood assays and are acceptable alternatives to tuberculin skin tests (TST).

a. These blood assays are more specific for TB infection than is the TST and can be used in all circumstances in which TST is currently used.

b. They are used to help diagnose *M. tuberculosis* infection by measuring the patient's immune reactivity to *M. tuberculosis* antigens.

c. A positive IGRA indicates the person has been infected with the TB bacteria.

d. Additional tests are required to determine if the person has latent TB infection or TB disease.

e. There is no reason to follow a positive IGRA with a TB skin test.

f. A negative IGRA indicates the person's blood did not react to the test and latent TB infection or TB disease is not likely.

2. IGRAs detect a cell-mediated immune response to *M. tuberculosis* to two proteins that are not present in BCG vaccines and are absent from the majority of non-tuberculosis mycobacterium.

a. IGRAs are capable of distinguishing between the sensitization caused by *M. tuberculosis* infection and that caused by BCG vaccination.

b. Previous vaccination with BCG will not cause a false positive result.

c. IGRAs are less affected by the presence of atypical mycobacteria that may cause a false positive skin test.

d. IGRAs should be preferred over the skin test for testing individuals who have received BCG, either as a vaccine or for cancer therapy.

3. Blood samples require prompt processing, usually within 8 to 30 hours after collection.

a. Incorrect collection technique or delays in transporting the blood sample may decrease the accuracy of the results.

b. Caution is advised when interpreting negative IGRA results in persons who have HIV/AIDS, are receiving immunosuppressive drugs, including those used for managing organ transplants, have diabetes mellitus, silicosis, CKD, and certain hematologic disorders.

4. Using an IGRA has several advantages.

a. In addition to being more specific for *M. tuberculosis* than the TST, use of the IGRA only requires one patient visit to conduct the test.

b. In many cases the results can be available in 24 hours.

c. It eliminates the need for an initial two-step TST in settings where periodic skin testing is planned.

d. It is less likely to have incorrect reading and interpretation of the results compared to the TST (CDC, 2010; Lardizabal, 2011).

VII.   Symptom screen.

A. A symptom screen or individual TB risk appraisal is a screening process using a standardized tool to help detect patients who might be candidates for medical follow-up to rule out either active TB disease or latent TB infection (LTBI).

Table 6.13

Classification of TB Skin Test Results

An induration of 5 mm or more is considered a positive reaction in the following high risk groups. Persons should be treated for LTB1 regardless of age:	An induration of 10 mm or more is considered positive in the following persons:	An induration of 15 mm is considered positive for persons who do not have any risk factors for TB.
Persons infected with HIV.	Persons with TST or BAMT conversions.	Persons with no known factors for TB disease. HCW who are otherwise at low risk for TB disease and who received baseline testing at the beginning of employment as part of a TB screening program.
Recent contacts of a person with TB disease.	Persons born or who have lived in developing countries with high incidence of TB disease.	
Persons with fibrotic changes on chest x-ray consistent with previous TB disease.	Persons who inject illicit drugs.	
Organ transplant recipients.	Residents and employees in congregate facilities and LTCFs (e.g., hospices, skilled nursing facilities), hospital and other healthcare facilities. Personnel from microbiology labs. Persons with any of the following clinical conditions that place them at high risk: • Silicosis • Diabetes mellitus • Chronic kidney failure • Certain hematologic disorders (e.g., leukemias and lymphomas) • Other specific malignancies (e.g., carcinoma of the head, neck and lung) • Unexplained weight loss of ≥ 10% of ideal body weight • Gastrectomy or jejunoileal bypass Persons living in areas with high incidence of TB disease. Children ≥ 4 years of age. Infants, children, and adolescents exposed to adults with high risk for developing TB.	

Adapted from Centers for Disease Control and Prevention (CDC). (2005). Guidelines for preventing the transmission of *M. tuberculosis* in health-care settings. *MMWR, 54,* RR-17.

Table 6.14

Infectiousness of People Known to Have or Suspected of Having TB Disease

Factors Associated with Infectiousness	Factors Associated with Noninfectiousness
Presence of cough	No cough
Cavity in the lung	No cavity in the lung
TB disease of lungs, airway, or larynx	Extrapulmonary (non-respiratory) TB
Patient not covering mouth or nose when coughing	Patient covering mouth or nose when coughing
Not receiving adequate treatment	Receiving adequate TB treatment for 2 weeks or longer
Undergoing cough-inducing procedures	Not undergoing cough-inducing procedures
Positive sputum cultures	Negative sputum cultures

Source: CDC (2008) Self-Study Modules on tuberculosis (1-5).

B. Per the CDC, it is a procedure in which patients are asked if they have experienced any departure from their normal function, appearance, or sensation related to TB disease.

C. Although people with TB disease may or may not have symptoms, most patients with TB disease will have one or more symptoms.

D. In most published series, fever, weight loss, and malaise are the most common symptoms of active TB disease in patients with kidney insufficiency.

E. The CDC recommends administering a symptom screen as a vital adjunct to the TB skin test or IGRA.

VIII. Infectiousness and precautions.

A. Infectiousness of a TB patient with untreated active pulmonary or laryngeal TB is directly related to the number of bacilli released into the air whenever that person coughs, talks, sings, or sneezes.
   1. Most patients with active TB disease are considered infectious if:
      a. They are coughing.
      b. They are receiving cough-inducing or aerosol-generating procedures.
      c. They have sputum smears that show presence of acid-fast bacilli (AFB) and are not receiving therapy.
      d. They have just started therapy.
      e. They have poor clinical or bacteriologic response to therapy.
   2. It is important to realize a negative sputum smear for AFB does not rule out the possibility of TB.

   a. AFB could be present in the smear but may not have been visualized by the laboratory personnel examining the slide under the microscope.
   b. All specimens should be sent for culture, regardless if the smear was negative or positive for AFB.
   c. Many patients with TB disease have negative AFB smears with a subsequent positive culture.
   3. When acid-fast bacilli are seen in a smear, they are counted; the greater the number of AFB, the more infectious the patient (CDC, 2008).

B. Airborne precautions prevent transmission of pulmonary TB disease and include preferred placement of the patient in an airborne-infection isolation room (AIIR) in the hospital until the patient is no longer considered potentially infectious (Siegel et al., 2007).
   1. It is expected that patients with active TB disease or suspected of having active TB disease will be dialyzed in the hospital setting where appropriate isolation is available.
   2. An airborne-infection isolation room is beyond the capacity of an outpatient dialysis facility and not required in the outpatient setting.

C. Infectiousness may persist for weeks or even months in patients with drug-resistant TB (see Table 6.14). Once effective therapy is begun, patients are no longer considered infectious as long as they meet all the following criteria.
   1. They have been receiving adequate drug therapy for 2 to 3 weeks.

2. They demonstrate favorable clinical response to therapy.
3. Demonstrate three consecutive negative sputum smears for acid fast bacilli (AFB) that have been collected at least 8 to 24 hours apart.

IX. Drug therapy.

A. Antituberculosis chemotherapy is designed to kill bacilli rapidly, minimize the potential for organisms to develop drug resistance and sterilize the host's tissues. Poor follow-through with the drug regimen is one of the primary reasons for the increases in drug-resistant strains.

B. Treatment of latent TB infection (LTBI) is prescribed to prevent progression to active clinical TB disease at a later date.
1. The preferred drug regime to treat LTBI is isoniazid (INH) daily for 9 months.
2. Alternative drug regimens are available.
3. Completion of treatment for LTBI may reduce the likelihood of TB reactivation up to 90%.
   a. It is recommended persons receiving treatment for LTBI receive baseline evaluation for liver disease and be assessed monthly for medication side effects and adherence to prescribed drug therapy.
   b. Side effect of INH may include drug-induced hepatitis and neurotoxicity (such as peripheral neuropathy or paresthesias of the hands and feet). Peripheral neuropathy occurs in less than 0.2% of people taking INH.
   c. Vitamin B6 or pyridoxine may be prescribed to minimize this possible side effect that is more often associated with conditions such as chronic kidney disease, diabetes, HIV, and alcoholism.
   d. Less than 1% of people taking INH develop hepatitis but as many as 10 to 20% will have temporary mild abnormal liver function tests (CDC, 2008).

C. Treatment of TB disease includes use of multiple drugs that the organisms are sensitive to, provision of the safest most effective therapy in the shortest time possible, and ensuring the patient adheres fully to the treatment regimen.
1. TB disease must be treated for a minimum of 6 months.
   a. There are several FDA-approved drugs available that can be used.
   b. First-line drugs include isoniazid (INH), rifampin (RIF), ethambutol (EMB), and pyrazinamide (PZA).
2. Treatment regimens for TB disease typically include an initial phase of four first-line drugs for the first 8 weeks followed by a continuation phase with at least two drugs.
3. Therapy modification may be indicated depending on special circumstances (i.e., drug resistance).
4. Both first-line and second-line drugs have potential adverse reactions, but toxicities are greater when using second-line drugs. Because of this, second-line drugs are only used for patients with drug resistance or drug intolerance.

D. Extra pulmonary TB, which occurs in places other than the lungs (e.g., pleura, lymph nodes, kidneys), is treated following the basic principles for treating pulmonary TB. A 6- to 9-month course of therapy is prescribed, except for TB meningitis that requires 9 to 12 months of therapy.

E. Drug-resistant TB diagnosis requires drug-susceptibility testing and prolonged treatment regimens.

X. Directly observed therapy (DOT).

A. Treatment of TB is lengthy and adherence to the prescribed TB treatment must be ensured. Direct observed therapy (DOT) has been shown to improve adherence and completion of therapy.
1. DOT is a public health strategy which helps patients take their medication as prescribed and helps patients complete the full course of treatment, achieving cure, and preventing the development of drug resistance.
2. The CDC defines DOT as an adherence-enhancing strategy in which a trained health-care professional or other trained person observes a patient swallow each dose of medication and records the dates that the medication was taken.
3. DOT facilitates timely recognition of treatment nonadherence, adverse drug reactions, and issues with medication tolerance. DOT should be done at a time and place convenient for the patient (CDC, 2008).

B. DOT should be considered for patients who may be a transmission risk or may have a challenge with treatment adherence. These persons include those with the following.
1. Pulmonary disease with positive sputum smears.
2. Previous treatment failure.
3. Drug resistant TB.
4. HIV infection.
5. Previous TB treatment.
6. Substance abuse.
7. Psychiatric illnesses.
8. Memory impairment.
9. Children and adolescents (parents should not be relied on to supervise DOT).

XI. Chronic kidney disease (CKD). Implications for TB.

A. Kidney disease complicates the management of TB. Antituberculosis medications may be cleared by the kidney and also by hemodialysis.

B. Drugs cleared by the kidneys in patients with creatinine clearance less than 30 mL/min and those receiving hemodialysis treatments are managed by changing dosing intervals (see Table 6.15).

C. Patients with CKD have additional clinical concerns, such as gastroparesis that may affect absorption of TB drugs and medications that interact with these drugs.

D. There is no data for peritoneal dialysis (PD) patients. Drug removal mechanisms differ between hemodialysis and PD, so it cannot be assumed that hemodialysis medication dosing precautions apply to PD.

E. Persons with LTBI and CKD in general should be treated, regardless of age, especially those with new TB conversion.

SECTION N
Immunizations

I. Overview of immunizations for CKD patients.

A. Background information.
1. Data show that immunization rates for chronic dialysis patients for seasonal influenza, pneumococcal disease, and hepatitis B fail to reach published goals.
2. Seasonal influenza immunization.
   a. The Department of Health and Human Services' Healthy People 2020 initiative has a 90% target for annual influenza vaccination of non-institutionalized, high risk adults ages 18 to 64 years.
   b. Per the United States Renal Data System (USRDS) 2012 Annual Data Report, only 65.4% of patients with CKD stage 5 received influenza vaccination, but that is increased from 58% in 2005.
3. Pneumococcal vaccination.
   a. Healthy People 2020 has set a target of 60% for pneumococcal vaccination of noninstitutionalized, high risk adults ages 18 to 64 years by 2020.

Table 6.15

TB Drug Frequency Changes for Adult Patients with Reduced Renal Function and Adult Patients Receiving Hemodialysis

Drug	Change in Frequency?
Rifampin	No change
Pyrazinamide	Yes
Ethambutol	Yes
Levofloxacin	Yes
Cycloserine	Yes
Ethionamide	No change
p-Aminosalicylic acid	No change
Streptomycin	Yes
Capreomycin	Yes
Kanamycin	Yes
Amikacin	Yes

Adapted from Centers for Disease Control and Prevention (CDC). (2005). Guidelines for preventing the transmission of *M. tuberculosis* in health-care settings. *MMWR, 54,* RR-17.

---

   b. The USRDS 2012 data reflects that only 25.6% of patients with CKD stage 5 received pneumococcal vaccine in the years 2009 to 2010.
4. Hepatitis B vaccination.
   a. The Centers for Medicare & Medicaid Services (CMS) Conditions for Coverage require that all susceptible patients be offered hepatitis B vaccine.
   b. The Healthy People 2020 target for hepatitis B vaccination of patients on long-term hemodialysis is 90%.
   c. However, according to the USRDS 2012 data, only 7.4% of all patients with CKD stage 5 received all three hepatitis B vaccinations in a year.
5. All of these vaccines are recommended by the Centers for Disease Control and Prevention (CDC) for patients on dialysis and persons with chronic kidney disease because of a higher risk of infection and/or disease severity due to altered immunocompetence.
6. Table 6.16 contains the current Healthy People 2020 goal recommendations for these vaccinations. Also, refer to Table 6.17 and Table 6.18 for additional information.

B. Hepatitis B.
1. In 2009, CDC estimated that:

Table 6.16

Healthy People 2020 Goals and Current Status of Immunizations

Hepatitis B Vaccine				
Objective	Increase in hepatitis B vaccine coverage in high-risk groups	2020 Target (unless noted)	1995 Baseline	Opportunity to Improve
IID-15.1	Long-term hemodialysis patients	90% (2010)	35%	55%
IID-15.3	Healthcare personnel	90%	64% (2008)	26%
Influenza and Pneumococcal Disease				
Objective	Increase in adults vaccinated NOTE: Healthy People 2020 did not set separate ESRD Goals	2020 Target	Baseline %, Year	Opportunity to Improve
IID-12.9	Healthcare personnel – Influenza	90%	45% (2008)	45%
Noninstitutionalized adults aged 65 years and older				
IID-12.7	Influenza Vaccine	90%	67% (2008)	23%
IID-13.1	Pneumococcal vaccine	90%	60% (2008)	30%
Noninstitutionalized high-risk adults aged 18–64 years				
IID-12.6	Influenza Vaccine	90%	39% (2008)	51%
IID-13.2	Pneumococcal Vaccine	60%	17% (2008)	43%
Institutionalized adults aged 18 and older (persons in long-term or nursing homes)				
IID-12.8IID-12.8	Influenza Vaccine	90%	62% (2005–2006)	28%
IID-13.3	Pneumococcal Vaccine	90%	66% (2005–2006)	24%

Data compiled from Healthy People 2020. http://www.healthypeople.gov/2020/topicsobjectives2020/objectiveslist.aspx?topicId=23#578823

Table 6.17

Vaccinations in Dialysis Patients

Vaccination in Dialysis Patients	Percent of patients who received vaccination
Influenza	69% (2009)
Pneumococcal	30% (2008-2009)
Hepatitis B	28% (2009)

Source: USRDS Annual Report, 2011

a. 38,000 persons were newly infected with hepatitis B in the United States.
b. Chronic hepatitis B infection leads to an estimated 2,000 to 4,000 deaths each year.
c. Between 800,000 and 1.4 million people in the United States have chronic hepatitis B infection.
2. It is recommended that patients with chronic kidney disease receive hepatitis B vaccination before they begin dialysis therapy, as they have been shown to have higher seroprotection rates and antibody titers.
a. All susceptible patients on chronic

Table 6.18

List of Vaccines and Their Use for Dialysis or CKD Patients

Vaccine	Recommended for Patients on Dialysis or Patients with CKD	Recommended for All Adults	May Use if Otherwise Indicated*	Contraindicated
Anthrax			X	
DTaP/Tdap/Td		X	X	
Hib			X	
Hepatitis A			X	
Hepatitis B	X			
Human papillomavirus			X	
Influenza (TIV)		X		
Influenza (LAIV)				X
Japanese Encephalitis			X	
MMR		X	X	
Meningococcal			X	
Pneumococcal	X			
Polio (IPV)			X	
Rabies			X	
Rotavirus			X	
Smallpox			X	
Typhoid			X	
Varicella		X	X	
Yellow Fever			X	

*No specific ACIP recommendation for this vaccine exists for patients on dialysis or patients with chronic kidney disease.

Source: Centers for Disease Control and Prevention (2006a). Guidelines for vaccinating kidney dialysis patients and patients with chronic kidney disease. (Available from http://www.cdc.gov/vaccines/pubs/downloads/dialysis-guide-2012.pdf)

hemodialysis should receive hepatitis B vaccination.

b. Patients on peritoneal or home hemodialysis should also receive hepatitis B vaccination because it is possible that they will require in-center hemodialysis at some point.

3. Hepatitis B vaccine is given in a three or four dose series, depending on the brand of vaccine being administered. Table 6.19 shows the dose schedules for both hepatitis B vaccine brands.

4. Testing should be performed 1 to 2 months after the final dose of the vaccine series is administered to determine the response to the vaccine.

a. Patients found to have anti-HBs levels of < 10 mIU/mL after receiving the first vaccine series should be revaccinated with a second hepatitis B vaccine series and retested 1 to 2 months after receipt of the final dose of the second vaccine series.

b. Those who do not demonstrate protective levels of anti-HBs after the second full vaccine series should be considered vaccine nonresponders and tested monthly for HBsAg. These patients require counseling regarding precautions to take to prevent hepatitis B infection.

c. Patients who respond to the vaccine with a

Table 6.19

Dose Schedules for Hepatitis B Vaccine for Patients

Group	Recombivax HB			Engerix B		
	Dose	Volume	Schedule	Dose	Volume	Schedule
≥ 20 years of age: predialysis	10 μg	1.0 mL	3 doses at 0, 1, 6 months	20 μg	1.0 mL	3 doses at 0, 1, 6 months
≥ 20 years of age: dialysis dependent	40 μg	1.0 mL	3 doses at 0, 1, 6 months	40 μg	Two 1.0 mL doses at one site	4 doses at 0, 1, 2, 6 months
< 20 years of age	5 μg	0.5 mL	3 doses at 0, 1, 6 months	10 μg	0.5 mL	3 doses at 0, 1, 6 months

Modified from Centers for Disease Control and Prevention (CDC). (2001a).

protective level of anti-HBs are considered immune. They should have annual anti-HBs testing. A booster dose of vaccine should be administered whenever the anti-HBs result is < 10 mIU/mL.

C. Influenza.
1. It is estimated that influenza causes more than 200,000 hospitalizations and 3,000 to 49,000 deaths annually in the United States. Most severe illnesses and deaths that are influenza-related occur in persons with chronic medical conditions, infants, young children, seniors, and pregnant women.
2. Routine annual influenza vaccination is recommended for all persons aged 6 months and older.
3. Vaccination is emphasized for persons who are at increased risk of severe complications due to influenza; this includes persons who have chronic kidney disease stage 5.
4. Influenza complications include pneumonia, bronchitis, sinus infections, and ear infections, and the person may experience worsening of chronic health problems.
5. Inactivated influenza vaccine is generally recommended for persons with chronic kidney disease.
6. Live attenuated influenza vaccine is contraindicated in persons with kidney dysfunction.
7. Persons with egg allergy who have experienced only hives after exposure to egg should receive the influenza vaccine. A recombinant hemagglutinin vaccine is now available for use in persons aged 18 through 49 years and can be administered to persons with egg allergy if they have no other contraindications to the vaccine.
8. Development of antibodies that provide protection against influenza takes about 2 weeks after vaccine administration.
9. CDC recommends influenza vaccinations each year as soon as influenza vaccine is available in the community. Influenza seasons can be unpredictable and can begin as early as October.

D. Pneumococcal.
1. Pneumococcal disease can cause serious illness and may lead to pneumonia, meningitis, bacteremia, and death.
a. In the United States, more than 50,000 cases of pneumococcal bacteremia occur each year, and approximately 3,000 to 6,000 cases of pneumococcal meningitis are diagnosed annually.
b. Vaccination is recommended for immunocompromised adults who are at risk of pneumococcal disease or its complications, including persons with chronic kidney failure.
2. Two types of vaccine are available for adults.
a. The 23-valent pneumococcal polysaccharide vaccine (PPSV23) is indicated for all adults.
b. The 13-valent pneumococcal conjugate vaccine (PCV13) is indicated for those age 50 years and older.
c. CDC recommends both vaccines for adults age 19 and older with immunocompromising conditions, including chronic kidney disease.
3. See Tables 6.20 and 6.21 for guidelines pertaining to these pneumococcal vaccines.

II. Immunization of healthcare workers.

A. Overview.
1. Because of their contact with patients or infective material from patients, healthcare workers are at risk for exposure to and potential transmission of infectious diseases.

Table 6.20

Guidelines for Administering PCV13 and PPSV23 Vaccines to Adults Aged 19 to 64 with Chronic Kidney Disease
Pneumococcal Vaccine Administration for Patients with Chronic Kidney Disease

Adults (ages 19 to 64)			
Vaccination History	**Recommended Regimen**		**Notes**
Never vaccinated with PCV13 or PPSV 23	Administer 1 dose of PCV13 now	Administer 1 dose of PPSV 23 ≥ 8 weeks later	Administer 1 dose of PPSV23 ≥ 5 years later	ACIP recommends that adults aged ≥ 19 years with immunocompromising conditions, functional or anatomic asplenia, CSF leaks, or cochlear implants, and who have not previously received PCV13 or PPSV23, should receive a dose of PCV13 first, followed by a dose of PPSV23 at least 8 weeks later. Subsequent doses of PPSV23 should follow current PPSV23 recommendations for adults at high risk. Specifically, a second PPSV23 dose is recommended 5 years after the first PPSV23 dose for persons aged 19–64 years with functional or anatomic asplenia and for persons with immunocompromising conditions. Additionally, those who received PPSV23 before age 65 years for any indication should receive another dose of the vaccine at age 65 years, or later if at least 5 years have elapsed since their previous PPSV23 dose.
Previously vaccinated with 1 dose PPSV23 ≥ 1 year ago; never vaccinated with PCV13	Administer 1 dose of PCV13 now	Administer 1 dose of PPSV23 ≥ 8 weeks after PCV13, which must be ≥ 5 years after first dose of PPSV23		
Previously vaccinated with 2 doses of PPSV23 (last dose was ≥ 1 year ago); never vaccinated with PCV13	Administer 1 dose of PCV13 now			
Previously vaccinated with ≥ 1 dose PCV13 (≥ 8 weeks ago); never vaccinated with PPSV23	Administer 1 dose of PCV13 now	Administer 1 dose of PPSV23 ≥ 5 years later		
Previously vaccinated with ≥ 1 dose of PCV13 (≥ 8 weeks ago) and 1 dose of PPSV23	Administer 1 dose of PPSV23 ≥ 5 years after first PPSV23 dose			

Source: Centers for Disease Control and Prevention (2006a). Guidelines for vaccinating kidney dialysis patients and patients with chronic kidney disease. (Available from http://www.cdc.gov/vaccines/pubs/downloads/dialysis-guide-2012.pdf)

2. Many of these diseases are vaccine preventable, and healthcare workers have the responsibility to take all reasonable precautions to prevent the spread of diseases, including participation in recommended immunizations.
3. The CDC Advisory Committee on Immunization Practices (ACIP) (2011a) has provided recommendations for specific vaccines for all healthcare workers.

B. Hepatitis B vaccination.
  1. The risk of acquiring hepatitis B virus (HBV) infection in the healthcare setting depends on the frequency of percutaneous and mucosal exposure to blood or body fluids containing HBV.
  2. The Occupational Health and Safety Administration (OSHA) require that hepatitis B vaccine be offered to susceptible healthcare workers with occupational exposure to blood and body fluids.

C. Influenza vaccination.
  1. Healthcare workers are exposed to persons with influenza in the workplace and are at risk of acquiring the disease and transmitting it to others.

Table 6.21

Guidelines for Administering PCV13 and PPSV23 Vaccines for Adults (ages 65 and over) with Chronic Kidney Disease

Adults (ages 19 to 64)		
Vaccination History	**Recommended Regimen**		**Notes**
Never vaccinated with PCV13	Administer 1 dose of PCV13 now	Administer 1 dose of PPSV23 ≥ 8 weeks after PCV13, which must be ≥ 5 years after last dose of PPSV23	All persons should be vaccinated with PPSV23 at age 65 years. Those who received PPSV23 before age 65 years for any indication should receive another dose of the vaccine at age 65 years or later if at least 5 years have passed since their previous dose. Those who receive PPSV23 at or after age 65 years should receive only a single dose.
Previously vaccinated with ≥ 1 dose PCV13 (≥8 weeks ago)	Administer 1 dose of PCV23 now		

Source: Centers for Disease Control and Prevention (2006a). Guidelines for vaccinating kidney dialysis patients and patients with chronic kidney disease. (Available from http://www.cdc.gov/vaccines/pubs/downloads/dialysis-guide-2012.pdf)

2. It is recommended for healthcare workers to receive the seasonal influenza vaccine each year.
3. Many organizations within the healthcare community (e.g., Infectious Diseases Society of America, National Foundation for Infectious Diseases, Society for Healthcare Epidemiology of America) have issued position papers supporting mandatory influenza vaccinations for healthcare workers.

D. Measles, mumps, and rubella (MMR).
   1. Due to declining vaccination rates and importation of virus from other countries where measles remain endemic, outbreaks in the United States have increased in the last few years.
   2. Healthcare workers should have documentation of adequate vaccination against measles, rubella and mumps or other acceptable evidence of immunity to these diseases (i.e., laboratory evidence of immunity or laboratory evidence of disease).

E. Varicella (chickenpox).
   1. Healthcare workers should have adequate documentation indicating immunity.
   2. This can include documentation of vaccination with two doses of varicella vaccine, laboratory evidence of immunity or laboratory confirmation of disease, diagnosis or verification of a history of varicella disease by a healthcare provider, or diagnosis or verification of a history of herpes zoster by a healthcare provider.

F. Tetanus, diphtheria, pertussis.
   1. Healthcare workers are not at greater risk for diphtheria or tetanus than the general population.
   2. However, healthcare workers should be able to provide evidence of immunization with a one-time dose of Tdap (tetanus toxoid, reduced diphtheria toxoid, and acellular pertussis vaccine), regardless of their most recent tetanus diphtheria (Td) vaccination status.
   3. Tdap vaccination can protect healthcare personnel against pertussis and help prevent transmission to patients (CDC, 2011b).

III. Measures to increase immunization rates.

A. Strategies for increasing immunization rates have been published.
   1. Strategies include standing orders, computerized record reminders, chart reminders, mailed or telephoned reminders, nurse-initiated reminders, as well as general and targeted education campaigns.
   2. Strategies have advantages and disadvantages and may be more appropriate to use based on the setting.

B. Resources. Many resources are available. Examples include:
   1. CDC's National Center for Immunization and Respiratory Diseases (NCIRD) (2014) website provides access to vaccination recommendations of ACIP, vaccination schedules, automated child

schedulers, an adult immunization scheduler, vaccine safety information, publications, provider education and training, and links to other vaccination-related websites (http://www.cdc.gov/ncird).

2. Immunization Action Coalition (IAC) (2014) provides a variety of free provider and patient information, including translations of vaccine information statements into multiple languages via their website http://www.immunize.org/

3. The National Network for Immunization Information (2014) is an affiliation of the Infectious Diseases Society of America, the Pediatric Infectious Diseases Society, the American Academy of Pediatrics, the American Nurses Association, the American Academy of Family Physicians, and others. This source provides current, scientifically valid information to the public, health professionals, policy makers, and the media via their website http://www.immunizationinfo.org/

SECTION O

Infections Related to Water, Reuse, and/or Machine Contamination

Most infections related to water, reuse, and/or machine contamination are caused by organisms either in the water distribution system, dialysate, or the dialysate effluent. These organisms primarily consist of gram-negative bacteria frequently found in dialysis fluids and fungi. With the current state of the art and technology, virus (HBV, HCV, and HIV) transmission either through errors in reuse or contamination of machines is a rare event in the United States (see Table 6.22).

I. Transmission of bloodborne pathogens.

A. Reuse.
   1. No documented transmission of HBV, HCV, or HIV among facilities that reprocess hemodialyzers in the United States.
   2. Transmission of HIV has occurred in Latin America due to reuse of access needles and reuse of hemodialyzers. In both cases these devices were inadequately disinfected between uses and shared among different patients.
   3. Strategies for preventing the transmission of bloodborne pathogens in a reuse program include:
      a. Exclusion of HBsAg+ patients from participating in a reuse program.
      b. Follow the Association for the Advancement of Medical Instrumentation (AAMI) recommended

Table 6.22

Organisms Typically Associated with Infections Related to Water, Dialysate, Reuse, and/or Machine Contamination

Bacterial Pathogens
Members of the Pseudomonaceae
Pseudomonas aeruginosa, Pseudomonas putida/fluorescens
Delftia acidovorans (previously *Pseudomonas acidovorans* and *Commamonas acidovorans*)
Brevundimonas diminuta, Brevundimonas vesicularis
Burkolderia cepacia complex
Ralstonia pickettii, Ralstonia mannitolytica, Ralstonia paucula, Ralstonia gilardii
Stenotrophomonas maltophilia
Members of the Enterobacteriaceae
Enterobacter cloacae
Klebsiella pneumoniae
Serratia marcescens, Serratia liquefaciens
Nontuberculous Mycobacteria
Mycobacterium fortuitum, Mycobacterium abscessus, Mycobacterium mucogenicum
Fungi
Candida parapsilosis
Phialemonium curvatum
Fusarium spp.

practices for the reuse of hemodialyzers.
      c. Label and assign each patient's dialyzer with a unique identifier and place warnings on dialyzers with patients with similar names.
      d. Do not reuse access needles.

B. Machine contamination.
   1. There has been at least one outbreak of HBV at a dialysis facility associated with the failure to use external transducer protectors to protect pressure monitoring equipment in hemodialysis machines. Transducer protectors can also fail when wetted, and some have suggested this as a possible route for HCV transmission.
   2. Contamination of frequently touched external surfaces of the hemodialysis machine can be a potential environmental reservoir for HBV and HCV. HBV can persist in an infectious state for at least 7 days while HCV has been demonstrated to persist in such a state for 24 hours.

II. Bacteremia/fungemia.

A. Reuse.
   1. Errors in dialyzer reprocessing have historically been associated with both pyrogenic reactions and

bacteremia. These errors have frequently occurred in facilities performing manual or semi-automated reuse. The typical errors that have been associated with these adverse events included:

  a. Failure to prepare dialyzer disinfectant to the correct concentration.

  b. Failure to fill the dialyzers with sufficient concentration of disinfectant.

  c. Failure to mix dialyzer disinfectant.

  d. Using disinfectant that is not compatible with the dialyzer membrane.

  e. Using water that did not meet AAMI recommended microbial and endotoxin limits.

  f. Accidentally not refilling the dialyzer with dialyzer disinfectant.

  g. Removing dialyzer header caps without disinfecting the O-rings, dialyzer header, and caps.

  h. Not reprocessing the dialyzer in a timely manner so that disinfectant has an appropriate contact time.

2. Bacteremia/fungemia can be prevented by:

  a. Following AAMI recommended practice for the reuse of hemodialyzers.

  b. Reprocessing dialyzers as soon as possible after the completion of a treatment session.

  c. Preparing dialyzer disinfectant per manufacturer's labeled instructions.

  d. If manually reprocessing dialyzers, ensuring that the dialyzers use at least 3 compartment volumes of disinfectant to fill the blood compartment with an adequate amount of dialyzer disinfectant. Most outbreaks investigated by the Centers for Disease Control and Prevention have been associated with manual reuse.

  e. To prevent sepsis caused by header removal during dialyzer reprocessing, there are several steps that could be taken.

    (1) If clots cannot be removed from the header spaces of the dialyzer, then consider discarding it.

    (2) If one removes the head caps from the dialyzer, then rinse the end of the fibers with a stream of RO water to remove clots, and then dip the O-ring, end of the dialyzer, and end cap in disinfectant before reassembling the dialyzer.

    (3) Use an automated process for removing clots from the header spaces.

    (4) Reevaluate heparinization protocols.

B. Machine contamination.

1. With single-pass hemodialysis equipment today, infections due to contamination of machines are not frequent. Patients may be infected either through the hands of healthcare workers, or by direct contact of the blood lines with the dialysate circuit (as in a dialysis machine's waste-handling option).

2. There are several sources of contamination of the internal fluid pathways of the machine: water delivered to the machine, powdered bicarbonate concentrates that are prepared with treated water at the facility, and retrograde growth up the effluent line from the drain.

3. Preventing bacteremia/fungemia associated with contaminated machines.

  a. Follow AAMI recommended practices for the microbial quality of water and dialysate.

  b. Disinfect water distribution system and hemodialysis machines at regular time intervals. This should be conducted at least monthly. Hemodialysis machines may need to be disinfected more frequently. Some equipment allows for heat disinfection to be performed on a daily basis.

  c. Conduct routine environmental monitoring of water and dialysate (e.g., microbiology and endotoxin testing).

  d. Perform preventive maintenance and quality assurance checks on equipment per manufacturer's recommendations.

  e. If using equipment with the ports to dispose of the dialyzer priming solution, follow manufacturer's recommendations with regards to preventive maintenance (routine changing of check valves), disinfection, and assessment of check valve competency.

Section P
Hemodialysis Precautions

I. General considerations.

A. Infection control precautions recommended for all patients on chronic hemodialysis are designed to prevent the transmission of bloodborne viruses as well as the transmission of and colonization with potentially pathogenic bacteria. Per the CDC, these precautions are more stringent than the Standard Precautions routinely used in hospitals (CDC, 2001a).

B. Implementation of the CDC Recommendations for Preventing the Transmission of Infections Among Chronic Hemodialysis Patients will reduce opportunities for patient-to-patient transmission directly or indirectly via contaminated equipment, supplies, medical devices, environmental surfaces and hands of dialysis personnel (CDC, 2001a).

C. Standard precautions are designed to protect health-care workers and service users from occupational exposure to blood or other potentially infectious materials. All human blood and certain human body fluids are treated as if known to be infectious for HIV, HBV, and other bloodborne pathogens.

D. The Occupational Safety and Health Administration mandates that each employer having an employee(s) with occupational exposure establish a written exposure control plan designed to eliminate or minimize employee exposure. The components of the plan must include, but are not limited to, the following.
1. Engineering and work practice controls to eliminate or minimize employee exposure (i.e., safety needles, needleless systems).
2. Personal protective equipment (PPE) (e.g., gowns, gloves, face shields).
3. Hepatitis B vaccination and postexposure evaluation and follow-up.
4. Communication of hazards to employees.

E. According to the CDC (2001a), "Standard precautions are the system of infection control precautions recommended for the inpatient hospital setting. Standard precautions are used on all patients and include use of gloves, gown, or mask whenever needed to prevent contact of the health-care worker with blood, secretions, excretions, or contaminated items."

F. In addition to standard precautions, more stringent precautions have been recommended by the CDC for the hemodialysis setting due to the increased potential for contamination with blood and pathogenic microorganisms and are the focus of this section on infection control.

II. Recommendations for infection control in the hemodialysis setting.

A. The CDC Recommendations for Preventing Transmission of Infections Among Chronic Hemodialysis Patients were published in *MMRW* (*Morbidity and Mortality Weekly Report*) in 2001. These recommendations provide measures for a comprehensive infection control program and include the following:
1. Infection control measures specifically designed to prevent transmission of bloodborne viruses and pathogenic bacteria.
2. Routine serologic testing for hepatitis B and C.
3. Vaccination of susceptible patients and staff.
4. Isolation of patients who test positive for hepatitis B surface antigen (HBsAg).

B. Must be carried out routinely for all patients in the hemodialysis center.

C. Includes additional measures to prevent HBV transmission.

D. Pages 18 to 28 of the April 27, 2001, *MMWR* including the "Recommended Infection Control Practices for Hemodialysis Units at a Glance" incorporated by reference into the ESRD Conditions of Coverage (42 CFR Part 494) are mandatory, must be adhered to, and must be demonstrated within the dialysis facility. In addition, CMS provided guidance for facilities (CMS, 2008).

III. Infection control precautions for all hemodialysis patients.

A. Wear gloves whenever caring for a patient or touching the patient's equipment at the dialysis station. No exceptions are made for when the equipment is presumed to be clean.

B. Gloves must also be worn while performing procedures that have the potential for blood, dialysate, or body fluid exposure, including but not limited to:
1. Performing procedures such as caring for the patient's vascular access.
2. Setting up reprocessed dialyzers pretreatment.
3. Inserting or removing the vascular access needles.
4. Touching blood lines, dialyzer, or machine during or after the hemodialysis treatment.
5. Administering medications.
6. Removing the blood lines and dialyzer post treatment.
7. Cleaning and disinfecting the dialysis machine and chair posttreatment.

C. Remove gloves, perform hand hygiene (hand washing or use of waterless alcohol-based antiseptic hand gel), and apply fresh gloves between patients or stations.
1. Examples of when gloves should be changed include, but are not limited to, whenever gloves are soiled (e.g., with blood, dialysate, body fluid), after touching a patient or their machine, before caring for another patient or touching another patient's machine, and when moving from a "dirty" area or task to a "clean" area or task.
2. The CDC defines a "dirty" area as an area where there is a potential for contamination with blood or body fluids and areas where contaminated or used supplies, equipment, blood supplies, or biohazard containers are stored or handled. A "clean" area is an area designated only for clean and unused equipment and supplies and medications (CMS, 2008).

D. Wash hands after gloves are removed and between patient contacts, as well as after touching blood, body fluids, secretions, excretions, and contaminated items. If hands are not visibly contaminated, a waterless, alcohol-based, antiseptic hand rub with 60% to 90% alcohol content can be substituted for hand washing.

E. Hand hygiene must be performed before entering and on exiting the patient treatment areas.

F. Items taken to a patient's dialysis station, including those placed on top of dialysis machines or on the dialysis chair, should either be disposed of, dedicated for use only on a single patient, or cleaned and disinfected before being returned to a common clean area or used for other patients.

G. Nondisposable items that cannot be cleaned and disinfected (e.g., adhesive tape, cloth-covered blood pressure cuffs) must be dedicated for use only on a single patient.

H. The medication preparation area should be away from the individual patient stations and designated as a clean area.

I. Unused medications or supplies (e.g., syringes, alcohol swabs) taken to the patient's station should not be returned to a common clean area or used on other patients.

J. Multiple-dose vials must not be carried from station to station.

K. Common carts should not be used to prepare or distribute medications.

L. If trays are used to distribute medications, the tray must be cleaned before using for a different patient.

M. Common supply carts that are used to store clean supplies in the treatment area should remain in a designated area at a sufficient distance from patient stations to avoid contamination with blood.

N. Single use vials/ampoules must be used for only one patient and should not be entered more than once.

O. Residual medication from two or more vials should not be pooled into a single vial.

P. Staff members should wear gowns, face shields, eye wear, or masks when performing procedures during which exposure to blood might occur.
   1. When a mask is needed, the mask must cover the caregiver's nose and mouth.

   2. Lab coats or gowns used as PPE must cover the arms and must be completely closed in the front.

Q. After each patient treatment, a low-level disinfectant should be used to clean environmental surfaces at the dialysis station, including the bed or chair, countertops, equipment, blood pressure cuffs, clamps, external surfaces of the dialysis machine, and containers used for prime waste. Special attention should be given to cleaning the control panels on the dialysis machine and other frequently touched surfaces, as well as the treatment chair that has the potential for contamination with the patient's blood.

R. Blood spills must be immediately cleaned with a cloth soaked with a tuberculocidal disinfectant or a 1:100 dilution of household bleach.

S. Venous pressure transducer protectors should be changed between patients and not reused.

T. External transducer protectors that become wet should be replaced immediately and inspected.
   1. If fluid is visible on the side of the transducer protector that faces the machine, qualified personnel should open the machine after the hemodialysis treatment is completed and check for blood contamination of the internal pressure tubing set and pressure sensing port.
   2. If contamination has occurred, the machine must be taken out of service and disinfected, using either 1:100 dilution of bleach or EPA-registered tuberculocidal germicide before further use.

U. Wastes generated by the hemodialysis treatment should be considered infectious.
   1. Place in leakproof containers with a secure lid.
   2. Remove from the patient treatment area throughout the day.
   3. Dispose according to local and state regulations. Clearly label and store in area protected from casual access.

SECTION Q

Regulations, Recommendations, Guidelines, and Quality Improvement

I. Overview.

A. To maintain inclusion in the federal Medicare program, dialysis and kidney transplant facilities are required to meet specific regulatory criteria (known as Conditions for Coverage) set by the Centers for

Medicare and Medicaid Services (CMS). They are also required to meet applicable state licensing rules and Occupational Safety and Health Agency (OSHA) regulations, and be aware of recommendations and guidelines provided by professional associations and state and federal agencies.

II. Regulations are mandatory requirements that must be met for the facility to practice within the "law."

A. Implement statutes passed by legislative bodies and signed into law by the governor (for state laws) or the president (for federal laws).

B. The public can influence the content and structure of the law during the legislative process by contacting their congresspersons to educate and influence the vote.

C. Once a bill has been passed and signed into statute, the applicable state or federal agency is charged with developing regulations to implement the law.

D. Statutes are typically broad, outlining the intent of the legislation. The specifics are usually found in regulation.

E. Regulations are subject to public influence as well.
1. Proposed state and federal regulations are published for public comment before being finalized.
2. Comments received are taken into consideration in developing the final regulations.
3. Examples of current regulations include Federal regulations that require end-stage renal disease (ESRD) facilities to prevent the transmission of infection. This regulation requires that facilities follow the recommendations issued by the Centers for Disease Control and Prevention (CDC) for infection control in hemodialysis facilities. These recommendations were discussed in Section P of this chapter.

III. Recommendations are voluntary and are often developed as the result of critical incidents or research evidence, rather than law.
Recommendations, by themselves, do not carry the weight of "law."

A. May be developed as a consensus process.
1. May be incorporated into regulations by reference.
2. Examples of professional organizations that have developed recommendations addressing infection control topics include:
   a. ANNA: *Nephrology Nursing Scope and Standards of Practice.*
   b. National Kidney Foundation (NKF): *Kidney Disease Outcomes Quality Improvement (KDOQI) Practice Guidelines.*
   c. Association for the Advancement of Medical Instrumentation (AAMI) has developed hemodialysis standards that have implications for infection control in dialysis.
   d. Association for Professionals in Infection Control and Epidemiology (APIC): *Guide to the Elimination of Infections in Hemodialysis.*

B. The federal agency that provides direction in the area of infection control is the Centers for Disease Control and Prevention (CDC). Their documents are designated as either "Guidelines" or "Recommendations."
1. Recommendations are based on findings from CDC investigations of critical incidents, research, or review of data and developed via expert opinion. There is an internal review process and public comments may be solicited, but there is no requirement to incorporate such comments into the final recommendation.
2. Guidelines are usually developed by CDC and external partners, based on evidence, and require public review and are published in the federal register for comment. Public comments have to be addressed by incorporation into the guideline or by providing a reason why the comment was not accepted. The completed document undergoes a final peer review process before being published as a guideline.
3. Recommendations may sometimes be formally adopted as regulations.
   a. This allows the state or federal government agency to use the work of professional organizations and other agencies, preventing the potential development of conflicting standards and reducing duplication of efforts.
   b. For example, CMS adopted the CDC document, *Recommendations for Preventing Transmission of Infections Among Chronic Hemodialysis Patients,* as part of the federal Conditions for Coverage, mandating that facilities comply with the "voluntary" recommendations developed by CDC. CMS surveyors are instructed to use the CDC document as the standard by which facilities are audited for infection control purposes.

IV. Practice guidelines and standards are more often being used as a way to organize and prioritize care delivery, and to evaluate the care delivered.

A. Recommendations and guidelines are sometimes used as an expected standard.

B. For example, Fistula First is an initiative to increase arteriovenous fistula use in all appropriate hemodialysis patients. It is an outgrowth of the KDOQI quality improvement recommendations. Every End-Stage Renal Disease Network participates in this initiative, and the Fistula First data has been incorporated into the CMS Measures Assessment Tool, the tool used by CMS surveyors to determine if a facility is meeting specific quality outcomes. When evaluating a facility's rate of fistulas, the benchmark used by CMS surveyors is the rate of fistulas recommended by Fistula First.

V. CMS Interpretive Guidance Manual and Frequently Asked Questions (FAQs).

A. Interpretive guidance manual was developed to provide additional information to surveyors and facility staff regarding the interpretation and application of the regulations found in the federal Conditions for Coverage.

B. FAQs are used by CMS to provide details and clarification and address commonly asked questions regarding the Conditions for Coverage and/or the interpretive guidance manual.

VI. CDC dialysis safety initiatives.

A. Dialysis patients have an increased risk of getting infections. Bloodstream infections are a particular risk because of the vascular access to the bloodstream that is required for hemodialysis.

B. In an effort to decrease the incidence of infections in dialysis patients, CDC has developed specific resources to educate dialysis personnel and patients (available at www.cdc.gov/dialysis).
   1. Training video and print resources for preventing infections in outpatient hemodialysis patients. These materials were sent to all dialysis facilities and demonstrate best practices for preventing bloodstream and other infections in outpatient hemodialysis settings.
   2. Observation tools and checklists were developed to promote CDC-recommended practices for infection prevention in hemodialysis facilities. These tools can be used to assess individual staff practices or to help the facility define its best practice.
   3. Observation tools should be used to determine if dialysis staff adheres to CDC-recommended practices. Results of observations should be regularly shared with staff to improve practice and direct quality improvement processes.
   4. Dialysis checklists are intended to be used as a simple reference tool and can be used for staff

training or orientation of new staff. They can also be used to remind staff of recommended practices.

C. CDC's Core Interventions for Dialysis Bloodstream Infection (BSI) Prevention – the CDC Dialysis Bloodstream Infection Prevention Collaborative developed a set of interventions that facilities can implement to decrease patient bloodstream infections (CDC, 2014h).
   1. The BSI Prevention Collaborative is a voluntary partnership between CDC and outpatient dialysis facilities in the United States. Participating facilities measure BSIs using the dialysis event surveillance modules in the National Healthcare Safety Network (NHSN) and a package of evidence-based practices to prevent these infections.
   2. CDC's National Healthcare Safety Network is the nation's most widely used healthcare-associated infection (HAI) tracking system. NHSN provides facilities, states, regions, and the nation with data needed to identify problem areas, measure progress of prevention efforts, and ultimately eliminate healthcare-associated infections. More information on NHSN may be found at http://www.cdc.gov/nhsn/
      a. NHSN is a secure, Internet-based surveillance system.
      b. Public health surveillance is the ongoing, systematic collection, analysis, interpretation, and dissemination of data regarding health-related events for use in public health action to reduce morbidity and mortality and improve health.
      c. NHSN is a surveillance system that allows facilities to track infections. These resources are critical for tracking and preventing infections and for evaluating the effectiveness of a specific infection prevention effort.
      d. NHSN data collection, reporting, and analysis are organized into three components: Patient Safety, Healthcare Personnel Safety, and Biovigilance. All use standardized methods and definitions in accordance with specific module protocols. For the purpose of ESRD reporting, the only component used at the time of this publication is the Patient Safety Component.
      e. NHSN can summarize what has been reported to date and display infection rates that can be used.
         (1) Track infections.
         (2) Evaluate and improve performance.
         (3) Evaluate specific infection prevention interventions.
         (4) Identify other areas for improved performance.

VII. Quality Incentive Program (QIP).

A. The Centers for Medicare and Medicaid Services (CMS) published a final rule encouraging all ESRD facilities to track quality indicators through NHSN by following the Dialysis Event Protocol.

B. Facilities must comply with the rule to receive full payment through the CMS Prospective Payment System (PPS).

C. ESRD QIP was designed by CMS to improve the quality of care provided to patients with CKD stage 5.

D. This first pay-for-performance program in any Medicare fee-for-service payment system has affected payments for dialysis services since January 1, 2012.

E. CMS will pay the facility based on the care that it provides to patients, as defined by QIP data.

F. The ESRD QIP includes the reporting of Bloodstream Infections in Hemodialysis Outpatients through the National Healthcare Safety Network (NHSN). For example, to meet the CMS ESRD QIP NHSN Reporting requirements, outpatient hemodialysis clinics had to submit their 2013 dialysis event data by April 15, 2014, to receive credit for Payment Year 2015.

G. For the most current information on the ESRD QIP refer to http://www.dialysisreports.org/ESRDMeasures.aspx

VIII. Continuous Quality Improvement (CQI) and Quality Assessment and Performance Improvement (QAPI).

A. The Conditions for Coverage specific to quality assessment and performance improvement require dialysis facilities to maintain and demonstrate evidence of its quality improvement and performance improvement program for review.

B. The facility QAPI program must measure, analyze, and track quality indicators or other aspects of performance that the facility adopts or develops that reflect processes of care and facility operations.

C. The QAPI program monitors the assessment and improvement of care in the facility, and aggregate patient data should be used in QAPI to evaluate the facility patient outcomes.

D. The QAPI encompasses all aspects of patient care, including in-center, home hemodialysis, home

peritoneal dialysis and self-care, as well as support services to provide that care.

E. The dialysis facility must develop, implement, maintain and evaluate an effective, data driven, quality assessment and performance improvement program with participation by the professional members of the interdisciplinary team.

F. The facility QAPI Committee establishes priorities, develops and implements improvement projects based on established priorities, and monitors these projects for effectiveness.

G. QAPI performance measures include all of the following, as identified by V-tags found in the CMS interpretive guidelines.
    1. Adequacy: Kt/V, URR (V629).
    2. Nutrition: Albumin, body weight (V630).
    3. Bone disease: PTH, Ca+, Phos (V631).
    4. Anemia: Hgb, Ferritin (V632).
    5. Vascular access: Fistula, catheter rate (V633).
    6. Medical errors: Frequency of specific errors (V634).
    7. Reuse: Adverse outcomes (V635).
    8. Patient satisfaction: Survey scores (V636).
    9. Infection control: Patient Care Outcomes (V637).

H. QAPI requirements for infection control under the Conditions for Coverage, Interpretive Guidelines, V637, require the dialysis facility to do the following.
    1. Analyze and document the incidence of infection to identify trends and establish baseline information on infection incidence.
    2. Develop recommendations and action plans to minimize infection transmission and promote immunization.
    3. Take actions to reduce future incidents.

I. The intent of QAPI in addressing infection control is to minimize the number of patients and staff who are exposed to or acquire infectious diseases at the facility.
    1. All patient infections must be recorded and followed up on.
    2. Surveillance information should include but not be limited to:
        a. Patients' vaccination status (hepatitis B, pneumococcal pneumonia, and influenza vaccines).
        b. Viral hepatitis serologies and seroconversions for HBV (and HCV and ALT, if known).
        c. Bacteremia episodes.
        d. Pyrogenic reactions.
        e. Vascular access infections.
        f. Vascular access loss due to infection.
    3. At a minimum, the surveillance information must

include the date of infection onset, site of infection, full identification of infecting organism(s), and antimicrobial susceptibility results.

4. There must be a periodic review of recorded episodes of bacteremia, vascular access infections, soft tissue infections, and other communicable diseases to aid in tracking, trending, and prompt identification of potential environmental/staff practice issues or infection outbreaks among patients.

5. Whenever possible, identify the method of transmission as well as the immune status of affected and at-risk patients. Ongoing tracking of infections must be done to ensure the safety of the patients.

6. Develop actions to be taken that are appropriate to the degree of risk to patients and staff. These actions could include in-service in infection control, implementation of different protocols for cleaning equipment between uses, and audits of practice regarding infection control precautions for dialysis. As infection control indicators are developed, refer to the CMS Measures Assessment Tool (MAT) for the current standard of practice.

IX. Surveillance.

A. Collection of surveillance data requires a systematic approach to data collection, including the use of standardized definitions for the identification and classification of events, indicators, and outcomes.
1. Collect and compile data that is relevant to the population, device, or procedure.
2. Use data from other agencies if available: NHSN, CMS, and CDC.

B. Compile and review data.
1. Determine the incidence of the healthcare-associated infection.
2. Use basic statistical techniques to describe the data: mean, standard deviation.
3. Determine the prevalence of epidemiologically significant findings.
4. Monitor antibiotic resistance patterns.

C. Reporting is the collection, aggregation, and analysis of data that are essential to improving patient outcomes.
1. Data must be used for further analysis and research and as a guide to the design of safer systems of care.
2. Many government and private entities collect and evaluate data, including federal and state agencies, national accrediting and certifying bodies, professional organizations, insurance companies, and individual healthcare delivery systems.

a. No standardized framework currently exists for classifying data despite the considerable effort and resources now being devoted to collecting and reporting these data.
b. The lack of such a framework is a major barrier to the systematic understanding of where and how these adverse events occur, and most important, how to prevent them.
3. Mandatory and public reporting initiatives significantly affect surveillance activities. Many states have enacted legislation and other mandates that require reporting data on HAIs, epidemiologically significant organisms such as MRSA, and related quality measures.

X. Patient and staff education.

A. Education and training of dialysis providers as well as patients with CKD and their caretakers is crucial to effective infection control and prevention.

B. Infection control priorities should be implemented in conjunction with a plan of appropriate education and training programs as well as methods to test staff competencies to help ensure consistency of desired practices.

C. A continual program for patient and caretaker education and training is a key requirement to promote self-care methods for infection prevention and to empower patients and families to report concerns about staff adherence to infection control practices.

D. Identify opportunities to access and provide educational resources. Use and adapt the expertise and educational programs developed by professional organizations such as the Association for Professionals in Infection Control, the Society for Healthcare Epidemiology of America, and the National Kidney Foundation.

E. There is a need for development of new continuing education programs and other training resources that address infection prevention issues specific to dialysis.
1. Collaborate with ESRD networks for infection control training and education.
2. Incorporate and sustain a culture of safety through infection control and prevention.
3. Establish and maintain a dialogue with organizations such as the national certification boards, technician certification groups, and others, to promote licensing and certification standards and competencies that reflect knowledge of recommended infection-prevention priorities as well as an adequate level of skill.

References

AIDS.gov. (2013). *Kidney disease.* Retrieved from http://aids.gov/hiv-aids-basics/staying-healthy-with-hiv-aids/potential-related-health-problems/kidney-disease/

Alliance for the Prudent Use of Antibiotics (APUA). (2013). http://www.tufts.edu/med/apua/about_issue/about_antibioticres.shtml

American Society of Microbiology (ASM). (2005). *Manual of susceptibility testing.* Retrieved from http://www.asm.org/ccLibraryFiles/FILENAME/000000002484/Manual%20of%20Antimicrobial%20Susceptibility%20Testing.pdf

Aminov, R.I. (2010, December 8). A brief history of the antibiotic era: Lessons learned and challenges for the future. *Frontiers in Microbiology.* (Review Article). doi: 10.3389/fmicb.2010.00134

Antimicrobial Resistance Learning Site (AMRLS). (2014). Contributors: Michigan State University, the University of Minnesota, and the Centers for Disease Control and Prevention. Retrieved from http://amrls.cvm.msu.edu/overview/sitemap-2

Arduino, M.J., & Tokars, J.I. (2005, June). Why is an infection control program needed in the hemodialysis setting? *Nephrology News & Issues.* National Institutes of Health. http://www.ncbi.nlm.nih.gov/pubmed/16008023

Arnold, A.S., Thom, K.A., Sharma, S., Phillips, M., Johnson, J.K., & Morgan, D.J. (2011). Emergence of *Klebsiella pneumoniae carbapenemase* (KPC)-producing bacteria. *Southern Medical Journal, 104*(1), 40-45. doi:10.1097/SMJ.0b013e3181fd7d5a http://www.ncbi.nlm.nih.gov/pmc/articles/PMC3075864/

Association for Professionals in Infection Control and Epidemiology (APIC). (2010). *Guide to the elimination of multidrug-resistant* Acinetobacter baumannii *transmission in healthcare settings.* Washington, DC: Author. http://www.apic.org/resource_/eliminationguideform/b8b0b11f-1808-4615-890b-f652d116ba56/file/apic-ab-guide.pdf

Association for Professionals in Infection Control and Epidemiology (APIC). (2013). *Guide to preventing* Clostridium difficile *infections.* Retrieved from http://apic.org/Resource_/EliminationGuideForm/59397fc6-3f90-43d1-9325-e8be75d86888/File/2013CDiffFinal.pdf

Ayliffe, G. (1997). The progressive intercontinental spread of methicillin-resistant *Staphylococcus aureus. Clinical Infectious Diseases, 24*(Suppl. 1), S74-79. Retrieved from http://cid.oxfordjournals.org/content/24/Supplement_1/S74.full.pdf

Barlow, M. (2009). What antimicrobial resistance has taught us about horizontal gene transfer. *Methods in Molecular Biology, 532,* 397-411. doi:10.1007/978-1-60327-853-9_23

Baron, E., Miller, M., Weinstein, M.P., Richter, S., Gilligan, P.H., Thomson, R.B., … Pritt, B.S. (2013). A guide to utilization of the microbiology laboratory for diagnosis of infectious diseases: 2013 recommendations by the Infectious Diseases Society of America (IDSA) and the American Society for Microbiology (ASM). *Clinical Infectious Diseases, 57*(4), e22-121. http://www.idsociety.org/uploadedFiles/IDSA/Guidelines-Patient_Care/PDF_Library/Laboratory%20Diagnosis%20of%20Infectious%20Diseases%20Guideline.pdf

Bickel, M., Marben, W., Betz, C., Khaykin, P., Stephan, C., Gute, P., … Jung, O. (2013). End-stage renal disease and dialysis in HIV-positive patients. Observations from a long-term cohort study with a follow-up of 22 years. *HIV Medicine, 14*(3), 127-135. http://www.medscape.com/viewarticle/779621

Boozer, J., Erwin, K., Gregory, A., & Thompson, S. (2014). Evolution of antibiotic resistance. PowerPoint presentation from University of Tennessee. Retrieved from https://notes.utk.edu/.../Evolution%20of%20Antibiotic%20Resistance.ppt

California Tuberculosis Controllers Association. (2007). *Guidelines for tuberculosis (TB) screening and treatment of patients with chronic kidney disease(CKD), patients receiving hemodialysis (HD), patients receiving peritoneal dialysis (PD), patients undergoing renal transplantation and employees of dialysis facilities.* Retrieved from http://www.ctca.org/fileLibrary/file_40.pd.

Centers for Disease Control and Prevention (CDC). (2000). Targeted tuberculin testing and treatment of latent tuberculosis infection. *Morbidity and Mortality Weekly Report, 49*(RR06);1-54. Retrieved from http://www.cdc.gov/mmwr/preview/mmwrhtml/rr4906a1.htm

Centers for Disease Control and Prevention (CDC). (2001a). Recommendations for preventing transmission of infections among chronic hemodialysis patients. *Morbidity and Mortality Weekly Report, 50*(RR05), 1-43.

Centers for Disease Control and Prevention (CDC). (2001b). Updated U.S. Public Health Service guidelines for the management of occupational exposures to HBV, HCV, and HIV and recommendations for postexposure prophylaxis. *MMWR Recommendations and Reports, 50*(RR-11), 1-52. http://www.cdc.gov/mmwr/PDF/rr/rr5011.pdf

Centers for Disease Control and Prevention (CDC). (2002). *Staphylococcus aureus* resistant to vancomycin – United States, 2002), *Morbidity and Mortality Weekly Report, 51*(26), 565-588. Retrieved from http://www.cdc.gov/mmwr/preview/mmwrhtml/mm5126a1.htm

Centers for Disease Control and Prevention (CDC). (2005). Guidelines for preventing the transmission of *M. tuberculosis* in health-care settings. *Morbidity and Mortality Weekly Report, 54,* RR-17.

Centers for Disease Control and Prevention (CDC). (2006a). *Guidelines for vaccinating kidney dialysis patients and patients with chronic kidney disease.* Retrieved from http://www.cdc.gov/vaccines/pubs/downloads/dialysis-guide-2012.pdf

Centers for Disease Control and Prevention (CDC). (2006b). Revised recommendations for HIV testing of adults, adolescents, and pregnant women in health-care settings. *Morbidity and Mortality Weekly Report, 55*(RR14), 1-17. http://www.cdc.gov/mmwr/preview/mmwrhtml/rr5514a1.htm

Centers for Disease Control and Prevention (CDC). (2007). Invasive methicillin-resistant *Staphylococcus aureus* infections among dialysis patients – United States, 2005. *Morbidity and Mortality Weekly Report, 56*(9), 197-199.

Centers for Disease Control and Prevention (CDC). (2008). *Self-study modules on tuberculosis (1-5).* Retrieved from http://www.cdc.gov/tb/education/ssmodules/pdfs/module1.pdf

Centers for Disease Control and Prevention (CDC). (2010). Updated guidelines for using interferon gamma release assays to detect Mycobacterium tuberculosis Iinfection – United States, 2010. *Morbidity and Mortality Weekly Report, 59*(RR-5). Retrieved from http://www.cdc.gov/mmwr/pdf/rr/rr5905.pdf

Centers for Disease Control and Prevention (CDC). (2011a). Immunization of health-care personnel: Recommendations of the Advisory Committee on Immunization Practices (ACIP). *MMWR Recommendations and Reports, 60*(RR-7), 1-45. http://www.cdc.gov/mmwr/pdf/rr/rr6007.pdf

Centers for Disease Control and Prevention (CDC). (2011b). Making healthcare safer: Reducing bloodstream infections. *CDC Vital Signs.* Retrieved from http://www.cdc.gov/vitalsigns/pdf/2011-03-vitalsigns.pdf

Centers for Disease Control and Prevention (CDC). (2011c). Vital signs: HIV prevention through care and treatment – United States. *Morbidity and Mortality Weekly Report, 60*(47), 1618-1623. Retrieved from http://www.cdc.gov/mmwr/preview/mmwrhtml/mm6047a4.htm?s_cid=mm6047a4_w

Centers for Disease Control and Prevention (CDC). (2012a). Healthcare-associated infections (HAIs). Frequently asked questions about *Clostridium difficile* for healthcare providers. Retrieved from http:// www.cdc.gov/hai/organisms/cdiff/ cdiff_faqs_hcp.html

Centers for Disease Control and Prevention (CDC). (2012b). Hepatitis B, epidemiology and prevention of vaccine-preventable diseases In CDC's *The pink book:* Course textbook (12th ed., 2nd printing, pp. 115-138). http://www.cdc.gov/vaccines/pubs/pinkbook/downloads/hepb.pdf

Centers for Disease Control and Prevention (CDC). (2012c). Reducing bloodstream infections in an outpatient hemodialysis center – New Jersey, 2008-2011. *Morbidity and Mortality Weekly Report, 61*(10), 169-173.

Centers for Disease Control and Prevention (CDC). (2012d). 2012 CRE Toolkit – *Guidance for control of carbapenem-resistant Enterobacteriaceae (CRE).* Retrieved from http:// www.cdc.gov/hai/organisms/cre/cre-toolkit/introduction.html

Centers for Disease Control and Prevention (CDC). (2013a). *Antibiotic resistance threats in the United States, 2013.* Retrieved from http://www.cdc.gov/drugresistance/threat-report-2013/index.html

Centers for Disease Control and Prevention (CDC). (2013b). CDC grand rounds: Preventing unsafe injection practices in the U.S. health-care system. *Morbidity and Mortality Weekly Report, 62*(21), 423-425. Retrieved from http://www.cdc.gov/mmwr/preview/mmwrhtml/mm6221a3.htm

Centers for Disease Control and Prevention (CDC). (2013c). *Core curriculum on tuberculosis: What the clinician should know* (6th ed.). Retrieved from http://www.cdc.gov/tb/education/corecurr/pdf/corecurr_all.pdf

Centers for Disease Control and Prevention (CDC). (2013d). Guidance for evaluating health-care personnel for hepatitis B virus protection and for administering postexposure management. *Morbidity and Mortality Weekly Report, 62*(rr10), 1-19. Retrieved from http://www.cdc.gov/mmwr/pdf/rr/rr6210.pdf

Centers for Disease Control and Prevention (CDC). (2013e). *Latent tuberculosis infection: A guide for primary health care providers.* Retrieved from http://www.cdc.gov/tb/publications/ LTBI/pdf/TargetedLTBI.pdf

Centers for Disease Control and Prevention (CDC). (2013f). Reported tuberculosis in the United States, 2012. Atlanta: U.S. Department of Health and Human Services. Retrieved from http://www.cdc.gov/tb/statistics/reports/2012/default.htm

Centers for Disease Control and Prevention (CDC). (2013g). Testing for HCV infection: An update of guidance for clinicians and laboratorians. *Morbidity and Mortality Weekly Report, 62*(18). Retrieved from http://www.ncbi.nlm.nih.gov/pubmed/23657112

Centers for Disease Control and Prevention (CDC). (2013h). *Trends in tuberculosis, 2012.* Retrieved from http://www.cdc.gov/tb/ publications/factsheets/statistics/Trends2013.pdf

Centers for Disease Control and Prevention (CDC). (2013i). Vital Signs: Carbapenem-resistant enterobacteriaceae. *Morbidity and Mortality Weekly Report, 62*(09), 165-170. Retrieved from http://www.cdc.gov/mmwr/preview/mmwrhtml/mm6209a3.htm

Centers for Disease Control and Prevention (CDC). (2014a). *Hepatitis B information for health professionals.* Retrieved from http://www.cdc.gov/hepatitis/HBV/

Centers for Disease Control and Prevention (CDC). (2014b). *Injection safety. Frequently asked questions (FAQs) regarding safe practices for medical injections.* Retrieved from http://www.cdc.gov/injectionsafety/providers/provider_faqs.html

Centers for Disease Control and Prevention (CDC). (2014c). *New CDC vital signs: Hepatitis C testing.* Retrieved from http://www.cdc.gov/vitalsigns/pdf/2013-05-vitalsigns.pdf

Centers for Disease Control and Prevention (CDC). (2014d). *One and only campaign.* Retrieved from http://www.oneandonlycampaign.org

Centers for Disease Control and Prevention (CDC). (2014e). *Viral hepatitis statistics & surveillance –Surveillance for viral hepatitis – United States, 2012.* Retrieved from http://www.cdc.gov/hepatitis/Statistics

Centers for Disease Control and Prevention (CDC). (2014f). *Viral hepatitis statistics & surveillance. – Incidence of acute hepatitis C by year United States, 1982-2011.* Retrieved from http://www.cdc.gov/hepatitis/Statistics/index.htm

Centers for Disease Control and Prevention (CDC). (2014g). *Methicillin-resistant Staphylococcus aureus (MRSA) infections.* Retrieved from http://www.cdc.gov/mrsa/

Centers for Disease Control and Prevention (CDC). (2014h). *CDC approach to BSI prevention in dialysis facilities (i.e., the Core interventions for dialysis bloodstream infection (BSI) prevention).* Retrieved from http://www.cdc.gov/dialysis/prevention-tools/core-interventions.html

Centers for Disease Control National Center for Immunization and Respiratory Diseases (NCIRD). (2014). Retrieved from http://www.cdc.gov/ncird/

Centers for Medicare & Medicaid Services (CMS). (2008). Center for Medicaid and State Operations/Survey & Certification Group CMS, ESRD Interpretive Guidance to the 42 CFR Part 494 Conditions of Coverage for ESRD Facilities. Retrieved from http://www.cms.gov/Medicare/Provider-Enrollment-and-Certification/SurveyCertificationGenInfo/downloads/SCletter09-01.pdf

Cohen, S.H., Gerding, D.N., Johnson, S., Kelly, C.P., Loo, V.G., McDonald, L.C., … Wilcox, M.H. (2010). Clinical practice guidelines for *Clostridium difficile* infection in adults: 2010 Update by the Society for Healthcare Epidemiology of America (SHEA) and the Infectious Diseases Society of America (IDSA). *Infection Control and Hospital Epidemiology, 31*(5). Retrieved from http://www.cdc.gov/HAI/pdfs/cdiff/Cohen-IDSA-SHEA-CDI-guidelines-2010.pdf

Collins, A. (2008). Preventing health care-associated infections. In R.G. Hughes (Ed.), *Patient safety and quality: An evidence-based handbook for nurses.* Rockville, MD: Agency for Healthcare Research and Quality. Retrieved from http://www.ncbi.nlm.nih.gov/books/NBK2683

Davies, J., & Davies, D. (2010). Origins and evolution of antibiotic resistance. *Microbiology and Molecular Biology Reviews, 74*(3), 417-433. doi:10.1128/MMBR.00016-10 Retrieved from http://mmbr.asm.org/content/74/3/417.full

Einollahi, B. (2012). Therapy for HBV infection in hemodialysis patients: Is it possible? *Hepatitis Monthly, 12*(3), 153-7. doi:10.5812/hepatmon.834. Retrieved from http://hepatmon.com/?page=article&article_id=5081

Esforzado, N., & Campistol, J.M. (2012).Treatment of hepatitis C in dialysis patients. In J.M. Morales (Ed.), *Hepatitis C in renal disease, hemodialysis and transplantation* (pp. 54-63). Basel, Switzerland: S. Krager AG.

Evans, B.A., Hamouda, A., & Amyes, S.G.B. (2013). The rise of carbapenem-resistant Acinetobacter baumannii. *Current Pharmaceutical Design, 19*(2), 223-238.

Food and Drug Administration (FDA). (2014a). *Antibiotics and antibiotic resistance.* Retrieved from http://www.fda.gov/Drugs/ResourcesForYou/Consumers/BuyingUsingMedicineSafely/AntibioticsandAntibioticResistance/UCM2007092

Food and Drug Administration (FDA). (2014b). *Battle of the bugs: Fighting antibiotic resistance.* Retrieved from http://www.fda.gov/drugs/resourcesforyou/consumers/ucm143568.htm

Fraser, S., Lim, J., Donskey, C.J., & Salata, R.A. (2014, August 15).

Enterococcal infections. *Medscape*. http://emedicine.medscape.com/article/216993-overview

Giske, C.G., Monnet, D.L., Cars, O., & Carmeli, Y. (2008). Economic impact of common multidrug-resistant gram-negative bacilli. *Antimicrobial Agents and Chemotherapy, 52*(3), 813-821. Retrieved from http://aac.asm.org/content/52/3/813

Healthy People 2020. Retrieved from http://www.healthypeople.gov/2020/topicsobjectives2020/objectiveslist.aspx?topicId=23#578823

Holmes, R. & Jobling, M. (1996). Genetics. In S. Baron (Ed.), *Medical microbiology* (4th ed.). Galveston, TX: University of Texas Medical Branch at Galveston. Retrieved from http://www.ncbi.nlm.nih.gov/books/NBK7908/

Hughes, S.A., Wedemeyer, H., & Harrison, P.M. (2011). Hepatitis delta virus. *Lancet, 378*(9785), 73-85. doi:10.1016/S0140-6736(10)61931-9. Epub 2011 Apr 20.

Immunization Action Coalition (IAC). (2014). Retrieved from http://www.immunize.org/

Ingham, B. (2014). Safe and healthy: Federal government to fight antibiotic resistance. Retrieved from http://fyi.uwex.edu/safepreserving/2014/09/24/safe-healthy-federal-goverment-to-fight-antibiotic-resistance/

Jao, J., & Wyatt, C.M. (2010). Antiretroviral medications: Adverse effects on the kidney. *Advances in Chronic Kidney Disease, 17*(1), 72-82. doi:10.1053/j.ackd.2009.07.009

Johannsson, B., Beekmann, S.E., Srinivasan, A., Hersh, A.L., Laxminarayan, R., & Polgreen, P.M. (2011). Improving antimicrobial stewardship: The evolution of programmatic strategies and barriers. *Infection Control and Hospital Epidemiology, 32*(4), 367-374. doi:10.1086/658946.

Johnson, E.A., Summanen, P., & Fiengold, S.M. (2007). Clostridium. In P.R. Murray (Ed.), Manual of clinical microbiology (pp. 889-894). Washington DC: ASM Press.

KDOQI Kidney Disease Quality Outcome Initiative (2006). National Kidney Foundation. *2006 updates, clinical practice guidelines and recommendations, Vascular access*. Retrieved from http://www.kidney.org/professionals/kdoqi/pdf/12-50-0210_JAG_DCP_Guidelines-VA_Oct06_SectionC_ofC.pdf

Kuhar, D., Henderson, D.K., Struble, K.A., Heneine, W., Thomas, V., Cheever. L.W.E., Gomaa A., Panlilio A.L., and the US Public Health Service Working Group (2013). Updated US Public Health Service Guidelines for the management of occupational exposures to human immunodeficiency virus and recommendations for postexposure prophylaxis. *Infection Control and Hospital Epidemiology, 34*(9), pp. 875-892. Retrieved from http://stacks.cdc.gov/view/cdc/20711

Lai, C.F., Liao, C.H., Pai, M.F., Hsu, S.P., Chen, H.Y., Yang, J.Y., ... Wu, K.D. (2011). Nasal carriage of methicillin-resistant Staphylococcus aureus is associated with higher all-cause mortality in hemodialysis patients. *Clinical Journal of the American Society of Nephrology, 6*(1),167-74. doi:10.2215/CJN.06270710

Lardizabal, A. (2011). Interferon-Y release assay for detection of tuberculosis infection – Chapter update in 2011. In *Guidelines for the diagnosis of latent tuberculosis infection in the 21st century* (2nd ed., pp. 57-61). Newark, NJ: New Jersey Medical School Global Tuberculosis Institute.

Laxminarayan, R., Duse, A., Wattal, C., Zaidi, A., Wertheim, H., Sumpradit, N., ... Cars, O. (2013). Antibiotic resistance – The need for global solutions. *The Lancet Infectious Diseases, 13*(12), 1057-1098. Retrieved from http://download.thelancet.com/pdfs/journals/laninf/PIIS1473309913703189.pdf?id=baa3DXYZLZvAFbflXDivu

Lee, G.C. (2012, February 17). Epidemiology and treatment of KPC'S ... What's the news? Review of current evidence.

Pharmacotherapy Rounds 2012. Retrieved from http://www.utexas.edu/pharmacy/divisions/pharmaco/rounds/lee02-17-12.pdf

Liu, C.H., & Kao, J.H. (2011). Treatment of hepatitis C virus infection in patients with end-stage renal disease. *Journal of Gastroenterology and Hepatology, 26*(2), 228-239. doi:10.1111/j.1440-1746.2010.06488.x

Malcolm, B. (2011, July). The Rise of Methicillin-Resistant *Staphylococcus aureus* in U.S. Correctional Populations. *Journal of Correctional Health Care, 17*(3), 254-265. doi:10.1177/1078345811401363

Martinez, J.L. (2012, January 13). Natural antibiotic resistance and contamination by antibiotic resistance determinants: The two ages in the evolution of resistance to antimicrobials. *Frontiers in Microbiology* (Opinion Article). doi:10.3389/fmicb.2012.00001

Muto. C (2005). Why are antibiotic-resistant nosocomial infections spiraling out of control? *Infection Control and Hospital Epidemiology, 26*(1), 10-12.

Nair, R., Ammann, E., Rysavy, M., & Schweizer, M.L. (2014). Mortality among patients with methicillin-resistant *Staphylococcus aureus* USA300 versus non-USA300 invasive infections: A meta-analysis. *Infection Control and Hospital Epidemiology, 35*(1), 31-41. doi:10.1086/674385.

Nassar, G.M., & Avus, J.C. (2001). Infectious complications of the hemodialysis access. *Kidney International, 60*(1), 1-13.

The National Network for Immunization Information (NNii). (2014). Retrieved from http://www.immunizationinfo.org/

Neu, H., & Gootz, T. (1996). Antimicrobial chemotherapy. In S. Baron (Ed.), *Medical microbiology* (4th ed.). Galveston, TX: University of Texas Medical Branch. Retrieved from http://www.ncbi.nlm.nih.gov/books/NBK7986

O'Grady, N.P., Alexander, M., Burns, L., Dellinger, E.P., Gardland, J., Heard, S.O., ... Healthcare Infection Control Practices Advisory Committee (HICPAC). (2011). 2011 guidelines for the prevention of intravascular catheter-related infections. Retrieved from http://www.cdc.gov/hicpac/bsi/bsi-guidelines-2011.html

Ohl, C.A., & Luther, V.P. (2011). Antimicrobial stewardship for inpatient facilities. *Journal of Hospital Medicine, 6*(Suppl. 1), S4-15. doi:10.1002/jhm.881

Oldfield, E.O., Oldfield, E., & Johnson, D.A. (2014). Clinical update for the diagnosis and treatment of Clostridium difficile infection. *World Journal of Gastrointestinal Pharmacology and Therapeutics, 5*(1), 1–26. doi:10.4292/wjgpt.v5.i1.1 Retrieved from http://www.ncbi.nlm.nih.gov/pmc/articles/PMC3951810/

Panlilio, A.L., Cardo, D.M., Grohskopf, L.A., Heneine, W., Ross, C.S. (2005). Updated U.S. Public Health Service guidelines for the management of occupational exposures to HIV and recommendations for postexposure prophylaxis. *MMWR Recommendations and Reports, 54*(RR-9), 1-17. Retrieved from http://www.ncbi.nlm.nih.gov/pubmed/16195697

Pascarella, S., Negro, F.. (2011). Hepatitis D virus: An update. *Liver International, 31*(1), 7-21. doi:10.1111/j.1478-3231.2010.02320.x. Epub 2010 Sep 29.

Patel, P.R., Yi, S.H., Booth, S., Bren, V., Downham, G., Hess, S., ... Kallen, A.J. (2013). Bloodstream infection rates in outpatient hemodialysis facilities participating in a collaborative prevention effort: A quality improvement report. *American Journal of Kidney Disease, 62*(2), 322-330. doi:10.1053/j.ajkd.2013.03.011

Paterson, D.L., & Bonomo, R.A. (2005). Extended-spectrum β-Lactamases: A clinical update. *Clinical Microbiology Reviews, 18*(4), 657-686. doi:10.1128/CMR.18.4.657-686.2005. http://www.ncbi.nlm.nih.gov/pmc/articles/PMC1265908/

Peacock, E. (2006). Infections in the hemodialysis unit. In A.E. Molzahn & E. Butera (Eds.), *Contemporary nephrology nursing: Principles & practice* (2nd ed., pp. 419-453, 565-570). Pitman, NJ: American Nephrology Nurses' Association.

Pegues, D., Hoffman, K., Perz, J., & Stackhouse, R. (2011). Unsafe injection practices: Outbreaks, incidents, and root causes. From *Medscape Safe Use, Medscape Education*. Retrieved from http://www.medscape.org/viewarticle/745695_transcript

Pol, S., Vallet-Pichard, A., Corouge, M., & Mallet, V.O. (2012). Hepatitis C: Epidemiology, diagnosis, natural history and therapy. In J.M. Morales (Ed.), *Hepatitis C in renal disease, hemodialysis and transplantation* (pp.1-9). Basel, Switzerland: S. Krager AG.

Rao, S. (2006). *Bacterial genetics*. Retrieved from http://www.microrao.com/micronotes/genetics.pdf

Rice, L.G., & Bonomo, R.A. (2007). Mechanisms of resistance to antibacterial agents. In P.R. Murray (Ed.), *Manual of clinical microbiology* (pp. 1114-1136). Washington DC: ASM Press.

Schmid, H., Romanos, A., Schiff, H., & Lederer, S.R. (2013). Persistent nasal methicillin-resistant staphylococcus aureus carriage in hemodialysis outpatients: A predictor of worse outcome. *BMC Nephrology, 14*(93). doi:10.1186/1471-2369-14-93

Siegel, J.D., Rhinehart, E., Jackson, M., Chiarello, M. & the CDC Healthcare Infection Control Practices Advisory Committee. (2007). *Guideline for isolation precautions: Preventing transmission of infectious agents in healthcare settings*. Retrieved from http://www.cdc.gov/hicpac/pdf/isolation/isolation2007.pdf

Silva, E., Da Hora Passos, R., Beller Ferri, M., Poli de Figueiredo, L. (2008). Sepsis: From bench to bedside. *Clinics, 63*(1), 109-120. Retrieved from http://www.ncbi.nlm.nih.gov/pmc/articles/PMC2664172/

Society of Critical Care Medicine. (2013). *International guidelines for management of severe sepsis and septic shock: 2012, 41*(2). Retrieved from http://www.sccm.org/Documents/SSC-Guidelines.pdf

Turabelidze, B., Lin, M. Wolkoff, B., Dodson, D., Gladbach, S., & Zhu, B.P. (2006). Personal hygiene and methicillin resistant *Staphylococcus aureus* infection. *Emerging Infectious Diseases, 12*(3), 422-427. Retrieved from http://wwwnc.cdc.gov/eid/article/12/3/pdfs/05-0625.pdf

United States Renal Data Systems (2011). *2011 USRDS annual report*. Chapter 10. Retrieved from http://www.usrds.org/2011/view/v2_10.asp#c

U.S. Department of Labor, Occupational Health & Safety. (2014). *Bloodborne Pathogens Standard Title 29 of the Code of Federal Regulations at 29 CFR 1910.1030*. Retrieved from https://www.osha.gov/pls/oshaweb/owadisp.show_document?p_id=10051&p_table=STANDARDS

World Health Organization (WHO). (2014a). *Antimicrobial resistance*. Retrieved from www.who.int/drugresistance/

World Health Organization (WHO). (2014b). *Hepatitis C*. Retrieved from http://www.who.int/mediacentre/factsheets/fs164/en/

World Health Organization (WHO). (2014c). *Hepatitis D*. Retrieved from http://www.who.int/csr/disease/hepatitis/whocdscsrlyo20022/en/index3.html

World Health Organization (WHO). (2014d).*Tuberculosis fact sheet*. Retrieved from http://www.who.int/mediacentre/factsheets/fs104/en/

Yurdaydın, C., Idilman, R., Bozkaya, H., & Bozdayi, A.M. (2010). Natural history and treatment of chronic delta hepatitis. *Journal of Viral Hepatology*. doi:10.1111/j.1365-2893.2010.01353.x. Epub 2010 Aug 15.

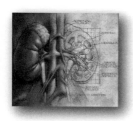

SELF-ASSESSMENT QUESTIONS FOR MODULE 2

These questions apply to all chapters in Module 2 and can be used for self-testing. They are not considered part of the official CNE process.

Chapter 1

1. Generalist and advanced practice nurses who desire to become credentialed as a Certified Genetics Nurse must submit a portfolio that includes which of the following?
   a. Pass a certification exam in advanced nursing genetics.
   b. Pass a certification exam on the Human Genome Project.
   c. Submit a portfolio to the American Nurses Credentialing Center (ANCC) that documents skills, knowledge, abilities, and career accomplishments in genetics
   d. Submit an essay describing your knowledge of genetics and pass an oral exam provided by the American Nurses Credentialing Center (ANCC).

2. Recent research an "association" between apolipoprotein L1 (APOL1) gene alleles with development and/or the progression of
   a. polycystic kidney disease.
   b. Alport's syndrome.
   c. hypertensive associated kidney disease in African Americans.
   d. medullary cystic kidney disease (MCKD).

3. The body's total blood supply circulates through the kidneys approximately
   a. 12 times an hour.
   b. 60 times an hour.
   c. 12 times a day.
   d. 60 times a day.

4. A normal first sign of kidney dysfunction is
   a. hypertension.
   b. proteinuria with normal GFR.
   c. hyperphosphatemia.
   d. decreased Hg.

5. Diagnosis of acute kidney injury (AKI) is made based on
   a. symptoms exhibited by the patient.
   b. changes in urine output.
   c. changes in laboratory parameters.
   d. b and c.
   e. a and b.
   f. a and c.

6. CKD is a process that involves multiple strikes or insults to the body and it usually progresses in a linear fashion. True or False?

7. Which of the following are good clinical indicators of kidney function?
   a. Serum creatinine levels.
   b. Serum potassium levels.
   c. Glomerular filtration rate.
   d. Plasma renin levels.

8. Postprocedure care for a patient following renal biopsy includes
   a. keeping head of bed elevated 90 degrees.
   b. decreasing fluid intake.
   c. encourage walking.
   d. collecting serial urines to assess hematuria.

9. Incidence of CKD is higher in which of the following? (Select all that apply.)
   a. Females.
   b. Males.
   c. Young adults.
   d. Older adults.

10. One of the most efficient means of reducing the burden of kidney disease is to do the following:
    a. Prevent development of kidney disease.
    b. Screen everyone for kidney disease.
    c. Reduce any potential for public alarm about kidney disease by providing education after diagnosis.
    d. Reduce the complications of kidney disease by promoting the use of herbal medications.

Chapter 2

11. KDIGO defines chronic kidney disease stage G2 A1 as which of the following?
    a. An eGFR between 60 and 89 mL/min without evidence of proteinuria.
    b. An eGFR between 45 and 59 mL/min without evidence of proteinuria.
    c. An eGFR between 33 and 44 mL/min without evidence of proteinuria.
    d. An eGFR between 15 and 29 mL/min without evidence of proteinuria.

12. Risk factors for CKD include all but
    a. diabetes.
    b. hypertension.
    c. overweight.
    d. ethnic minority.

13. The USTSPF recommends that routine screening for CKD be done for (choose all that apply)
    a. those with diabetes.
    b. people diagnosed with hypertension.
    c. men with an abdominal girth < 40 inches.
    d. an elderly person with no symptoms.

14. Interventions that are focused on improving outcomes of CKD include which of the following?
    a. Achieve improved blood pressure control.
    b. Increase hemoglobin levels to 13.5 g/dL.
    c. Delaying treatment by referring to nephrology at stage 3.
    d. A single caregiver system.

15. What do nursing strategies for management of complications of CKD all have in common? (Select all that apply.)
    a. A coordination of care services to assure that needs are met.
    b. A nurse involved in the treatment and decision making for patient care.
    c. Involved and active patient participation.
    d. Medications that are universal to all patients.

16. Education for those with CKD must be provided by a qualified professional. True or False

Chapter 3

17. Patients with CKD often become depressed, which must be distinguished from
    a. anger.
    b. adjustment disorder.
    c. normal behavior.
    d. family conflict.

18. Cultural competence of nephrology nurses involves recognizing that
    a. CKD occurs equally in all genders and nationalities.
    b. illegal immigrants are disproportionately diagnosed with CKD.
    c. treatment guidelines are primarily based on research primarily involving Caucasian subjects.
    d. the profession of nursing is increasingly diverse.

19. The best objectively clear way to know that learning has taken place is by which of the following?
    a. A change in behavior or abilities to engage in self-care by the patient.
    b. Determining that the teaching plan includes behavioral objectives.

    c. Having the patient read a brochure and asking questions.
    d. Using a posttest to test the patient's knowledge after the session.

20. An important reason for nephrology nurses to be involved in working to gain patient and family engagement is that
    a. it will increase the patient's likelihood for educating and mentoring others with kidney disease.
    b. patients and family are more likely to understand the process of their health care.
    c. the effects of illness are going to be less disruptive.
    d. complications are less likely to occur when the patient and family are engaged.

21. Families of military members diagnosed with kidney disease may denote coping problems that are related to the following:
    a. PTSD.
    b. TBI.
    c. CMV.
    d. a and b.
    e. a, b, and c.

22. Transplant recipients who also have a disability other than kidney failure and continue to work may be eligible for which form of assistance?
    a. QWDI.
    b. An MA plan.
    c. Medicare Part B.
    d. SSDI.

23. Increased activity was found to
    a. decrease muscle mass.
    b. increase the need for need for iron.
    c. increase aerobic capacity.
    d. decrease HDL.

24. The national Physician Orders for Life-Sustaining Orders (POLST) is defined as (choose all that apply)
    a. treatment preferences.
    b. medical orders.
    c. instigated by the patient and their family.
    d. should be begun once diagnosed with a terminal illness.

Chapter 4

25. Which of the following should not be used as a marker of protein energy wasting (PEW) for a patient with chronic kidney disease?
    a. Albumin.
    b. C-reactive protein.
    c. Pre-albumin.
    d. Cholesterol.

26. Which of the following is a safe choice for treating hypoglycemia for a patient with diabetes receiving hemodialysis?
    a. ½ cup apple juice.
    b. ½ cup orange juice.
    c. ½ cup milk.
    d. ½ cup regular cola.

27. Inadequate protein and energy intake in older patients on hemodialysis is associated with which of the following?
    a. Lower markers of nutrition.
    b. Better survival.
    c. Lower comorbidities.
    d. Higher functional status.

28. Which of the food sources of dietary phosphorus has the highest phosphorus absorption?
    a. Vegetables.
    b. Milk.
    c. Meat.
    d. Processed foods.

29. What is the recommended protein intake for a patient on peritoneal dialysis?
    a. 0.8 to 1.0 g/kg/day.
    b. 1.0 to 1.1 g/kg/day.
    c. 1.2 to 1.3 g/kg/day.
    d. 0.8 to 1.3 g/kg/day.

30. Triceps skinfold thickness is used to measure which of the following nutritional parameters?
    a. Muscle.
    b. Subcutaneous fat.
    c. Body mass index.
    d. Frame size.

Chapter 5

31. Which of the following is an effect of kidney disease on drug pharmacokinetics?
    a. Usually do not experience any accumulation of metabolites.
    b. Volume of distribution (Vd) may be decreased with increased fluid accumulation.
    c. Loading doses of drugs are always required.
    d. Risk for drug toxicity is increased.

32. In patients with CKD with anemia, iron therapy is used to achieve which of the following goals?
    a. To increase the quality of life and prevent complications related to anemia.
    b. To achieve hemoglobin levels of 12–13 mg/dL.
    c. To minimize the need for blood transfusion and ESA therapy.
    d. Both a and c are goals for iron therapy.

33. Which of the following antihypertensive agents is recommended as a first-line therapy in patients with CKD and hypertension?
    a. Metoprolol.
    b. Clonidine.
    c. Lisinopril.
    d. Hydralazine.

34. Which class of diuretics is recommended to be used as an initial therapy for the treatment of hypertension in patients with CKD stages 1 through 3?
    a. Loop diuretics.
    b. Aldosterone antagonists.
    c. Thiazide diuretics.
    d. Potassium sparing diuretics.

35. Which of the following statements regarding phosphate binders is true?
    a. Aluminum-based binders should be reserved for short-term use in patients with persistently high serum phosphorus levels.
    b. The use of calcium-based phosphate binders does not result in hypercalcemia.
    c. Sevelamer is the only noncalcium-containing product that is chewable.
    d. Lanthanum is the least potent phosphate binder.

36. Which of the following is a cation-exchange resin used to treat hyperkalemia?
    a. Famotidine.
    b. Sodium polystyrene sulfonate.
    c. Gemfibrozil.
    d. Aliskiren.

37. Which of the following is true regarding the dialyzability of drugs?
    a. Drugs primarily excreted by the kidney are often removed by hemodialysis.
    b. Drugs with a larger molecular weight are more likely to be removed by dialysis.
    c. Drugs that are highly protein bound are more likely to be removed by dialysis.
    d. Drugs with a small volume of distribution are less likely to be removed by dialysis.

Chapter 6

38. The most effective way to prevent an infection in a vascular access is to (choose all that apply)
    a. follow strict aseptic cannulation technique.
    b. train staff in infection control.
    c. encourage use of catheters for access.
    d. use proper hand washing.

39. One of the factors that contributes to the development of drug-resistant organisms is
    a. nonadherence to handwashing procedures.
    b. completing the full course of antibiotics as prescribed.
    c. prescribing antibiotics based on culture and sensitive reports.
    d. using antibiotics to treat viral infections.

40. Isolation in a separate room for treatment is required for which of the following viral infections?
    a. HBV.
    b. HCV.
    c. HIV.

41. Which work practices assist in prevention of occupational exposure? (Select all that apply.)
    a. Adhere to OSHA's standards.
    b. Follow the CDC recommendations.
    c. Ask the patient when his/her last shower was.
    d. Use safety-needles.

42. Which of the following apply to someone who has latent TB infection rather than active TB disease? (Select all that apply.)
    a. Should wear a mask when in public until the completion of antituberculin therapy.
    b. Will have negative sputum smears and cultures.
    c. The chest x-ray will usually be normal.
    d. The QFT-G will be positive.
    e. Will have a positive TB skin test.

43. The Centers for Disease Control and Prevention (CDC) recommends that persons with chronic kidney disease receive which vaccines?
    a. Hepatitis A, hepatitis B, and influenza.
    b. Influenza, hepatitis B, and pneumococcal.
    c. Hepatitis B., influenza, and whooping cough.
    d. Pneumoccal, MMR, and influenza.

44. To prevent infections related to the dialysis unit's water, the water system should be disinfected at minimum
    a. daily.
    b. weekly.
    c. monthly.
    d. yearly.

45. The facility QAPI team in the dialysis center should include:
    a. professional members of the interdisciplinary team.
    b. only the persons involved in addressing each specific problem.
    d. just the center's governing body.
    c. only the nurse manager and medical director.

Answer Key

Chapter 1
1. c
2. c
3. a
4. b
5. d
6. False
7. c
8. d
9. a, d
10. a

Chapter 2
11. a
12. c
13. a, b
14. a
15. a, b, c
16. True

Chapter 3
17. b
18. c
19. a
20. d
21. d
22. a
23. c
24. a and b

Chapter 4
25. b
26. a
27. a
28. d
29. c
30. b

Chapter 5
31. d
32. d
33. c
34. c
35. a
36. b
37. a

Chapter 6
38. a, b, d
39. d
40. a
41. a, b, d
42. b, c, d, e
43. b
44. c
45. a

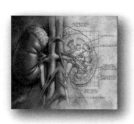

INDEX FOR MODULE 2

Page numbers followed by **f** indicate figures.
Page numbers followed by **t** indicate tables

glycosuria in, 103
Hematologic system
  in chronic kidney disease, 122
  examination of, 96t
Hematuria in calculi, 84
Hemodialysis
  annual cost of, 226
  daily, 263
  dyslipidemia in, 280
  exercise in
    benefits of, 235, 236
    limitations to, 238
    recommendations on, 238–239, 241t
  immunizations in, 381
  and infections, 385–388
    CDC recommendations on, 387, 390
    Ebola virus, 363–364
    hepatitis B, 348, 352t, 353, 387
    hepatitis C, 354, 355, 387
    HIV, 360
    occupational exposure to, 387
    prevention and control of, 386–388, 389
    risk factors for, 334
    tuberculosis, 324t, 379, 379t
    vascular access and catheter-related, 337–340, 390
  intermittent, 364
  machine contamination in, 385, 386
  medication management in, 322–325, 323t–325t
  nocturnal, 263
  nutrition in, 262–263
    minerals in, 283, 284
    sodium in, 278–279
  in pregnancy, 275–276
  reuse programs in, 385, 386
Hemoglobin, in anemia and CKD, 130, 131t, 132, 133, 162, 165
  in ESA therapy, 166, 167, 303
  in iron supplementation, 167
Hemoglobin A1C in diabetes mellitus, 130, 138–139, 161, 262, 270
Hemolytic uremic syndrome, 118
Hemorrhage, gastrointestinal, in acute kidney injury, 68
Hepatitis B, 346–354
  acute, 349
  CDC recommendations on, 387
  characteristics and structure of virus, 346, 347f
  chronic, 349
  clinical features in, 348
  and hepatitis D infection, 358
  incidence of, 347, 348f
  isolation precautions in, 353
  in machine contamination, 385
  occupational exposure to, 365, 366
  risk factors for, 347–348
  screening for, 350–351
  serologic tests and markers in, 349t, 349–351, 351t
  transmission of, 348
  treatment of, 353–354, 354t
  in unsafe injection practices, 367
  vaccination, 347, 350, 351t, 351–352, 352t, 353
    in chronic kidney disease, 379–382, 380t, 381t, 382t
    in dialysis, 380t, 380–381

dose and schedule in, 352t, 382t
  in healthcare workers, 350, 352t, 366, 367t, 383
  in susceptible patients, 351t, 351–353
Hepatitis C, 354–358
  acute, 355
  CDC recommendations on, 387
  characteristics and structure of virus, 354
  chronic, 355
  clinical features of, 355
  incidence and prevalence of, 354, 354f
  in machine contamination, 385
  occupational exposure to, 365, 366
  risk factors for, 355
  seroconversion, 357
  serologic tests and markers in, 351t, 355–357, 356f, 357t
  transmission of, 355
  in unsafe injection practices, 367
Hepatitis D, 358–359
Hepatorenal syndrome, acute kidney injury in, 54–55, 55t, 63–64
Herbal remedies, 267
  in Ayurvedic therapy, 277–278
Heterozygosity loss, 10
Hispanics, 203
  chronic kidney disease in, 156, 158
  communication of, 206
  health beliefs of, 206
  kidney failure in, 203
  religion and spirituality of, 208
Histamine H1 receptor antagonists, 316–317
Histamine H2 receptor antagonists, 302
Historical aspects, of genetics and genomics, 4–5
History taking, 91, 92t–100t
  in acute kidney injury, 53–54
  on family health history, 13–14, 20, 93t
  in nutrition assessment, 258
  on spirituality, 200
HIV infection, 359–360
  acute renal injury in, 54, 63
  cultural risk factors for, 203
  dialysis in, 359–360, 385
  glomerulonephritis in, 82
  nephropathy in, 359
  occupational exposure to, 365, 366
  tuberculosis in, 372, 374, 376t
HMB CoA reductase inhibitors, 137, 178–179, 313–314
Homeostasis, 30, 30f
Horseshoe kidney, 77
Hospice, 245
Human Genome Project, 5
Human immunodeficiency virus infection, 359–360. See also HIV infection
Hyaline casts, urinary, 102t, 107
Hydrogen ions, 48–50
Hydronephrosis, 84–85
  physical examination in, 91
  physiologic, in pregnancy, 64
Hydrostatic pressure
  Bowman's capsule, 30, 35, 36
  definition of, 35t
  glomerular, 30, 34–35, 36, 37, 43
  in renal pelvis, 50
Hypercalcemia, in hyperparathyroidism, 64
Hypercoagulation in chronic kidney disease, 122
Hyperglycemia

in diabetes mellitus, 87, 174, 270
  in dialysis, 270
  and glycosuria, 103, 270
Hyperkalemia, 172–173
  in acute kidney injury, 68
  cation-exchange resin in, 173, 312–313
  in dialysis, 264
Hypernatremia, 46
Hyperosmotic solutions, 35t
Hyperparathyroidism
  calcimimetics in, 312
  primary, acute kidney injury in, 64
  secondary, in chronic kidney disease, 121, 124, 168, 169
Hyperphosphatemia in chronic kidney disease, 121, 135, 168
  phosphate binders in, 318–319
Hypertension, 87–90
  adherence to treatment in, 129
  in African Americans, 18, 87, 89, 175, 176, 177, 203
  alcohol consumption in, 178
  and apolipoprotein L1 mutation, 18
  borderline, 88
  and chronic kidney disease, 73t, 87–90, 119, 127–129, 156, 161–162, 175–178
    drug therapy in, 175–176
    lifestyle factors in, 176–178
    in pregnancy, 183
    screening in, 157–158
    treatment goals in, 175, 176
  classification of, 162, 162t
  cultural risk factors for, 203
  in diabetes mellitus, 86, 175, 176
  drug therapy in, 88–89, 175–176, 304–308
  emergency or urgency in, 89
  essential, 88
  exercise benefits in, 235
  in kidney transplantation, 266, 267
  lifestyle factors in, 88, 127, 176–178
  malignant, 89
  nutrition in, 129, 177–178, 266, 267
  primary, 18–19, 88
  pulmonary, 235
  renovascular, 89–90
  secondary, 88
  smoking cessation in, 178
Hypertriglyceridemia, 137
Hyperuricemia
  in acute kidney injury, 62
  in chronic kidney disease, 171
  in familial juvenile nephropathy, 18
  in gout, 62, 171
Hyperuricosuria, 105
Hypoalbuminemia in malnutrition, 173
Hypocalcemia in chronic kidney disease, 121
Hypoglycemia
  in diabetes mellitus, 270, 271
  in exercise, 236
Hypoglycemic agents, oral, 271, 325t
Hypokalemia
  in acute kidney injury, 67
  in distal renal tubular acidosis, 79
Hyponatremia, 46
  in syndrome of inappropriate ADH secretion, 45
Hypoplasia, renal, 77
Hyposmotic solutions, 35t